Alzheimer's Disease

Alzheimer's Disease

Life Course Perspectives on Risk Reduction

Amy R. Borenstein, Ph.D., M.P.H.
and
James A. Mortimer, Ph.D.

University of South Florida
Department of Epidemiology and Biostatistics
Department of Neurology
Tampa, FL, USA

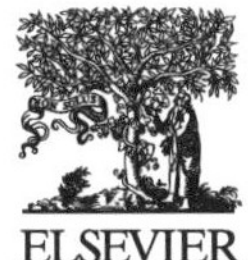

AMSTERDAM • BOSTON • HEIDELBERG • LONDON
NEW YORK • OXFORD • PARIS • SAN DIEGO
SAN FRANCISCO • SINGAPORE • SYDNEY • TOKYO

Academic Press is an imprint of Elsevier

Academic Press is an imprint of Elsevier
125 London Wall, EC2Y 5AS.
525 B Street, Suite 1800, San Diego, CA 92101-4495, USA
50 Hampshire Street, 5th Floor, Cambridge, MA 02139, USA
The Boulevard, Langford Lane, Kidlington, Oxford OX5 1GB, UK

Notices

Knowledge and best practice in this field are constantly changing. As new research and experience broaden our understanding, changes in research methods, professional practices, or medical treatment may become necessary.

Practitioners and researchers must always rely on their own experience and knowledge in evaluating and using any information, methods, compounds, or experiments described herein. In using such information or methods they should be mindful of their own safety and the safety of others, including parties for whom they have a professional responsibility.

To the fullest extent of the law, neither the Publisher nor the authors, contributors, or editors, assume any liability for any injury and/or damage to persons or property as a matter of products liability, negligence or otherwise, or from any use or operation of any methods, products, instructions, or ideas contained in the material herein.

ISBN: 978-0-12-804538-1

British Library Cataloguing-in-Publication Data
A catalogue record for this book is available from the British Library.

Library of Congress Cataloging-in-Publication Data
A catalog record for this book is available from the Library of Congress.

Publisher: Nikki Levy
Acquisition Editor: Emily Ekle
Editorial Project Manager: Timothy Bennett
Production Project Manager: Julie-Ann Stansfield
Designer: Victoria Pearson Esser

Typeset by MPS Limited, Chennai, India

Dedication

For my brave and loving parents, Lucia and Israel Borenstein, who encouraged me to do anything I wanted to do. I also dedicate this book to my loving and brilliant husband who is the best colleague I could hope to have.

—A.R.B.

For my intellectual and life partner, Amy Borenstein.

—J.A.M.

Contents

Section IV
Epidemiologic and Biologic Markers

Section V
Future Steps

Preface

Alzheimer's disease (AD) is rapidly becoming a major public health challenge in the United States and around the world. The largest segment of the US population, the baby boomers, are just beginning to enter the age at high risk for AD. If effective methods for preventing this illness are not found and implemented, this demographic transition will lead to an epidemic of AD with huge economic, personal, and societal costs in the coming decades. Although the epidemiology of AD is still relatively young compared with the epidemiology of cardiovascular disease and cancer, knowledge about the risk factors for AD, and ways in which it might be prevented has exploded in the last 30 years.

The aim of this book is to provide students, researchers, clinicians, and the general public with a critical review of what is currently known about the distribution of AD in populations, its risk factors, and promising avenues for its early detection and ultimately its prevention. Given the enormous number of studies that have been published in this area, no review can claim to be comprehensive. We have endeavored to focus on epidemiologic investigations that provide the most valid and reliable data, while also including provocative viewpoints based on animal and human studies. Because we want the material in this book to be accessible to a more general audience, we begin with a primer on epidemiologic concepts to familiarize nonepidemiologists with the basic tools of the field, including the types of study designs that are used in epidemiology, the interpretation of study data, and methodological problems that may be encountered.

Although scientists continue to debate when AD begins, it is clear that genes are critical to its causation. It also is becoming clear that factors encountered in early- and midlife can either hasten or delay the appearance of clinical symptoms. Because the seeds of this illness are present at conception and risk is modified throughout life, we will take a life course approach in describing the risk and protective factors for the disease. The prevention of AD lies in our ability to either slow down the rate of accumulation of pathology through biologically modifying pharmaceutical drugs or by delaying onset of clinical symptoms through brain-healthy modifiable behaviors.

The book is divided into five main sections. In the first section, we begin with a description of the first recognized case of the disease as described by Dr Alois Alzheimer at the beginning of the twentieth century. This is followed by chapters on the clinical appearance, progression, diagnosis, and neuropathology of AD. The final chapter in this section considers the threshold model that provides the context for interpreting the association of brain pathology and reserve with the clinical manifestation of dementia. In Section 2, we summarize the descriptive epidemiology of AD with regard to its prevalence, incidence, survival, and mortality. In Section 3, we introduce the concept of two types of risk factors: those for the underlying neuropathology of the disease and those for the expression of its clinical symptoms. The remainder of this third section is devoted to a critical summary of the large body of literature concerning contributions of genetic and environmental factors to the causation of this disease. In Section 4, we review biomarkers for this condition that can be observed during the preclinical phase of AD. Because the pathology is already advanced at the time a case can be diagnosed, effective prevention will likely require identification of the individuals at risk for this illness years or decades in advance of the initial symptoms. In Section 5, we address the science of preventing AD from an epidemiologic perspective, including how prevention might occur at the individual and population levels.

Amy R. Borenstein
James A. Mortimer

Acknowledgments

This book is the result of many years of collaboration and discussion about Alzheimer's disease and related neurologic diseases, epidemiology, statistics, genetics, and biology between the coauthors. It also is the culmination of many interactions with those who have been our teachers, colleagues, friends and students. Dr Borenstein first thanks her parents for supporting her through school and always encouraging her to reach her goals. She thanks her father for giving her the love of data from his profession as a Ph.D. economist with the United Nations. She also thanks Dr Ann Stromberg of Pitzer College, Claremont, CA, for introducing her to the field of epidemiology in 1976. Professor Emily White at the University of Washington School of Public Health and Community Medicine and Fred Hutchinson Cancer Research Center played a critical role in Dr Borenstein's academic development, serving as her mentor through her dissertation research. Professor White introduced Dr Borenstein to Alzheimer's disease in 1983 and proposed that Dr Borenstein pursue her dissertation in this area. She is particularly grateful to Dr Leon Thal (1945–2007), who awarded her a Neurosciences Education and Research Foundation Merit Award for most promising new investigator in Alzheimer's disease research in 1992. The greatest thanks are given to her coauthor, professional partner, and husband, Dr James A. Mortimer, for his constant professional advice and collaboration, his patience and love.

Dr Mortimer thanks his many mentors as well as collaborators that he has worked with over the past 40 years. His initial interests in neuroscience were sparked by the founders of this field, including Dr Rodolfo Llinas, as well as Dr Gardner Quarton, who served on his doctoral committee at the University of Michigan and provided direction in his early career. Later at the National Institutes of Health, he developed techniques for recording from single neurons in awake animals with Dr Edward Evarts, a prelude to his later interests in diseases of the nervous system. He thanks his collaborators in the Department of Neurology at the University of Minnesota, where he spent 20 years as a faculty member, in particular, Dr David Webster, who facilitated the development of a research center devoted to Alzheimer's disease and Parkinson's disease. Other important collaborators included Drs David Snowdon and Bill Markesbery at the University of Kentucky, his coprincipal investigators on the Nun Study, and Dr Margaret Gatz of the University of Southern California with whom he worked on the Swedish Twin Study of Dementia. His most important influence over the past 20 years has been his wife, Dr Amy Borenstein, with whom he has shared this intellectual journey and without whom the ideas in this book would not have evolved.

Both of us would like to thank our friends and colleagues, most notably Drs Lon White, Peter Schofield, Lorene Nelson, and Lenore Launer for their many hours of insightful discussions and heated debates about the nature and causes of Alzheimer's disease and other neurodegenerative disorders.

Our gratitude goes to the many Alzheimer patients and their families, as well as people without the disease, who participated in the many research studies that are represented in this book. The altruism that goes into participating in observational studies and clinical epidemiologic trials represents the pinnacle of the subject-researcher connection. Despite their own uphill battles, they selflessly donated their time and effort to help others to move science forward and help solve the mysteries of our time.

Finally, we are incredibly fortunate to have our children, Rebecca Anna Graves and Kent Mortimer, and his wife and daughter, Diane and Eileen, without whose love and support this book would not have been possible.

Prologue

A Primer on Epidemiologic Concepts and Methods

Epidemiology is the basic science of public health that examines the distribution of diseases in human populations by person, place, and time (descriptive epidemiology), and the causes or etiology of these diseases (analytic epidemiology). Epidemiologic methods are used in both observational studies and clinical research investigating the effects of drugs or other interventions in the treatment and prevention of disease. In this primer, we explain the basic concepts of epidemiology for those who are not trained in public health.

While the ultimate goal of epidemiologic research is to identify potential causes of diseases and to use this information for prevention, its starting point is to describe the occurrence of disease by characteristics related to person, place, and time by answering the following questions: Who gets the disease? Where does the disease occur more or less frequently? What are the disease trends over time? These descriptive questions can be answered by looking at *rates* of disease among defined populations, across geographic locations, and over time. More detailed questions regarding risk or protective factors for the disease, such as having a particular exposure, can be addressed by analytic studies that compare individuals' histories who have the disease to those who do not have the disease. Alternatively, one can begin with individuals who are disease-free and follow those who are exposed to a risk or protective factor and those who are not exposed to the same risk factor over time to see whether those with the exposure develop the disease more often than those not exposed. In experimental epidemiology, a group of people are randomized to receive a drug or intervention of some kind (exposure) or not to receive it and are followed over time to test whether those who received the intervention develop the disease less frequently than those who did not receive the intervention.

DESCRIPTIVE EPIDEMIOLOGY

Incidence

The most important measure for understanding causation is the incidence rate, the number of new disease events divided by the number of people who are at risk in a defined population for a specified period of time. For example, in a study of Alzheimer's disease (AD), let's assume that a population of 1,000 people known to be free of AD at the start of the study (baseline) is carefully followed over the ensuing 10 years. If everyone in the study survived for the entire 10 years, the denominator for the incidence rate would be 1,000 × 10 = 10,000 person-years. However, some participants will not complete the 10 years of follow-up. Some may refuse to continue their participation because of sickness or another reason, others may be lost to follow-up because they leave the area in which the study is being conducted, and still others may die. The denominator of the incidence rate takes such losses into account. The numerator is a count of the number of people who did not have the disease of interest at the beginning of the study, but developed the disease over the 10 years. If the incidence rate is say, 2% per year, then over 10 years of complete participation, 200 people will get the disease (20 per year if all characteristics stayed the same for all years of the follow-up). Because the denominator will be smaller than 10,000, the true incidence rate will be a little larger than 2%. For example, if the denominator is 8,986, the incidence rate will be 200/8,986 or 2.23%. We can look at the incidence rate in any subgroup of the population we wish. For example, we can divide up or "stratify" the population of 1,000 people into men and women, different age groups, different exposure groups (e.g., people who eat fish three or more times a week and those who eat fish two or fewer times a week); or any other variable that we measure at baseline in the "cohort" we decide to follow. This allows us to look at the incidence rate by characteristics related to person. For example, we might find that people who eat fish three or more times per week have a lower incidence rate of the disease than those who eat fish two or fewer times per week.

To compare disease incidence according to place or geographic location, we could compare incidence rates by age groups in men and women in different countries or states. It is important to note that such comparisons will only be valid if the disease is defined in the same way in different places. To determine whether the frequency of the disease has been changing over time, we would need to measure the disease the same way over many years, and compare the incidence rates at the two (or more) time points, taking into account differences by other characteristics that may have changed in that time period, like the age structure in the population. It is important to recognize that there are reasons that we might see changing incidence rates over time that may not be related to real changes in the incidence rate (the speed of developing new disease). For example, the disease may become better recognized in the medical community or the stigma associated with the disease may lessen over time increasing the likelihood that doctors make a diagnosis. There also may be changes made in the diagnostic criteria for the disease that will lead to apparent increases or decreases in the incidence rates of a disease. Epidemiologists first consider whether such methodological changes could be responsible for differences in incidence rates by person, place and time. Only after such explanations can be excluded or adjusted for is it possible to make a valid statement about differences related to etiology of disease.

Prevalence

The prevalence rate differs from the incidence rate in that it counts the number of *existing* cases of disease in a defined population *at a specified time*, rather than the number of new or incident cases, and divides this by the size of the population that is living and at risk (including those who are living with the disease). Another way of expressing the prevalence rate is that it measures the proportion of people in a defined population that has a disease at a specified point in time (Rothman, Greenland, & Lash, 1998). The prevalence rate provides a good measure of the burden of the disease. Going back to our example, if we followed 1,000 people for 10 years, and 20 people developed the disease each year, then by year 3, we should have approximately 60 people who are living with the disease, provided no one has died from the disease during that period. The prevalence rate (P) at year 3 would be 60/1,000 = 6%. The prevalence rate is heavily influenced by the duration of survival after disease onset and is generally equal to the incidence rate (I) multiplied by the mean duration (D) of the disease ($P = I \times D$). For AD, mean survival is about 7 years. Thus, a new case is expected to live on average 7 years. For some diseases in which the duration of disease is short, for example, pancreatic cancer, the incidence rate will be approximately equivalent to the prevalence rate. For other diseases such as multiple sclerosis with very long durations, the prevalence rate or burden of the disease in the population will be much higher than the incidence rate.

The prevalence rate generally is not of interest in studies of etiology. If we examine risk factors for prevalence, we will mix risk factors for incidence (true disease rate) with those for duration. The incidence rate is appropriate for studying risk factors related to the speed or rate of developing a disease.

Mortality

The mortality rate uses as its numerator the number of deaths from the disease of interest in a specified time period divided by the number of people at risk of dying in the population. In our example, in the cohort of 1,000 people, let's assume that 3% died the first year. Because the closed cohort is growing older each year, we would expect the percent of deaths to increase a little in subsequent years and we could use actuarial data to estimate the expected death rates each year, which would depend on the cohort members' sex and age distributions. We can examine the mortality rate among people with AD and compare that to the mortality experience in the rest of the cohort to see whether AD increases the probability of death.

Unless we enumerate observed deaths within a defined study cohort in a rigorous manner, enumerating deaths from AD in large populations is extremely inaccurate. Most commonly, this would be done using death certificate data. For AD, these are highly unreliable due to variability in who is reporting and how much they know about the deceased person, as well as standards in reporting and how AD is assigned to a code on the certificate. Comparing mortality rates for AD between different countries is highly questionable, since the measurement of whether someone had AD or a related dementia varies from country to country, as does the practice and quality of maintaining death records.

ANALYTIC EPIDEMIOLOGY

Epidemiologic tools include two main types of analytic designs from which an estimate of risk can be derived. Using the scientific method, epidemiologists develop a hypothesis regarding potential causation and then analyze data to test this hypothesis. The presence of an association is determined by the ability to refute or not to refute the null hypothesis of no association between an exposure and an outcome. In epidemiology, we seek the same result over many studies (consistency) conducted with differing methodologies and in different populations, before we apply other causal criteria to infer a cause-and-effect relationship between a putative exposure and an outcome.

Randomized Clinical Trials

Scientists have long considered randomized clinical trials (RCTs) the gold standard of study designs, the design that "proves" whether an exposure causes an outcome. In such a trial, the exposure is manipulated by the investigator by randomly assigning a defined group of people to receive or not receive a drug, behavioral, dietary, or other intervention. The relative risk (RR) compares the incidence rate of disease among those randomized to the treatment or intervention to those randomized not to receive the treatment or intervention. The goal of randomization is for the two groups to resemble one another in all respects except for the intervention. Successful randomization depends on the size of the sample and proper implementation of the randomization scheme. RCTs can only be conducted using interventions that will putatively lower the incidence rate of the disease over the follow-up period. Risk factors for disease, such as smoking or exposure to chemicals, cannot ethically be randomly allocated to individuals. Although RCTs offer the best level of evidence for an exposure-outcome relationship, there are several methodological issues that can bias the results and many challenges that must be carefully considered.

Observational Cohort Studies

Observational cohort studies are generally considered to provide the next best level of scientific evidence to support causal inferences. It is important to note that null findings in a randomized trial do not prove that a risk factor does not cause a disease. Null findings may be the result of low statistical power from a small sample size or an inadequately long duration of the trial. As we shall see in this book, AD evolves over several decades. Therefore, relatively brief RCTs may not be the optimum design to examine risk factors that exert their effects over years or decades. Randomized controlled trials and observational cohort studies for AD *answer different questions*, rather than provide different levels of evidence.

When potentially harmful exposures are examined and when potentially protective exposures that have their effects over many years are of interest, the observational cohort study is the study design of choice. Epidemiologists typically assemble a cohort of individuals that can be defined geographically, ethnically, or by specific characteristics, such as religion or occupation, examine each person for the presence or absence of the disease of interest at the start of the study, and then follow the population carefully to document incident cases of disease.

In studies of dementia or AD, potential cohort participants are usually first screened with a cognitive test and are asked to participate in a full neurologic and neuropsychological examination if they meet specified screening criteria or if they are otherwise deemed to be at high risk for dementia or AD. Because a cohort study aims to identify new or incident cases of dementia or AD, only those judged not to be demented at initial evaluation (baseline) are included in the cohort to be followed. At the baseline examination, these nondemented participants are questioned using a highly structured questionnaire about a large number of risk factors, such as their family and medical histories, their educational background, diet, exercise, and other personal habits including smoking and alcohol consumption. Typically every 2–3 years, the cohort is seen again, and the cognitive screening test is readministered, with individuals meeting study criteria for going on to the clinical evaluation being tested in depth for the presence of incident dementia. This is called a two-phase, or multiphase case-finding procedure. Each potential case is discussed by the study consensus diagnostic committee in which physicians and neuropsychologists fill out diagnostic criteria for dementia and for dementia subtype, for example, AD, vascular dementia, or dementia due to another cause. The study may continue for many years or may end, usually depending on funding. The investigators can then examine risk factors from the baseline or from any examination during the study follow-up period as they relate to incident cases of the prespecified outcomes. The RR is typically calculated, by dividing the incidence rate of dementia or AD among individuals exposed to a factor by the incidence rate of dementia or AD among individuals who were not exposed. If this RR exceeds 1.0 and the probability of this happening by chance is smaller than 5% ($p<0.05$) (which is equivalent to saying that the 95% confidence interval or 95% CI does not include 1.0), the risk factor is said to be "statistically significant" with respect to its association with increased risk for the outcome. If the RR is less than 1.0 and $p<0.05$, the risk factor is said to be inversely associated with or protective for the outcome. If the p-value is >0.05 (the 95% CI includes 1.0), the factor is said not to be significantly associated with the risk for disease. There are multiple forces that can falsely elevate or decrease the RR estimate, which we will deal with briefly in the sections on Validity, Bias and Confounding.

One type of RR that we will use in the book is the hazard ratio (HR). Simply put, the HR is the true ratio of two incidence rates, in which the estimated measure of effect (the RR) takes time into account. Thus the HR not only tells us the magnitude of the RR (how strong the RR is comparing exposed to unexposed individuals) but also tells us that people with the factor will get the disease earlier (risk factor) or later (protective factor) in time than those without the factor.

The attributable risk, or the risk difference, is the rate of disease that would be eliminated if we could eliminate a causal exposure. This measure subtracts the incidence rate among unexposed individuals from the incidence rate among exposed individuals. The population attributable fraction estimates the proportion of the disease that is due to the exposure if the exposure is causally related to the incidence of disease. This proportion depends on the prevalence of the exposure in the population of interest.

Case-Control Studies

While cohort studies (and experimental clinical trials) can measure the speed of acquiring the disease of interest, case-control studies cannot. The only exception is when a case-control study is nested within a cohort study. Case-control studies are considered the next best analytic design with regard to study design quality. In a case-control study, all or a representative sample of cases of the disease are found, preferably in a known population, and controls (people without the disease) are selected from the same or a similar population as the cases. It is very important to use the same criteria to select cases and controls, the single exception being presence of the outcome. For example, if the disease criteria require that cases be free of vascular disease, controls must also be selected from among those free of vascular disease. Otherwise, vascular disease may be found to be a protective risk factor for the disease. Controls may be matched to cases on characteristics like age, sex, or education to increase the power to examine other factors, or they may be selected at random from the same population as the cases. If matched, the factors used to match cannot be examined for their association with the disease. Once the cases and controls have been identified, they may be interviewed about their exposures before the disease began in the cases, and DNA and other biospecimens may be obtained. To identify risk factors, the two groups are compared. Since incidence rates are not available, the odds ratio (OR) is used. The OR is the odds that cases (people with the disease) have been exposed to the risk factor divided by the odds that controls (persons without the disease) have been exposed to this factor, that is, the OR compares the proportion of cases who have been exposed to the factor with the proportion of controls who have been exposed. The OR is interpreted the same way as the RR or HR. If the OR exceeds 1.0 and $p<0.05$ (the 95% CI does not include 1.0), the factor significantly increases the risk for disease; if the OR is less than 1.0 and $p<0.05$, the factor decreases the risk for disease.

Case-control studies are the preferred study design for diseases that are sufficiently rare (less than 5% of the population at risk) that a cohort study would not easily generate a sufficient number of cases for meaningful analysis (the concept of statistical power). Because their memory for past events and exposures is impaired, we cannot interview AD cases after they present with dementia. For this reason, case-control studies of AD have traditionally utilized proxy informants, including spouses, children, or other knowledgeable informants, to gather past exposure histories by interview. This intrinsically lowers the quality of data that can be used in the estimation of risk. Because proxy informants respond less reliably than cases would if they were able to, interviewing only case proxy informants and not control proxy informants creates a bias that is mitigated somewhat if control proxy informants are also interviewed (Nelson et al., 1990). A validation substudy can be implemented within the case-control study such that controls are interviewed about themselves and control proxy informants are interviewed about the controls and their responses compared to check for data quality.

Cross-Sectional Studies

This study design uses a defined population or group of people to measure exposures and outcomes at the same time. While exposures may also be measured from the subjects' past mimicking a case-control or case-cohort design, the traditional cross-sectional study measures both at the same time. Therefore, no incidence rates are available and prevalence is usually the only measure available of the occurrence of the disease. Prevalence studies are cross-sectional studies in that they provide a snapshot of the population at a certain time. In this sense, this study design is considered descriptive rather than analytic. However, because we can calculate ORs and prevalence ratios (the proportion of exposed with the disease divided by the proportion of unexposed with the disease, used when the disease is not rare or when we are not sure of the temporal sequence of the exposure and the disease), cross-sectional studies can give us valid data regarding *possible* causation, particularly for exposures that do not change with time, such as genes.

Because an exposure must precede the onset of the disease in time to be considered a cause of the disease and cross-sectional studies do not allow for the temporal sequence of the exposure-disease association to be determined, they provide a lower level of scientific evidence than case-control studies. It is important to note that with regard to AD cohort or case-control studies also may have difficulty in establishing temporal sequence between exposure and outcome. Even though we try to establish that the exposures occurred before clinical disease onset, if the disease is characterized by pathological changes that precede clinical symptoms, the exposure may represent a marker of the underlying disease pathology and may not be causally associated with the disease. This issue is considered in Chapters 21 and 22 of this book.

Ecologic Studies

Studies that are based on average levels of an exposure in populations rather than specific levels in individuals and in which the outcome of interest is prevalence or incidence of a disease in those populations are called ecologic studies. For example, mean dietary fat intake in different countries can be studied with regard to AD prevalence or incidence. While the mean level of exposure in a population may be associated with the incidence or prevalence of a disease, this does not necessarily imply that the exposure in individuals within the population is associated with the disease. Studies comparing mean exposures in populations can be subject to the ecologic fallacy, whereby patterns observed at the aggregate level are not seen at the individual level. Therefore, ecologic data cannot be used to support a statement of association. Because of this caveat, we will not consider this study design in this book.

Case Reports and Case Series

These types of reports provide the weakest level of scientific evidence, and fall into the descriptive study design category. A case report is a description of clinical and/or histologic observations for a single patient, and a case series describes such observations for a small group of patients. Because these reports do not include a comparison or control group, such data cannot be used to support the existence of an association between an exposure and an outcome. Often, when a disease is first seen by a physician, it is described in the literature as a case report. A small group of cases may then be assembled to see if there are commonalities among the cases. This occurred with the first case series report of Kaposi's Sarcoma in eight homosexual men in New York City, which heralded recognition of the AIDS syndrome (Hymes et al., 1981). Case reports are often used to generate a hypothesis to be tested later using an analytic study design, such as a case-control or a cohort study. Because case series and reports do not provide reliable data with regard to causation, they will not be considered in this book.

CASE DEFINITION

What is critically important about case reports and case series as well as analytic designs is the definition of a case. In epidemiology, explicit case definition criteria are of paramount importance to the uniform measurement of the outcome. If the outcome is misclassified (there are people in the case group without the disease or the control group is contaminated with some cases), the observed measure of effect from analytic studies may be falsely underestimated.

ASSOCIATION VERSUS CAUSATION

Epidemiologic methods can sometimes directly address causation if the exposure of interest is suited for an experimental study (randomized controlled trial or RCT). This is because at baseline, neither group has been exposed to the intervention and no one has had the outcome. When one group is experimentally exposed and shows a difference in outcome over time, assuming all other methodological issues are addressed, we can infer that the exposure occurred before the outcome (temporal sequence) and is likely a cause, at least in some of the participants in the trial.

In cohort and case-control studies, once an association has been found, there are three main questions that need to be addressed. Is the association *precise*, that is, could the study findings be due to chance alone? Second, is the association *valid*, that is, do the study findings reflect the true relation between the exposure and the outcome? Third, is the association *causal*, that is, is there sufficient evidence to infer a causal association between the exposure and the outcome? We will address each of these briefly.

PRECISION

Since each study uses a new sample of people from the population, there are natural errors associated with the selection process. In epidemiology it is important to minimize such errors. A "Type I" error occurs when one concludes that there is an association between the exposure and the disease, whereas in fact there is no association. These errors can occur because of poor study design or analysis or be due to chance. A "Type II" error occurs when the study fails to find an association, but in fact there is one in the natural world. This type of error can be due to bias or to other methodological shortcomings, such as the need to use proxy informants or designing the study with too few subjects. Precision refers to the size of the random error that can occur in the estimate of the OR or RR. Low precision is reflected by wide CIs around the estimate of risk. Precision of the estimate can be increased by increasing sample size. Samples that are too small may lead to wide CIs that include 1.0, leading to a Type II error (failure to reject the null hypothesis of no association when an association is actually present). It is important to add that while we use an α-value (size of permissible Type I error) of $p \leq 0.05$ as our default setting to declare a "statistically significant finding" (corresponding to a 95% CI that is statistically significant if it excludes the null value of 1.0 and not statistically significant if it includes the null value of 1.0), we should not dismiss p-values that are a bit higher than 0.05. For example, if the p-value for a result is 0.06 or 0.07, this means that the inclusion of a few more people in the sample might have made the difference between being statistically significant or not statistically significant. Thus, we might give such a p-value more consideration than if the p-value is clearly larger.

VALIDITY

Other errors in epidemiology fall under the umbrella term "validity," which refers to the extent to which the findings from a study reflect the true underlying situation in nature. These errors can be broadly grouped under two subheadings: internal validity and external validity. Internal validity refers to the degree to which the two groups being studied—the cases and the controls or the exposed cohort and the unexposed cohort—are like one another in all ways except the disease (case-control study) or the exposure (cohort study) permitting a *fair* comparison to be made. In a case-control study, the cases and controls should be selected from the same underlying population such that if the control became a case, s/he would be diagnosed in the same way with the disease as the cases in the study. External validity refers to the generalizability of the studied groups to the outside world. A study must be internally valid first, and then can be judged for its ability to extrapolate to the general population (external validity). An example of an internally valid study is the Nun Study (Snowdon et al., 1996), a study of 678 American Roman Catholic nuns who were members of the School Sisters of Notre Dame and were ages 75–102 at the beginning of the study. One inclusion criterion into the study was that the nuns were required to agree to donate their brain to the study when they died. This made the study unique, as it was the first to be able to examine neuropathologic lesions in the brain in an unbiased population of individuals who either became demented during the follow-up or remained cognitively intact. Before the Nun Study, autopsy case series were highly biased because only certain individuals who die are selected for autopsy, with dementia patients being over-represented. While the Nun Study has high internal validity, some scientists have questioned whether the study's findings can be generalized to other populations (external validity), for example, to men, or to individuals of different race/ethnicities living in the community.

In order for a study to be internally valid, the two groups being compared will ideally be similar to one another with regard to all characteristics of person, place and time except for the disease (in a case-control study) or the exposure (in a cohort study). This is why the randomized controlled trial has traditionally been considered the gold standard of epidemiologic study design. Successful randomization will result in intervention groups that match each other on both measured (and unmeasured, such as all genes) variables. In an observational study, we may have to adjust for differences between the groups on measured variables that differ between the groups and are also related to the outcome of interest (confounding). In order for the groups to be similar to one another, epidemiologists pay a great deal of attention to the selection of participants. In a case-control study, for example, a group of cases that come from a clinic or hospital may have some biases that are not immediately measurable. If the clinic or hospital is known for its work in an area, for example, it may have an Alzheimer's Disease Research Center, then it may attract highly educated caregivers who want their loved one who is developing dementia to be clinically evaluated by expert doctors. When investigators conduct a case-control study using these cases, they may select controls that come from the same geographic area as the cases but are less educated. The cases may be found to have more education than controls, which in fact is the reverse of the truth. This finding would have been generated by referral bias and led to the wrong conclusion about the association between education and AD. Such biases are known in epidemiology as *selection bias*. Epidemiologists are trained to choose comparison groups that minimize selection bias such that fair comparisons can be made between them.

Another important source of bias in epidemiologic studies is called *observation bias*, which has to do with the way in which variables are defined and measured in the study. When a variable is measured with a large degree of random error, the RR or OR is reduced toward the null value of 1.0. This increases the chance of making a Type II error and erroneously concluding that an association is not present when in reality it is. Conversely, the effect measure (the RR or OR) can be erroneously overestimated if cases and controls are compared with regard to an exposure, and proxies for cases either over-recall the exposure, proxies for controls under-recall the exposure, or both occur simultaneously. This will result in a RR or OR that is overestimated relative to the underlying truth and may cause the investigator to conclude that an association exists when in fact it does not exist in the underlying population (a Type I error). Biases can work in different ways, and although cohort studies are thought to be superior to case-control studies, there are biases that apply to cohort studies that do not apply to case-control studies. For example, in a cohort study, individuals who at baseline do not have AD but present with clinical symptoms in the first few years of follow-up will likely already have some memory loss. When these individuals are interviewed for the study, they may selectively under-recall their past exposure histories. Individuals who are not destined to get AD will not under-recall such exposures. The net effect of this error is that the RR for positive risk factors will be attenuated toward the null value of 1.0, making a true effect more difficult to detect. In this book, we will have many opportunities to discuss different forms of bias and how the study results may be distorted by them.

One of the most important forms of bias is *confounding*. This occurs when a third variable associated with both the exposure and the outcome of interest explains some or all of the association that is seen between the exposure and the disease. We might be interested in the effect of a higher or lower education on the risk for AD. If we were just to examine the association between higher education and AD, we might find that there is a strong inverse association (people with higher education levels have lower risk for AD) but when we look at age, we find that the younger people in the sample have a higher education level than the older people in the sample. Since age is related to education level and also is related to the risk for AD, a subsequent adjustment for age would give more "credit" to older people for low education and less "credit" to younger people, therefore leveling the playing field so that a fair comparison can be made between the two education groups. We might still find an inverse association between education and risk for AD, but it will likely be weaker than we observed before we adjusted for age (the "crude" RR). In this example, age is a confounder of the education–AD association and it is necessary to adjust for it to estimate an internally valid RR. Most of the time, we have many confounders that must be dealt with simultaneously and statistical modeling is used to for such adjustment.

Related to the topic of confounding is another concept we will deal within the book where a variable may seem on the surface to be a confounder, but is instead an "intermediate" or a "mediating" variable. This means that it may meet the criteria for confounding (it is associated with the exposure and is an independent risk factor for the outcome), but it is in the causal pathway between the exposure and the outcome. In this case, the exposure is causally related to the intermediate variable, which in turn causes the outcome. An example of this might be that physical exercise causes an increase in whole brain volume as measured by magnetic resonance imaging, which in turn determines if a person has clinical dementia or not. Brain volume in this example is not a confounder that needs to be adjusted, but is instead a stepping stone in the causal pathway between physical exercise and the probability of developing dementia.

A third variable in addition to the exposure and the outcome can be a confounder, an intermediate variable or an effect-modifier. *Effect-modification* refers to the magnitude of an association between an exposure and an outcome being different for different levels of a third variable. For example, if a person has a genetic predisposition to AD, for example, carries an Apolipoprotein E-ε4 allele, and has a low education level, it might be hypothesized that their risk for AD would be much higher than if they had the genetic susceptibility gene alone or they had a low education level alone. Do the two risk factors biologically interact to produce a much higher risk? Effect-modification is defined as a process in which an exposure acts with another factor to increase or decrease the risk for disease. There are two kinds of effect-modification: multiplicative (sometimes called synergistic) and additive. The first type is where the combined effects of the exposure and the third variable exceed the *product* of each effect alone. The second type is where the combined effects of the exposure and the third variable exceed the *addition* of each effect alone. We will have an opportunity to discuss both types of effect-modification in the ensuing chapters.

As we enter the age of personalized medicine, scientists are concerned with defining subgroups of individuals who have multiple genetic risks for AD (G–G interactions), or who have genetic risks and environmental risks (G–E) that interact with one another. As AD is a highly complex disease, there are likely to be multiple genetic and environmental risk factors that act together to modify its risk.

CAUSATION

If a statistically significant association has been demonstrated between an exposure and an outcome and the investigator has controlled for potential biases, causal criteria can be applied to evaluate whether an exposure is likely to "cause" the outcome. These generally include the strength of the association; consistency of the association across studies; specificity of the cause leading to a single effect; temporality, that is, the cause must precede the effect in time; biologic gradient, that is, when the exposure increases, there should be a proportional increase or decrease in incidence of the disease depending on whether the exposure is positively or inversely related to the outcome; as well as biologic plausibility (Hill, 1965). Not all criteria need to be fulfilled to conclude that a risk factor is likely to be causally associated with an outcome. For example, a cause-and-effect association may be clear even in the absence of a known biologic mechanism (Herbst, Ulfelder, & Poskanzer, 1971; Kehrberg et al., 1981).

In observational cohort studies, when an association exists independently of other factors and bias does not distort the observed measure of relative effect (HR/RR/OR), the causal criteria specified above are carefully considered one-by-one. If the weight of the evidence in the literature favors a causal conclusion, then one can be made, at least tentatively. There is no quantitative way to assess the probability of whether an exposure causes an outcome. This judgment is based on a qualitative evaluation of the information available. Therefore, bold causal statements are rarely made by epidemiologists. Commonly a systematic review and/or a meta-analysis is written to summarize the body of evidence for a given research question. Systematic reviews are qualitative summaries of the evidence, whereas meta-analyses are quantitative summaries of the RR/ORs across studies. In meta-analyses, the summary measure of effect might be stratified by study design, geographic location or another effect-modifier. In addition, meta-analyses analyze the heterogeneity of studies and often estimate the probability of publication bias, the tendency to publish more positive findings in the medical literature than null ones.

PREVENTION

Medicine and public health aim to promote, preserve, and restore health and to lessen suffering. Prevention implies that we want to stop something from happening. Prevention is currently thought of in a broader sense than it was in the past. Not only should prevention apply to those at imminent risk; it also should apply to those at elevated risk and to those who currently appear to be risk-free but who might benefit from interventions that impact their future risk. Traditionally, epidemiology has classified three levels of prevention. Primary prevention targets the reduction of risk factors or causes of disease by focusing on modifying the stage of susceptibility to disease to prevent development of the underlying pathology. Secondary prevention targets subclinical disease (underlying pathology) in an effort to prevent the clinical manifestations of disease. Tertiary prevention attempts to reduce complications from a clinical disease that would limit a patient's function and disability (Oleckno, 2008). The concept of prevention is changing as we learn more about how to characterize diseases before they manifest themselves clinically and will continue to evolve in the coming decades. Because of improvements in biomarkers for many diseases allowing clinicians and researchers to visualize pathology before clinical symptoms arise, the lines between the different types of prevention are becoming blurred.

Section I

Defining a Case

Chapter 1

The "First" Case

The initial recognition of the disease that was later named after him was made by a German psychiatrist, Dr Alois Alzheimer, at the beginning of the twentieth century. The case he described was Auguste Deter, or Auguste D. (Figure 1.1), who was admitted at age 51 to the insane asylum in Frankfurt am Main on November 25, 1901 and placed under the care of Dr Alzheimer (Maurer, Volk, & Gerbaldo, 1997). Auguste D.'s presentation included both psychiatric and cognitive symptoms. From the initial symptom of jealousy of her husband, she was observed to progressively lose her memory and become disoriented in her home, misplacing and hiding items and becoming paranoid that someone was going to kill her. In the asylum, she exhibited signs of confusion interspersed with times of rationality, and would become delirious, aggressive, and sometimes suffer from auditory hallucinations. Dr Alzheimer reported that she often screamed for many hours, and that she was unable to understand her situation (Stelzmann, Schnitzlein, & Murtagh, 1995). At times, it was impossible to examine her due to her erratic behavior. Over time, her memory became seriously impaired, and while she could still name objects shown to her, she forgot them as soon as they were removed from view. She developed problems reading and writing and called things by their wrong name, such as "milk-pourer" instead of "cup." She could not understand questions or follow a conversation. Although her gait and reflexes were normal, her cognition continued to decline as her illness progressed. In the end, Auguste D. "was lying in bed in a fetal position completely pathetic, incontinent. In spite of all nursing care, she had developed bedsores" (Stelzmann, Schnitzlein, & Murtagh, 1995). Auguste D. lived for 4½ years after her first symptoms began. Her causes of death included septicemia due to bedsores and pneumonia.

Alois Alzheimer was born in 1864 near Wűrzburg, Germany. In 1888, he was a medical resident at the Hospital for the Mentally Ill and Epileptics in Frankfurt am Main and later became a senior physician there. His interests were wide-ranging, from dementia of degenerative and vascular origins to epilepsy, forensic psychiatry, and psychoses (Maurer, Volk, & Gerbaldo, 1997). In 1903, Alzheimer moved to Munich, where he worked with Dr Emil Kraepelin, the founder of modern scientific psychiatry who proposed that the origins of psychiatric disease were biological changes in the brain. Dr Franz Nissl, the leading

Alzheimer's Disease. DOI: http://dx.doi.org/10.1016/B978-0-12-804538-1.00001-8

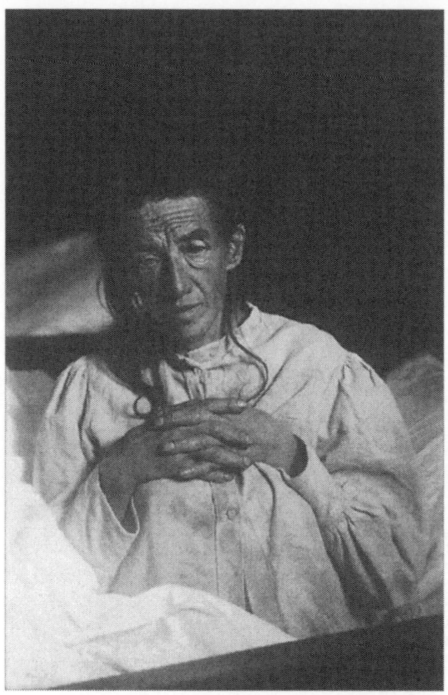

FIGURE 1.1 Auguste Deter. Dr Alzheimer's first case, described in 1906. Photograph dated 1902.

neuropathologist of his day, taught Alzheimer new histopathologic techniques to study disorders of the nervous system. These two influences were key to Alzheimer's discovery and description of the disease that would bear his name.

Alzheimer continued to follow Auguste D.'s case until her death on April 8, 1906 and subsequently studied the neuropathology of her disease using brain autopsy tissue. On November 4, 1906, Dr Alzheimer gave a lecture describing Auguste D.'s case. In the first case report published in 1907 (Alzheimer, 1907), he described the histopathologic findings of peculiar changes in the neurofibrils (neurofibrillary tangles) and neuritic (amyloid) plaques. Using Bielschowsky's silver method of staining, he reported that inside a cell that appeared normal were one or more fibrils that were unusually thick. Many fibrils that were adjacent to one another had similar changes. These appeared as thick bundles or clumps. Sometimes, bundles of fibrils occurred outside cells, at locations of once healthy neurons that had degenerated. He called these fibrils "neurofibrillary degeneration." Alzheimer also described minute "miliary foci" distributed throughout the cortex now known as amyloid plaques that were caused by the deposition of a "special substance in the cortex." He reported that the plaques were extremely numerous and that almost one-third of the cortical cells had degenerated and died. Accompanying these findings were observations that the brain had significantly atrophied (shrunk) and that the larger vascular tissues showed arteriosclerotic changes (Stelzmann, Schnitzlein, & Murtagh, 1995). In recognition of his pioneering work, his colleague Dr Kraepelin suggested the disease be named after Dr Alzheimer. By 1911, there were several case series published of cases similar to Auguste D.'s (Kraepelin, 1910; Perusini, 1909).

Auguste D.'s case is remarkable for her young age at onset and her rapid decline. Some have debated whether her case was really Alzheimer's disease (AD) or another illness, such as Pick's disease (known today as frontotemporal dementia). However, most experts agree that Auguste D. displayed the hallmarks of AD and that her disease was correctly diagnosed. The neuropathologic findings supporting the diagnosis of AD were important at the time because they showed that mental disorders could have an organic substrate. Prior to this time they were considered functional disorders. The findings fit well with Kraepelin's view that psychiatric diseases have a biological basis.

Auguste D. was certainly not the "first" case of the disease. By the early 1900s, senile dementia (meaning losing one's mental faculties in advanced age) was a recognized clinical entity. What was new was the relatively young age at which Auguste D. presented with clinical symptoms. Kraepelin described the newly named "Alzheimer's disease" as a "particularly serious form of senile dementia…that sometimes starts as early as in the late forties" (Kraepelin, 1910). In fact, we know today that familial forms of AD can lead to extremely early disease presentations with some beginning as early as the 20s (Wisniewski et al., 1998). However, these cases are very rare as we shall discuss in Chapter 10. AD is predominantly a disease of old age.

The initial description of AD as a presenile dementia to be distinguished from senile dementia persisted until the late 1960s, when pioneering neuropathologic studies of normal and demented individuals (Tomlinson, Blessed, & Roth, 1968, 1970) led to the recognition that the same disease was responsible for much of the more common form of dementia occurring in later life as well. While early-onset cases are of interest, this book focuses primarily on the more common later-onset cases of AD and the potential for preventing them.

Chapter 2

Clinical Appearance, Progression, and Classification

Although memory loss is the hallmark and one of the earliest signs of Alzheimer's disease (AD), problems with language, personality changes, aggression, insight and understanding, confusion, hallucinations and delusions, as well as loss of ability to perform activities of daily living are common clinical characteristics of the disease as it progresses. In this chapter, we will describe the clinical research criteria that have been used as the "gold standard" for this disease over the last 30 years. In Chapter 3, we will discuss how these criteria have been applied in epidemiologic studies to identify prevalent and incident cases of the disease. We will then examine the neuropathologic basis for this illness in Chapter 4 and review the clinicopathologic correlation or degree to which the neuropathologic findings explain the clinical disease. Finally, in Chapter 5, we will discuss the emergence of clinical symptoms in the context of the threshold model of brain reserve in dementia and AD.

WHAT IS DEMENTIA?

The term "dementia" has connotations of lunacy from its Latin derivation from *de-* meaning "without" to *ment*-meaning "mind." In the eighteenth century, the term dementia had legal implications, indicating a lack of competence to care for oneself physically and mentally. During the first six decades of the twentieth century, dementia when it occurred in old age was frequently considered a normal consequence of aging and used synonymously with the term "senility." Alternative terms used to describe dementia were "organic brain syndrome" and "arteriosclerotic brain disease," the latter term implying a specific cause, arteriosclerosis, for the condition. Early prevalence studies from Scandinavia and the United Kingdom used the term "chronic organic brain syndrome" interchangeably with dementia (Mortimer, Schuman, & French, 1981). Dementia when it occurred in individuals above age 65 was referred to as "senile brain disease" and "senile dementia," to separate it from presenile dementias occurring before this age. The distinction between presenile and senile dementia has now largely

Alzheimer's Disease. DOI: http://dx.doi.org/10.1016/B978-0-12-804538-1.00002-X

been dropped because the pathologies responsible for dementia are known to be similar regardless of age.

Dementia is an umbrella term that refers to an acquired loss of intellectual function that features a disturbance in memory, but is also accompanied by impairment in at least one other cognitive domain, including language disturbance (aphasia), impaired ability to perform motor activities despite intact motor function (apraxia), failure to recognize or identify objects despite intact sensory function (agnosia), or disturbance in executive functioning (planning, organizing, sequencing, or abstracting information and activities) (American Psychiatric Association, 2000). These domains can be measured neuropsychologically by assessing performance on tests of language, attention/executive function, and visuospatial skills (Petersen, 2004). The memory impairment usually presents as a problem in the ability to learn new information or to recall recently learned information. This loss in short-term memory may begin innocuously with what many equate with "senior moments" like forgetting where something is located, forgetting to turn off the stove or lock the doors. In individuals who are developing dementia, memory lapses progress to significant impairments in short-term memory. Problems with recall of information learned more remotely in time, e.g., getting lost while driving to a familiar place or remembering the names of the past four US presidents, generally occurs later in the progression of dementia or AD.

Other typical signs around the beginning of the disease include problems with following a story or conversation and naming objects or people. A person also may have trouble when faced with a new or complex task or have problems with calculation, such as in balancing a checkbook. Inappropriate behavior linked to the loss of judgment and a "personality change" can be one of the first signs or can occur later in the disease. Personality changes may accentuate already existing traits. For example, a person who was conscientious may become rigid, a guarded person may become suspicious or paranoid, and a usually content person may become oblivious and docile. Fear and agitation understandably result from the insight a person may have at the beginning of their illness. This usually occurs independently of behavioral problems, such as hallucinations and delusions, which are likely due to more advanced disease pathology and occur somewhat later in the disease course (Harwood, Barker, Ownby, & Duara, 2000). As illustrated by Alzheimer's first patient, visual and auditory hallucinations, delusions involving stolen items the patient has hidden himself, or delusions of jealousy are characteristics of moderate-to-severe disease.

Because the first signs of AD are often mild and can be confused with normal forgetfulness, it is frequently difficult to accurately date the clinical onset of disease. In the community, family physicians, internists, and neurologists may assess short-term memory by asking patients to remember three words after a delay or by giving them a brief test like the Mini-Mental State Examination (MMSE) (Folstein, Folstein, & McHugh, 1975). Both of these approaches lack sensitivity to the earliest signs of AD, but are useful for detecting a case of dementing illness that has progressed to a more advanced stage. Because it is not specific to dementia, the MMSE cannot be used by itself to diagnose dementia (Tombaugh & McIntyre, 1992).

Neuropsychological test batteries are more sensitive and reliable than screening tests, but are not routinely administered in private clinical settings in the community, particularly in general practice. In the research setting, longitudinal studies that administer a brief screening test like the MMSE set a score on this test below which a detailed neuropsychological battery is given. Screening is done prior to neuropsychological testing primarily to save money in large population-based studies. A few studies are able to conduct clinical, neurological, and neuropsychological examinations on all subjects (Ding et al., 2014; Roberts et al., 2008). When these research populations are followed prospectively, it is possible to observe the year in which performance on neuropsychological testing begins to deviate from normal, i.e., from that expected for a person of the same age and education. Studies where representative populations are all given complete clinical examinations are the exception rather than the rule, and even when it can be done, each person in the population can only be observed every year or two. If a subject was normal for his age at one exam and abnormal in the next, one must infer the time point at which he converted from one state to another. Consequently, dating the onset of the illness is imprecise, particularly when the information must be obtained from a routine clinical examination.

COURSE AND PROGRESSION OF DEMENTIA

The course of dementia varies with the underlying cause. In rare cases like dementia due to B_{12} vitamin deficiency, the course is potentially reversible. In one case series at the Alzheimer's Disease Research Center in Pittsburgh, PA, 6% of individuals diagnosed with possible AD had vitamin B_{12} deficiency, and none of these cases developed a progressive dementia leading to nursing home admission or death over a 17-year follow-up period after appropriate therapy was given (Lopez et al., 2000). Other potentially reversible causes of dementia include other dietary deficiencies, alcoholism, depression, drug abuse, acute head injury, hormonal imbalances, inflammatory conditions, infections, medication side effects, normal-pressure hydrocephalus, subdural hematoma, thyroid disease, and tumors. Blood testing and imaging are needed to rule out these causes of dementia.

In degenerative dementia such as AD, a progressive decline is observed. The decline can be quantified clinically using an instrument such as the Clinical Dementia Rating Scale (CDR; Hughes, Berg, Danziger, Coben, & Martin, 1982) or the Global Deterioration Scale (GDS; Reisberg, Ferris, de Leon, & Crook, 1982). The CDR is usually completed by a physician and is based on an interview with the patient and informant(s). The domains include Memory, Orientation, Judgment and Problem Solving, Community Affairs, Home and

Hobbies, and Personal Care. Memory is rated 0 if there is no memory loss or slight, inconstant forgetfulness, and 3 if memory loss is severe. Orientation is rated 0 if the patient is fully oriented to time and place and 3 if the person is oriented to person only. If the patient can solve everyday problems well, judgment and problem-solving are rated 0; if the patient is completely unable to make judgments or solve problems, the rating is severe (3). Independent function in everyday life, including work, shopping, business and finances, and usual participation in volunteer and social groups is rated 0 for Community Affairs, and a severe rating of 3 is given if there is no semblance of independent function outside of the home. Home and Hobbies are rated 0 if the patient is participating in their prior intellectual interests and hobbies as before, and severe (3) if they have withdrawn from all of their home activities and hobbies. Personal care is rated 0 if the patient can do all of their usual hygiene, dressing, and keeping of personal effects, and 3 if they require a great deal of help with personal care and are frequently incontinent. Scores between 0 and 3 include no dysfunction (CDR score of 0), questionable dysfunction (0.5), mild dementia (1.0), moderate dementia (2.0), and severe dementia (3.0). Scores of 4 and 5 are assigned when there are profound (4) and terminal (5) functional deficits. Profound changes include speech that is usually unintelligible or irrelevant, inability to follow simple instructions or comprehend commands, and only occasional recognition of the spouse or caregiver. A person in a profound CDR state will use his fingers more than utensils when eating and will require help eating, toileting, and grooming. They will only be able to walk a few steps with assistance and will not venture outside of the home. A person in a terminal CDR state will not comprehend any speech or recognize anyone. They will need to have complete help with feeding, often requiring a nasogastric tube. In addition, they will often be incontinent and bedridden, frequently with contractures. The cause of death is often from aspiration, bronchopneumonia, or decubiti. The condition directly responsible for death will usually be listed as the cause on the death certificate, and dementia may be listed as the underlying or contributing cause. There are no standards in the field for coding of the death certificate within or across countries, so death certificates are usually considered a poor choice for documenting outcomes in epidemiologic studies of dementia.

To calculate the global CDR score, an automated algorithm has been developed that scores ratings of 0–3 for the six domains described above (Baty & Morris, 2011). Another measure that is commonly used to quantify the severity of dementia is the CDR Sum of Boxes. For this measure, the scores are summed for a total possible score of 0–18.

For the GDS, seven stages are defined. Stage 1 is normal, and includes individuals at any age who are free of objective and subjective symptoms of cognitive and functional decline and also free of behavioral and mood changes. Stage 2 is "normal aged forgetfulness." Stage 3 is consistent with mild cognitive impairment (MCI), defined below. Stage 4 is mild AD, manifested by a reduced ability to manage complex activities of daily living (commonly referred to as "instrumental activities of daily living" or IADLs). Stage 5 is characterized as moderate AD, in which the patient needs assistance in selecting appropriate clothing for the weather and with daily hygiene. Stage 6 is associated with moderate-to-severe AD in which the patient is unable to dress themselves correctly without assistance. Finally, Stage 7 is that of severe AD, which includes loss of speech and the ability to walk. With excellent nursing care, the transition from Stage 6 to 7, or the transition to death, may be delayed.

CLINICAL RESEARCH CRITERIA FOR DEMENTIA

The diagnosis of dementia in epidemiologic studies relies on a set of clinical research criteria that are applied as uniformly as possible to all participants. Although several sets of criteria exist, the ones most commonly used in epidemiologic studies of dementia and AD are the criteria of the Diagnostic and Statistical Manual (DSM) of the American Psychiatric Association and the criteria for the International Classification of Diseases (ICD). It is important to recognize that the research criteria for dementia provide guidelines for diagnosis, not hard and fast rules. In epidemiologic studies, the determination of whether a participant is demented or not is a clinical decision reached after discussion in a clinical consensus conference. The reason this is necessary is that individual differences unrelated to dementia diagnosis can influence the decision of whether or not a particular individual is classified as demented. For example, a participant may perform poorly on a specific neuropsychological test due to unfamiliarity with test-taking procedures related to low education or may be impaired in an activity of daily living because of a physical impairment unrelated to cognitive ability. The decision of whether he or she is demented relies on taking such issues into account.

The most frequently used clinical research criteria for dementia are from the DSM of the American Psychiatric Association (American Psychiatric Association, 2000). These criteria have undergone several revisions over the past 60 years. The initial versions of this manual (I and II) published in 1952 and 1968 recognized chronic brain syndrome due to arteriosclerosis and senile brain disease. The third edition published in 1980 introduced the term dementia (Spitzer, Williams, & Skodol, 1980) and produced the first workable criteria for this syndrome. Subsequent editions (III-R, IV) have maintained the general criteria for dementia with seemingly minor, but possibly important, changes. Epidemiologic studies have used versions III-R and IV, so these are the criteria we shall review here.

In both DSM-III-R and DSM-IV, the following criteria must be satisfied for a diagnosis of dementia to be made:

1. There must be demonstrable evidence of impairment in memory that includes impaired ability to learn new information (short-term memory) *and* impairment in the recall of previously learned information (long-term memory) in DSM-III-R. In DSM-IV, this criterion can be satisfied if either impairment in short-term memory or long-term memory is demonstrated.

2. There must be demonstrable evidence of impairment in at least one other domain. In DSM-III-R, these include impairment in abstract thinking, impaired judgment, other disturbances of higher cortical function such as language and constructional ability, and personality change. In DSM-IV, these include aphasia, agnosia, apraxia, and executive functioning.
3. The cognitive deficits in (1) and (2) must each cause significant impairment in social or occupational functioning and must represent a significant decline from a previous level of functioning. The operationalization of this criterion is sometimes difficult, as the interpretation of "significant" is at the discretion of the diagnosing physician and based on reports from informants, usually the patient's family. When there is no family or an informant is not knowledgeable of the patient's personal life, the validity of such reports is questionable. Also, when dementia occurs in older age, many patients no longer work so a decline in occupational functioning may not be relevant. A number of instruments have been developed to address this problem, such as the CDR described above (Hughes et al., 1982) and the Informant Questionnaire on Cognitive Decline in the Elderly (IQCODE; Jorm & Jacomb, 1989), which are sometimes used in research as adjuvants to screening (IQCODE) or to diagnostic classification (CDR). The CDR is the most common instrument used in epidemiologic studies of dementia, either to grade the severity of the dementia syndrome or to examine transitions from one severity grade to the next.
4. The deficits observed must not occur exclusively during the course of a delirium. Delirium is an acute confusional state that develops rapidly and often fluctuates in intensity. This syndrome is accompanied by deficits in attention and severe disorganization of behavior. In contrast to dementia that usually develops over months and is caused by pathologies in the brain, delirium is frequently the result of a condition outside the brain, such as a urinary tract infection or other organ dysfunction. It also is a common side effect of medications that affects the function of the brain, particularly anticholinergics and benzodiazepines. While delirium can occur *in* dementia, dementia can only be diagnosed in the absence of delirium. When family informants are questioned retrospectively about the presence of dementia before death, an acute episode of delirium is often confused with dementia.

Criterion 1 in DSM-III-R calls for deficits in short- *and* long-term memory, while in DSM-IV, short- *or* long-term memory deficits are required. This change should produce higher sensitivity in detecting dementia using the DSM-IV criteria in comparison with the DSM-III-R criteria.

The difference in which domains to consider for impairment between DSM-III-R and DSM-IV (criterion 2) has led some to propose that studies employing the DSM-III-R criteria should be interpreted differently from those using the DSM-IV criteria (Erkinjuntti, Ostbye, Steenhuis, & Hachinski, 1997). This is true when the sets of criteria are applied rigidly. However, it is likely to be much less of a problem when potential cases are reviewed in a clinical consensus conference (Erkinjuntti et al., 1997).

Subtypes of dementia can be diagnosed by individual sets of criteria described in the DSM-IV manual. However, for epidemiologic studies subtyping more commonly utilizes additional sets of clinical research criteria as discussed below. Recently, a revision of the DSM was published (DSM-V) (American Psychiatric Association, 2013). In DSM-V, the term "dementia" has been replaced with the term, "major neurocognitive disorders" in light of perceived stigma of the term "dementia," and a new addition has been made: "minor neurocognitive disorder." Because DSM-V criteria have not been used in epidemiologic studies to date, we will not consider its definitions.

The DSM-IV subclassification of "Dementia of the Alzheimer's Type" is reached if five criteria are fulfilled, in addition to those for dementia: (1) the course is characterized by gradual onset and continuing cognitive decline, (2) the cognitive deficits are not caused by another condition that causes progressive deficits in memory and cognition (e.g., cerebrovascular disease, Parkinson's disease, Huntington's disease, subdural hematoma, normal-pressure hydrocephalus, or brain tumor), (3) there are no systemic conditions that can cause dementia, for example, urinary tract infection, (4) the deficits are not caused by substance-induced conditions, and (5) the deficits are not caused by another Axis I disorder, such as major depressive disorder or schizophrenia.

Vascular dementia (VaD) by DSM criteria is another possible subdiagnosis of the dementia syndrome. VaD is diagnosed when "focal neurologic signs and symptoms are present or when laboratory evidence indicative of cerebrovascular disease is judged to be etiologically related to the disturbance" (American Psychiatric Association, 2000). Focal signs include exaggeration of deep tendon reflexes, extensor plantar response, pseudobulbar palsy, gait abnormalities, or weakness of an extremity. Laboratory evidence includes evidence from imaging, e.g., infarcts involving the cortex and underlying white matter or extensive microvascular disease.

CLINICAL RESEARCH CRITERIA FOR OTHER DEMENTIAS

Other dementias, such as dementia due to Parkinson's disease, frontotemporal dementia, and HIV/AIDS, can be diagnosed by DSM criteria when there is "evidence from the history, physical examination or laboratory findings that the cognitive deficits are due to the direct physiological consequence of another general medical condition" (American Psychiatric Association, 2000). There is a vast literature on what is commonly termed "non-AD dementias" that is beyond the scope of this book. In addition, an individual can have more than one subtype of dementia. In fact it is common for multiple pathologies to be present together. Some studies suggest that most dementia patients have a mixed AD-vascular disease pathology (Neuropathology Group of the Medical Research Council Cognitive Function and Aging Study (MRC-CFAS), 2001; White et al., 2005).

A representative autopsy study in Chicago (Schneider, Arvanitakis, Bang, & Bennett, 2007) demonstrated that, of 80 cases fulfilling neuropathologic criteria for AD, 46% had AD with no other pathology and 39 (49%) had two pathologies (25 AD with vascular infarcts, 12 with AD and Parkinson's disease or Lewy body disease, and 2 with AD and another pathology, such as a brain tumor or amyloid angiopathy with multiple hemorrhages). In addition, 5% of patients had all three pathologies (AD, infarcts, and Parkinson's disease/Lewy body disease). It is also important to note that the probability of concurrent pathologies increases with age, making it harder to diagnose one particular subtype in the old-old (age 85 and over). The DSM criteria therefore allow for dementia due to multiple etiologies.

CLINICAL RESEARCH CRITERIA FOR AD (NINCDS-ADRDA)

For AD, the National Institute of Neurological and Communicative Disorders and Stroke (NINCDS) and the AD and Related Disorders Association (ADRDA) Work Group diagnosis, known as the NINCDS-ADRDA criteria (McKhann et al., 1984) have been used for almost three decades. New criteria were published in 2007 (Dubois et al., 2007) and 2011 (McKhann et al., 2011) that update the NINCDS-ADRDA clinical guidelines and incorporate imaging biomarkers into the diagnostic process. Because of the significant expense involved in acquiring imaging on all individuals from a population-based study, the implementation of these criteria in epidemiologic studies has not yet occurred, and it remains to be seen whether this can be realistically done or whether the new criteria will be implemented principally into clinical research studies and trials. Since the studies described in this book have all used the 1984 and not the 2007/2011 criteria, when we refer to the NINCDS-ADRDA criteria in subsequent chapters, we will be referring to the 1984 criteria.

The NINCDS-ADRDA criteria (McKhann et al., 1984) have much in common with DSM-IV criteria for dementia of the Alzheimer type, but also permit the diagnosis of AD to be considered as possible, probable, or definite. The 1984 criteria for *probable AD* are: (1) there are impairments in memory and at least one other domain (orientation, language, judgment and problem-solving, or personality); (2) these deficits lead to impairment in the ability of the individual to carry out their daily activities in comparison with their performance in the past; (3) the cognitive deficits have a gradual onset with progression over at least 1 year; (4) delirium is not present; and (5) there are no systemic disorders or other brain diseases that could, by themselves, cause these progressive deficits in memory and cognition. In the original guidelines, there was a last criterion that an individual could not be younger than age 40 or older than age 90 to be diagnosed with AD. Because it has been established that pathologic AD does not look different in very young or very old individuals, this criterion has generally been ignored in epidemiologic studies.

If the criteria for probable AD are not met, we can consider whether an individual meets *possible AD* criteria. This will be the diagnosis if the individual meets most criteria for probable AD, but presents with variations in onset or course or has unusual symptoms like major language or motor function impairments. When there are other disorders that could result in dementia like a coexisting vascular component or Parkinson's disease, but it is thought that AD causes the dementia, or when there is a single, gradually progressive cognitive deficit in the absence of another identifiable cause, the diagnosis of possible AD may be made.

Finally, if an individual meets criteria for possible or probable AD during life and is found to have histopathologic evidence for AD on brain autopsy or biopsy, she or he is considered to have *definite AD*.

CLINICAL RESEARCH CRITERIA FOR VaD (NINDS-AIREN)

Research criteria were published in 1993 to diagnose dementia due to vascular causes (Roman et al., 1993). As before, we start with the presence of dementia. The individual must then meet both of the following criteria: (1) cerebrovascular disease must be present. This is defined by the presence of focal neurologic signs, such as hemiparesis, lower facial weakness, Babinski sign, sensory deficit, hemianopia, and dysarthria consistent with stroke (with or without a clinical history of stroke); and (2) evidence of relevant cerebrovascular disease by brain imaging (by CT or magnetic resonance imaging (MRI) scan) is required, demonstrating multiple large vessel infarcts or a single strategically placed infarct (in the angular gyrus, thalamus, basal forebrain, or PCA or ACA territories), as well as multiple basal ganglia and white matter lacunes or extensive periventricular white matter lesions, or some combination of these. The third criterion is very important and sometimes difficult to establish. There should be a temporal relationship between the cerebrovascular disease and the onset of clinical symptoms of dementia specifically, with (1) onset of dementia within 3 months after a recognized stroke, or (2) with abrupt (stepwise) declines in cognitive function, or fluctuating stepwise progression of cognitive deficits (Figure 2.1). Failure to accurately document the timing of the vascular event with respect to the onset of cognitive decline can result in misclassification of the VaD outcome. Some clinical signs may be documented in conjunction with these observations. For example, *probable* VaD may be accompanied by gait disturbance (small-step or marche-à-petit-pas or magnetic, apraxic–ataxic, or parkinsonian gait); history of unsteadiness and frequent, unprovoked falls; early urinary frequency, urgency and other urinary symptoms not explained by urologic disease; pseudobulbar palsy and personality and mood changes; abulia; depression; emotional incontinence; or other subcortical deficits, including psychomotor retardation and abnormal executive function (Roman et al., 1993). If both criteria 1 and 2 (vascular disease) and criterion 3 (temporal relation between vascular events and cognition) are met, the physician can make the

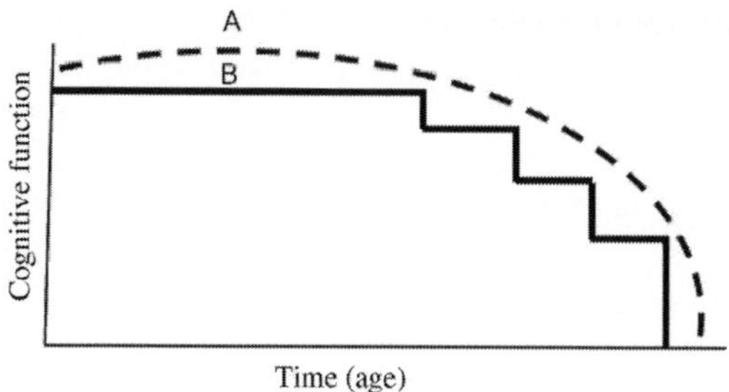

FIGURE 2.1 Clinical courses of Alzheimer's disease and vascular dementia. Alzheimer's disease has an insidious onset and progressive course (line A), while vascular dementia has an abrupt onset and stepwise progression (line B).

diagnosis of *probable* VaD. If the individual does not meet such criteria, the diagnosis of *possible* VaD is considered. If dementia occurs in the presence of focal neurologic signs and one or more of the following questions are answered "Yes," the individual may meet NINDS-AIREN criteria for possible VaD: (1) brain imaging studies to confirm cerebrovascular disease are missing; (2) there is not a clear temporal relationship between dementia and stroke/vascular signs; (3) there is a subtle onset and variable course that does not follow the distinct patterns shown in Figure 2.1 (such as cognitive improvement following a vascular event).

Several potential problems are associated with the application of disease criteria in epidemiologic studies. Individuals may meet a possible AD diagnosis by NINCDS-ADRDA criteria and at the same time, meet NINDS-AIREN criteria for possible VaD. The method used in an epidemiologic study for classifying "AD" and "VaD" may vary between studies, because of differences in operationalization of the criteria and potential overlap between these diagnoses. This complicates our ability to get a clear understanding of the frequency of dementia subtypes. In addition, the classification of dementia subtypes with the older criteria is based primarily on clinical findings. Criteria for "definite" subclassifications in the past 30 years have only been made at autopsy. More recent criteria (Cummings, Dubois, Molinuevo, & Scheltens, 2013; Dubois et al., 2007; McKhann et al., 2011) have incorporated imaging biomarkers, including positron emission tomography (PET) for Alzheimer lesions and MRI for regional brain volumes, in addition to assays of cerebral spinal fluid, to increase the specificity of a diagnosis of AD. This approach will reduce misclassification in the clinic setting, but applying such criteria in the population-based setting is at present unlikely because of the high cost. It is likely that most population-based studies will continue to rely on the NINCDS-ADRDA and NINDS-AIREN criteria, which are based largely on clinical observations.

Vascular Cognitive Impairment

It was recognized in the beginning of the 2000s that cerebrovascular effects on the brain were far broader than the concept that was defined by "multi-infarct dementia" or "VaD." Many cases of AD have concomitant vascular cognitive impairment (VCI). It also is recognized today that vascular pathology plays at least an additive role in the expression of dementia due to other causes. The field of VCI has developed significantly over the last decade, and the reader is referred to some excellent reviews of this area of the literature (Gorelick et al., 2011; O'Brien et al., 2003; Rincon & Wright, 2013).

ICD9/10: ANOTHER METHOD OF CLASSIFYING DEMENTIA

Another classification scheme for dementia that is used in epidemiologic studies, particularly for medical record-based and death certificate data, is the ICD. This system has gone through several revisions since being introduced originally in 1900 to classify causes of death. In the 1950s, the ICD was expanded to include morbidity statistics. "Senility and ill-defined diseases" first appeared in ICD-7 published in 1955, and presenile and senile dementia in ICD-8 published in 1965. In ICD-9 published in 1975, under "Hereditary and degenerative diseases of the central nervous system," specific codes for AD, Pick's disease, dementia with Lewy bodies, and other etiologies were introduced. In the ICD-10 published in 1993, the list of etiologies was expanded with subcategories of dementia in AD and VaD as well as additional causes added. Most countries in the world have been using the ICD-10 system for reporting of health events, with a notable exception being the United States. In October 2014, the Department of Health and Human Services in the United States mandated that ICD-10 codes be used in place of ICD-9 codes. The nonuniform adoption of ICD-10 has made comparisons of rates between countries more difficult.

Whether DSM-IV and ICD-10 provide comparable data has been addressed in studies comparing dementia diagnoses using these two sets of criteria. A study examining the discrepancy of results between ICD-10 and DSM-IV dementia diagnostic schemas found a 100% agreement between the two sets of criteria when applied to 207 patients presenting to a primary health care clinic in Norway (Naik & Nygaard, 2008). In this study, a broad interpretation of the ICD-10 criterion addressing "decline in other cognitive abilities such as abstraction, judgment, and problem-solving" was employed. In another, population-based study in Germany (LEILA75+) (Riedel-Heller, Busse, Aurich, Matschinger, & Angermeyer, 2001), a two-phase study (cognitive screening and clinical evaluation) assessed 1692 individuals and compared the annual incidence rates using DSM-III-R and ICD-10 criteria. The resulting incidence rates were similar, 45.8 (95% CI = 35.0–59.0) for DSM-III-R and 47.4 (95% CI = 36.1–61.2) for ICD-10. In a survey of 205 psychiatrists from 66 countries, the ICD-10 diagnoses were found to be valued more for diagnostic and training purposes, and the DSM-IV for research purposes (Mezzich, 2002).

Clinical criteria define a phenotype, and the accuracy of the clinical diagnosis can be judged using the neuropathologic diagnosis as the gold standard. When a clinical diagnosis is made, how well does it predict the actual neuropathologic diagnosis? This requires the quantification of the positive predictive value (PPV), the probability of having the neuropathologic diagnosis given a clinical diagnosis. The PPV is quite high (80–90%; Corey-Bloom et al., 1995), but varies depending on where the diagnosis is made (a highly specialized dementia clinic will have higher figures), what criteria are used, and how old the person is. Individuals aged 85 and over are more likely to have multiple brain pathologies. Therefore, defining a single cause for dementia will be more difficult than it is in younger people. These concepts are covered more thoroughly in Chapter 4. For our discussion here, the main point is that the clinical diagnosis can be misclassified, even in the hands of seasoned diagnosticians. This is due to the complexity of the disease and the need to sometimes follow a patient in time in order to feel more comfortable with the initial diagnosis.

MILD COGNITIVE IMPAIRMENT

As we shall show in this book, there is considerable evidence that the pathologic process of AD develops over many years and more likely decades. We will argue that it is a lifelong process, with risk reduction possible at all ages. Because of the long preclinical period associated with AD, by the time the disease is clinically expressed, the damage done in the brain may be irreversible (Petersen, 2009). To address this concern and the need for earlier diagnosis, a new diagnostic entity, MCI, representing an earlier, preclinical period of AD was introduced in 1999 (Petersen et al., 1999) and updated in 2004 (Petersen, 2004). Since that time, many studies have been conducted to describe the prevalence and incidence rates of MCI and to identify its risk factors. The distinction between MCI and dementia is important, because, as we shall see in the section on Descriptive Epidemiology, the frequency of the disease in populations is highly dependent on the methods used to define cases. In addition, it is important to determine whether risk factors differ for the clinical transition from normal cognition to MCI and for the transition of MCI to dementia or AD. If MCI is a mediating state between normal cognition and AD, it is possible that risk factors for AD, for example the genotype APOE-ε4, may influence the onset of MCI, but not the transition from MCI to AD. Our ultimate goal is to advance the detection of AD to an earlier time, preferably in the asymptomatic period when brain pathology is accumulating but there are no or few clinical symptoms.

Although the term "MCI" was coined in 1999, awareness of cognitive decline in old age prior to dementia had been recognized for decades. What was unclear was whether this transition from normal to abnormal was something that happened to all people as they aged, or whether memory and/or cognitive impairment represented the beginnings of a malicious process in only some people. "Benign senescent forgetfulness" was said to be distinct from "malignant senescent forgetfulness," which was thought to be a precursor of AD as early as 1962 (Kral, 1962). "Age-associated memory impairment" and "age-related memory impairment" referred to the normal changes in memory expected with increasing age. This type of memory loss was not considered to be malignant and could occur as the result of declines in older people's ability to assemble single units of information during the encoding process and to later retrieve them within their proper episodic context. One alternative explanation of this phenomenon is the "use-it-or-lose-it" hypothesis, which maintains that cognitive abilities decline as they are used less and less. Another theory maintains that older people have a lower attentional ability, which causes them to encode more poorly, and yet another posits that older people have less "self-esteem" about their memory as they age, which leads to poorer memory performance (Light, 1991). Other terms used for MCI have included "incipient" or "questionable" dementia, "isolated memory impairment," and "cognitive impairment-no dementia."

The original criteria for MCI (Petersen et al., 1999) included: (1) a memory complaint on the part of the patient or a family member; (2) documentation of normal activities of daily living (no decline in "social and occupational functioning" as described by the DSM criteria); (3) normal general cognitive function (within 1.5 standard deviations of the norms expected for the age and education of the individual); (4) abnormal memory for age (1.5 or more standard deviations below age and education norms); and (5) does not meet dementia criteria. In 2004, these criteria were modified to encompass a broader definition of impairment in cognitive domains other than memory, as it became apparent that subtypes of MCI exist (Petersen, 2004). MCI was divided into amnestic MCI (aMCI) and nonamnestic MCI (naMCI) depending on whether or not memory is impaired. Each of these subtypes can have one or multiple domains affected. In aMCI, if memory is the only domain affected, it is called "aMCI-single domain." If memory and at least one other domain are affected, it is called, "aMCI-multiple domain." For naMCI, if only one nonmemory domain is affected, it is called "naMCI-single domain" and if multiple nonmemory domains are affected, it is called "nonamnestic MCI-multiple domain." It has been shown that each of these subtypes is associated with different outcomes. aMCI-single domain is predictive of AD and depression, aMCI-multiple domain predicts AD, VaD, and depression, and naMCI-multiple domain predicts future development of dementia with Lewy Bodies and VaD. naMCI-single domain, the least common type, is associated with frontotemporal dementia and dementia with Lewy bodies (Petersen, 2004). Therefore, the MCI sub-diagnosis may assist the physician and patient in determining what the eventual outcome will be.

What was viewed in the 1980s and 1990s as a dichotomous state (demented or not demented) and later as three distinct states (normal, MCI, and AD) is now recognized as a *continuous cognitive trajectory*. While in case–control comparisons, AD cases looked quite different from controls, MCI cases' cognition (and,

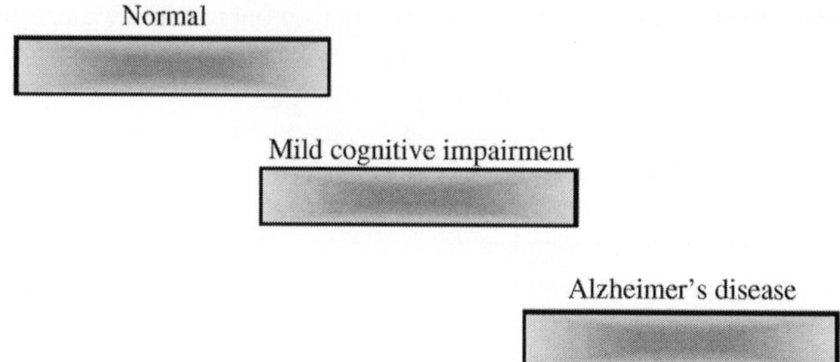

FIGURE 2.2 Cognitive continuum showing the overlap between normal aging, mild cognitive impairment, and Alzheimer's disease. *Adapted from Petersen (2004).*

pathology, if they died before becoming demented or were given an amyloid PET scan while in this clinical state) fall in the middle between normal and AD, with substantial overlap between the two (Figure 2.2).

This pathologic and clinical continuum is now accepted in the scientific literature, and the field is close to reaching some consensus on the order in which events take place. Amyloid deposition is thought to occur first, with neuronal injury, atrophy, and cognitive dysfunction following (Jack et al., 2010). The cascade of events leading to AD is discussed in more detail later in this book.

CLASSIFICATION OF MCI AND DEMENTIA USING NEUROPSYCHOLOGICAL TESTING

Although formal neuropsychological testing is not required for the diagnosis of dementia, the clinical classification of MCI depends in large part on the results of detailed cognitive assessment. The subtypes of MCI, for example, depend on which neuropsychological domains are affected. After a neuropsychological test is developed, norms are developed for it, which may be specified for different age, sex, and education strata. This means that the way the test behaves in a large, cognitively normal population, preferably representative of the general population, is documented. Most neuropsychological tests are sensitive to age and education level, which, as we shall see in later chapters, also are risk factors for AD. The best tests are those that are free of such biases, but such tests are uncommon. Once the test has been normed, performance can be quantitatively judged against the norms in standard deviations. Therefore, when memory is being judged as being normal or not, only those performing more than 1.5 standard deviations below the mean may be considered to fulfill criteria for MCI and only those scoring two or more standard deviations below the mean are considered for inclusion as possible dementia cases. Of course, as long as we specify what the cutoff is between normal and abnormal, we can define "abnormal" performance in different ways. Using one standard deviation below the mean as a cutoff score will result in more MCI suspects (Liepelt-Scarfone et al., 2011; Pendlebury, Mariz, Bull, Mehta, & Rothwell, 2013) than using 1.5 standard deviations below the mean. If high sensitivity is desired, 1.0 standard deviations can be used as the cutoff. If higher specificity is desired, 1.5 standard deviations would be more appropriate.

Neuropsychologists divide cognitive function into several domains. Most of these domains correspond to damage in particular regions or circuits in the brain. For example, episodic memory depends heavily upon the integrity of the hippocampal formation and other closely linked regions, such as the entorhinal cortex and medial temporal lobe. These regions associated with episodic memory are among the first to accumulate neurofibrillary tangles, one of the two principal brain lesions that characterize AD. As the disease progresses, other areas of the brain, including much of the cerebral cortex, develop similar lesions. Because diagnosis of AD requires an impairment of memory in addition to one or more deficits in other cognitive functions, it is necessary to assess multiple cognitive domains. Early in the disease course, at the MCI stage, it is possible for the only domain to be affected to be that of episodic memory. The following are the major domains that are usually assessed in evaluating whether an individual has AD (Weintraub, Wicklund, & Salmon, 2012).

Episodic Memory

A deficit in the ability to learn and remember new information (episodic memory) is frequently the earliest recognized sign of an Alzheimer process. Episodic memory tests may include free recall or recognition of objects, words, or locations that are learned.

Language and Semantic Knowledge

Relatively early in the disease course, individuals with AD can show impairment in naming objects and in rapid recall of information from long-term storage (e.g., the names of animals). These deficits likely reflect the loss of semantic memory that accompanies the disease.

Executive Function and Attention

These tasks are strongly associated with function of the frontal lobe of the brain. Performance on tests that require mental manipulation of information (executive function) and allocation of attention, particularly that needed to remember new information (working memory), begin to be affected fairly early in the course of AD and worsen as the disease progresses.

Visuospatial Function

Much of the early compromise in visuospatial function appears to be due to control of visual attention. In this regard, the deficit is similar to those seen on verbal executive or attentional tasks. A rare form of AD (posterior cortical atrophy) begins with compromise to several higher order visual functions. Because of this and the high sensitivity of visuospatial tests to AD pathology, neuropsychological batteries aimed at detecting AD generally include one or more tests of complex visual construction or perception.

NEED FOR STANDARDIZATION

The manner in which the criteria are operationalized in the clinical research setting is critical to the identification of cases of dementia. For example, there has long been heated debate about how "a decline from a previous level of social or occupational functioning" should be interpreted. Also of concern is how to apply the criteria in the same manner in different cultural and ethnic groups, in which "decline" from a previous, higher level may be interpreted differently, given the cultural expectations of what older people should be doing. There have been attempts to harmonize the criteria across cultures (Larson et al., 1998; Mayeux et al., 2011), but no consensus guidelines exist. As we will describe in the chapters on the frequency and occurrence of AD and dementia in population-based studies, in addition to the differing interpretations of the clinical criteria for dementia and AD, there are differences between populations studied (age and education distributions, socioeconomic status, access to medical care, distribution of vascular risk factors and other characteristics), sampling strategies, participation and attrition rates, availability of proxy informants who know the putative cases well, and the ways that information is gathered for the diagnoses. The inability to standardize methods to diagnose dementia cases across studies may underlie some discrepancies in the estimates of its prevalence and incidence rates, leaving open the question of whether differences in prevalence and incidence rates across studies are real or due to methodological variations. Even studies that were designed to examine cross-cultural differences, which attempted to standardize all protocols and procedures across study sites, can experience differences in rates that are due to different competing risks and mortality rates between populations and other methodological differences that were not able to be controlled. Therefore, determining true differences in the incidence rates is not always possible (Graves, Larson, White, Teng, & Homma, 1994; Osuntokun et al., 1992).

Other issues surrounding the concept of MCI are evolving over time as more information becomes available. In addition to VaD criteria, criteria for VCI have been introduced, which cover all forms of cognitive impairment from MCI of vascular origin through VaD (Gorelick et al., 2011). There is a need to define earlier manifestations of non-AD dementias, such as vascular or Lewy body dementias. Thus, newer definitions of MCI require a change in cognition and impairment in one or more cognitive domains, which does not have to include memory (Albert et al., 2011). At the same time, it is recognized that impairment in episodic memory (the capacity to learn and retain new information) will be the main feature of MCI patients who later develop AD. The idea of subclassifying the cause or etiology of the MCI has also gained favor (Albert et al., 2011). For "MCI due to AD," some experts have proposed the use of the term, "prodromal AD" to get at the concept of the continuum, rather than discrete categories of clinical diagnoses. With this intepretation, the term, "conversion" to a clinical state has been replaced with the term "progression."

Revised criteria for MCI (Albert et al., 2011) allow for MCI patients to have some mild problems in the performance of their daily functional tasks, whereas the early interpretation of this criterion for MCI required documentation of normal activities of daily living (ADLs) (Petersen et al., 2001, 1999). This small change in the operationalization of this criterion for MCI could increase misclassification between the diagnoses of MCI and dementia, which would increase the prevalence and incidence rates for MCI and reduce those for dementia (Morris, 2012). In a study examining this misclassification, Morris (2012) argues that the diagnosis of MCI might best be restricted to non-AD dementias, while those who have "MCI due to AD" be called "preclinical," "prodromal," or "early" AD. These concepts are evolving as we learn more about the underlying pathologic processes and adapt our clinical terminology to new ways of thinking.

Chapter 3

Epidemiologic Definition of a Case

In epidemiologic studies, the need for standardized definitions of what constitutes a case is of paramount importance in order to decrease the probability of misclassification of outcome, which in turn can contribute to over- or underestimation of the magnitude of the effect measure. The earliest studies of prevalence in the 1960s and 1970s used cases that were diagnosed by physicians in the community or were found in hospital medical records, but definitions were not standardized. In descriptive or cross-sectional studies of prevalence or in case–control studies of dementia or AD, it is important for a case that has already been diagnosed to be reviewed using standardized definitions that are explicitly described by the investigators carrying out the study. Inclusion and exclusion criteria and the method by which standard criteria like the DSM or NINCDS-ADRDA are operationalized should be specified so that all cases are defined the same way. In case–control studies, some investigators have taken steps to screen out controls who score below a certain cutoff on an overall test of cognition to reduce misclassification of controls, because in older age AD is not a rare disease, as we shall see in Chapter 6.

Investigators may decide to conduct clinical examinations or identify cases using a standardized definition to rediagnose cases to ensure that they meet the inclusion criteria for the study, or at least review the medical records to document whether the criteria used in the study are met. It is rare in the epidemiologic literature that study investigators will simply accept diagnoses made in the community by family practitioners, internists, or even neurologists not affiliated with the study, because considerable clinical judgment and interpretation goes into the diagnosis.

Studies that do not take the extra steps to carefully examine the eligibility of each case are considered to be methodologically less rigorous and potentially less internally valid than those that do. Exceptions do exist, and "passive" case-finding can be acceptable when the method used is validated within the population studied, such as has been done in the Rochester Epidemiology Project in Rochester, MN and at Group Health Research Institute in Seattle, WA

Alzheimer's Disease. DOI: http://dx.doi.org/10.1016/B978-0-12-804538-1.00003-1

(Knopman, Petersen, Rocca, Larson, & Ganguli, 2011). Passive case ascertainment of course has its advantages, especially in the new age of the electronic medical record, because it is much less expensive for epidemiologic studies than active case-finding. Depending on the target population, it may be important to assure that the records cover all or a majority of the individuals living in a geographic catchment area. Additionally, the records must be detailed and complete enough to produce diagnoses that are valid and that minimize missing data. One problem with passive ascertainment is that the case must be severe enough to result in the individual seeking medical attention. Therefore, this method is relatively insensitive for milder cases of dementia, AD, or MCI. In the Mayo Clinic Study on Aging, a study was undertaken to determine the sensitivity of the passive method using an in-person evaluation as the gold standard to detect prevalent dementia. This comparison showed that 30% of prevalent dementia cases found in the in-person (active) case ascertainment were missed by the passive method (Knopman et al., 2011). Also, this study did not include milder forms of cognitive impairment (MCI or prodromal AD). These are the cases most likely to be missed because they have a higher chance of remaining undetected by the medical care system.

The United States currently has no registry for AD, as exists for cancer (Surveillance and Epidemiology End Results; http://seer.cancer.gov/registries/list.html). Moreover, only one national study exists that clinically evaluated its sample and is representative of the US population: the Aging, Demographic, and Memory Study (ADAMS; Langa et al., 2005) based on the Health and Retirement Survey of more than 30,000 individuals across the United States age 50 and over. ADAMS sampled 1,770 people age 70 and over to participate in a focused study of memory, with the goal of conducting clinical evaluations in 850 individuals. Of 856 ADAMS participants assessed, only 252 participated in a follow-up evaluation 18 months after the baseline. While these data can give us valuable prevalence figures that represent all people in the United States aged 70 and over, the small numbers and potentially biased follow-up preclude valid estimates of incidence rates by region of the United States or by race or ethnicity. A large, national cohort study of AD and other dementias is sorely needed that would examine risk factors for incidence within multiple racial/ethnic and cultural groups with a standardized methodological framework. As we shall discuss in Chapters 6 and 7, most current data come from studies conducted in one geographic region on one population subgroup, with a few of these individual studies enrolling multiple racial or ethnic groups.

Studies that examine individuals in-person became the norm in prevalence and longitudinal studies of the incidence of and risk factors for dementia or AD in the late 1980s. Because the process of screening and clinically evaluating many subjects is time-consuming and personnel-intensive, the standard methodology used was a "two-phase design." In the first phase, the population was screened with a relatively short global cognitive test, such as the Mini-Mental Screening Examination. Those who scored below a predetermined cutoff point on the test were referred to a more comprehensive assessment, typically involving a complete clinical history and evaluation, neurologic examination, administration of a detailed neuropsychological battery, blood tests to rule out reversible causes of dementia, and imaging to rule out tumors and to observe markers of cerebrovascular disease and other contributing factors. An interview with an informant was frequently conducted during the clinical assessment phase, often involving acquisition of information to compute a CDR or IQCODE score and to complete behavior and neuropsychiatric checklists. The consensus diagnostic committee then met, and using all available data and laboratory results, filled out the DSM criteria for dementia and other criteria to subtype the dementia.

There are three major designs that have been used to count prevalent and incident cases of dementia or AD. The first is to validate the global cognitive screening test in the population in which it will be used (this is a critical first step that many studies overlooked), select the cut-point with the highest sensitivity and specificity and invite participants who "fail" the test (at or below the selected cut-point) for more detailed clinical and neuropsychological evaluations. This ignores those who "pass" the test and assumes there are no cases in this group, often an erroneous assumption. The second method is essentially the same as the first, but this method is not considered a pure "screening method" because a number of those who pass the test are sampled for the clinical evaluation to see if there are any "missed" cases (false-negatives, those who scored well on the test but who truly have clinical disease). This method yields a higher and more accurate prevalence or incidence rate, because, as shown in Figure 3.1, the true prevalence in the population is a + c/N. When cells *c* and *d* are ignored, the prevalence is estimated as a/N, which can underestimate the true rate. One possible problem with the sampling technique is that if an insufficient number of participants are sampled from those who passed the screen (screen-negatives) and a very small number of true cases are detected in this group one would have little confidence in the rate observed, since the confidence interval around the false-negative rate can be very wide and therefore statistically unstable. This must be kept in mind in studies that used this design and discovered false-negatives.

	True cases	True non cases	
Screening test			
Positive	a	b	
Negative	c	d	
Total	a + c	b + d	N

FIGURE 3.1 Two-by-two table for a cognitive screening test.

In a modification of this sampling technique, among screen-negatives, sampling probabilities are defined based on the rates of cognitive impairment expected, e.g., by age and score on the cognitive test. Because we expect that people age 85 and over have a high probability of being cognitively impaired, this group might be oversampled or all of them may be invited to be clinically evaluated. People who score below the cut-point are automatically sampled with a 100% probability. Those who score in other strata of the cognitive test, for example, in a middle "gray zone," are sampled at intermediate rates.

Investigators directing large population-based cohort studies have selected different ways to screen or sample for the discovery of incident cases. In one of our studies, the *Kame* Project, a sampling technique was used for the prevalence phase (Graves, Larson, et al., 1996) but screening only without sampling for false-negatives was used for the incidence waves (Borenstein et al., 2014). Another group used a sampling technique to detect both prevalent and incident cases in studies conducted in east Boston (Hebert et al., 1995) and Chicago (Evans et al., 2003). The sampling approach is preferred over the screening methodology in that persons from all cognitive strata are sampled, producing less bias, and the results are then weighted back to the original target population to estimate prevalence or incidence rates. However, if the screening methodology is used and a high cut-point is selected on the cognitive screen, one may argue that there are few true cases to be detected above the cut-point, and if they are there, they would not meet dementia criteria. Therefore, the success of the screening methodology depends on the cut-point set for test positivity. Most studies of dementia must screen or sample a large number of false-positives to detect each true-positive case. In a study conducted in Chicago, for example, of 835 individuals sampled for the clinical evaluation, 139 had AD, with a ratio of 6 false-positives for every true-positive found (Evans et al., 2003). Because there is no diagnostic marker for AD that can be readily applied in populations, the process of detecting AD and other dementias is time- and cost-intensive.

Other ways to detect cases in populations include the use of large national databases that are available in some countries. In Scandinavia, for example, the universal health care system allows cases to be identified by ICD codes. In the United States, HMOs like Kaiser Permanente in California and Group Health Cooperative in Washington state maintain large databases with excellent medical records on its members. With this method, individuals do not have to be screened and a sample worked up clinically. Disadvantages of this method include the possible lack of uniformity in the application of diagnostic criteria (at the physician level, depending on the extent of standardization required by the organization) and the likelihood of undiscovered cases who remain in the population and never come to medical attention.

Epidemiologic studies have used a wide array of different cognitive tests to screen populations for dementia. Since performance on these tests is highly sensitive to education and culture, each study uses the test that is most appropriate for its population and ideally one that has been validated in that population. The association between educational attainment and scores on mental status tests has long been appreciated (Gurland, 1981; Kahn, Pollack, & Goldfarb, 1961; Pfeiffer, 1975). In the mid-1980s, around the time of the first systematic funding of prospective cohort studies of dementia by the National Institutes of Health (NIH), the role of education in screening was questioned (Kittner et al., 1986). It was suggested that poorer cognitive performance by lower educated people may be due to impaired ability to take tests, and that people with higher education could compensate for early deficits and so were more likely to "pass" the test. To control for this test bias, Kittner et al. (1986) proposed that cut-scores be stratified by education level to allow the test to be more difficult for more educated persons to pass and easier for more poorly educated persons (improving test specificity). Around the same time, evidence was accumulating to support an inverse association between educational attainment and the prevalence (Bonaiuto et al., 1995; Dartigues, Gagnon, Michel, et al., 1991; Fratiglioni, Grut, Forsell, et al., 1991; Zhang, Katzman, Salmon, et al., 1990) and incidence of dementia (Li, Shen, Chen, et al., 1991), as well as with cognitive decline (Colsher & Wallace, 1991; Evans et al., 1993). Therefore, it can be argued that, while stratification by education would improve test validity, it would partially or completely reduce the ability to study education as an etiologic factor for dementia and AD (Mortimer & Graves, 1993). Most investigators have decided not to stratify the cut-scores by education in an effort to allow the association between education, cognition and the occurrence of AD to be examined.

Before concluding this chapter, a few words should be mentioned about the detection of prevalent versus incident cases and about detecting MCI or prodromal dementia versus AD in epidemiologic studies. Because prevalent disease is a representation of everything that has happened up to a particular point in time, we can view it as a robust outcome, albeit for etiologic studies, it is tainted by the duration of the disease. When a prevalent case of dementia is found, the case will likely have a global cognitive score that is well below normal for his or her age, and the case will meet all research criteria, regardless of which criteria are used. In prospective studies, prevalent cases are found at the baseline (the first evaluation of the cohort) and only nondemented cohort members are followed over time for incident dementia.

Epidemiologists usually view incident cases as the "gold standard" for the study of etiologic factors in the causation of disease. However, incident cases may meet all of the research criteria at any follow-up wave, but may do so only marginally, exceeding thresholds for cognitive impairment by only a small amount. The diagnosis of incident dementia therefore is less secure than that for prevalent dementia. One way this is dealt with in epidemiologic studies is to require the person to be as or more impaired in subsequent assessment waves. However, if the newly diagnosed incident case dies before the next assessment, this is not possible.

Chapter 4

Neuropathology of Alzheimer's Disease

Pathology is often considered the gold standard of disease. However, at autopsy the presence of disease pathology, even severe pathology, is detected frequently when no symptoms are present prior to death. This situation certainly applies to Alzheimer's disease (AD) where about a third of those who meet stringent neuropathologic criteria for this illness at autopsy are not demented during life (Mortimer, Borenstein, Gosche, & Snowdon, 2005; Neuropathology Group of the Medical Research Council Cognitive Function and Aging Study (MRC-CFAS), 2001; Schneider et al., 2007; Snowdon et al., 1997). Understanding why this occurs and what it means for epidemiologic studies of the disease is important to our understanding of the risk factors for AD as well as the role played by brain reserve in the prevention of the dementia of AD.

Figure 4.1 shows the two principal brain lesions that characterize the pathology of AD, the neurofibrillary tangle, and the neuritic plaque. The presence of large numbers of these microscopic lesions throughout much of the brain is the basis for the neuropathologic diagnosis of this illness. However, as we shall see, many individuals fulfill various sets of neuropathologic criteria for this condition, but fail to meet clinical criteria for dementia or even for mild cognitive impairment. The presence of plaques and tangles at autopsy therefore appears to be necessary, *but not sufficient*, to cause the clinical outcomes of interest. In this chapter, we will consider the association between the severity of these lesions and the presence of cognitive impairment and dementia. In addition, we will examine what other types of neuropathology may be important in modifying this association. Finally, we will consider the findings to date of longitudinal epidemiologic studies that have access to neuropathologic data on their participants.

CLINICOPATHOLOGIC STUDIES

To understand the relationship between cognitive status during life and brain pathology, a number of studies have obtained brain autopsies from individuals studied prospectively for cognition and dementia during life. Ten of these

Alzheimer's Disease. DOI: http://dx.doi.org/10.1016/B978-0-12-804538-1.00004-3

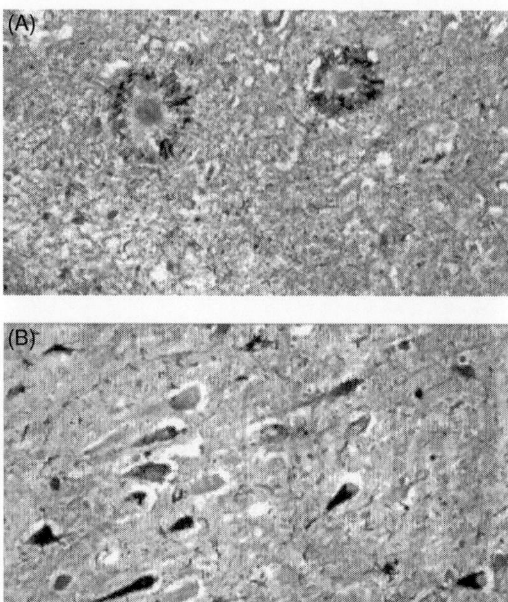

FIGURE 4.1 Principal neuropathologic lesions in Alzheimer's disease showing amyloid plaques outside the cell bodies (A) and neurofibrillary tangles inside the cell bodies (B).

prospective clinicopathologic cohort studies (Bennett et al., 2012; Bennett, Schneider, Buchman, et al., 2012; Brayne et al., 2009; Fujimi et al., 2008; Gelber, Launer, & White, 2012; Montine, Sonnen, Montine, Crane, & Larson, 2012; Mortimer, 2012; O'Brien et al., 2009; Oinas et al., 2009; Richardson et al., 2012) have collected more than 200 brains each (Table 4.1). These studies differed greatly in the degree to which they were representative of the general population. Therefore, several questions relating to potential selection bias must be considered when reviewing their findings. First, how representative was the population from which the samples were taken and to what extent were these studies those of volunteers who may have agreed to participate because of specific characteristics *including cognitive impairment*? Second, what proportion of the group that was approached agreed to participate in a study that involved brain donation? Finally, what percentage of the population who agreed to brain donation actually had autopsies performed at the time of death?

Those studies that focused on relatively small samples with distinctive characteristics, including religious congregations (Bennett et al., 2006; Bennett, Schneider, Arvanitakis, & Wilson, 2012; Mortimer, 2012) and small isolated communities (Fujimi et al., 2008; Oinas et al., 2009) had the highest participation rates. Studies from more representative populations, for example, the Adult Changes in Thought Study (Montine, Sonnen, Montine, Crane, & Larson, 2012) had lower participation rates and were potentially subject to greater selection bias.

TABLE 4.1 Clinicopathologic Cohort Studies That Collected More Than 200 Autopsied Brains

Study	Number Autopsied to 2012	Description of Sample
Vantaa 85+ Study	304	Older residents of city in Finland who agreed to autopsy
Nun Study	606	All members of a specific congregation (School Sisters of Notre Dame) living in the United States who agreed to autopsy
Baltimore Longitudinal Study of Aging	211	Volunteer cohort of well-educated persons
Honolulu-Asia Aging Study	559	Survivors of the Honolulu Heart Program, a large cohort study of Japanese American men born 1900–1919
Cambridge City Over-75s Cohort Study	225	Original cohort was largely representative of people older than 75 living in Cambridge, UK
MRC Cognitive Function and Ageing Study	456	Participants from a random sample of about 8000 older residents of 6 regions in England. Relatively high initial participation rate (85%)
Religious Orders Study	539	Volunteer cohort encompassing more than 30 Catholic religious congregations who agreed to autopsy
Hisayama Study	281	Study of almost all older residents of Japanese rural community
Rush Memory and Aging Project	424	Volunteer cohort from continuing care retirement communities, retirement homes and subsidized housing in Chicago area
Adult Changes in Thought Study	438	Cohort of participants in large HMO over 65 at entry. High initial refusal rate: >50%

The Vantaa 85+ Study's first publication on neuropathology (Polvikoski et al., 1995) concerned the association between the Apolipoprotein E gene, deposition of beta amyloid, and dementia. The following year in 1996, the initial publication from the Nun Study showed that characteristics of autobiographic essays written by Catholic sisters while they were in their early 1920s predicted

Alzheimer neuropathology 60 years later (Snowdon et al., 1996) (Chapter 11). A series of publications in the beginning of the twenty-first century from the Honolulu-Asia Aging Study (White, 2009) focused on clinicopathologic correlations, as did the Religious Orders Study (Bennett et al., 2006; Bennett, Schneider, Arvanitakis, & Wilson, 2012), the Rush Memory and Aging Project (MAP; Bennett et al., 2012), and two studies in the United Kingdom (Brayne et al., 2009; Richardson et al., 2012). The studies listed in Table 4.1 as well as a number of smaller clinicopathologic studies have contributed greatly to our understanding of the pathological bases for dementia as well as the association of risk factors for the disease with the neuropathologic outcomes.

CRITERIA FOR NEUROPATHOLOGIC AD

Epidemiologic studies rely on the existence of uniform criteria for internal and external comparisons. Criteria for the diagnosis of neuropathologic AD are therefore critical. To assert that a patient has definite AD, he or she needs to fulfill two sets of criteria, clinical criteria for AD during life and neuropathologic criteria for AD at autopsy. AD is a clinicopathologic entity, that is, it is defined by a combination of neuropathologic changes in the brain and dementia symptoms during life.

Historically, several sets of neuropathologic criteria have been developed to define AD. The initial attempt to develop a consensus set of criteria for neuropathologic AD occurred in 1985 (Khachaturian, 1985) shortly after the NINCDS-ADRDA diagnostic criteria for clinical AD (McKhann et al., 1984) were published. These criteria, frequently referred to as the Khachaturian criteria after the first author of the article, were developed by a panel of neuropathologists who met to develop "minimal microscopic criteria" for AD that could be used in general hospital autopsies. The Khachaturian criteria specified the areas of the brain that had to be stained and examined for the diagnosis to be made and the number of plaques and tangles that had to be seen in sections taken from the neocortex to establish the diagnosis. The approach was to develop age-specific criteria, with different numbers of plaques and tangles needed depending on the age of the decedent. With increasing age, the number of plaques needed for diagnosis increased and the number of neocortical neurofibrillary tangles decreased.

In the early 1990s, a second consensus conference led to the Consortium to Establish a Registry for Alzheimer's Disease (CERAD) criteria for neuropathologic AD. The CERAD criteria (Mirra et al., 1991) added degrees of certainty to the diagnosis, that is, possible, probable, or definite, similar to the NINCDS-ADRDA clinical criteria and dropped the requirement entirely for there to be neurofibrillary tangles in the neocortex in order to make the diagnosis. In addition, they required that only individuals with a clinical history of AD be given a diagnosis, acknowledging the general practice of neuropathologists of using the clinical description in addition to their observations to arrive at neuropathologic diagnoses. Instead of counting plaques, they provided pictures to rate the severity of plaques in one of three semiquantitative categories: sparse, moderate, or severe. Again, age-dependent criteria were used with greater plaque density required for diagnosis at older ages.

Both of these sets of criteria suffered from the fact that the pathologic diagnostic criteria changed with age. In this regard, they differed from pathologic criteria for heart and cancer diagnoses, which are the same regardless of age. Because the criteria made it more difficult for older people to be given a neuropathologic diagnosis of AD, they had the effect of blunting the apparent exponential increase in the frequency of this illness with age. Finally, at advanced ages, neither set of criteria required the presence of neurofibrillary tangles in the neocortex to reach the diagnosis.

By the mid-1990s, data began accumulating showing that neocortical neurofibrillary tangles were more strongly related to cognitive impairment than were plaques (Bierer et al., 1995). These data contributed to the development of the Reagan criteria in 1997 (Hyman & Trojanowski, 1997), in which the presence of neocortical neurofibrillary tangles was considered necessary for the diagnosis of high likelihood of neuropathologic AD and in which age at death did not play a role in the diagnosis. The main difference between these criteria that divided the diagnosis into "high," "intermediate," and "low" likelihoods of AD and the CERAD criteria was the requirement that in addition to plaques, tangles must be present in the cortex for high and in the limbic system for intermediate likelihoods of neuropathologic AD. Furthermore, it was strongly recommended that Braak staging techniques (Braak & Braak, 1991) be used for determination of the location and presence of neurofibrillary tangles. Like the CERAD criteria, the Reagan criteria required that the patient have dementia during life. Specific criteria for a diagnosis of high likelihood of AD included a severe neocortical neuritic plaque rating according to the CERAD criteria and the presence of neocortical tangles (stage V/VI according to Braak staging). For intermediate likelihood, neocortical plaques were rated as moderate and Braak stage was III or IV, indicating the presence of neurofibrillary tangles in the limbic system, but not the cerebral cortex.

Ideally, clinical and neuropathologic criteria for AD should be applied without regard for satisfaction of the other set of criteria. In clinicopathologic studies of individuals unselected for cognitive status, the Reagan criteria have been applied without the requirement for preexisting dementia. Presently, the Reagan criteria represent the gold standard for neuropathologic diagnosis of AD and are used both for their traditional purpose of identifying individuals with this disease who were demented during life and in research studies to identify people who meet the neuropathologic criteria, but may or may not meet clinical criteria for dementia during life.

From an epidemiologic point of view, what are the problems of requiring that clinical dementia criteria be fulfilled in order to say that someone met neuropathologic criteria for AD? The most important consequence is that we are not able to look at risk factors for the pathology independently of risk factors

Neuropathologic AD	Clinical dementia: Yes	Clinical dementia: No
Yes	184	80
No	69	169

False-positive rate = 30%
Positive predictive value = 70%

Clinical dementia	Neuropathologic AD: Yes	Neuropathologic AD: No
Yes	184	69
No	80	169

False-positive rate = 27%
Positive predictive value = 73%

FIGURE 4.2 Positive predictive values and false-positive rates for neuropathologic and clinical diagnoses in The Nun Study. AD, Alzheimer's disease.

for clinical expression of dementia, since the former condition requires the presence of the latter. Another issue to consider is one of potential bias. If the neuropathologist knows that an individual was demented prior to death, he or she may be more likely to interpret the neuropathologic findings, which are semiquantitative, as consistent with neuropathologic AD. Conversely, if he or she knows the individual was cognitively intact prior to death, he or she may be more likely to interpret the neuropathologic findings as not consistent with neuropathologic AD. The solution to this problem is to blind the neuropathologist to the clinical status of the patient prior to death and ask them to render their opinion regarding the presence of neuropathologic AD independently of whether the patient was demented or not. Many clinicopathologic research studies, including the Nun Study, the Religious Orders Study, the MAP, and the Cambridge City over 75s Cohort Study have followed this protocol, allowing these studies to examine risk factors for neuropathologic AD independently of risk factors for dementia. Although blinding of the neuropathologist was not specified in the Adult Changes in Thought Study, this study used the Reagan criteria without the requirement for dementia prior to death to categorize autopsied participants into high, intermediate or low likelihood of neuropathologic AD.

Criticisms of neuropathologic criteria have centered on the lack of a one-to-one relationship between neuropathologic diagnosis and clinical diagnosis. This is illustrated by the Nun Study, where the presence or absence of dementia was assessed annually and the neuropathologist was blinded to the clinical diagnosis at the time of death. Figure 4.2 shows the number of decedents in the Nun Study who met neither, one, or both clinical and neuropathologic AD criteria at the time of death. The positive predictive value of a diagnosis of neuropathologic AD was 0.7; that is, only 70% of the individuals whose autopsy results were consistent with neuropathologic AD were demented in the year prior to death. This implies that 30% of these decedents were not demented despite the presence of neuropathologic AD. Similarly, 73% of individuals with a clinical diagnosis of dementia fulfilled Reagan criteria for AD, while 27% did not. These findings are consistent with those obtained in other clinicopathologic studies

TABLE 4.2 Percentages of Study Participants in Cohort Studies Meeting Criteria for Neuropathologic AD Who Were Not Demented Prior to Death

Study	Number of Nondemented Participants	Mean Age at Death	Percent with Neuropathologic AD (Reagan Criteria, Intermediate or High)
Nun Study	249	89.1	30.3
Galvin et al. (2005)	41	84.6	31.7
Bennett et al. (2006)	134*	83.3	37.3
All studies (weighted average)			32.6

Excludes participants with mild cognitive impairment.

(Table 4.2). In studies that used the Reagan criteria for AD, about one-third of individuals satisfying these criteria at autopsy were not demented prior to death. The condition of satisfying the neuropathologic criteria, but not clinical dementia criteria, has been referred to as asymptomatic AD (Iacono et al., 2009).

CONTINUOUS MEASURES OF NEUROPATHOLOGIC SEVERITY

A second approach to studying the association between Alzheimer lesions and dementia has been to examine the associations between continuous or staged measures of neuropathologic severity and dementia or cognition. As the disease progresses, the distribution of neurofibrillary tangles in the brain expands (Braak & Braak, 1997) (Figure 4.3). This pattern observed in autopsied brains from nondemented and demented people is characterized by seven Braak neurofibrillary stages (0, I–VI), with the pathology becoming more severe with increasing stage. Lateral views of the brain (Figure 4.3) show expansion of affected regions with darker areas being those containing larger numbers of neurofibrillary tangles. With increased progression of the disease, the affected portions of the brain spread from the transentorhinal and entorhinal regions (stages I and II) to the hippocampus and surrounding areas (stages III and IV) and subsequently to the neocortex (stages V and VI).

Data from 130 participants in the Nun Study (Riley, Snowdon, & Markesbery, 2002) show that Braak neurofibrillary stage as a measure of neuropathologic severity of AD is strongly correlated with the severity of cognitive impairment, ranging from intact cognition to dementia (Figure 4.4). None of the participants without appreciable neurofibrillary tangle formation (Braak stage 0) was demented, while 70% of those with severe Braak stages V and VI were. Although this association

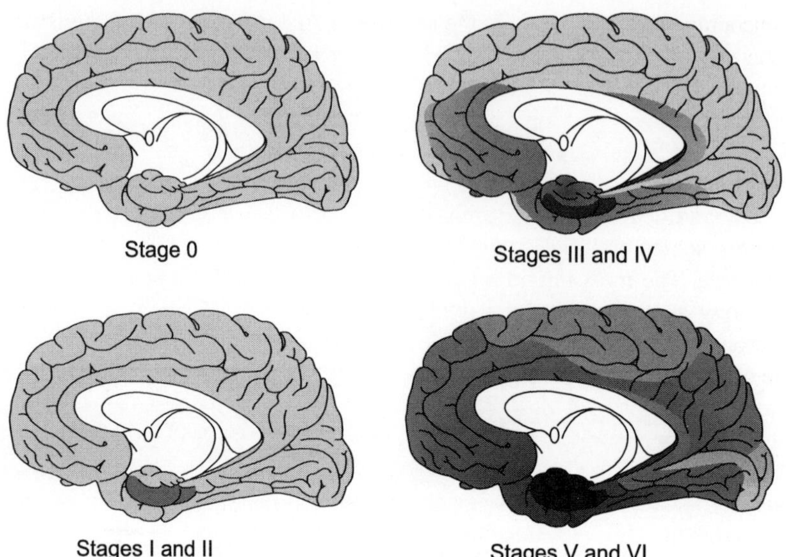

FIGURE 4.3 Braak neurofibrillary stages. Increased density of neurofibrillary tangles shown by darker shading. *Adapted from Braak and Braak (1997).*

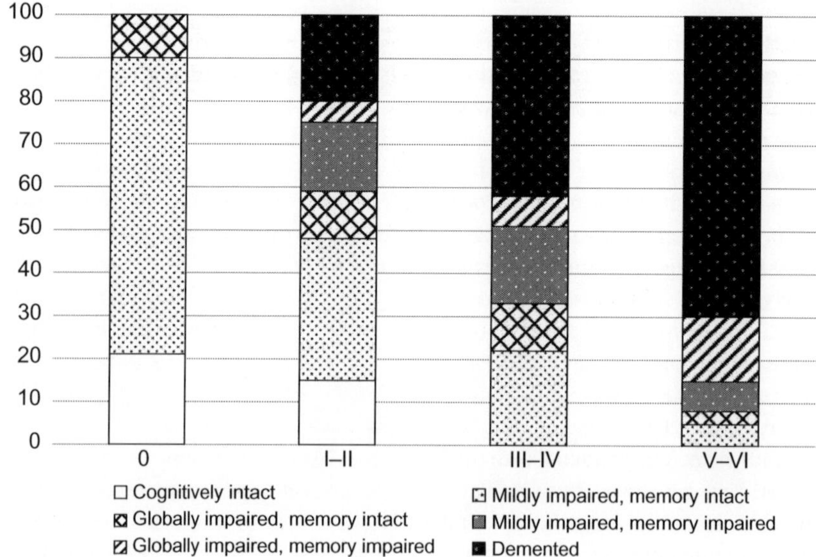

FIGURE 4.4 Percent of decedents with specified cognitive status just prior to death by category of Braak neurofibrillary stage. *Adapted from Riley et al. (2002).*

is encouraging in showing that the severity of Alzheimer lesions in the brain is associated with the risk of dementia, 30% of those with the most severe Alzheimer changes were not demented at the time of death and those in Braak stages III and IV were almost evenly split between demented and not demented, and even those in Braak stages I and II included over 20% who were demented.

What explains the lack of strong correspondence between AD lesions at autopsy and dementia at the time of death? Two factors appear be important: the presence of brain lesions other than plaques and tangles, and the amount of reserve. The most important brain lesions in addition to Alzheimer neuropathology are large and small strokes and vascular disease in small vessels (microinfarcts) serving the brain. One of the first publications to explore the role of vascular disease in modifying the effects of Alzheimer pathology compared four groups of autopsied sisters from the Nun Study, one with neither AD pathology nor vascular brain infarcts, one with AD pathology only, one with vascular infarcts but without AD pathology, and one with both types of lesions (Snowdon et al., 1997). Considering the final cognitive assessment in the year prior to death, AD by itself led to marked loss in cognitive function with a mean of 15/30 points on the Mini Mental State Exam. The combination of AD pathology and vascular infarcts was associated with more severe cognitive impairment with a mean score of 3/30. Interestingly, the presence of one or more vascular infarcts *in the absence of AD pathology* had little influence on cognitive performance, which was very similar to that found in people with neither AD nor vascular lesions. Among those nuns satisfying neuropathologic criteria for AD, those with one or two small infarcts in the basal ganglia or deep white matter had a 20-fold increased dementia risk compared to those without such lesions. A strong modifying effect of vascular lesions increasing the strength of association between Alzheimer pathology and dementia also has been reported in other studies, notably the Religious Orders Study (Arvanitakis, Leurgans, Barnes, Bennett, & Schneider, 2011), the MAP (Schneider et al., 2007), and the Adult Changes in Thought Study (Montine et al., 2012).

Another important modifier of the effect of Alzheimer lesions on the presence of dementia are Lewy bodies found in the brainstem of persons with Parkinson's disease and more widely in the cortex in Lewy body dementia. Lewy bodies by themselves are rarely associated with dementia (Schneider et al., 2007; Weisman et al., 2007), but increase the risk for dementia among those satisfying neuropathologic criteria for AD likely through an acceleration of cognitive decline (Boyle, Wilson, et al., 2013; Boyle, Yu, Wilson, Schneider, & Bennett, 2013). One additional pathology that appears to increase the rate of cognitive decline in those with Alzheimer neuropathology is the presence of Transactive response DNA-binding protein 43 (TDP-43) with high density in the brain (Wilson et al., 2013). This protein, which is associated with frontotemporal lobar degeneration, was identified in 46% of autopsied brains from the Religious Orders Study, but appeared to exert its effects only when present at very high levels, which occurred in relatively few brains.

Are individuals with AD pathology more likely to have vascular lesions or Lewy bodies? Several studies have shown an association between clinically determined stroke and clinical AD, individuals with clinically determined strokes having higher risk for AD. In the Nun Study, the presence of large or lacunar brain infarcts was not associated with Alzheimer neuropathology ($\chi^2 = 0.005$, $p = 0.94$). This finding was confirmed in other large clinicopathologic studies, including the Religious Orders Study (Schneider, Wilson, Bienias, Evans, & Bennett, 2004) and the Honolulu-Asia Aging Study (Launer, Petrovitch, Ross, Markesbery, & White, 2008). For the latter study, no statistical association with the severity of Alzheimer lesions was found for any type of vascular brain infarct, including microinfarcts. Why then did some studies show a statistically significant association between the presence of stroke and AD? As we have seen, strokes greatly increase the risk that an individual with neuropathologic AD will become demented and can be labeled as having clinical AD. This disclosing effect would lead to an apparent association between stroke and AD, which is not present when the underlying neuropathology is examined.

In summary, strokes and Lewy bodies *by themselves* usually do not lead to significant global cognitive impairment of dementia. However, prevention of strokes would very substantially reduce the incidence of clinical dementia *among people who fulfill neuropathologic criteria for AD.* Reduction of risk factors for stroke therefore has great promise for decreasing the incidence of clinical, but not pathologic AD.

POPULATION ATTRIBUTABLE FRACTION OF PATHOLOGIES IN THE CAUSATION OF DEMENTIA

The population attributable fraction (PAF), or the percent reduction that would occur if the risk factor was not present, for dementia in relation to Alzheimer, vascular, and Lewy body lesions can be estimated from population-based studies with autopsy confirmation. When this was done in the Adult Changes in Thought Study, high Braak neurofibrillary stage (V or VI) was associated with a PAF of 45%, while microvascular lesions had a PAF of 33% and Lewy bodies a PAF of 10% (Montine et al., 2012). Similar PAFs (38.5% for Alzheimer's neuropathology and 25.6% for vascular pathology) were reported from the Nun Study (Mortimer and Borenstein, 2014). However, in the latter analysis, a third factor related to brain reserve was included and had a comparable PAF to Alzheimer lesions. Brain reserve reflects the size of the brain at full development, education, and IQ. People with larger brains and higher education and/or IQ appear to be able to buffer the effects of Alzheimer and other lesions and remain nondemented at levels of AD pathology that would produce dementia in persons with smaller brains or lower education and/or IQ. The effect of brain reserve on the risk for dementia is considered in more detail in the next chapter.

IS NEUROPATHOLOGIC AD AN INEVITABLE OUTCOME OF AGING?

The question of whether neuropathologic AD is an inevitable outcome of aging is of considerable interest as the number of individuals living to age 100 and beyond continues to increase. Most studies suggest that the incidence of dementia continues to increase to age 100 (Corrada, Brookmeyer, Paganini-Hill, Berlau, & Kawas, 2010; Edland, Rocca, Petersen, Cha, & Kokmen, 2002; Hall et al., 2005; Ruitenberg, Ott, van Swieten, Hofman, & Breteler, 2001). However, assessment of Alzheimer lesions at autopsy among people who were not demented at death shows that the frequency of individuals satisfying criteria for neuropathologic AD peaks in the early 1990s and declines thereafter (Figure 4.5). Moreover, densities of neurofibrillary tangles in the neocortex in the same individuals begins to decline slightly earlier (Figure 4.6). Given that plaques and tangles once established are unlikely to be removed from the brain, these data suggest that those who survive beyond age 90 are likely to have a lower *rate* of accumulation of neurofibrillary tangles over the life course. These findings are consistent with AD lesions playing a smaller role in dementias occurring after age 90 in comparison to other causes (Middleton, Grinberg, Miller, Kawas, & Yaffe, 2011). Furthermore, they suggest that neuropathologic AD, while common through age 100, may *not* be an inevitable consequence of aging given present life expectancies.

If the entire population developed AD lesions across the life course at the same rate and if these lesions once developed remained for the lifetime of the individual, the frequency of individuals satisfying neuropathologic criteria for AD would continue to rise with age. However, if the *rate* of accumulation of Alzheimer's lesions were distributed, for example, as a normal distribution, the frequency of neuropathologic AD would rise to a certain age and decline thereafter. One way a normal distribution for rate of accumulation of lesions might

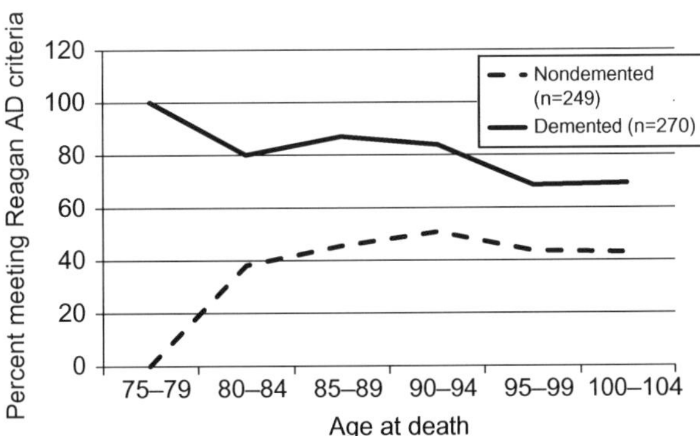

FIGURE 4.5 Percent of decedents in the Nun Study meeting Reagan high likelihood criteria for Alzheimer's disease at autopsy by age at death.

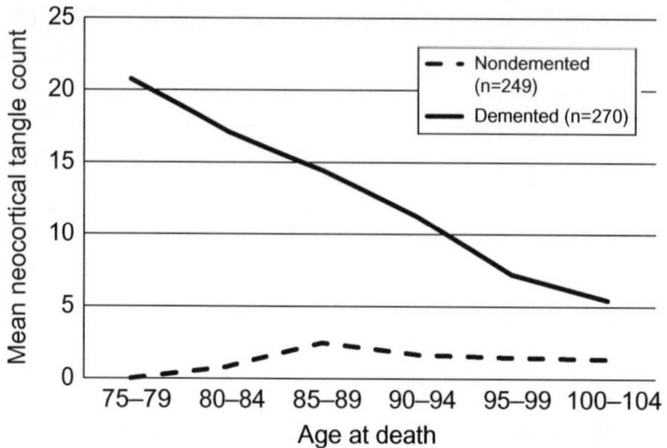

FIGURE 4.6 Mean neurofibrillary tangle count per section of the neocortex in the Nun Study by dementia status at death.

arise would be if the rate of accumulation of AD pathology were determined by many genes with small effects. Inclusion of one gene with a major effect, such as Apolipoprotein E, in addition to many with small effects would result in a more skewed distribution, with an earlier peak. As long as everyone accumulated AD lesions at a nonzero rate, everyone would eventually satisfy the criteria for neuropathologic AD if they lived long enough. However, for slow accumulation rates, they may have to live hundreds of years for this to occur!

DO WOMEN HAVE MORE ALZHEIMER'S PATHOLOGY THAN MEN?

The role of sex in the causation of Alzheimer neuropathology is controversial. One study (Corder et al., 2004) based on a large autopsy series from German hospitals found that women in Braak neurofibrillary stages I–III (mild pathology) had a slightly elevated neuritic plaque stage in comparison to men in these NFT stages. Although the autopsy series was large, factors important to the selection of autopsied cases may have differed by sex, given the larger numbers of men compared to women who were autopsied. Because the autopsy sample presumably included patients with and without cognitive impairment, differences in the frequency of cognitive impairment by sex could have been responsible for the small sex differences observed in this study. While several studies have found that female carriers of the ε4 susceptibility allele for Apolipoprotein E have a higher risk of developing AD than males with this allele (Bretsky et al., 1999; Farrer et al., 1997; Payami et al., 1994), analyses of biomarkers for AD in the CSF that reflect the severity of Alzheimer neuropathology in the brain have revealed few significant differences in the relation of these biomarkers to Apolipoprotein E genotype between men and women (Altmann, Tian, Henderson, Greicius, &

Alzheimer's Disease Neuroimaging Initiative, 2014). The finding that women carriers of apoliproprotein E-ε4 are at higher risk for dementia than male carriers could be explained alternatively by sex differences in reserve capacity and brain volume discussed in Chapter 5.

CLINICOPATHOLOGIC STUDIES PROVIDE INFORMATION ABOUT THE PATHOGENESIS OF DEMENTIA

Autopsy studies also can be used to investigate the pathogenesis of AD. Bennett and his coworkers (Bennett, Schneider, Wilson, Bienias, & Arnold, 2004), using data from the Religious Orders Study, examined the pathologic transition from amyloid load to neurofibrillary tangles. With multiple logistic regression adjusted for age, sex, and education, these authors showed that adding counts of neurofibrillary tangles to a model for percent area occupied by Aβ eliminated the association between amyloid load and dementia, but the converse was not true. Adding amyloid load to a model of neurofibrillary tangles predicting dementia had little effect on the association with neurofibrillary tangles. This is consistent with a *sequence* of pathologic events where the effect of amyloid deposition on dementia is mediated by neurofibrillary tangles, implying that β-amyloid develops first and gives rise to neurofibrillary tangles.

Using a similar set of analyses in the Nun Study, we addressed the question of whether the major susceptibility genotype for AD, Apolipoprotein E-ε4 affects dementia through Alzheimer neuropathology, vascular pathology or microinfarcts (Mortimer, Snowdon, & Markesbery, 2009). Addition of Alzheimer neuropathology to a model with Apolipoprotein E-ε4, age and education eliminated the association with Apolipoprotein E-ε4, whereas addition of either vascular pathology or microinfarcts had no effect on the association between ε4 and dementia. These findings suggest that the effect of ε4 on dementia is largely mediated by the severity of AD pathology, and not through other pathologies or mechanisms.

MRI–NEUROPATHOLOGIC ASSOCIATIONS

Because autopsy data are frequently difficult to obtain, it is useful to know how structural MRI findings are correlated with neuropathologic findings at autopsy. Two studies (Gosche, Mortimer, Smith, Markesbery, & Snowdon, 2001; Jack et al., 2002) have examined the correlation between Braak neurofibrillary stage and the volume of the hippocampus, a region of the brain strongly affected in AD. Results from the Nun Study are shown in Figure 4.7 for left hippocampal volume and Braak neurofibrillary tangle stage, both determined after death. A strong correlation ($r = -0.68$, $p<0.01$) was evident, suggesting that the volume of the hippocampus obtained from a structural MRI scan can be used to estimate the severity of Alzheimer pathology in the brain. A smaller correlation

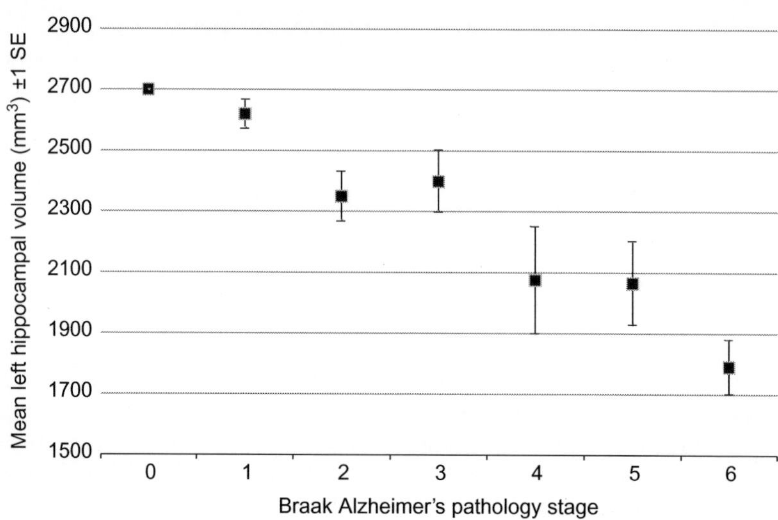

FIGURE 4.7 Correlation between Braak neurofibrillary stage and mean left hippocampal volume, The Nun Study.

($r = -0.39$, $p<0.01$) between hippocampal volume and Braak neurofibrillary stage was obtained in the second study, in which hippocampal volume determined from an antemortem scan (mean 1.8 years before death) was compared with Braak stage determined postmortem.

Recently, it has become possible to radiologically image amyloid plaques in the brain during life using positron emission tomography (PET) scans with compounds that bind to plaques containing fibrillar β-amyloid. As shown in Figure 4.8, the correlation between the regional density of plaques found at autopsy and the amount of PIB retention, a PET measure of aggregated brain amyloid, in the same regions is very high (Ikonomovic et al., 2008), confirming that the premortem imaging findings reflect amyloid plaques well.

From the viewpoint of epidemiologic studies, it is important to consider which imaging biomarker of underlying Alzheimer pathology is more sensitive, and therefore is more useful to detect the disease earlier. Two approaches have been taken to this issue: (i) calculations of cut-off scores for abnormal values of fibrillar amyloid beta (Aβ) on PET scans and MRI-determined hippocampal volumes by comparison of subjects with normal cognition and dementia followed by determination of when in time before the onset of dementia each measure becomes abnormal (Jack et al., 2011); and (ii) comparison of the timing of initial changes in fibrillar Aβ and hippocampal volume in carriers versus noncarriers of dominantly inherited genes (Bateman et al., 2012). The first approach (Jack et al., 2011) depends critically on the selection of cutpoints for the two measures. The authors used an independent sample of 53 participants

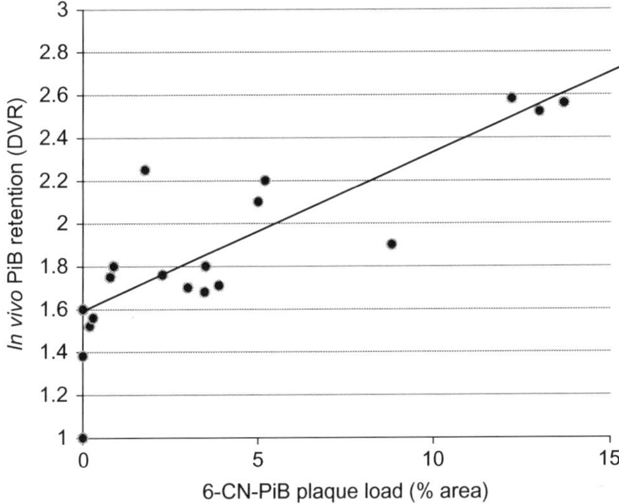

FIGURE 4.8 Association between retention of PiB, a PET ligand for aggregated beta amyloid, and plaque load for similar regions of the brain. *Adapted from Ikonomovic et al. (2008).*

at the Mayo Clinic who had an MRI performed within 3.5 years of death and selected the hippocampal volume cutpoint that best distinguished high from low fulfillment of Reagan neuropathologic criteria. However, published data from the Nun Study suggests that hippocampal volume distinguishes intermediate from low fulfillment of Reagan neuropathologic criteria and that a more sensitive cutpoint for hippocampal volume would have been appropriate to detect the earliest changes of Alzheimer pathology. In a head-to-head comparison of fibrillary Aβ PET scans and hippocampal volume, hippocampal volume appeared to be a little better in distinguishing normal cognition from MCI and dementia (Jack et al., 2008). While the authors of this paper argue that the two methods provide complementary information, the gain in diagnostic accuracy from the combination was only very slightly better when fibrillary Aβ imaging was added to hippocampal volume (2%), whereas the diagnostic accuracy was improved more by the addition of hippocampal volume to fibrillary Aβ PIB (11%). Comparison of the timing of initial changes in fibrillar Aβ and hippocampal volume in carriers of dominantly inherited genes (Bateman et al., 2012) suggest that changes in these imaging markers both became significant 15 years prior to dementia onset.

Considering the relative costs of the two techniques, hippocampal volume is likely the preferred imaging measure of Alzheimer neuropathologic severity early in the illness. Despite its lack of specificity for the illness, hippocampal volume is strongly associated with the density of neurofibrillary tangles and appears to be sensitive to differences in Braak stage as early as stage II (Figure 4.7) (Gosche, Mortimer, Smith, Markesbery, & Snowdon, 2002).

Because fibrillary Aβ PET scans provide more specificity for the underlying illness, combinations of these two imaging measures is likely to give the most sensitive and specific indication of impending disease.

IS ATROPHY THE FINAL COMMON PATHWAY LINKING BRAIN PATHOLOGY WITH DEMENTIA?

Given that shrinkage of the brain is associated with both Alzheimer and vascular lesions, the question can be asked whether atrophy of the brain is the final common pathway linking brain lesions to dementia. Clinicopathologic data from the Nun Study suggest that while brain atrophy is an independent predictor of dementia, Braak neurofibrillary tangle stage remains an important predictor when both are included in the same model (Riley et al., 2002). In the Honolulu-Asia Aging Study, brain weight controlled for brain volume (a measure of atrophy) partially mediated associations between microinfarcts and cognitive performance in demented subjects, suggesting that atrophy secondary to vascular disease may contribute to the expression of dementia (Launer, Hughes, & White, 2011). When microinfarcts, neurofibrillary tangles and neuritic plaques were included as independent variables in the same regression model predicting brain weight, neurofibrillary tangles and microinfarcts, but not neuritic plaques, were significantly associated with this outcome. Finally, microinfarcts, neurofibrillary tangles, and brain weight were all significant independent predictors of cognitive performance. The cascade of events leading to dementia is depicted in Figure 4.9, showing the model proposed by Jack et al. (2010). It is important to understand that the events overlap, e.g., that the beginning of brain atrophy (Brain structure) closely follows the beginning of neurodegeneration secondary

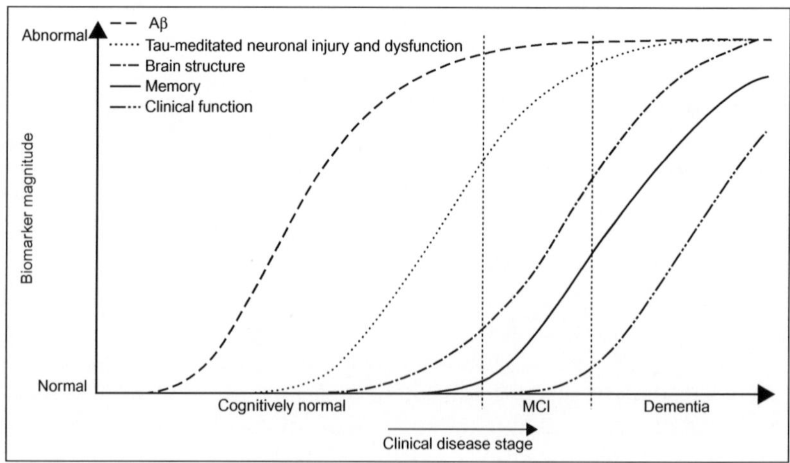

FIGURE 4.9 Dynamic biomarkers of the Alzheimer's pathological cascade. Aβ, aggregated beta amyloid. *Adapted from Jack et al. (2010).*

to neurofibrillary tangles (Tau-mediated neuronal injury and dysfunction), and that both of these processes proceed in parallel. Given the dynamic nature of this process, it should not be surprising to see that both neurofibrillary tangles and atrophy independently contribute to cognitive dysfunction when groups of subjects at different disease stages are included in the analyses. Although Jack considers only Alzheimer lesions in his model, one can easily envisage a parallel vascular model in which microinfarcts accumulate and dynamically lead to progressive atrophy, which contributes to additional cognitive impairment. In answer to the question of whether atrophy is the final common pathway leading to dementia, therefore, it must be acknowledged that dementia results in part from functional impairments directly related to Alzheimer and vascular lesions and in part from the subsequent shrinkage and loss of neurons resulting from these lesions.

COMMENTS

Because neuropathology in the form of lesions or atrophy is necessary to produce dementia, understanding its risk factors is important to the eventual prevention of this outcome. AD appears to be the most important neuropathology resulting in dementia. Vascular and Lewy body lesions greatly increase the chances a person will be demented when they have AD lesions, but rarely cause dementia by themselves. There is an association between pathologic severity and cognitive status, but the relationship is not one-to-one, with many individuals with established AD neuropathology never becoming demented, while others with relatively mild pathology do. This lack of strong correspondence can be attributed to the joint contributions of several pathologies as well as to brain reserve, which we review in the next chapter.

Chapter 5

The Threshold Model of Dementia

As noted in Chapter 4, approximately one-third of individuals meeting strict criteria for neuropathologic AD at autopsy were not demented at the time of their death. In addition, study participants with comparable levels of neuropathology at autopsy had a very wide distribution of cognitive presentations before death, ranging from intact cognitive function to severe dementia. The ability of people to maintain a high level of cognitive function in the presence of substantial Alzheimer pathology is often attributed to brain (Mortimer, 1995) or cognitive reserve (Stern, 2002).

Mortimer (1995) proposed that "clinical expression of AD requires two conditions to be met: first, a propensity, which is largely genetically determined, to accumulate Alzheimer lesions over the life course at a sufficiently rapid rate to meet neuropathologic criteria for AD at death; and second, the attainment of a critical threshold of brain reserve beyond which normal cognitive function cannot be maintained." In this context, brain reserve is considered to reflect the amount of functional brain tissue that remains at any given time, which is related to its maximum value attained in early adulthood and loss since that time. Theoretically, brain or cognitive reserve could reflect structural characteristics including the number and size of neurons and the density and pattern of their interconnections or the collection of cognitive strategies for solving problems or taking neuropsychological tests. The latter view could be considered in terms of the ways in which existing brain networks are used. Having a larger or more well-connected brain or computer would enable faster information processing, but actual performance would depend critically on the way brain networks are utilized (in the case of a computer, its software).

THE THRESHOLD MODEL OF DEMENTIA

In 1986, a threshold model of dementia was proposed by Roth (1986), who noted that dementia would not occur until a critical number of Alzheimer lesions or brain softening secondary to infarcts is reached (Figure 5.1). The problem with this model is that individuals can start out adult life with larger or more

Alzheimer's Disease. DOI: http://dx.doi.org/10.1016/B978-0-12-804538-1.00005-5

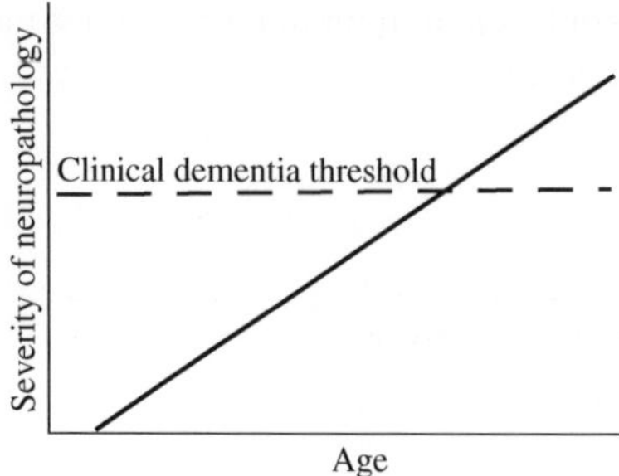

FIGURE 5.1 Early concept of the threshold hypothesis.

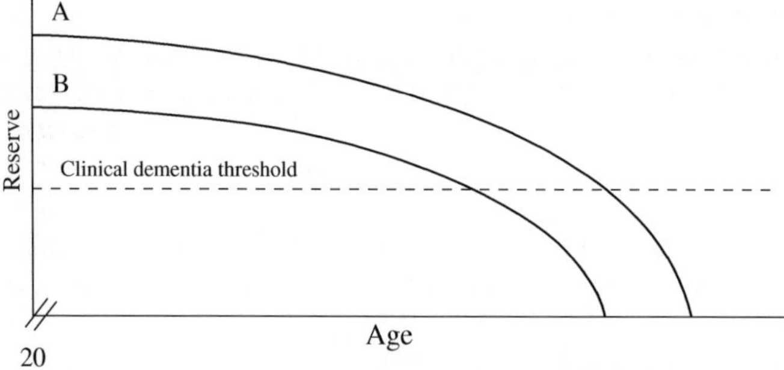

FIGURE 5.2 Reformulated concept of the threshold model for dementia.

well-connected brains and those with similar numbers of Alzheimer lesions may cross the critical threshold for dementia at different times depending on their reserve. A reformulation of the model (Figure 5.2) was proposed by Mortimer (1988) in which the amount of functional brain tissue present early in life constitutes the initial level of brain reserve (curves A and B in Figure 5.2), and a threshold for dementia is reached when the level of brain reserve is reduced to a critical level with the loss of functional brain tissue. The presence of varying amounts of reserve buffering the onset of dementia is now widely accepted as the explanation for the dissociation between the severity of Alzheimer neuropathology at death and cognitive status immediately before death.

An understanding of one's risk of becoming demented *involves measurement of both pathology and reserve*. Measures of Alzheimer neuropathology during life are available through PET assessment of the amount of aggregated amyloid-beta in the brain (Lowe et al., 2014), but the ability of this measure to predict *if or when* one will become demented is limited (Knopman et al., 2012). Better prediction is provided by the volume of the hippocampus, which is highly correlated with Braak neurofibrillary stage (Gosche, Mortimer, Smith, Markesbery, & Snowdon, 2001; Gosche, Mortimer, Smith, Markesbery, & Snowdon, 2002), but again this single measure is variably correlated with cognitive ability.

Adequate prediction requires at a minimum combining measures of Alzheimer and other brain pathologies with reserve.

WHAT IS RESERVE AND HOW CAN WE MEASURE IT?

A succinct definition of reserve provided in a recent review is "the hypothesized capacity of an adult brain to cope with brain damage in order to minimize symptomatology" (Morbelli & Nobili, 2014). The key word in this definition is "hypothesized." Although most Alzheimer scientists acknowledge the existence of reserve, measurement and quantification of reserve represents a major challenge. Ideally, we would like to have a single measure of reserve that captures the relationship between neuropathology and clinical expression of AD. However, to date, reserve has been measured indirectly through education, literacy, IQ, occupational characteristics, brain volume, or head circumference.

One way to assess the presence of reserve is to compare individuals at similar levels of cognitive impairment with respect to their occupation and education. Using regional cerebral blood flow techniques to assess the underlying level of neuropathologic damage, Stern, Alexander, et al. (1995) found that comparably impaired Alzheimer patients who had had occupations associated with higher interpersonal skills had markedly reduced blood flow in the parietal lobe compared with patients with previous occupations characterized by lower interpersonal skills. Therefore, they reasoned that patients with occupations associated with higher interpersonal skills must have greater reserve to compensate for their more severe pathology. Otherwise, such patients would have been considerably more impaired. When education levels of all participants in the Nun Study who remained nondemented at death were examined, those with low education had considerably milder neuropathology compared to those with high education, suggesting that participants with more reserve (higher education) were able to remain nondemented with much higher levels of Alzheimer neuropathology (Figure 5.3) (Mortimer et al., 2005).

Most studies that have considered reserve have used years of education as a surrogate for this concept. These studies have generally found that lower education is a strong risk factor for dementia of the Alzheimer type and that higher education protects one from becoming demented (Mortimer and Graves, 1993; Sharp & Gatz, 2011). Although years of education is a variable that is easily obtained, it is unclear what this number is actually measuring. Years of education is more likely a surrogate for other risk factors, such as having a higher IQ, learning strategies for problem-solving, or experiencing greater cognitive activity during life with consequences for brain growth and development. In addition, the quality of the schools attended and involvement of the students with their educational experience is not captured by simple enumeration of the number of years of education. Alternative measures, such as literacy (Manly, Touradji, Tang, & Stern, 2003) and IQ (Fritsch et al., 2005; Schmand, Smit, Geerlings, & Lindeboom, 1997), while correlated with years of education, have been shown

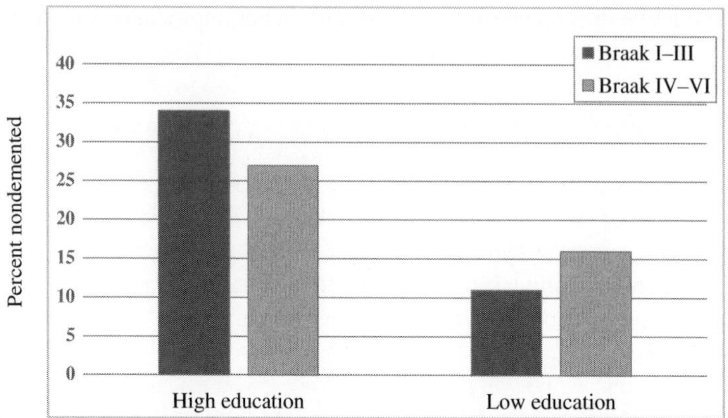

FIGURE 5.3 Percent of nondemented deceased Catholic sisters by educational attainment (high education = Bachelor's degree or higher; low education = less than a Bachelor's degree) and Braak neurofibrillary stage at autopsy. *Adapted from Mortimer, Borenstein, Gosche, and Snowdon (2005).*

to be more strongly associated with dementia risk. In addition, access to higher education may be limited in some populations by low socioeconomic status. In such populations, educational attainment may reflect poor early nutrition, which could be associated with brain development.

Another reserve factor that has been associated with cognitive impairment and dementia is maximal attained brain size (Mortimer, 2009). This variable is usually measured as total intracranial volume on MR scans or indirectly through determination of head circumference. The role of education and brain size as indicators of reserve offering prevention of dementia is covered in more detail in Chapter 11.

Although years of education, IQ, and maximum brain size are associated with dementia risk, these indicators of reserve are established early in life and are usually static after attaining adulthood. Therefore, while they are associated with cognitive function late in life, they do not reflect the effects of risk factors that operate during adult life and influence reserve. Dynamic measures related to reserve include regional and total brain volumes, which change over the lifespan and are affected by numerous pathologies as well as growth in response to exercise, hormones and other factors. A correlate of brain volume, brain weight at autopsy, has been studied and found to strongly influence risk of dementia (Launer, Hughes, & White, 2011). Another measure of reserve is reaction time, which has been shown in many studies to strongly correlate with IQ (Deary & Caryl, 1997). Because reaction time increases with aging and is increased in Alzheimer's and cerebrovascular diseases, it may provide a more dynamic index of reserve than IQ, especially when combined with static measures of reserve established early in life, such as years of education, IQ, and head circumference (Borenstein, Dahlquist, Wu, Larson, Teng, 2007).

The relative importance of reserve and brain pathology in predicting the risk for dementia has been explored in factor analyses of neuropathologic and clinical risk factors (Borenstein, Mortimer & Larson, 2014; Mortimer & Borenstein, 2014). In these analyses, we found that the amount of reserve is *as important* as the severity of Alzheimer pathology in predicting who becomes demented. We were able to characterize reserve by a single factor that included whole brain volume (brain weight) and education in an autopsy study and IQ, simple reaction time, and education in a cohort study. The fact that reserve plays such an important role may help to explain the dissociation between severity of neuropathology and cognitive function and the finding that about one-third of those with severe Alzheimer lesions at autopsy remain nondemented at the time of their death.

Because reserve is related to early brain development (Chapter 11) as well as to risk factors in adult life, prevention of Alzheimer's disease through maintenance and growth of functional brain tissue (reserve) remains an important target throughout the life course.

Section II

Descriptive Epidemiology

Chapter 6

The Prevalence of Alzheimer's Disease

The number of Alzheimer's disease (AD) cases worldwide, estimated to be almost 27 million in 2006, is expected to quadruple by 2050, with one in every 85 people having AD at that time if interventions that reduce incidence are not implemented (Brookmeyer, Johnson, Ziegler-Graham, & Arrighi, 2007). The increase in the crude prevalence rate or the number of AD cases divided by the population size is driven by two factors, precipitous declines in both the fertility rate and the mortality rate. As might be expected, these declines differ by country. In the last 50 years, the fertility rate has been cut in half around the globe and is expected over the next 50 years to drop to replacement level (2.1 children per woman) (Population Division Department of Economic and Social Affairs, 2002). In developed countries, this drop in the fertility rate has already been achieved, with 1.5 children per woman in 2000–2005. Interestingly, the rate of fertility decline over the last 30 years is more pronounced in the developing regions of the world. Despite this, differences remain among developing countries. The fertility rate is 5.5 children per woman in Africa, but is 2.5 or lower in Asia, South America, and the Caribbean.

Drops in fertility have generally preceded declines in mortality. The less developed regions of the world are making the largest strides today in decreasing their mortality rates, but they have further to go, since they are starting life with lower life expectancies (a person born in developed countries will live an average of 12 years longer than a person born in the less developed countries). Over time, this gap will decrease as the developing nations catch up to the more developed nations (Population Division Department of Economic and Social Affairs, 2002). With respect to prevalence rates for AD, other important demographic trends include the fact that not only are people living longer, but increases in life expectancy are more pronounced among those who already survived to age 60. Life expectancy at age 60 was 18.8 years in 2000–2005, and this will increase to 22.2 years in 2045–2050. Larger increases are seen at successively older attained ages. In addition, the sex disparity in survival (women outliving men) is expected to decrease gradually in the next 50 years in developed countries; while in developing countries, it will continue to widen.

Alzheimer's Disease. DOI: http://dx.doi.org/10.1016/B978-0-12-804538-1.00006-7

With the global population successively achieving the rectangularization of the population pyramid (Figure 6.1), there will be more old people with dementia and AD who require care from a younger, shrinking population. In parallel with the demographic transition, the epidemiologic transition, in which infectious diseases are slowly replaced by chronic diseases (Omran, 2005) is still underway in developing countries, resulting in greatly increased numbers of dependent older people suffering from chronic diseases like Alzheimer's. Globally, 13.2% of people aged 60 and over are in need of care, representing over 100 million, and by 2050, this number is expected to reach 277 million, most of whom will be in low- and middle-income countries (Prince, 2013). In population-based surveys conducted in Latin American, China, India, and Nigeria, about half of all dependent people have dementia.

The annual price tag of dementia care in the world was $604 billion in 2010 (Prince, 2013), with an estimated $200 billion being spent in the United States alone (Alzheimer's Association, 2012). By 2050, without a reduction in incidence, the annual cost is estimated to be $1.1 trillion. In developing countries, most public health efforts have focused on infectious diseases. AD is still seen in many countries as a normal part of aging. Although mental illnesses have been recognized as an important public health priority, AD is not included as contributing to these disorders and is largely ignored (Shafqat, 2008). While only 46% of dementia cases live in Western Europe and North America, these regions account for 89% of the total costs. The main reason that costs for dementia care are so much lower in low- and middle-income countries is that the formal social care sector barely exists and care is given by unpaid, informal caregivers. In the West, much of the care is provided by professional social, medical, and nursing home care providers. Secular trends in aging and the dementia epidemic are considered by economists to present a significant threat to global economic stability around the world (Prince, 2013).

CASE DEFINITION AND DETECTION

The most important problems that epidemiologists face in developing valid estimates for the number of prevalent AD cases around the world is case definition and detection. While combinations of biomarkers, including cognitive performance, have the ability to provide a high degree of classification accuracy to separate cognitively normal individuals from those with abnormal cognition due to aMCI and AD (area under the curve = 0.93, 95% CI = 0.91–0.95) (Schmand, Eikelenboom, & van Gool, 2011; Weiner et al., 2013), translation of this ability to classify individuals in populations remains a major challenge. Measuring biomarkers is expensive and invasive and is likely not going to be accessible to global populations in the short-term.

There are many challenges to comparing prevalence rates for AD and dementia across countries. Cultural expectations of older people and referral to medical care for a disease that currently has no effective treatment are uneven

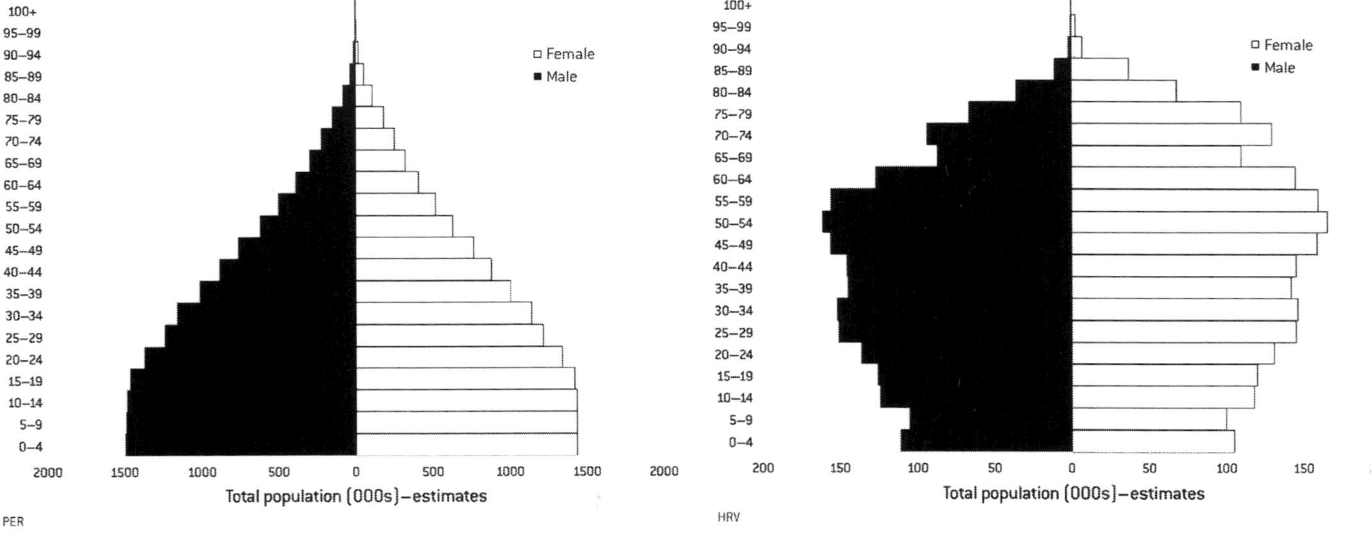

FIGURE 6.1 Rectangularization of the population pyramid. As a defined population grows older, the pyramid characterizing a young population (left panel) changes to a rectangle (right panel).

around the world. Lifestyle factors and poverty also may attenuate the motivation to seek medical attention. Because of these and other social, cultural, and economic issues, epidemiologic studies that use active case-finding techniques within defined populations provide the best estimates of prevalence and incidence rates, and our discussion will be limited to these.

AD is a disease affecting older people. Therefore, current age distributions and life expectancies coupled with cause-specific mortality rates that vary across populations will greatly affect the proportion of people found to have AD in different countries or regions of the world. The frequency of AD may also differ based on educational attainment in different populations, as reviewed in Chapter 11. More educated populations likely can delay the clinical presentation of disease to later ages, resulting in higher prevalence rates in older age strata and lower prevalence rates at younger ages (Gatz, Prescott, & Pedersen, 2006; Mortimer, Borenstein, Gosche, & Snowdon, 2005). In general, a population's mean brain reserve, including its genetic propensity for attaining a larger mean brain size as well as the many socioeconomic and cultural impacts affecting growth and loss of the brain across the life course, will affect how many people in that population have AD. In addition, as secular changes occur in education and increasing westernization brings improved early-life conditions to developing countries, prevalence may vary depending on the time frame that is being examined. Therefore, early prevalence estimates published in the 1960s and 1970s may be less relevant today. In this chapter, we seek to identify the best current estimates of the prevalence of AD and dementia and predict future rates if the disease cannot be curtailed over the next 30–40 years.

Epidemiologic studies of prevalence are difficult to compare because of variation in numerous aspects of study design that affect the final numbers. First, the population source must be considered. *Does the population source include community-dwelling as well as institutionalized individuals?* Including institutionalized persons will increase the prevalence estimates. In some countries, institutionalization is rare. In those regions, access to all older people living in the community is critical to obtaining valid dementia rates. When older people live with younger generations, gate-keepers may prevent study personnel from accessing all older people, resulting in underestimates of the frequency of dementia. *What is the youngest age included in the prevalence survey (60, 65, 70, 75)?* Clearly, crude prevalence rates will be lower if the lowest age included in the study denominator is 60 and higher if this age is 75.

Participation rates in prevalence studies may differ by country and by culture, and studies with low participation rates may not give us valid estimates. When prevalence studies have relatively small sample sizes, investigators may choose to report age-specific rates using 10-year age intervals, whereas larger studies will commonly use 5-year age intervals, rendering comparison of age-specific rates difficult. Comparison among studies using age-standardized rates depends on which standard population is used, limiting the utility of this technique in comparing rates across several different countries.

Second, the choice of the cognitive screening instrument can impact the final numbers in a significant way, depending on the sensitivity and specificity of that test in relation to the clinical diagnosis. Few studies use the same cognitive screening test(s), and even when they do, different cut-points are often applied, making comparison difficult. Nevertheless, it is important that each study establish the best cut-point for use in their population. The need to conduct each study in the most efficient and cost-effective manner usually overrides the concern of methodological standardization across studies. Additionally, some population-based studies invite only those participants who fail the cognitive screen for a clinical evaluation, while others sample screen negatives, and still others use a sampling approach. The ability to detect false-negatives is a critical step in correctly enumerating the prevalence or incidence rate, as we have already discussed.

Third, the clinical diagnosis may be based on different neuropsychological tests selected by the investigators and, while the same clinical research criteria may be used (e.g., the DSM criteria for dementia and the NINCDS-ADRDA criteria for AD), they may be applied and interpreted in different ways. For example, how is "a decline in social and occupational function" (one of the DSM criteria) defined? How are very mild cases classified—as "cases" or "controls"? Nonstandard operationalization of MCI, DSM, and NINCDS-ADRDA criteria may occur.

The burden of AD on individuals, caregivers, and society is related to its prevalence. However, this burden may differ greatly depending on the distribution of the severity of dementia within populations. Individuals with mild dementia generate much less burden than those with moderate to severe dementia. Unfortunately, information on the severity of dementia is rarely available in population-based studies. Prevalence rates of the disease may mask very different distributions of AD severity in different studies and regions of the world, which are critical to determining burden of the illness.

Because prevalence is equal to the incidence rate multiplied by the duration of disease, the incidence rate is more germane to the question of how frequently the disease occurs in populations and whether this rate is changing over time. Changes in incidence will reflect not only changing contributions of risk factors to disease incidence, but also the effects of improved recognition and diagnosis of the disease as technology to identify the disease improves.

PREVALENCE OF AD IN THE UNITED STATES

The debate about how many people have AD in the United States began in the late 1980s and early 1990s, when a landmark paper was published in the *Journal of the American Medical Association* (JAMA), which claimed that the prevalence of AD was "higher than previously reported" (Dysken et al., 2014; Evans et al., 1989). Specifically, the paper, based on a study of the residents of East Boston, MA, reported a prevalence rate of AD of 10.3% (95% CI 8.1–12.5%), which increased from age 65–74 (3.0, 95% CI 0.8–5.2%) to age 75–84 (18.7%, 95% CI 13.2–24.2) to age 85+ (47.2%, 95% CI 37.0–63.2). Additionally, 84.1% of the demented population was considered to have AD as the cause of their dementia. This was one of the first modern prevalence studies in the United States that used standard research criteria for the diagnosis of probable AD in a total population. The claim that the rates were higher than suspected was discussed in a series of letters to the Editor in the months following the paper's publication (Bowden et al., 1990). Points that were raised included the homogeneity of the sample (mostly Italian Caucasian), the relatively low educational achievement of the population, the reliance on mostly psychometric testing for diagnosis, the lack of application of the DSM-III criterion for dementia of a "loss of intellectual abilities sufficient to interfere with social or occupational functioning," the classification of very mild cases as cases of AD (which may today have been classified as MCI instead), and the underestimation of other causes of dementia besides AD. An average of 16 months elapsed between the screening phase and the clinical evaluation phase, which means that additional subjects could have developed the disease during this lag time, and also that prevalent cases could have died and not been counted in the clinical evaluation phase.

The East Boston Study's prevalence figures were later extrapolated by the Alzheimer's Association to determine the number of AD cases in the United States, which in 1990, was estimated to be around 4 million. In 1998, the General Accounting Office submitted a report to the Secretary of Health and Human Services in which 18 prevalence studies of AD were reviewed. In that report, the number of AD cases in the United States was estimated to be 1.9 million (United States General Accounting Office, 1998). Many of the studies used in this analysis were from Europe and therefore included mostly Caucasians (as in the East Boston Study). The most recent prevalence estimates used by the Alzheimer's Association are based on a second population-based study conducted by the same authors in a geographically delimited population of blacks (54%) and whites (46%) (Chicago Health and Aging Project, CHAP; Hebert, Weuve, Scherr, & Evans, 2013). Their analysis, projected to the 2010 US Census, showed an overall prevalence of AD in 2015 of 5.1 million people. Brookmeyer et al. (2011) reported prevalence proportions from the only nationally representative sample that exists in the United States, the Aging, Demographics and Memory Study (ADAMS) described in Chapter 3. The overall prevalence of dementia from this study was 13.7% (corresponding to 3.7 million Americans), and of AD, 9.5% (2.5 million Americans), consistent with the earlier estimate by the General Accounting Office. The variability in the estimated numbers of people with AD in the United States appears to depend more on the methodologies used in individual studies to identify cases than on the statistical techniques used to estimate them. According to Brookmeyer et al. (2011), the strongest determinant of this number is the case definition used and the clinical threshold used to determine caseness.

The National Health and Aging Trends Study (NHATS; Kasper, Freedman, & Spillman, 2013) also reported prevalence rates that are nationally representative of the Medicare population in the United States. This study began in 2011 and collected in-person interviews of individuals enrolled in Medicare sampled by counties and zip codes with oversampling of the oldest-old and of Black non-Hispanics. Seventy-one percent of the targeted group (N = 8,245) participated. The presence of dementia was not clinically evaluated. Instead, an individual was classified as demented if (i) the sampled person or their proxy responded that the sampled person was diagnosed by a doctor with dementia or AD; (ii) a cut score on a dementia screening interview (the AD8) administered to the proxy respondent indicated "probable dementia"; or (iii) cognitive test performance (memory, orientation, and executive function) was at least 1.5 standard deviations below the mean. Nursing homes were not sampled, but in the study areas, half of nursing home respondents were counted as having probable dementia and half were counted as not being impaired. Compared with participants age 71 and higher from ADAMS (Kasper et al., 2013), the rate for probable dementia in NHATS was 14.8% (vs 13.9% for dementia in ADAMS), and the rate for possible dementia in NHATS was 10.6% (vs 22.0% for CIND in ADAMS). However, ADAMS clinically evaluated participants for dementia, whereas NHATS did not, so this comparison is tenuous.

The occurrence of dementia or AD must be viewed within the context of the methodological challenges described earlier in this chapter, and the limits of the technology that we have to detect the disease. As pointed out by the Alzheimer's Association, newer criteria for AD that incorporate biomarker results to detect people in the "preclinical" phase of AD or MCI would result in much higher estimates of prevalence (Gaugler et al., 2013).

WORLDWIDE PREVALENCE RATES OF AD AND DEMENTIA

In 2010, the global impact of dementia was examined by Alzheimer's Disease International (Wimo & Prince, 2010). They reported an age-standardized prevalence rate of dementia for people age 60 and over of 5–7% worldwide in 2009, resulting in an estimated 34.4 million people with dementia. Others have forecast a doubling of this number every 20 years, with estimates in 2030 being 66 million and in 2050, 115 million (Prince et al., 2013). The number in 2030 represents an 85% increase over 2010 figures, increasing to 225% for the 2050 numbers compared with 2010. According to a meta-analysis of standardized prevalence rates around the world, rates for all dementias range from 4% in East Asia to about 8.5% in Latin America, a relatively narrow band given the many methodological challenges involved in estimating the frequency of the disease.

It has been known for many years that at least half of elderly in nursing homes have some form of dementia, with some estimates even higher (Magaziner et al., 2000). In one study conducted in Glasgow, Scotland among residents of 48 participating nursing homes, 58% had a dementia diagnosis and an additional 13.6% were cognitively impaired (Lithgow, Jackson, & Browne, 2012). In a total population study of Japanese Americans in Seattle, WA (The *Kame* Project), the prevalence of all dementias among community-dwelling participants was 2.9% (95% CI = 1.9–4.0), but among those living in institutions, 66% had dementia (Graves, Larson, et al., 1996). This is not surprising, but must be kept in mind when we consider prevalence rates in different regions around the globe, since customs related to caring for elderly dementia patients vary in terms of informal versus formal care. Therefore, low-to-middle-income countries that have few long-term care facilities should have a community prevalence rate that is relatively higher than that in Western countries with large numbers of nursing homes.

PREVALENCE OF MCI

The prevalence of MCI in older people varies substantially between studies, from about 15–25% of those age 70 and above (Petersen, 2009). In the Mayo Clinic Study of Aging, among 2000 nondemented participants, the prevalence rate of MCI between the ages of 70 and 89 was 16.3%. These authors found that the ratio of amnestic to nonamnestic MCI was 2:1 in this age range. Other studies have generally shown a range of prevalence rates of MCI between 14% and 18% among people age 70 and older (Petersen et al., 2009). In younger populations age 60+ or 65+, the prevalence of MCI is lower. When prevalence rates are needed for resource allocation such as future needs for nursing homes or health care, rates for MCI must be considered in addition to those for dementia.

METHODOLOGICAL ISSUES IN PREVALENCE STUDIES

In a meta-analysis of 22 studies of dementia conducted between 1945 and 1985, Jorm, Korten, and Henderson (1987) found important differences in the prevalence rates of dementia among studies meeting specific inclusion criteria. Three characteristics were statistically significant predictors of these differences: (i) Higher rates were found in urban areas compared to rural areas, which could have reflected the inclusion of more severe cases only in rural-based studies or could have been due to differences between urban and rural communities in life expectancy after disease onset. (ii) Studies of whole populations produced lower rates than those of random samples, likely due to more intensive examination of individuals in random samples where more detailed information was collected. (iii) Studies that included "mild" cases had fewer "moderate and severe" cases than those including only "moderate and severe" cases (Seshadri et al., 2011).

One investigator (Launer, 2011) commenting on the range of prevalence estimates concluded that: "There is no simple answer to the question, 'What is the prevalence of dementia in a particular community?' The answer varies depending on how we wish to define and measure (it)." She went on to note that the purposes of estimating prevalence will dictate the amount of information and rigor necessary. These purposes include etiologic research to suggest novel risk factors, surveillance to document secular trends, planning for resources necessary to care for people with dementia, or estimating the number of people who might be eligible to take a new medication or another intervention relevant to treatment of patients with a particular severity of disease. The main point made in this article is that in order to conduct etiologic research, we must "go deep," i.e., collect in-depth information on each individual in the study. If our main purpose is to plan for resources, we must "go-wide," that is, obtain broad phenotypic data and provide increased coverage of the population. In dementia research, the "go-wide" option requires the random selection of a large enough population to include adequate numbers of people belonging to heterogeneous groups. In the United States, sufficient numbers of minority, urban/rural, poor/wealthy populations must be included to provide stable and representative rates. The only "nationally representative" study we have in the United States is the ADAMS study, which is too small to fairly represent the US population. Therefore, we have had to rely on a variety of studies conducted in different population segments to estimate prevalence of dementia and AD in the United States. In the absence of a sufficiently large and representative study, this piecemeal approach to estimating prevalence has been the basis for the numbers used by funding bodies such as the NIH and organizations such as the Alzheimer's Association.

PREVALENCE RATES BY AGE

As the epidemiology of AD evolved over the last 30 years, two common sentences could be found in many papers. The first was "Only age and family history are known risk factors for AD." We will examine family history of dementia in more detail in Chapter 10. The second was "The prevalence rate doubles every 5 years." The earliest recognition of doubling in the rate every 5 years came from the meta-analysis reported by Jorm et al. (1987). In that paper, estimated age-specific prevalence rates were, for age 60–64: 0.7%; 65–69: 1.4%; 70–74: 2.8%; 75–79: 5.6%; 80–84: 10.5%; 85–89: 20.8%; and 90–95: 38.6%. The approximate doubling trend of dementia rates with every 5 years of additional age has been repeatedly reported in many subsequent studies and is widely accepted (Borenstein Graves, 2004).

An interesting problem that is common to many prevalence studies conducted to date is that the rates for the highest age strata are based on very small sample sizes and as a result are statistically unstable. This has led to uncertainty regarding prevalence rates in those above age 90. The oldest-old (defined as 85 and over) is the fastest growing segment of the population in many developed countries. Do the prevalence rates in this age group continue to increase with age, do they plateau or do they decrease? These questions can begin to be answered by studies that focus on very old samples. One example is the 90+ Study, which enrolled 91 individuals age 90 and over (Corrada, Brookmeyer,

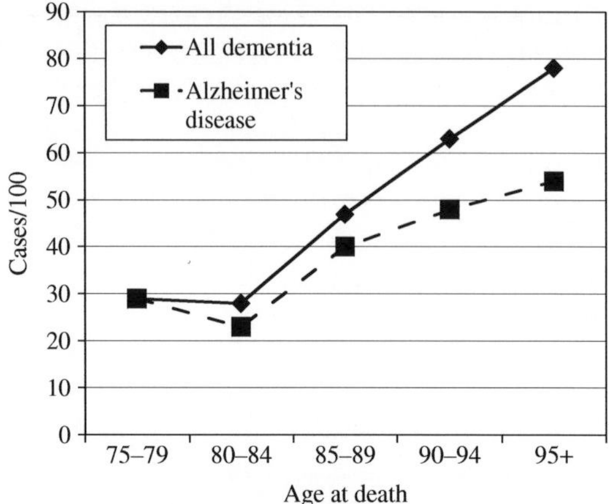

FIGURE 6.2 Prevalence of dementia by age at death, the Nun Study.

Berlau, Paganini-Hill, & Kawas, 2008). This sample was 77% female and 99% White, with a mean age of 94. More than half of the participants lived at home (56%); the remainder lived in a nursing home or in a group home. The overall prevalence of dementia was 41.2% (95% CI = 38.0–44.4) among all participants age 90 and over and rates beyond age 90 continued to double every 5 years, suggesting that the prevalence of this condition continues to rise in very old age.

Some debate exists as to whether the age-specific prevalence rates of AD above age 90 continue to increase. The original NINCDS-ADRDA criteria (McKhann et al., 1984) excluded a diagnosis of AD in people under the age of 40 and over the age of 90. This has been revised in more recent criteria (McKhann et al., 2011), in which it was recognized that the disease pathophysiology is not different in rare young cases or in common very old cases. What has also become clear is that it may be harder to diagnose very old people with AD, because of the multiple pathologies that accumulate, making the exact cause of the dementia hard to pinpoint. Several autopsy studies have reported a *decline* in the association between neurofibrillary tangle pathology and clinical dementia in the oldest-old (Gardner, Valcour, & Yaffe, 2013), suggesting that other pathologies act together to push people over the dementia threshold at advanced ages. In the Nun Study, we observed that while the prevalence of clinical dementia continued to increase with age into the 95+ age group, the prevalence of neuropathologically confirmed AD increased less steeply, diverging from the curve for clinical dementia starting at age 80–84 (Figure 6.2).

In addition, we found that the pathology that is most closely aligned with cognitive symptoms, cortical neurofibrillary tangles, *decreased* among both dementia cases and nondemented participants with increasing age above 90 (Figure 6.3), suggesting an increasing role of other pathologies in causing dementia in the oldest-old.

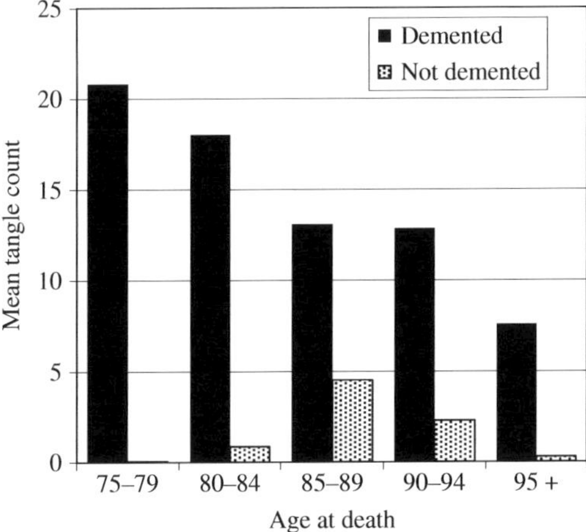

FIGURE 6.3 Mean number of neocortical neurofibrillary tangles by age at death in demented and nondemented participants in the Nun Study.

PREVALENCE RATES BY SEX

Although some studies have found higher prevalence rates for AD among women (Bachman et al., 1992; Graves, Larson, et al., 1996; Seshadri et al., 2002), others found no differences when adjusted for age, and still others reported lower rates in women in the young-old (60–74) and marginally higher rates in women in the old-old (85+) (Hofman et al., 1991). Because of differences in life expectancy between men and women, it is possible that women with the disease live longer than men with the disease, which would increase the prevalence in women versus men. This issue is better addressed by incidence data (Chapter 7), which are not contaminated by differences in disease duration.

Even in the oldest-old, studies have been equivocal in finding higher prevalence rates in women (Gardner et al., 2013), and when there is a difference, it is of marginal importance. One exception is the 90+ study, where the rates continued to double among women, but were relatively flat among men (Corrada et al., 2008). In addition, prevalence rates were associated with lower education levels among women, but not among men. It is possible that women's prevalence rates are more subject to the effects of low brain reserve in very old ages, while men's are not. It also could be that incidence rates plateau for men over age 90, as has been shown in the Rotterdam Study and in the Bronx Aging Study (Corrada et al., 2008). Finally, if men die more rapidly after becoming demented, women can have higher prevalence rates, regardless of differences in incidence rates. It is widely known that women live longer than men on average and that dementia reduces survival differentially by sex (see Chapter 8). Our discussion on incidence in Chapter 7 should help to clarify which of these explanations is most likely.

PREVALENCE OF AD AND OTHER SUBTYPES

There is general agreement that AD is the "most common" of the dementias. Despite this assertion, the frequency of AD in comparison with other dementias likely depends on age, race, and ethnicity. In the United States, AD constitutes about 60–80% of the dementia diagnoses.

Figure 6.4 shows the proportion of clinical dementia that may be attributed to each subtype, but these are just estimates, and change with characteristics of person and place. For example, we have seen that the oldest-old have more mixed pathologies of dementia than younger persons, and as we shall see in "Prevalence and Place" section below, the proportions may vary by place as well.

Clinical diagnoses depend on the existence of key markers and characteristics of dementing diseases. For example, a person is more likely to be diagnosed with vascular dementia if he or she has focal neurologic signs, has MRI evidence of cerebrovascular disease and presents with a step-like declines in cognitive function (Chapter 3, Clinical research criteria for vascular dementia). This does not mean that AD neuropathology is not present. In a study that examined 483 autopsied participants from the Religious Orders Study and the Rush Memory and Aging Project in Chicago, 179 persons who were on average 87 years old had probable AD clinically. Of these, 87.7% had pathologic AD and 45.8% had mixed pathologies. Thirty percent had AD with macroscopic infarcts and 10.6% had AD with neocortical Lewy Body disease; and 4.5% had all three pathologies (Schneider, Arvanitakis, Leurgans, & Bennett, 2009). Therefore, even among people with probable AD clinically, multiple pathologies contribute to the clinical picture.

In addition, the proportions of pathologic diagnoses may vary depending on the source of the cases, whether from the community or from dementia specialty clinics with more of the clinical diagnoses being explained by AD neuropathology in clinical versus community cohorts (Schneider, Aggarwal, Barnes, Boyle, & Bennett, 2009).

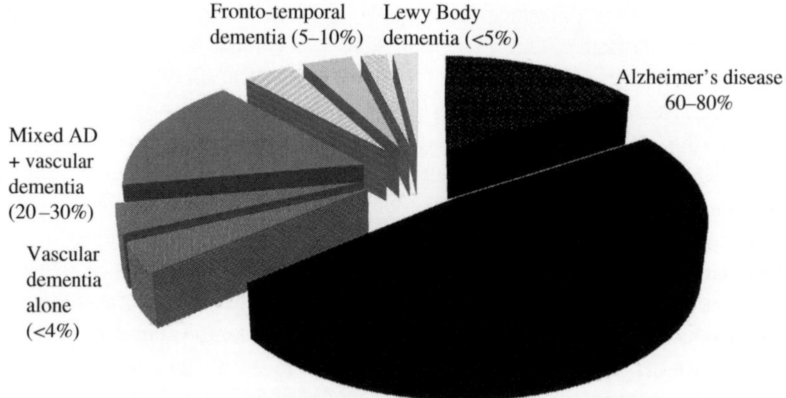

FIGURE 6.4 Estimates of the proportion of dementia subtypes.

PREVALENCE AND RACE OR ETHNICITY

Information on racial or ethnic differences in the prevalence of dementia and AD in the United States is limited. Changing demographics will result in the decline of the Caucasian population from 63% in 2011 to 47% in 2050. Conversely, the Hispanic population will grow from 17% to 29%, the Asian population from 5% to 9%, and the African-American population will remain relatively stable during the same period (Passel & Cohn, 2008). Racial and ethnic minorities remain underrepresented in epidemiologic research in general, and dementia research is no exception. The lack of information about minority health stems from multiple sources, including potential participants' lack of access to information and health care, fears about discrimination and stigma, and cultural mistrust of the medical establishment, stemming in part from historically unethical studies of African-Americans (George, Duran, & Norris, 2014).

A few US population-based studies have focused on dementia in different minority groups. These include studies of older African-Americans (Gurland et al., 1999; Hebert, Scherr, Bienias, Bennett, & Evans, 2003; Hendrie et al., 1995; Plassman et al., 2007). Two longitudinal studies have been conducted among Americans of Japanese origin: the Honolulu-Asia Aging Study (HAAS; White et al., 1996) and The *Kame* Project (Graves, Larson, et al., 1996). In addition, the Sacramento Area Latino Study on Aging (SALSA) study (Haan et al., 2003) provided estimates of dementia prevalence in a largely Mexican American population in California and the WHICAP study in New York City (Gurland et al., 1999) provided rates for Caribbean Hispanics. The Alzheimer's Association used data from the CHAP and ADAMS studies in their 2013 Report (Gaugler et al., 2013), citing a twofold higher risk among older African-Americans, with Hispanics having a 1.5-fold increased prevalence compared with older Whites. It is possible that the disparities in rates are due in part to the higher prevalence of vascular diseases, such as high blood pressure and diabetes, and lower levels of education in these population groups. With regard to etiology, incidence studies on racial disparities are more informative. These will be discussed in Chapter 7.

PREVALENCE AND PLACE

Given that differences in prevalence can be due to differing methodologies, it became clear in the late 1980s and early 1990s that there was a need to conduct methodologically standardized studies of prevalence, incidence, and risk factors for dementia and AD in different countries and ethnic groups. Three research groups set out to do so, supported by the National Institute on Aging (Chandra et al., 1998; Graves, Larson, White, Teng, & Homma, 1994; Osuntokun et al., 1992). In the first study, called the *Ni-Hon-Sea* Project (Larson et al., 1998), Japanese Americans aged 65 and over were compared between Seattle, WA (The *Kame* Project, N = 1985; Graves, Larson, et al., 1996) and Oahu, Hawaii

(The Honolulu-Asia Aging Study, HAAS, N = 3,734; White et al., 1996) and these populations were compared with Japanese living in Hiroshima, Japan (The Adult Health Study, conducted by the Radiation Effects Research Foundation, N = 2,222; Yamada et al., 1999). The motivation for this study was the observation in the late 1980s that it appeared that prevalence rates for what was then called "multiinfarct dementia" (known as "vascular dementia" today) were higher in Asia and those for AD were lower; while in the United States and in Western Europe, AD was more common than VaD (Graves, Larson, et al., 1996). We wanted to know whether the frequency of AD and VaD changed as populations of similar genetic ancestry migrated from Japan to Hawaii to the mainland United States. This hypothesis is illustrated in Figure 6.5 and follows a similar pattern to that seen for stroke (more common in Japan) and cardiovascular disease (more common in the United States) that sparked an earlier cross-cultural comparison called the "Ni-Hon-San" Study (Japan, Honolulu and San Francisco; Marmot et al., 1975). The *Ni-Hon-Sea* Project was designed so that the studies of dementia were methodologically standardized. The crude prevalence rates for all-cause dementia in the three studies were 7.2% in Japan, 9.3% in Hawaii, and 6.3% in Seattle, WA. For AD, they were 5.9%, 5.4%, and 3.5% respectively, and for VaD, 3.8%, 4.2%, and 1.4%.

Despite methodological standardization across the three studies, the included populations were of different ages (over 60 in Japan, over 70 in Hawaii, and 65+ in Seattle, WA). In addition, despite the uniform use of the Cognitive Abilities Screening Instrument as the cognitive screening instrument, different cut-points were used at the sites due to differing education distributions. In addition, the figures above do not take into account "other" or "unknown" types of dementia. The lack of completely standardized methodology was impossible because the studies were funded separately and each site had finite financial resources. Insufficient data were given in the published papers for us to compute age-standardized prevalence rates. Although Japanese populations have relatively

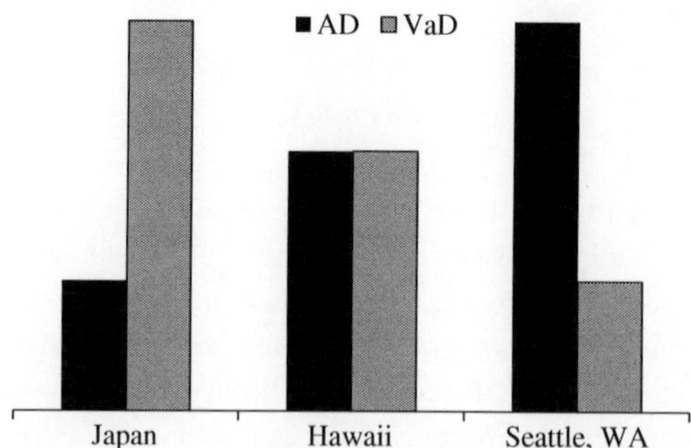

FIGURE 6.5 Hypothetical distribution of the frequency of AD and VaD in Japanese populations in Japan, Hawaii and mainland United States, with AD increasing and VaD decreasing with migration to the West.

low frequencies of the apolipoprotein E-ε4 allele (0.106 in the *Kame* Project) (Borenstein, Mortimer, & Larson, 2014), an established and strong risk factor for AD (see Chapter 10), the association between this allele and the risk of disease was extremely robust in these populations (Borenstein et al., 2014; Havlik et al., 2000). In summary, despite rigorous attempts to standardize methodologies across sites, differences in the underlying populations and in the applications of cut-points and clinical criteria remain, and the hypothesis of differences in the proportion of dementia related to Alzheimer's and vascular disease was not able to be reliably tested.

A second important study of AD in Africans in comparison with African-Americans was conducted by Hendrie and Osuntokun and their colleagues (Hendrie et al., 2001, 1995; Osuntokun et al., 1992). This study examined two populations aged 65 and over, a community-dwelling African population in Ibadan, Nigeria (where there are no nursing homes) (N = 2,494), and a sample of African-Americans living in the community and in nursing homes in a geographic area of Indianapolis, Indiana (N = 2,212). The motivating factor behind studying these two populations stemmed from the authors' observation that some of the African population in the United States forcibly migrated from West Africa during the slave trade era. The study used a cognitive screening instrument called the Community Screening Instrument for Dementia, the purpose of which was to minimize age, sex, and education influences on cognitive performance. The Indianapolis sample was statistically significantly older than the Ibadan sample (73.9 (SD = 7.0) vs 72.3 (SD = 7.5), $p < 0.001$). The samples had the same distribution by sex. The mean education of the US subjects was 9.6 years (SD = 3.1) and the Nigerian subjects, 0.8 years (SD = 2.3), with a literacy rate in the United States of 97.9% and in Nigeria, 15.2%. Screened participants were sampled for the clinical evaluation using a two-phase design. DSM-III-R and ICD-10 criteria were employed for diagnosis of dementia, the NINCDS-ADRDA criteria for AD, and the ICD-10 for diagnosis of vascular dementia. Consensus diagnoses were conducted by the principal investigators at both sites together, so that methodological standardization could be achieved. Age-adjusted prevalence rates for dementia were 2.3% (95% CI = 1.17–2.41) in Ibadan and 8.2% (95% CI = 7.09–9.40) in Indianapolis, and for AD, 1.4% (95% CI = 0.62–2.20) in Ibadan and 6.2% (95% CI = 5.13–7.34) in Indianapolis. The prevalence of AD was higher in Indianapolis in all age strata compared with Ibadan, but results were given only in 10-year strata. The authors proposed several explanations for these findings, including the influence of different risk factors for the disease in the two cultures, possible residual cultural bias in diagnosis despite strenuous efforts to standardize the clinical diagnostic process across the sites, higher mortality rates and shorter survival rates after dementia onset in Ibadan, and differential time from the screening phase to clinical diagnosis at the two sites (10 months in Ibadan, 5 months in Indianapolis). Another reason for the large difference in prevalence may be due to the differential effect of apolipoprotein E-ε4 on the risk for AD in the two populations. In Ibadan, despite a substantial number of participants carrying an apolipoprotein E-ε4 allele, there was no association between this allele and AD (Gureje et al., 2006), whereas in Indianapolis, there was a strong effect of apolipoprotein E-ε4 on the risk of AD (Murrell et al., 2006). Other studies have found less of an effect or an absence of an effect of apolipoprotein E-ε4 (particularly for heterozygotes) on cognitive outcomes and AD among African-Americans (Borenstein et al., 2006; Tang et al., 1996b).

The last study was a cross-national comparison (as opposed to a cross-cultural comparison) of a rural population in Ballabgarh in northern India with a rural population in southwestern Pennsylvania (Monongahela Valley). In Ballabgarh (Chandra, 1998), 4,450 individuals aged 55 and older in 27 villages in the study area were recruited door-to-door and enrolled. In the Monongahela Valley (MoVIES) cohort (Ganguli, Chandra, et al., 2000), 1,681 were identified from local voter registration lists. A cognitive test was developed for this comparative study, which used a two-phase design. The prevalence rates for dementia by DSM-III-R and AD by NINCDS-ADRDA criteria were 2.0% and 1.8%, respectively, of the Indian sample and 14.9% and 13% of the US sample, respectively (when comparing people only age 70 and over in both samples). Low overall life expectancy, short survival after disease onset and possibly the presence of protective lifestyle factors might explain these differences. The investigators also found a somewhat lower frequency of the apolipoprotein E-ε4 allele in the Indian sample (0.07) compared with the MoVIES sample (0.11).

Other attempts to estimate the number and proportion of the population with dementia in different geographic regions have been made. In one, a Delphi consensus approach was used. This method uses qualitative measures from published work to derive quantitative estimates using experts to reach a consensus about dementia prevalence in 5-year age strata found in population-based studies (Ferri et al., 2005). The study utilized the 14 regions of the world defined by the World Health Organization, which included the Americas, Europe, N. Africa and the Middle East, Africa, South Asia, the western Pacific. Using 10 expert groups, the investigators obtained 10 independent prevalence estimates for each 5-year age stratum, which were summarized as the mean prevalence estimate. The exercise was conducted in two rounds. The first set was sent to all 10 experts who were then asked to reconsider their own estimates based on the findings from the other nine groups in the second round. The areas of the world with prevalence rates based on good methodology were the United States and Canada, Western Europe, Iceland, the United Kingdom and Scandinavia, Israel, Japan, South Korea, and Australia. The areas with some studies but of a more moderate data quality included China, India, Bangladesh, Thailand, Malaysia, and New Zealand. Prevalence rates in Brazil, Nigeria, South Africa, Egypt, and Turkey were based on single studies. Other regions have no studies of dementia. Figure 6.6 presents a graphical representation of a table from this paper to show the mean prevalence rates in different regions of the world arrived at by consensus. What is clear is that the Americas has the highest age-specific rates, with

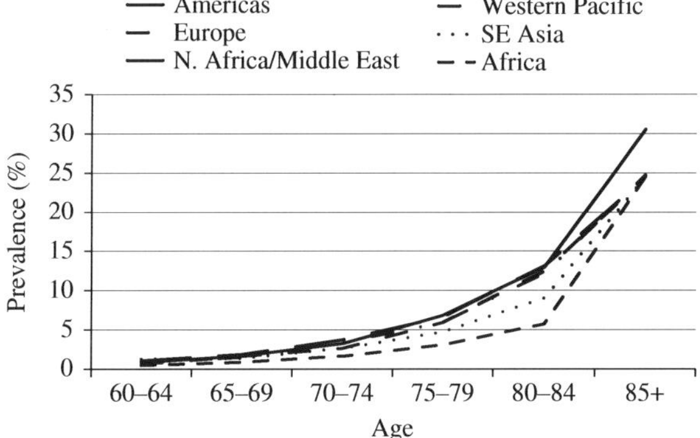

FIGURE 6.6 Average of group mean consensus estimates for prevalence of dementia (%) for each world region and age group (Ferri et al., 2005).

Europe, the Western Pacific, and North Africa/Middle East being next highest. The lowest rates are in Southeast Asia and in Africa. However, the lowest rates (in Africa) were also based on the fewest studies, with relatively low data quality.

Whether the differences in rates around the world are artifacts of methodology due to differing cultural expectations of older people, differential access to medical care or other characteristics specific to each population, or real differences in risk factors for incident AD, is not known. Risk factor epidemiology, including gene-environment interactions, will help us to understand geographic variation in incidence of AD and dementia, the subject of Chapter 7.

Chapter 7

The Incidence of Alzheimer's Disease

The incidence rate measures the speed of development of new disease. For etiologic studies, the incidence is a more accurate measure to use because it does not include duration of disease, which is implicit in the measure of prevalence and has risk factors that can be confused with those for disease incidence. When a person meets clinical criteria for Alzheimer's disease, we usually consider this to be an "absorbing state," that is, the diagnosis will not revert to normal or MCI unless the diagnosis is in error. Figure 7.1 shows all possible transitions that can occur up to the time of death. It is assumed here that all persons who develop AD must go through MCI first, even though this may not always be captured in prospective cohort studies. While it is beyond the scope of this book to discuss incidence rates to all clinical states and death, we will focus on the incidence of MCI and AD from normal cognition and also discuss briefly the incidence of the transition from MCI to AD.

For prevalent cases, the date of onset of AD is usually determined from information obtained from a knowledgeable informant. The accuracy of this date will depend on the extent to which the proxy informant is knowledgeable about the patient's day-to-day activities. For example, a spouse generally will have better knowledge than an adult child, but a spouse of a few years may not be as knowledgeable as an adult child. In addition, when a proxy informant is asked to recall the onset of disease symptoms, she or he may recall very early events that may or may not be directly related to the disease. For example, should disease onset be the time when the patient forgot the route to drive home or the time when he forgot where his car was when he came into the parking lot of the grocery store? Although "senior moments" are common, are they predictive of real dementia onset? There are clearly problems associated with retrospective determination of the time at which we should consider a prevalent case to have become demented.

In contrast with dating the onset of the disease in prevalent cases, dating onset of dementia is more straightforward in incident cases. Some studies use the date of first clinical examination that leads to a consensus diagnosis of

Alzheimer's Disease. DOI: http://dx.doi.org/10.1016/B978-0-12-804538-1.00007-9

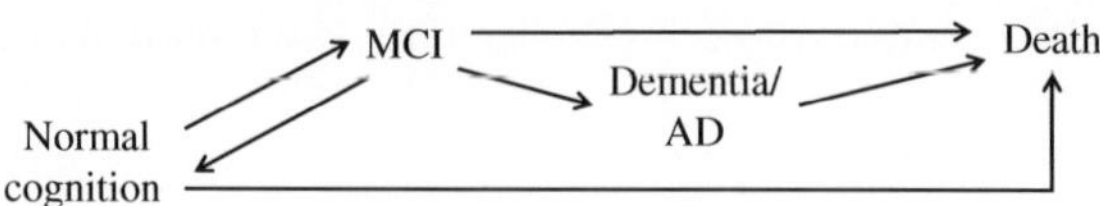

FIGURE 7.1. Clinical state transitions in incident cognitive disorders.

dementia or AD as the onset date. In epidemiologic studies, we are unable to conduct weekly or monthly surveillance. Nor would this necessarily be useful, since there can be great variability in symptoms of AD in the first year or two. When incidence waves are conducted 2 years apart, there is sufficient time for individuals to progress from one clinical state to another. In fact, we may miss some cases if they develop MCI and AD and then die of another cause, but it is usually financially infeasible to screen or sample a cohort every year. Because we cannot know the month in which a case transitions from one clinical state to another, we usually use an interval-censoring method to estimate the time of onset. For example, we may know that the last time the individual was seen, they were cognitively normal and did not meet criteria for MCI, dementia, or AD, and the next time they were seen (say, 2 years later), they met such criteria. From this information, we can estimate the age at onset using this method in a research study, and we do not have to depend on the proxy informant's memory of when the disease began.

Another issue that must be considered in a prospective cohort study is how to deal with participants who are lost from the cohort through death, refusal, or out-migration. The last time the participant was seen, they could have been cognitively normal, but we cannot assume that they remained so at the point at which they left the study. As we shall discuss in Chapter 8, people who die are at a pronounced increased risk of having dementia, and those who refuse may have different risk factors for the outcome than those who remain in the cohort through the end of the study. In some studies, the greatest attrition occurs in the period between baseline and the first incidence wave. In the *Kame* Project, 1,836 participants were followed for up to 10 years. Since it is culturally improper for older Japanese to refuse, there were many people who "delayed" their biennial visits for the four incidence waves that occurred after the baseline visit, such that at the end of the study, about three times as many people refused compared with the previous incidence waves. Therefore, depending on the population's culture, refusals may occur at the beginning or at the end of the study. Regardless of when attrition occurs, investigators usually build in procedures to query the next-of-kin to discover the cognitive status of the participant before death (excluding the last few months of life when end-of-life conditions such as delirium can be confused with dementia). Instruments such as the Dementia Questionnaire may be administered that would allow investigators to conduct a consensus diagnosis on these individuals similar to what was done for living incident cases (Kawas, Segal, Stewart, Corrada, & Thal, 1994). Analyses could then be conducted using the consensus diagnosis of the participant's status at or near the time of death.

In longitudinal studies, a small proportion of participants may miss one or more visits. In the case of a participant missing an incidence wave, the interval censoring has to take into account a longer period (say, 4 years instead of 2). In a two-phase design, individuals who are screened and invited to return for a clinical examination may choose not to come in. When this occurs, there are missing data for the clinical diagnosis. When a participant misses the baseline clinical evaluation, but they return to the study in the first incidence wave and are found to have dementia or AD, they may truly have prevalent, not incident, disease. This problem can also occur at any incidence wave. Investigators must take steps to take this into account statistically so as not to misestimate the incidence rates (Izmirlian, Brock, & White, 2000).

INCIDENCE RATES BY AGE AND SEX

Because studies vary in the methodology of case definition, which we discussed in previous chapters, incidence rates also vary. In Figure 7.2, we include studies that reported rates for AD alone in 5-year age groups from 65 to 89 (with the exception of the important study from East Boston (Evans et al., 2003) that only published data for 10-year age strata). For the Jorm 1998 meta-analysis (Jorm & Jolley, 1998), pooled rates for mild AD for three parts of the world (Europe, United States, and East Asia) are shown. Regardless of methodological variations among studies, the general pattern of increasing incidence with increasing age mirrors that of the prevalence figures: the rates approximately double every 5 years. From these and other studies, the overall incidence from normal cognition to dementia or AD for those over age 60 is usually cited as 1–2% per year.

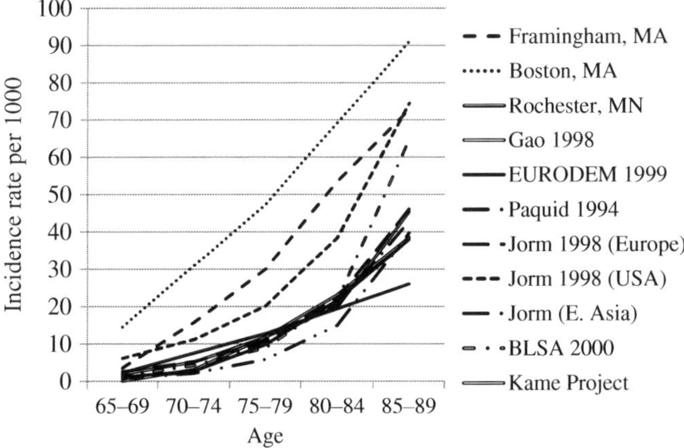

FIGURE 7.2 Age-specific incidence rates of Alzheimer's disease.

Cumulative Lifetime Risk

The cumulative incidence, a measure of disease risk during a period of time, can be termed the "lifetime risk" if the period of observation extends to the time of death. The Framingham Study, a study of heart disease and stroke in the population of Framingham, MA, has examined participants biennially since 1948. In 1976–1978, the investigators added a cognitive component with the addition of the Mini-Mental Status Examination to its evaluation. Because its participants were followed to death, this study provides a good source of data from which to estimate lifetime risk. For men, the lifetime risk of AD at age 65 was 6.3% (95% CI = 3.9–8.7), which increased marginally to 7.1% (95% CI = 0–15.1) at age 90; for women, the corresponding risks were 12.0% (95% CI = 9.2–14.8) and 8.2% (95% CI = 2.6–13.7) (Seshadri et al., 1997). These figures were compared by the authors with the estimates of lifetime risks of other diseases related to aging, such as fracture and cancer. The estimated lifetime risk for dementia in a 65-year-old woman from the Framingham study was 19% (95% CI = 15.4–22.5) (as opposed to 12.0% for AD), and for hip fracture in a comparably aged woman, it was 16%, and for cancer, 29%.

For a 65-year-old man, the lifetime risk for AD is about half that of a comparably aged woman, which can be attributed to women living longer than men. In the Framingham cohort, at age 65, women were expected to live another 22.7 years and men only 18.8 years (Seshadri et al., 1997). With regard to lifetime risks at different ages, the Framingham authors report that these do not increase with age as might be expected, but rather are fairly flat across age strata, because increases in risk with increasing age are counter-balanced by declining residual life expectancy. In particular, the decline in the lifetime risks in very old age is accounted for by steep increases in mortality. The authors of this paper caution that estimates of lifetime risk are based on the incident experience of the cohort and not of the individual. Individual risk depends on the person's individual life expectancy, as well as the presence of the whole spectrum of risk factors in that individual (Seshadri et al., 1997). The authors also state that subjects with very mild forms of dementia and those with dementia at time of death of less than 6 months' duration were excluded from their calculations. Therefore, their estimates of lifetime risk may be somewhat underestimated. Because the Framingham Study does not include large enough numbers of non-white participants, these projections also are limited in their generalizability to other racial groups.

Incidence of MCI

In France, the Personnes Agées QUID (PAQUID) cohort of 3,777 community-dwelling participants age 65 and over was followed between 1988 and 1998 for clinical transitions from normal cognition to amnestic MCI, normal cognition to dementia, normal cognition to cognitive impairment-no dementia, amnestic MCI to dementia, and amnestic MCI to normal (Larrieu et al., 2002).

The annual incidence rate for AD among 1,654 initially nondemented subjects age 70 and up at baseline was 1.7% (95% CI = 1.6–1.8); for transition from normal to amnestic MCI, it was about 1%; and for the transition from amnestic MCI to AD, 8.3% (95% CI = 6.9–9.7). The transition rate from cognitive impairment-no dementia, a group that would meet criteria for nonamnestic MCI, to AD was also elevated compared with individuals with normal cognition (7.1%, 95% CI = 6.4–7.7). For the combination of the three groups (normal, amnestic MCI, and other cognitive impairment-no dementia), the incidence rate to types of dementia other than AD was much lower (0.64%, 95% CI = 0.62–0.68).

Of 58 amnestic MCI subjects at baseline and 37 amnestic MCI patients at 2-year follow up in the PAQUID study, over 40% were normal at the 5-year follow-up. Therefore, a large proportion of people with amnestic MCI reverted back to normal cognition. Although this proportion is surprisingly high, it was based on performance on a single neuropsychological test, which could easily have fluctuated around the cut-point used to separate normal from abnormal, resulting in instability of the amnestic MCI diagnosis. Reversion to normal cognition from MCI was also studied in the Mayo Clinic Study of Aging (MCSA) (Roberts, Knopman, et al., 2014). In that study, 38% of participants with a diagnosis of amnestic or nonamnestic MCI reverted to normal. However, among those MCI patients who reverted back to normal, 65% later developed MCI or dementia (HR = 6.6 for dementia ($p < 0.0001$) compared with participants who were normal at enrollment without an MCI diagnosis) (Roberts, Knopman, et al., 2014). These findings suggest that MCI, a diagnosis largely based on cognitive performance, is less reliable than that of dementia, in which functional impairment secondary to cognitive deficits is required. However, the fact that many of those who reverted to normal later went on to develop AD and dementia suggests that MCI was frequently an indicator of chronic rather than transient impairment.

The MCSA has provided additional data about progression to dementia from MCI (Roberts, Knopman, et al., 2014), demonstrating that progression to dementia increases with age, is greater among women than men, and is greater among multiple-cognitive domain MCI patients than among single-cognitive domain MCI. The MCSA investigators also observed that the risk for reversion to cognitively normal status was lower among people who had amnestic MCI or multiple domain nonamnestic MCI as well as among carriers of the apolipoprotein E (APOE)-ε4 allele, a major risk factor for AD discussed in Chapter 10. Therefore, individuals diagnosed with MCI who had more severe cognitive impairment, especially on memory tests, or had increased genetic risk for AD were more likely to be in a true transition to AD or dementia than those with isolated nonmemory cognitive impairments who were not at higher genetic risk of AD.

Another cohort study that examined incidence of MCI was conducted in northern Manhattan, New York, in three contiguous census tracts in the Washington/Hamilton Heights and Inwood neighborhoods (the WHICAP study) (Manly et al., 2008). Individuals age 65 and over residing in this area were invited to participate in a cohort study of aging and cognitive function. The cohort was 28.4% non-Hispanic White, 32.6% non-Hispanic Black, and 39% Hispanic and was composed of 2,364 community-dwelling participants, 1,800 of whom were nondemented and did not have MCI at the first visit. The incidence rate of amnestic MCI among these 1,800 was 2.3% (95% CI = 1.9–2.6) and for nonamnestic MCI, 2.8% (95% CI = 2.4–3.2), for a total incidence of all MCI at 5.1% (95% CI = 4.6–5.6). The much lower incidence rate of MCI in the PAQUID study (1%) (Larrieu et al., 2002) is likely explained by the restriction of the definition of MCI in PAQUID, which was limited to amnestic MCI, whereas in the WHICAP study, all types of MCI were included. The incidence of single-domain (memory-impaired) MCI from WHICAP was 1.4% (95% CI = 1.1–1.7), similar to the PAQUID figures.

If They Live Long Enough, Will Everyone Get Dementia?

One of the most important questions that remains is, "Will everyone develop dementia or AD if they live long enough?" This question can be broken into two parts: (i) Will everyone develop dementia? and (ii) Will everyone develop AD? The supposition that most people will likely develop dementia if they lived to, say, 150, is supported by the ever-increasing age-specific incidence rates, which do not appear to level off or decline in the extremely old age groups. In the 90+ Study, a population-based sample of 330 nondemented subjects 90 years and over was followed for 5 years. Incidence rates of dementia doubled each 5.5 years, from 12.7% per year in the 90–94 age stratum, to 21.2% per year in those aged 95–99, and 40.7% per year in the 100+ age group (Corrada, Brookmeyer, Paganini-Hill, Berlau, & Kawas, 2010). Although studies rarely have statistically stable incidence rates for people over age 90, one study that has both very old women and neuropathology on all subjects is the Nun Study (Snowdon, 2001; Snowdon et al., 1996). Unpublished data from this study of 678 Catholic Nuns of the School Sisters of Notre Dame, which required brain donation upon death as an inclusion criterion for participation, show a continuing increase in the frequency of dementia at the time of death, with a less steep incline for the proportion of individuals with dementia who met Reagan neuropathologic criteria for probable AD (Figure 7.3). These findings suggest that non-AD pathologies and age-related changes likely play a larger role in causing dementia in the very old compared with younger cases. As we saw in figure 4.6, the mean number of neurofibrillary tangles in the neocortex decreases with advanced age in the very old in both demented and nondemented subjects, albeit the demented patients have higher means in all age strata.

The evidence points to the incidence of dementia continuing to rise in the very old, but the severity of AD pathology declining. There are two main interpretations for the continuing increase in the incidence of dementia but not AD. First, there is the issue of selective survival. Those who survive into extreme

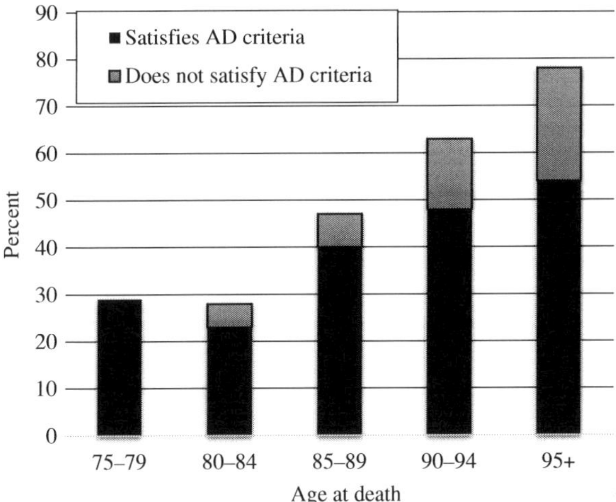

FIGURE 7.3. Percent of Nun Study participants who had dementia at death by satisfaction of Reagan AD neuropathologic criteria and failure to satisfy AD criteria. (n = 529).

old age may have fewer genes that increase the rate of AD pathology accumulation or alternatively may have genes that are protective for the development of pathology. A second explanation is the loss of reserve capacity with increasing age, which makes it more likely that people will develop dementia without fulfilling neuropathologic criteria for AD. In the Cognitive Function and Ageing Study, a multicenter, prospective population-based study of older people in the United Kingdom, 456 deceased individuals were examined at autopsy (Savva et al., 2009). Cortical and hippocampal atrophy were semiquantitatively rated and dichotomized into none or mild versus moderate or severe. In *both* demented and nondemented groups, the prevalence of moderate and severe atrophy increased with age (from 75 to 95), but the prevalence of atrophy was much higher in those who were demented. Since the attainment of the clinical threshold of dementia is largely predicted by atrophy (Jack et al., 2005), the continuous process of losing brain tissue with increasing age can be represented by the illustration in Figure 7.4. Here, each individual experiences their own trajectory, which is determined by genetic and environmental risk factors and the level of initial reserve. In extreme old age, most people will attain the clinical threshold, but some people with unusual protective factors such as larger brains may be able to "escape" cognitive impairment. For example, the longest-lived human, Jeanne Calment, who lived to the age of 122.5, was said to be mentally intact until her death (Wikipedia, The Free Encyclopedia). Therefore, while *most* people will likely attain the clinical threshold of dementia (not necessarily due to AD alone) at very old age, a minority of people may not.

What is age doing then? In 1986, Brody and Schneider defined *age-related diseases* as those that "have a temporal relationship to the host but are not

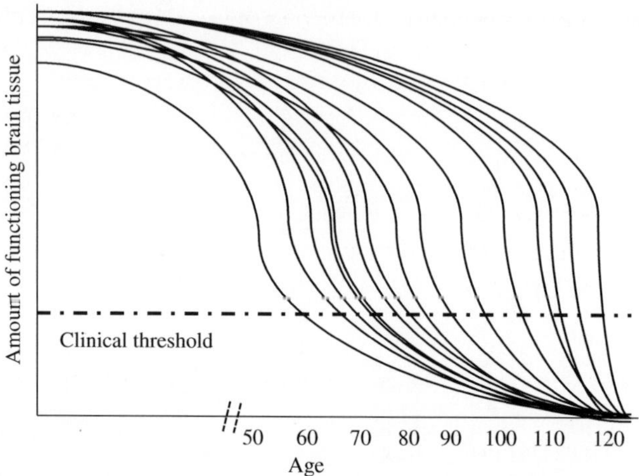

FIGURE 7.4. Illustration of different trajectories toward cognitive impairment.

necessarily related to aging processes," and *age-dependent diseases* as those "whose pathogenesis appear to involve the normal aging of the host" (Brody & Schneider, 1986). By these definitions, dementia appears to fall into the age-dependent category, but as we have just seen, if the prevalence of AD neuropathology *decreases* in extreme old age, AD may be age-related and not age-dependent. Increasing age is likely increasing risk for dementia by allowing the accumulation of increased neuropathology with the passage of time and by reducing reserve through loss of brain tissue. Aging involves the atrophy of many organ systems, and the concept of reserve capacity applies to more than just the brain (Calleja-Agius, Muscat-Baron, Brincat, 2007; Folkow and Svanborg, 1993).

Incidence by Sex

Do women have more reason to worry about becoming demented or getting AD compared to men? In Chapter 6, we suggested that women may have higher prevalence rates than men at older ages and that this may be due to increased survival after onset. Incidence rates should provide a clearer answer to the question. In 1998, two meta-analyses of incidence rates for dementia and AD were published (Gao, Hendrie, Hall, & Hui, 1998; Jorm & Jolley, 1998). In the meta-analysis of Gao, women had a slightly higher risk than men for dementia, which, however, did not achieve statistical significance (OR = 1.18, 95% CI = 0.95–1.46, but women did have a significantly higher risk for AD compared with men (OR = 1.56, 95% CI = 1.16–2.10). Jorm reported no sex difference in dementia incidence, but reported higher incidence rates for AD among women after age 85. Another paper from the Kungsholmen Project in Sweden (Fratiglioni et al., 1997), a population-based study of 1,473 residents aged 75 and higher, reported an age-adjusted RR for women of 1.9 for dementia and 3.1 for AD. Other studies have not found a significant sex effect for AD (Borenstein, Mortimer, Larson, 2014; Hebert, Scherr, McCann, Beckett, & Evans, 2001; Kukull et al., 2002). In the 90+ Study, women were not at increased risk for dementia compared with men (Corrada et al., 2010). However, no data were available from this study for AD incidence in very late life. Although the findings are mixed, they suggest that women may have higher risk for AD at advanced ages (over 85) than men. The findings for dementia, for the most part, do not show differences by sex.

One methodological issue that is difficult to resolve in the diagnosis of dementia in very old patients is the degree to which the DSM criterion of "decline in occupational and social life due to cognitive impairment" is met. The manner in which this criterion is operationalized will to some extent lead to differences in findings between studies. Other methodological differences also may contribute to varying rates found among studies, e.g., the interval between visits and the use of interval censoring, as well as differential loss-to-follow-up in various studies, which is higher among the very old. Finally, there could be residual confounding by age. Incidence rates are usually presented in 5-year age strata, so differences in survival among men and women could lead to higher rates in women that would be more apparent if 1-year age strata were examined. The combination of these methodological shortcomings, differential survival by sex, and few studies with large sample sizes in the 90s and 100s make the question of differential incidence rates of dementia between women and men difficult to answer.

In 2012, the largest incidence study in the world was published by the 10/66 Dementia Research Group (Prince et al., 2012). A population-based, cross-national study was undertaken in urban regions of Cuba, the Dominican Republic, and Venezuela, and in both urban and rural geographic regions of Peru, Mexico, and China using standardized methods (see "Incidence and Place" section for more details about this study). Incidence was assessed 3–5 years after the prevalence phase, and all 12,887 participants were clinically examined for dementia. In this study, men had a reduced risk for incident dementia compared with women using 10/66 criteria (Prince, Acosta, Chiu, Scazufca, & Varghese, 2003) (HR = 0.72, 95% CI = 0.61–0.84). The highest age group was ≥80; therefore, the answer to the question of whether incidence rates in women exceed those for men in the "young-old" may be "yes," particularly in low-to-middle income countries.

If women are at higher risk than men for AD, to what can this be attributed? The population cohorts that have been studied to date grew up at a time when women had less access to education. Women do have smaller brain volumes, in accordance with their generally smaller stature. Lower education, smaller head circumference, and shorter stature are risk factors for the clinical expression of AD (see Chapter 11). Men also are known to die of vascular causes more readily than women, resulting in a survival cohort of men with lower vascular risk in the older ages (Chapter 14). The APOE-ε4 genotype also may have a more detrimental effect among women (Chapter 10). Estrogen may play a neuroprotective role among women until menopause; and the lack of it, particularly many years after the cessation of estrogen production, may also explain higher incidence rates among women over the age of 80 (Chapter 19). We will explore these and other risk factors in later chapters.

INCIDENCE AND RACE

One of the earliest systematic studies of incidence by race examined individuals from the Duke Established Populations for Epidemiologic Studies of the Elderly (Duke EPESE) living in one urban and four mostly rural counties in North Carolina between 1986 and 1990 (Fillenbaum et al., 1998). Three-year incidence rates of dementia (rates for AD were not available) were generally higher in blacks for men and higher in Whites for women, but the overall crude rates were about the same (Whites = 6.2% (95% CI = 2.7–9.7); blacks = 5.8% (95% CI = 2.6–90)). This study used deceased subjects to retrospectively ascertain dementia status, and there was differential participation by race ($p = 0.049$) that could have biased the incidence rates. The Einstein Aging Study in the Bronx, NY (Katz et al., 2012) found somewhat higher rates among blacks aged 70 and over (3.54, 95% CI = 2.26–5.56) compared with comparably aged whites (2.16, 95% CI = 1.58–2.96), with most of the differences being present in those aged 80–89.

In the Cardiovascular Health Study (Fitzpatrick et al., 2004), a multisite study of risk factors for cardiovascular disease in over 5000 people age 65 and over, participants were recruited in 1989–1990 from Medicare eligibility rosters in four regions of the United States: North Carolina, Maryland, California, and Pennsylvania. In 1992–1993, 687 African-Americans were recruited and in 1998, the Cognition Study was initiated that included a test of global cognition and an MRI. Over 3,000 subjects, including 563 African-Americans, completed all tests and were classified by dementia status. Incidence rates for dementia (not AD) were higher among African-American women (58.8/1000 person-years) than White women (34.7 per 1000), and also higher among African-American men (53/1000) than White men (35.3/1000). Differences by race, but not by sex, were statistically significant ($p = 0.003$).

In the WHICAP study (Tang et al., 2001), participants were sampled from Medicare beneficiaries living in an area of three adjoining census tracts in the Washington Heights and Inwood neighborhoods of New York City. Six-hundred and ten African-Americans, 760 Caribbean Hispanics, and 418 whites were enrolled in the final sample that was followed for an average of 4 years. Of these participants, 156 developed probable or possible AD by NINCDS-ADRDA criteria. Incidence rates were higher for African-Americans than whites in every 10-year age stratum, with those for Caribbean Hispanics following between African-Americans and whites. Age-standardized incidence rate ratios compared to whites, adjusting for education, illiteracy, and cardiovascular and cerebrovascular conditions, were 2.4 (95% CI = 1.5–4.0) for African-Americans and 2.0 (95% CI = 1.2–3.4) for Caribbean Hispanics. The generalizability of these results to the US population is tenuous, as the Hispanics in this study were primarily Dominican and this subgroup was admixed with individuals of African descent. A paper from the same study also found that in people who did not carry an APOE-ε4 allele, the cumulative risk of AD to age 90 was four times higher among African-Americans (RR = 4.4, 95% CI = 2.3–8.6) and twice as high in Hispanics (RR = 2.3, 95% CI = 1.2–4.3) compared with whites; while among study participants who carried an ε4 allele, there were no significant differences in cumulative risk among the three racial groups.

INCIDENCE AND PLACE

The story about the prevalence rates of dementia and AD from cross-cultural studies is not complete without also discussing the incidence rates. Since the prevalence is strongly related to the duration of the disease, differential survival by geographic location could have an important effect on the resultant rates. In the *Ni-Hon-Sea* Project, the three studies of Japanese descent published their results independently. In Japan, the primary goal of the incidence rates was to investigate whether the dose of ionizing radiation sustained during the Hiroshima bombing in 1945 (the mandate of this study's funding) modified the risk for developing dementia (Yamada et al., 2009). The incidence rates were stratified by dose, but not by age. No association was present between radiation dose and risk for AD. The incidence rate in those at the lowest radiation dose for women was 12.9/1000 person-years (95% CI = 9.5–17.4), and for men, 5.7/1000 person-years (95% CI = 2.9–11.4). In the *Kame* Project (Borenstein et al., 2014), the crude incidence rate for women was 13.2/1000 person-years (95% CI = 10.5–15.9) and for men, 8.8/1000 person-years (95% CI = 6.3–11.3). The *Kame* cohort included participants aged 65 and over, while the Adult Health Study in Hiroshima included participants 60 and over. Therefore, the *Kame* cohort was expected to have somewhat higher incidence rates. In the Honolulu Asia-Aging Study (HAAS), which studied men only over the age of 70, the overall crude incidence rate of AD was 7.5/1000 person-years (95% CI 0.8–14.2) (Havlik et al., 2000), which is not statistically different from that obtained in the *Kame* Project or the Adult Health Study. Because all three studies used similar methodologies, the lack of differences between them in AD incidence suggests that similar risks for this condition may exist in Japan, Hawaii, and Seattle.

In another study, incidence rates among 2,459 Yoruba in Ibadan, Nigeria were compared with 2,147 African-Americans living in Indianapolis, IN after a mean follow-up of about 5 years (Hendrie et al., 2001). A prevalence study was followed by two incidence waves, one after 2 years and the other after 5 years. Age-specific incidence rates for AD were 3.6-fold higher among African-Americans than among Yoruba for those aged 65–74; 2.3-fold higher among those aged 75–84; and 1.4-fold higher among those 85 and older. The age-standardized incidence rate adjusted for mortality was 1.15% (95% CI = 0.96–1.35) among Yoruba and 2.52% (95% CI = 1.4–3.64) among African-Americans. Comparison of age-standardized prevalence and incidence rates show that age-standardized prevalence rates for AD (Chapter 6) differed by a factor of four between African-Americans and Yoruba, while age-standardized incidence rates for AD differed by a factor of two. These ratios suggest that lower incidence and higher mortality after onset (shorter disease duration) contributed about equally to the lower prevalence rates of AD among Yoruba as compared to African-Americans.

The same group reported that APOE-ε4 was a risk factor for AD in the Indianapolis cohort, but only among those who were homozygous for the allele (OR = 4.8 (95% CI = 1.7–13.6) vs OR = 1.2, (95% CI = 0.6–2.45) for those who were heterozygous) (Sahota et al., 1997). Among Yoruba, APOE-ε4 was not associated with AD (Osuntokun et al., 1995). The analyses among Yoruba were based on only 12 AD subjects (probable and possible AD) and 39 unaffected, cognitively normal individuals. Among these, only 3 AD subjects and 14 controls had one or two APOE-ε4 alleles; therefore, the null association in this group could be due to small numbers.

Another attempt to standardize methodology across continents for identification of incident cases compared two communities, one in the Monongahela Valley in Pennsylvania (MoVIES), and the other in a rural community in Ballabgarh, Northern India (Chandra et al., 2001). In MoVIES, 1298 dementia-free participants aged 65 and over were followed for 10 years, with 153 incident cases of probable and possible AD by NINCDS-ADRDA criteria (Ganguli, Dodge, Chen, Belle, & DeKosky, 2000). For AD, the incidence rate was 21.1/1,000 person-years (95% CI = 16.6–26.7) for men and 18.1/1,000 person-years (95% CI = 14.7–22.4) for women. Comparable rates in Ballabgarh were 3.7/1,000 person-years (95% CI = 1.4–8.0) for men aged 65 and over, and 2.59 (95% CI = 0.5–7.6) for women of the same age. The wide confidence intervals for the Ballabgarh cohort are due to the very few cases of probable and possible AD (n = 10) that were found in the incident cohort of 2,698 participants. After standardizing the rates to the 1990 US Census population, the incidence rate ratio was 3.7 times higher in the MoVIES cohort compared with the Indian cohort (17.5/1,000 person-years vs 4.5/1,000 person-years, respectively). Besides the small numerators in the Ballabgarh cohort, this cohort was followed for only 2 years for this publication. A longer follow-up would have been useful to obtain more stable rates.

We showed in Figure 7.2 that incidence rates are similar around the world in terms of the shape of the curve with increasing age. Brookmeyer, Johnson, Ziegler-Graham, and Arrighi (2007) updated the review of Jorm and Jolley (1998) to include more recent estimates of age-specific incidence rates for AD, and developed an equation that predicts a doubling of AD incidence every 5.5 years. Application of this equation to various geographic regions yielded no differences in the doubling times ($p = 0.3$). They concluded that geographic variations in incidence rates are likely due to methodological differences.

An important effort that sheds some light on whether incidence rates for AD vary around the world is the 10/66 Dementia Research Group's population-based cohort study (Prince et al., 2012). Baseline and 3- to 5-year incidence waves were conducted using a one-phase survey among individuals aged 65 and over in 7 countries (defined urban regions of Cuba, Dominican Republic, and Venezuela, and urban and rural areas in other countries). All 11,718 participants who were not demented in the prevalence phase (2003–2007) were clinically reexamined and had an informant interview in 2007–2010. Dementia diagnoses were made using two sets of criteria: the 10/66 and the DSM-IV (American Psychiatric Association, 2000). The former criteria use cognitive test and informant-based scores as well as diagnostic information from clinical interviews in a logistic regression analysis predicting the probability of being an incident case; while for DSM-IV, cases had to meet these criteria for cognitive impairment, including decline in social or occupational functioning and exclusion of another mental disorder and delirium. 10/66 diagnoses are used primarily in the paper to report incidence rates. 10/66 criteria were twice as likely to result in the definition of a case as the DSM-IV criteria. This could reflect in part the difficulty of applying the criterion for decline in social or occupational functioning in low- to middle-income countries, where there may be varied cognitive expectations of older people and there is more informal support for elders' daily activities. In this population-based study, 770 incident cases of 10/66 dementia were identified (2.22% per year); only 284 of these also met DSM-IV criteria (0.82% per year). The authors compared their findings with EURODEM DSM-III-R criteria (instead of using their own DSM-IV criteria), so the comparisons are likely unfair. The age-standardized rates from 10/66 were between 20 and 30/1000 person-years, compared with EURODEM's 18.4/1000 person-years. By 10/66 criteria, rates were highest in Venezuela, intermediate in China, and lowest in Peru (Prince et al., 2012). This study suggests that the incidence of dementia in middle-income countries is generally similar to that in high-income countries, although, as we shall see in Chapter 11, lifetime socioeconomic influences may differentially impact the risk for AD.

INCIDENCE AND TIME TRENDS

Because most systematic cohort studies did not begin until the early 1990s, there are few sources of data to assess secular trends in incidence of dementia and AD. The best estimates come from the Mayo Clinic's Rochester Epidemiology Project (REP) (Kokmen, Beard, O'Brien, et al., 1993; Rocca et al., 2011), which provides surveillance of the population of Olmsted County, MN. The REP maintains a medical records linkage system for the county in which the Mayo Clinic provides most of the care. Other healthcare providers in the community participate in the REP, leading to more complete ascertainment. A list of diagnostic codes suggesting dementia was sought in the records. It is important to note that the number of codes increased over time, from 112 in 1975–1984 (Rocca, Cha, Waring, & Kokmen, 1998) to 132 codes in the 1990–1994 period (Knopman, Petersen, Cha, Edland, & Rocca, 2006), which could increase the likelihood of finding cases. Each potential case's medical record was abstracted and rediagnosed by a neurologist using criteria similar to the DSM-III-R, although the criteria were not standardized due to the primary purpose of the records being for clinical, not research, purposes. The population of Olmsted County, MN, is constituted mostly of whites, with half being men and half women, 110,000 being enumerated in the 1990 US Census. Using cases identified in this manner and denominators from the US Census, incidence rates were calculated, unadjusted for sex, because no differences by sex were observed. Over the 20 years, trends in incidence inconsistently oscillated, and no statistically significant effects for calendar year were found, although there was a decrease between 1985 and 1994 (RR = 0.97 per calendar year, 95% CI = 0.95–0.99, $p = 0.004$), implying a 3% decline per year or a 30% decline over a decade (Rocca et al., 2011). The increase in effort over time to discover all cases in the population, including more sources in addition to the Mayo Clinic medical records, should have led to an *increase* in incidence over time. The observed *decrease*, if a true decline, is therefore best explained by a true drop in incidence rates over the last 10-year period examined.

In another examination of trends in incidence over time conducted within the Rotterdam Study (Schrijvers et al., 2012), two subcohorts, one begun in 1990 (N = 5,727) and the other in 2000 (N = 1,769), were followed for 5 years. Age-adjusted incidence rates for dementia (n = 286 and n = 49 incident dementia cases in the two subcohorts, respectively) were lower in the 2000 subcohort than in the 1990 subcohort (RR = 0.75, 95% CI 0.56–1.02), but this difference was not statistically significant. Nondemented subjects in 2005–2006 had larger brain volumes ($p < 0.001$) and fewer white matter lesions on MRI than nondemented subjects in 1995–1996. The latter finding may be related to lower stroke risk in the later cohort, which would have the effect of lowering the risk of dementia among those with AD pathology (Chapter 4). The differences observed could not be explained by differences in participation rates in the subcohorts (88.3% and 88.9%, respectively).

The issue of whether or not incidence rates for dementia and AD are declining over time (Filley, 2015) is very important, since a decline may have important prognostic significance. Because of secular increases for protective risk factors such as education, IQ, head and brain size, and decreases in stroke incidence, a decreasing incidence of dementia would be expected, possibly tempering the coming epidemic to a degree. However, this potential mitigation may be offset by increases in the incidence of obesity and diabetes, risk factors for the disease (Chapter 14). Because obesity and diabetes rates are increasing rapidly among young and middle-aged adults, we will not know the impact these will have on dementia incidence until these cohorts move into the age of high risk for dementia, which could take 30–50 years.

Chapter 8

Survival and Mortality in Alzheimer's Disease

As early as 1976, Dr Robert Katzman noted that the late-onset form of Alzheimer's disease (AD) "may rank as the fourth or fifth most common cause of death in the US ... yet the U.S. vital statistics tables do not list 'Alzheimer disease,' 'senile dementia,' or 'senility' as a cause of death, even in the extended list of 263 causes of death" (Katzman, 1976). The death certificates in the United States and many other developed countries have been poor sources of information regarding death from AD. Dementia and AD cause many deaths indirectly. For example, death may result from aspiration pneumonia in advanced AD patients who are unable to eat or decubitus ulcers among patients who are bedbound. It is therefore important that all causes of death—underlying, immediate, associated or contributing—be analyzed on the death certificates. Even then, the death certificate is a poor source of information due to the frequent lack of information available to the physician completing it.

In the first study of US mortality data taking into account all causes of death, Chandra, Bharucha, and Schoenberg (1986) examined causes of death in 1971 and 1973–1978 using International Classification of Diseases Adapted for Use in the United States (ICDA) (US Department of Health Education and Welfare, 1967) rubrics for "senile or presenile brain disease" (ICDA rubric 290) and "senility" (ICDA rubric 794). Data were analyzed separately for deaths due to dementia and those with dementia. The overall annual age-adjusted mortality rate was 0.41 and 2.19/100,000 for mortality due to and with senile and presenile dementia, respectively, and 0.52 and 12.21/100,000 for mortality due to and with senility, respectively. In this analysis, rates were higher among men and for whites for deaths due to and with senile and presenile dementia, and for nonwhites, the rates were higher for deaths due to and with senility. Among those who died with senile and presenile dementia, the most common underlying causes of death were coded as diseases of the heart (33.4%), senile and presenile dementia (18.2%), cerebrovascular diseases (12.9%), and influenza and pneumonia (4.5%). For those dying with senility, the top five underlying

Alzheimer's Disease. DOI: http://dx.doi.org/10.1016/B978-0-12-804538-1.00008-0

causes of death were diseases of the heart (41.7%), cerebrovascular diseases (14.6%), arteriosclerosis (9.3%), influenza and pneumonia (7.9%), and malignant neoplasms (4.4%). Only 18.2% of the death certificates listed senile and presenile dementia as the underlying cause of death, and 4.3% listed senility as the underlying cause among those who had died *with* these conditions (Chandra et al., 1986).

In a study using NCHS mortality data, age-adjusted annual mortality rates per 100,000 for AD for ages 65 and over increased from 2.5 in 1979 to 37.5 in 1995 (Hoyert & Rosenberg, 1997). This large increase likely reflects changing codes and diagnostic criteria, as well as increased awareness of the disease. The study by Hoyert and Rosenberg reported that 20,000 death certificates had AD as the underlying cause of death and another 20,000 as another cause of death. In a commentary, White (1997) estimated a conservative number of 100,000 deaths in the United States around this time from end-stage dementia, based on a prevalence of AD at the time between one and two million. Therefore, it would appear that in only 40% of cases were dementia diagnoses included on death certificates. Other studies have produced higher estimates. Among patients enrolled in studies reporting their findings to the Consortium to Establish a Registry for Alzheimer's disease (CERAD) (Raiford, Anton-Johnson, Haycox, et al., 1994), dementia was reported on about two-thirds of death certificates. It must be kept in mind that this group of patients was highly selected and that participation in a research study on dementia could increase the likelihood of dementia appearing on the death certificate. In a UK study (Martyn & Pippard, 1988), only 22% of demented patients had an ICD code of presenile or senile dementia on their death certificate. However, 58% of these death certificates mentioned the word "dementia" somewhere on the certificate. Frecker, Pryse-Phillips, and Strong (1995) reported their experience from Newfoundland, Canada, where they noted that 51/59 (86.2%) death certificates for probable AD cases by NINCDS-ADRDA criteria listed AD on the certificate. The place of death may make a difference in the degree of accuracy, because, for example, the clinical histories of patients dying in hospital are less known to physicians than those dying in nursing homes.

Data derived from the Chicago Health and Aging Project (CHAP) and extrapolated to the US population (Weuve, Hebert, Scherr, & Evans, 2014) estimated that 600,000 people with AD died in 2010 in the United States, including people who received medical care and those who did not. By 2030, these estimates are expected to increase to 900,000, and in 2050, to 1.6 million. In addition, due to the aging of the US population, the proportion of deaths with AD will increase rapidly. By 2050, 43% of all older adult deaths will occur among people with AD, up from 32% in 2010 (Weuve et al., 2014). While there is a trend for death certificates to increasingly include AD as a cause, there is consensus that only about half of existing AD cases are ever diagnosed (Thies & Bleiler, 2011).

AD IN THE TOP 10 LEADING CAUSES OF DEATH

In 2010, the top 10 leading causes of death among people age 65 and over listed AD as sixth, with 83,494 deaths (Murphy, Xu, & Kochanek, 2013). If there truly are 600,000 deaths per year from AD, AD would be regarded as the #1 cause of death in the United States, instead of heart disease (which, in 2010, was estimated to claim 477,338 lives). It is important to note that in national statistics, the numbers of deaths reported for AD are those for which the underlying cause of death is AD. Many patients with AD die from heart disease, stroke, pneumonia, and influenza, which would frequently be considered as the underlying causes of death. The degree to which AD contributes to such deaths is unknown. For example, would the person have died from stroke if they didn't have AD? This issue highlights the difficulty in pinpointing the individual contributions of various chronic diseases as well as acute illnesses, such as influenza, in causing death in the oldest segment of our population.

Given that about 50% of cases of dementia are not diagnosed before death, screening for incident dementia or AD in community-based studies and following cases over time is necessary to accurately enumerate deaths and to appreciate the importance of AD and dementia in increasing the risk for death. It also is important to start with incident cases, so that the time between onset and death can be counted properly. In addition, studies need to be relatively large so that there is a sufficient number of incident and mortality outcomes. Such data are available from a number of studies, and a few are selected here for illustrative purposes.

In the PAQUID study, begun in 1988, a cohort of 2,923 community-based elders age 65 and over living in southwestern France (Gironde and Dordogne) were randomly sampled from electoral rolls and followed for up to 8 years (Helmer, Joly, Letenneur, Commenges, & Dartigues, 2001). During this time, 281 incident cases were diagnosed with dementia (67% AD), with a mean age at onset of 80 ± 5.9 among men and 83.5 ± 6.1 among women. Mortality was analyzed using Cox proportional hazards models with delayed entry, adjusting for sex, education, comorbidities, and dependence in ADL/IADL at baseline. In the population, the RR for mortality associated with incident dementia was 1.80 (95% CI = 1.46–2.21), and about the same, 1.72 (95% CI = 1.34–2.21) for AD. The analysis also showed effect-modification by age, such that dementia had less of an impact on mortality with increasing age (RR= 0.95, 95% CI = 0.92–0.98 per year). For participants dying with dementia above age 85, the RR was elevated but not statistically significant (RR = 1.37, 95% CI = 0.91–2.04). In this study, there were no sex differences in the RR for dying with dementia. There was an increased risk for dying with respiratory disease among individuals with AD; and the risk for dying with cerebrovascular disease was statistically significant for dementia, but not for AD. The median survival time from onset of dementia to death was 4.5 years for all ages, being longer among women (7.3 years at age 75 compared with 4.5 for men; and 4.4 at age 85 compared with

3.5 for men), likely reflecting the survival advantage of women over men in the general population. Survival time also was modified by education, with those with more education having shorter survival times than those with less education (Amieva et al., 2010).

Modification of survival time by education was also reported in the WHICAP cohort. The RR for dying among AD patients was 1.9 (95% CI = 1.2–3.0) for those with 9 or more years of education in comparison with those with 8 or fewer years. Those with higher occupational attainment also experienced a higher risk for mortality compared with those with lower occupational attainment (RR = 2.2, 95% CI = 1.1–4.3) (Stern, Tang, Denaro, & Mayeux, 1995). This would be predicted by the threshold hypothesis, since AD patients with higher education and occupation would experience a later clinical onset of their disease, when AD-related neuropathology was more severe given their higher brain reserve. Such individuals would be expected to decline more rapidly and have a shorter duration of disease from onset to death (Stern, Alexander, Prohovnik, & Mayeux, 1992).

The WHICAP study also found a differential survival in AD by race/ethnicity (Helzner et al., 2008). Over a mean follow-up time of about 4 years, 323 incident AD cases developed, who were on average 87 years old at baseline and who had a median lifespan of 92.3 years. The median survival after AD onset among non-Hispanic whites was 3.7 years, 4.8 years among African-Americans, and 7.6 years among Hispanics. The findings were not explained by differences in overall lifespan by race/ethnicity. However, these differences could be explained by differences in education and occupational attainment, with the African-Americans and Hispanics being diagnosable at earlier ages.

Another way to look at mortality is to compare remaining life expectancy for AD patients in comparison to the general population. In the Adult Changes in Thought Study (ACT Study), an AD patient registry was set up in 1987 in the Seattle, WA regional area to identify all persons age 60 and over in the population of a health-maintenance organization of 23,000 members who developed AD (Larson et al., 2004). Between 1987 and 1996, incident cases were invited to participate in the study, and 970 with suspected dementia (521 AD: 431 probable and 90 possible by NINCDS-ADRDA criteria) were followed annually. Survival in AD in this sample did not vary by education and was longer for younger-onset patients and women. Poorer survival with AD was predicted by male sex, lower baseline cognitive score, poorer Dementia Rating Scale score, and by the existence of frontal release and extrapyramidal signs, history of falls, incontinence and history of heart disease and stroke. Survival time medians from diagnosis to death were 7.5 for AD cases ≤75 years old, 5.6 for those 76–80, 4.9 for those 81–85 years old, and 3.2 for those over age 85. A 70-year old woman with AD was expected to live 7.7 fewer years than a woman in the general US population, and a similarly-aged man, 8 fewer years. This gap narrowed with increasing age (3.3 years for an 80-year old woman and 3.1 years for an 80-year old man, and 1.8 and 0.5 years at age 90 for women and men, respectively). The Hazard Ratios for mortality by MMSE score, using scores of 25–30 as the reference group, were 1.4 (95% CI = 1.01–1.94) for MMSE scores 22–24, 1.69 (95% CI = 1.24–2.31) for MMSE scores 18–21, and 2.67 (95% CI = 1.94–3.66) for MMSE scores ≤17.

Two cohort studies that required autopsy consent for enrollment are informative for mortality. Both studies, the Religious Orders Study (ROS) and the Rush Memory and Aging Project (MAP), enrolled nondemented participants. In the ROS, the 1,168 subjects were Catholic nuns, priests, and brothers aged 65 and older from around the United States (Bennett, Schneider, Arvanitakis, & Wilson, 2012). The analysis of mortality in this cohort was conducted between 1994 and 2013 (James et al., 2014). In the Rush MAP, 1,574 people living in retirement communities and senior housing around Illinois (Bennett, Schneider, Buchman, et al., 2012) were enrolled between 1997 and 2013. The studies were conducted by the same research team, all measures were standardized, and the authors pooled the data assuming the populations were comparable. There were a total of 2,566 nondemented subjects 78 years old at baseline who were followed for an average of 8 years, 559 of whom developed incident AD over the study follow-up (mean age of AD diagnosis 86.5 ± 6.5). Six hundred and ninety-two (34.5%) of the nondemented participants died, versus 398 (71.2%) of those with incident AD. The median survival time from diagnosis of AD to death was 3.8 years and depended on the age of the subject at diagnosis: 4.4 years for those age 75–84 and 3.2 for those age 85 and over. After adjusting for age, sex, race, education, and study in the proportional hazards regression model, the HR for mortality associated with incident AD was 3.13 (95% CI = 2.74–3.58). The authors calculated the population attributable fraction (PAF) for mortality associated with AD, meaning the proportion of deaths in this population that were attributable to AD. These estimates were 37% for participants between the ages of 75–84 after adjustments for demographic variables, and 36% for those age 85 and older. When these PAFs were extrapolated to the number of deaths in the United States, the authors estimated that there were 503,400 excess deaths in 2010 associated with AD. This estimate is very close to the estimate of 600,000 obtain by Weuve et al. (2014). Importantly, the authors of the ROS and Rush MAP point out that their estimate of the number of people dying because of AD is 5–6 times higher than that acknowledged by the CDC in 2010 (83,494 deaths). This study has been criticized because no individual data were used to investigate the actual causes of death of cohort members and because the samples were not population-based. In contrast to the PAF published by the Rush group (James et al., 2014), the Alzheimer's Association report for 2013 states that the PAF for AD on mortality over a 5-year period in people age 65 and over ranges from 5% to 15% (Gaugler et al., 2013). This estimate was based on population cohort studies (in Sweden and in the United States).

In a review paper published in 2012 (Brodaty, Seeher, & Gibson, 2012), the authors calculated the number of years of life lost due to dementia by subtracting survival times from life-table data matched by age at diagnosis and sex ratio in countries in which 42 studies were published. They included studies from the United States (49%), Europe (44%), and Australia (7%). In young-onset disease, the absolute number of years of life lost was much higher (range 9.6–19.4 years) compared with late-onset disease (range 1.3–9.2 years). Years of life lost among young-onset cases was 60–94% of their average life expectancy, compared with 16–73% for later-onset patients. Among the eight studies that looked at differences in survival in men and women, women lost more years of life in absolute terms, but the relative loss of years of life was similar by sex, decreasing with increasing age.

COMPETING CAUSES OF DEATH

It is important to recognize that deaths from other chronic diseases are decreasing, while deaths due to AD are increasing. In the 2013 Alzheimer's Disease report (Gaugler et al., 2013), it was noted that deaths due to stroke decreased between 2000 and 2010 by 23%, due to heart disease by 16%, due to human immunodeficiency virus by 42%, and due to prostate cancer by 8%. During the same period, Alzheimer deaths increased by 68% (according to NCHS statistics). The changing picture of mortality suggests that in the future, AD will become a much more important contributor to mortality than it is today, unless effective preventions for this illness are discovered and employed.

Section III

Analytic Epidemiology

Chapter 9

Introduction to the Analytic Epidemiology of Alzheimer's Disease

When biologically modifying drugs become available to treat Alzheimer's disease (AD), these medications are likely to be most effective if given to people in the preclinical phase of the illness. Discovering who these at-risk people are is best approached using a multimodal strategy, including epidemiologic risk factors and markers, genetic markers, neuropsychological testing, imaging, and cerebrospinal fluid or blood markers.

Because we are interested in preventing AD in the general population, the methodology for identifying preclinical cases of the disease must be both cost-effective and acceptable. It is unlikely that we can afford to give everyone every test to detect AD early, even if they were to agree to a prolonged and often invasive set of measures. Therefore, we will need to prioritize markers to those with sufficiently high sensitivity and specificity that are both cost effective and acceptable.

Preventing the disease is an alternative option to "curing" the disease. Currently, funding for prevention represents a tiny fraction of the monies that have been invested in trying to find a cure. One estimate from the United Kingdom cites that ratio as 1 penny:1,000 pounds (D. Smith, 2013). Clinical trials of drugs to treat AD have generally failed, except for cholinesterase inhibitors and memantine (for an excellent review, see L. S. Schneider, Mangialasche, et al., 2014).

It is our view that we do not have to wait until an effective drug is developed to begin preventing AD. For example, there is abundant evidence that cardiovascular risk factors are associated with increased risk for AD and that physical and mental exercise as well as nutritional factors can influence its development. Most of these data come from observational studies, which represent the long-term effects of chronic exposures over the life course in a disease that develops over decades. In addition, a small number of clinical trials have been performed, showing that nutritional as well as physical and mental exercise interventions can influence the shrinkage of the brain that is related to AD expression. The

Alzheimer's Disease. DOI: http://dx.doi.org/10.1016/B978-0-12-804538-1.00009-2

remainder of this book will discuss factors that either increase the risk for AD or are inversely associated with this risk. Both observational and experimental studies will be considered. Again, our focus is not to include every study that has been conducted, but to give a critical and updated view of each risk or protective factor within the context of the best studies.

In 2004, we proposed that there are two major types of risk factors for AD (Borenstein Graves, 2004). The first type refers to those that increase the risk for the disease pathology. These include, but are not limited to, known major genetic mutations for the disease (including Chromosome 21 β-APP mutations, Chromosome 14 Presenilin 1 mutations, and Chromosome 1 Presenilin 2 mutations), the polymorphism for apolipoprotein E (APOE-ε4), other genes that contribute risk for AD; Down syndrome and head injury. The second type refers to risk factors for disease expression. These include factors that affect development, growth and shrinkage of the brain across the life course, as well as the development of cognitive strategies for optimum utilization of the brain in individuals who carry pathology for AD. Accumulating evidence shows that some of the factors that improve reserve also may have effects on neuropathology as well.

In Chapter 10, we will consider the genetic factors that have been shown to increase the risk of AD and consider how much of the illness is determined by genes. In Chapter 11, we will discuss known and possible links between perinatal and early-life family conditions, such as the intrauterine environment, birth weight, birth order and sibship size, and late-life cognition. Other conditions relevant to early life, including paternal social class, poverty and deprivation in childhood, have begun to be studied in a few cohorts with very long follow-up times. In discussing other influences on AD from early life, we will consider education, IQ, and linguistic ability as well.

The remaining chapters in Section 3 are devoted to adult life risk factors. We will consider head trauma, smoking and alcohol consumption, the role of vascular disease in AD, diet, physical and cognitive exercise, social engagement, and medications that might be inversely related to AD risk, focusing on nonsteroidal anti-inflammatory drugs, statins, hormone replacement therapy, and anticholinergic medications.

In the context of the threshold theory, we can view clinical expression factors that increase AD risk as *hastening* clinical onset to earlier ages given a fixed genetic risk, and those that decrease AD risk as *delaying* clinical onset to later ages given the same genetic risk. Brookmeyer, Gray, and Kawas (1998) calculated the potential effects on the prevalence of AD of interventions that would delay the age at which individuals clinically manifest symptoms. They report that an intervention (or set of interventions) that reduced the overall risk for AD by 25% would result in a mean delay of 2 years, while an intervention that reduced AD risk by 50% would result in a mean delay of 5 years. The latter intervention would decrease the prevalence of AD in the year 2027 by almost half (52.5%) (Brookmeyer et al., 1998). Clearly then, prevention across the lifespan is an avenue that should be pursued in addition to finding medications that can reduce the pathology of the disease.

HISTORY AND METHODOLOGICAL ASPECTS OF ANALYTIC STUDIES OF AD: CASE–CONTROL STUDIES

Case–control studies, by virtue of their generally lower costs and relatively fast completion, were conducted as the first step in the systematic investigation of the etiology of AD. This study design was most common in the 1970s and 1980s. There are surprisingly few reports in the literature summarizing the results and methodological shortcomings of these studies. The case–control study gave epidemiologists a jumping-off place, beginning with what is fondly and at the same time disparagingly termed "fishing expeditions." Fishing expeditions are done when little is known about a field. Investigators examine a large number of exposures in one case–control study. These may include risk and protective factors that already have some support from earlier studies (e.g., age and family history of memory problems), seem biologically plausible (e.g., head trauma, smoking), or that give rise to other diseases (e.g., pesticides in Parkinson's disease, diabetes for vascular disease). This in turn can produce spurious findings (Type I errors) if the number of comparisons is large and no correction for multiple comparisons is used. There was the danger in the case–control study era that a statistically significant finding may have been due to chance. One of many examples of this is the report from a case–control study that nose-picking was associated with later-onset AD ($OR_{matched}$ = 7.0 [7/1 discordant pairs, $p = 0.08$]), and physical underactivity was associated with earlier-onset AD ($OR_{matched}$ = not calculable due to a zero in the denominator [14/0discordant pairs, $p = 0.0005$]) (Henderson et al., 1992). At a meeting where these findings were presented, one of our colleagues joked to one of us, "To stop Alzheimer's, we just have to stop sitting around and picking our noses." Although this comment was obviously meant to be facetious, we must be cautious about interpreting results based on small numbers.

While the case–control studies likely produced some false-positive results, they may also have produced false-negative ones. In order to focus on the purest form of AD, most of these studies chose to exclude possible AD by NINCDS-ADRDA criteria, eliminating cases where the relatively common vascular lesions could be contributing to disease expression. By focusing on probable AD cases without evidence for stroke or cerebrovascular disease, individuals with vascular risk factors for these outcomes were excluded from the cases, but not from the controls. Consequently, risk factors such as hypertension, diabetes, and hypercholesterolemia were not identified as risk factors for AD in the case–control studies. When prospective cohort studies began, participants unselected for vascular risk factors at baseline were followed for development of incident AD, permitting the important role of vascular risk factors in the clinical expression of AD to be observed. In fact, prospective cohort studies sometimes obtained the opposite findings from case–control studies. For example, case–control studies suggested that cigarette smoking, a risk factor for stroke, might be inversely related to AD. Cohort studies gave us the opposite answer, that cigarette smoking was a risk factor (Chapter 13). Cohort studies have also permitted the examination of risk factors for other dementia subtypes, such as Lewy body dementia and frontal temporal dementia.

Most of the cases in case–control studies were identified from dementia clinics or through hospital records. A selection bias is likely present in cases who were brought to medical attention by their family members. If family members were in denial, the patients may not come to medical attention until a moderate-to-severe dementia is present. Other AD patients may not come to medical attention at all, because they lived alone and did not have close family members to observe their condition and bring them to medical attention. In addition, if a demented individual identified in a clinic had no identifiable proxy informant, they would usually have been excluded from case–control studies.

The use of proxy informants is necessary for dementia patients who cannot provide valid information about their own exposures. However, their use invites information bias. Case proxies may either overreport or underreport past exposures, depending on their own recall, level of background reading, and desire to pin the cause on an identifiable event, such as a head injury. Furthermore, recall bias can be aggravated by control proxies underreporting exposures. Proxies are frequently selected from the next-of-kin who brings the patient in. This will most often be a spouse or an adult child. For some types of remote information, such as information about early life and adolescence, siblings may be better informants. The proxy type was usually not matched in the cases and controls, which could result in odds ratios biased either toward or away from the null value of 1.0.

When proxy informants must be used for cases, they should also be used for controls (Nelson, Longstreth, Koepsell, & van Belle, 1990). In an attempt to evaluate the quality of the information obtained from proxy informants, some case–control studies of AD conducted a validation study of control and control–proxy informant pairs to measure the degree of agreement between the two sources of information. The assumption of such validation studies was that the agreement between case–case proxy informant pairs would be similar to control–control proxy informant pairs. This is not necessarily true. For example, in a case–control study matching on informant type (we only accepted spouse informants), we rated exposure to chemicals in the cases' and controls' occupations two ways by asking the spouse and by assessment by an industrial hygienist who was blinded to case–control status. Figure 9.1 shows the results for one chemical exposure (Graves, A. Borenstein, unpublished). Epidemiologists usually assume that case proxies over-recall exposures due to the natural instinct to identify a cause for the disease. In this study, the sensitivity of reporting positive exposure was higher (83%, compared to an objective and blinded assessment made by an industrial hygienist) among case spouses, than among control spouses (61.5%). The specificity of reporting exposures by spouses was the same for both cases and controls, implying that if the industrial hygienist rated the occupation as not exposed to a certain chemical, both case and control

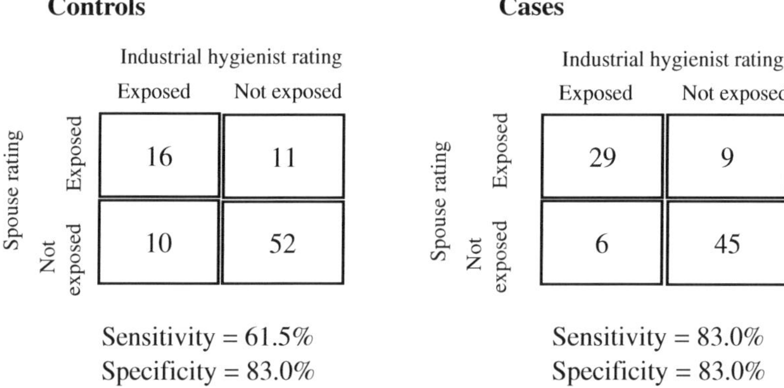

FIGURE 9.1 Sensitivity and specificity of case and control spouse rating of exposure against industrial hygienist ratings of exposure from a matched case–control study of occupational exposures and Alzheimer's disease. *Graves, A. Borenstein, unpublished data.*

spouse proxies were equally likely to rate it as nonexposed. These findings suggest that control informants may be more likely to under-recall exposures than case informants to over-recall exposures.

Most cases used in the case–control studies were prevalent cases. This implies that some of the identified risk factors may be associated with survival with AD, but not with incident AD. This problem is compounded by how long a case included in a case–control study is allowed to have had the disease. There usually were no limits placed on this in the inclusion criteria of most studies. Therefore, longer-duration cases were more likely to be included (this is called "length bias"). For example, if the case-fatality due to AD is modified by smoking status, smokers will be less likely to be identified as prevalent cases in case–control studies. This could result in an inverted odds ratio, suggesting that smoking is protective for AD (Graves and Mortimer, 1994).

The study base principle that cases and controls should be members of the same defined population (Wacholder, McLaughlin, Silverman, & Mandel, 1992) was often not met in case–control studies. Sometimes cases came from a specific hospital or clinic and controls were also selected from the same hospital. Other times, controls might have been identified from people living in the same neighborhoods as the cases. This is not because the investigators were not aware of the study base principle, but rather because before population-based studies of AD were established, ascertainment of all cases in a primary base was not possible. In these instances, the desire for cases and controls to resemble each other by characteristics other than the disease took precedence over representation of the study base. In some studies, for example, controls were selected from patients in the same hospitals in which the case was diagnosed. Although this may seem appropriate, it would have the effect of increasing the frequency of cardiovascular and other diseases in the control sample, making it less likely that these diseases would be found to be risk factors and possibly suggesting that such diseases in the controls were protective for AD.

After the first set of case–control studies was published, a reanalysis of raw data (a pooled reanalysis) was conducted (van Duijn, Stijnen, Hofman, 1991). This type of reanalysis is useful in increasing the power to observe significant associations that are not evident in individual studies, particularly for uncommon exposures. However, it also can amplify the effects of uncontrolled bias or confounding. This is not a problem in the traditional use of meta-analysis of randomized clinical trials (RCTs). If subtle Relative Risks (say for the sake of argument, a RR = 1.2) are not statistically significant because the individual trials are not sufficiently large, then pooling of trials can boost statistical power. Since RCTs are randomized to treatment status, confounding biases are minimized or eliminated, and if the RR = 1.2 becomes statistically significant, the only question remaining is whether or not the treatment effect is clinically significant (Clayton, 1991). The pooled reanalyses of case–control studies conducted in 1990 helped to advance knowledge about risk factors for AD by pointing to variables that were important to investigate in cohort studies, including family history of dementia, smoking, depression, early and advanced maternal age, alcohol consumption, and occupational exposures to chemicals such as lead and solvents.

PROSPECTIVE COHORT STUDIES

Teachers of epidemiology commonly place study designs in a hierarchical structure (Figure 9.2), with systematic reviews and meta-analyses at the top, and randomized controlled trials (experimental, or clinical epidemiology) second. This is followed by cohort studies and case–control studies, with cross-sectional studies near the bottom of the analytic part of the pyramid. The rationale behind this hierarchy is driven by the desire to establish the temporal sequence between the exposure and the outcome, and also because RCTs eliminate confounding, at least in theory. Given perfect application of methodology in all of these study designs, and assuming all exposures and outcomes operate similarly, this hierarchy is correct. However, the nature of the exposures and disease, as well as the problems that can arise in randomized controlled trials, must be taken into account in an imperfect and often idiosyncratic world. There are as many things can go wrong in a RCT in its design and conduct, as can go wrong in an observational study. For example, a trial may have substantial selection bias, can be implemented in the wrong population, can use the wrong intervention, can have too short a follow-up period, can have compliance rates that are too low, dropout rates that are too high, and can examine the wrong outcomes. Likewise, prospective cohort studies are not always better than case–control studies. Each student of epidemiology should consider carefully their exposure(s) and outcome(s) and critically assess under what circumstances a cohort study is, and is not, superior in design over another design.

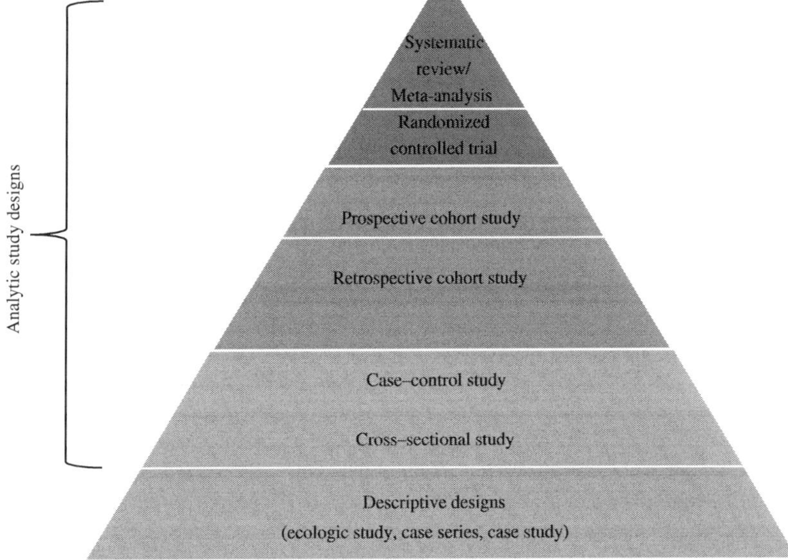

FIGURE 9.2 Hierarchy of analytic study designs in epidemiology.

One potential shortcoming of cohort studies of AD is the reliance on individuals who will become demented in the ensuing few years to provide accurate and complete information on their exposures that occurred in the past. Because many of these individuals will have memory impairments, despite not meeting prevalent dementia criteria, there is a strong likelihood that they will forget to report exposures in comparison to participants who do not become demented in the study. One could argue that a case–control study with data provided by cognitively intact proxy informants who are well-versed in the exposure histories of the index cases and controls could provide more valid exposure data than a cohort study where participants who are in the early stages of a dementing illness are asked to recall exposures. The issue is discussed in more detail in Chapters 10 and 12.

Another potential problem in prospective cohort studies is the definition of incident cases. Because AD diagnosis requires a decline from a previously higher level of functioning, absence of a knowledgeable informant may delay diagnosis until a further period of follow-up to determine whether the individual's cognitive impairment is progressing. If a study terminates before such individuals are reassessed, incident cases may be missed. Incident cases that are progressing rapidly will be more likely to be detected as an incident case (providing the time between study visits is sufficiently short to catch them before death) than slowly progressing cases, who may hover around the clinical border between MCI and dementia. Studies that, due to financial or other constraints, are able to examine the cohort only after 4–5 years have passed since the previous visit will have problems with cases being missed that became demented and died during the interval.

The validity of cohort studies can also be compromised by attrition. Given the advanced age and dependence of older populations studied for onset of AD, dropout due to disease, institutionalization, or death can produce a survivor cohort in which the risk factor associations with dementia are different from those in the baseline cohort. Attrition due to moving outside the study area to be closer to children and other relatives can also influence the characteristics of the remaining cohort. Investigators of cohort studies of dementia, of course, are well aware of these sources of attrition bias and make every effort to ascertain the status of participants who leave the study or try to determine whether the attrition affects risk factors for dementia by comparing individuals who continue participation in a study with those who leave. Most Cox proportional hazards models assume that participants who drop out during the follow-up of the cohort have the same baseline risk for the outcome as those who remain in the cohort. This is also untrue in most cohort studies of aging populations. Thus, more recent studies that take into account competing mortality in their analyses may be more valid than those that do not.

The era of large prospective cohort studies of dementia and AD funded by the US National Institutes of Health (NIH) began in the 1980s and early 1990s (Borenstein et al., 2014; Bennett, Schneider, Arvanitakis, & Wilson, 2012; Bennett, Schneider, Buchman, et al., 2012; Evans et al., 2003, 1989; Ganguli, Dodge, Chen, Belle, & DeKosky, 2000; Gatz et al., 1997; Graves, Larson, et al., 1996; Gurland et al., 1999; Haan et al., 2003; Hendrie et al., 2001; Katz et al., 2012; Kukull et al., 2002; Snowdon et al., 1996; Tang et al., 2001; Tschanz et al., 2005). Large cohort studies in the United States that followed thousands of participants for up to 10 years or longer, persisted until around the beginning of the 2010s. Although most of these studies have now terminated, a few remain active. Paralleling the US studies, large prospective studies of older populations have been conducted in a number of European countries, including the Personnes Agées QUID (PAQUID) (Dartigues, 1991) initiated in 1991 and the Three-City Study initiated in 1999 (The 3C Study Group, 2003) (both in France), the Rotterdam Study conducted in the Netherlands that started in 1990 (Hofman et al., 2013), and the Cognitive Function and Ageing Study I and II from the United Kingdom (Matthews et al., 2013) that began in the late 1980s. Another important cohort study was conducted in Kungsholmen, Sweden (Fratiglioni, Grut, Forsell, 1991). In addition to these studies designed specifically to study risk factors for AD and dementia, many studies were initiated during the middle to late half of the last century to study risk factors for incident cardiovascular and cerebrovascular diseases. Several of these studies, including the Framingham Heart Study (Bachman et al., 1992), the Honolulu Heart Program (White et al., 1996), and the Cardiovascular Health Study (Lopez et al., 2003) added cognitive evaluations during the 1980s and 1990s to capture potential cases of AD. Because they collected detailed information on vascular disease and risk factors, these studies have provided very important information concerning the vascular etiology of AD and other dementias.

Because valuable information has come from both cohort and case–control methodologies, our discussion of risk factors across the life course will include both of these types of studies.

A THIRD SET OF RISK FACTORS FOR AD

In 2004, we proposed that there are two different types of risk factors for dementia: one set for the pathology of AD, and another for the clinical expression of the disease (Borenstein Graves, 2004). Since then, we have added a third set, risk factors that are early markers for future disease onset. Examples of elements that form these three sets of risk factors are shown in Table 9.1. In Chapter 5, we discussed the concept of brain reserve and described a model in which individuals lose brain function at varying rates. Those who have autosomal dominant genetic mutations causing dysfunction in proteins related to ß-amyloid have the steepest loss throughout their lifetimes and the earliest onset of cognitive dysfunction. Those who have genetic polymorphisms for "risk genes" such as APOE-ε4, BIN1, and ABCA7 (Bertram, McQueen, Mullin, Blacker, & Tanzi, 2007) have trajectory slopes between those with familial AD and those with no apparent genetic risk, with clinical effects frequently dependent on gene dose (presence of 0, 1, or 2 alleles). Finally, those with no apparent genetic risk have the slowest underlying progression of pathology and latest disease onset. Other pathologic risk factors include Down syndrome and head injury, both of which are known to increase the amount of amyloid deposition in the brain (covered in Chapters 10 and 12, respectively). Other pathologies, such as vascular and Lewy body pathology, accelerate progression to reduce the time to achieve the clinical threshold of disease in those with Alzheimer pathology.

In addition to pathology, the maintenance of brain reserve can delay the onset of clinical disease expression, and factors that reduce brain reserve can hasten onset. Increasing or maintaining brain reserve, given a fixed genetic risk, provides an alternative way to reduce risk for AD. We have shown (Borenstein, Mortimer & Larson 2014; Mortimer & Borenstein, 2014) in two cohort studies (The Nun Study and The *Kame* Project) that the population attributable fraction for incident dementia is greater for brain reserve than it is for either Alzheimer or vascular pathology. In these two studies, between 40% and 47% of incident dementia could be explained by reserve, adjusting for factors related to AD and vascular pathology. Therefore, maintenance and growth of brain reserve is a promising avenue to pursue for reducing the incidence of this disease in the population. Decreased clinical expression of AD pathology can also be achieved through reduction of vascular comorbidities by modification of vascular risk factors. As we have discussed, many cases of dementia, particularly among people 85 years and over, have multiple brain pathologies. Which pathology is in the "driver's seat" is still being debated, but purely non-AD dementia without any AD pathologic contribution (e.g., "pure" vascular dementia, Lewy body dementia, Fronto-Temporal Dementia) is rare, in comparison with AD.

TABLE 9.1 Three Sets of Risk Factors for Dementia and AD

Pathogenic (Pathologic)	Clinical Expression	Early Markers (Prodromal)
Single gene mutations (APP, PS1, PS2)	Education	Atrophy of hippocampus and whole brain volume
Apolipoprotein E-ε4	IQ (frontal lobe function)	Imaging of amyloid plaques/tau
Family history (other genes with lower Odds Ratios)	Early brain development and early life factors	$A\beta_{42}$, $A\beta_{40}$ (plasma)
Down syndrome	Vascular diseases/diabetes	CSF $A\beta_{42}$/P-tau ratio and Total tau
Insulin-dependent pathways?	Depression	Depression
Head injury	Smoking	Subjective memory complaints
	Excessive alcohol consumption	Loss of olfaction
	Hormone replacement therapy	
	Physical activity	
	Cognitive activity	
	Social activity	
	Diet	
	Obesity	

The remainder of Section 3 focuses on analytic epidemiologic research that has occurred over the last 50 years. Genetic risks are discussed in Chapter 10. Genes can affect both pathologic and clinical expression risk factors. For example, head circumference and height (at birth) as well as vascular conditions, such as diabetes and hypertension, have associations with both genes and environmental influences (Carmelli, Cardon, & Fabsitz, 1994; Lunde, Melve, Gjessing, Skjaerven, & Irgens, 2007). In addition, although some exposures cannot be averted completely (such as head trauma, for which we can reduce the risk but not to zero), others are lifestyle choices, such as smoking, drinking alcohol, diet, and physical, cognitive, and social activities. By choosing healthy lifestyles, we also can reduce our probability of having hypertension and diabetes. Even though we can not yet change our genes, we do have control over our lifestyle choices, which can affect the time to clinical expression of underlying pathology leading to dementia.

Chapter 10

Family History, Genetics, and Down Syndrome

Outside of age, the strongest risk factor for Alzheimer's disease (AD) is family history of a similar illness in blood relatives. In addition to specific mutations in three genes, variants of more than 10 genes are now known to be related to the risk of this illness (www.alzgene.org). In addition, virtually all individuals with Down syndrome (DS) develop the neuropathology of AD if they live long enough, consistent with the location of the critical gene for the amyloid precursor protein (APP) on chromosome 21. In this chapter, we review the early studies suggesting the genetic association, the evolving view of the role of genetics in the causation of AD, and the connection between DS and AD and its possible significance for causation in sporadic AD. In addition, we discuss the three mutations that cause familial AD, the discovery of the major susceptibility apolipoprotein E (APOE) allele, and other genes discovered in genome-wide association studies (GWAS) that likely play a role in disease causation.

EARLY FAMILY STUDIES

Family history of AD is not only one of the most powerful risk factors for this syndrome, but also is the first risk factor outside of increased age to be described for this illness. Although individual pedigrees showing familial aggregation of AD in presenile cases (onset before age 65) were published as early as 1932 (Schottky, 1932), the first systematic study of familial aggregation in a series of presenile cases was published by Torsten Sjogren and his collaborators in 1952 (Sjogren, Sjogren, & Lindgren, 1952). This study, which was based on 18 autopsied cases of AD with an average age at onset of 53, showed increased risk of a similar disease in parents and to a lesser extent in siblings. Comparisons were made with the apparent incidence of this rare condition in the general population of Sweden.

The most important family study was performed by Leonard Heston at the University of Minnesota in the 1970s (Heston, Mastri, Anderson, & White, 1981). Heston began with a series of 2,204 brain autopsies performed at

Alzheimer's Disease. DOI: http://dx.doi.org/10.1016/B978-0-12-804538-1.00010 9

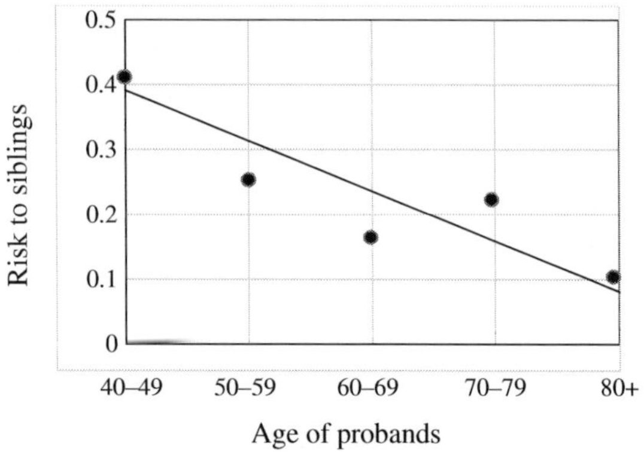

FIGURE 10.1 Empirical risk to siblings by age of probands. *Adapted from Heston et al. (1981).*

Minnesota State Hospitals between 1952 and 1972, of whom 304 had clinical evidence of a primary degenerative dementia. Reappraisal of the neuropathologic diagnosis yielded 231 cases of AD. All 30 cases with symptoms beginning before age 65 and 96 of the remaining 191 cases of dementia beginning after age 65 were selected for family study. For each of these cases, information about blood relatives (both first and second degree) was obtained through interviews with at least one, but more often multiple family members and through medical records and death certificates. Adjusted for age, 19% of parents and 12% of siblings were considered to be at risk for the condition. As shown in Figure 10.1, there was a strong relationship between the risk to siblings and the age at which the cases originally became symptomatic. The earlier the onset of the disease, the higher the risk to siblings. Affected siblings on average were almost 5 years older than the cases at the time of initial symptoms. While the method used to examine secondary cases among family members in Heston's study disclosed unexpected high risks for siblings of cases with onset before 70, the absence of proper controls for comparison limited the results to cases where onset was before this age. Table 10.1 from a later paper by Heston (1985) shows the increased risk for AD when onset in the proband was younger than 70 years old and particularly when more than one family member (a sibling plus a parent was affected: rightmost column).

CASE–CONTROL STUDIES AND FAMILY HISTORY OF DEMENTIA

Case–control studies of AD conducted primarily in the 1980s permitted comparison of cases of this illness with nondemented controls with regard to family history of dementia. The results from a pooled reanalysis of case–control studies in 1991 strongly supported the earlier findings of family studies in showing increased risk to blood relatives of patients with onset prior to age 70, and in

TABLE 10.1 Empirical Age-Specific Risks to Siblings by Characteristics of Their Family

Age Interval	Proband's Onset >70	Proband's Onset <70	Proband's Onset, <70 with Parent Demented
55–64	2.1 ± 1.4	5.6 ± 2.5	8.3 ± 4.6
65–74	4.2 ± 2.1	9.6 ± 3.3	20.6 ± 6.6
75+	8.5 ± 4.0	17.1 ± 3.9	46.4 ± 7.0

Source: Adapted from Heston (1985).
Values for proband's onsets are percentages± standard error.

TABLE 10.2 Family History of Dementia and Odds Ratios for Alzheimer's Disease, Findings from Pooled Reanalysis of Case–Control Studies

	Exposure Frequencies			
Study	Cases	Controls	OR[a]	95% CI
Australia	58/170	21/170	3.8	2.1–6.9
Italy	29/116	Dec-97	2.6	1.0–7.5
Netherlands	96/198	37/198	4.8	2.8–8.1
Bedford, MA, USA	21/103	9/162	4.4	1.8–10.7
Denver, CO, USA	21/54	18/50	1	0.5–2.2
Durham, NC, USA	25/44	14/87	7.2	2.7–19.1
Seattle, WA, USA	55/129	29/130	2.5	1.4–4.4
Overall analysis	305/814	140/894	3.5	2.6–4.6
Excluding USA, Denver	284/760	122/844	3.6	2.7–4.9

Source: Adapted from van Duijn (1991).
[a]*Adjusted for age, gender, number of siblings, and education.*

addition extended this risk to include those over this age (van Duijn, Clayton et al., 1991). Table 10.2 from the paper reporting the pooled reanalysis results was based on 1,119 cases and 2,034 controls and showed a pooled odds ratio of 3.5 (95% CI = 2.6–4.6) for history of dementia in first-degree blood relatives. Figure 10.2A and B show the percentages of Alzheimer cases and controls with a positive family history in the parents and in siblings. For family history of dementia in the parents (Figure 10.2A), there was little difference between cases and controls when the onset age was 70 or above. By contrast, a large

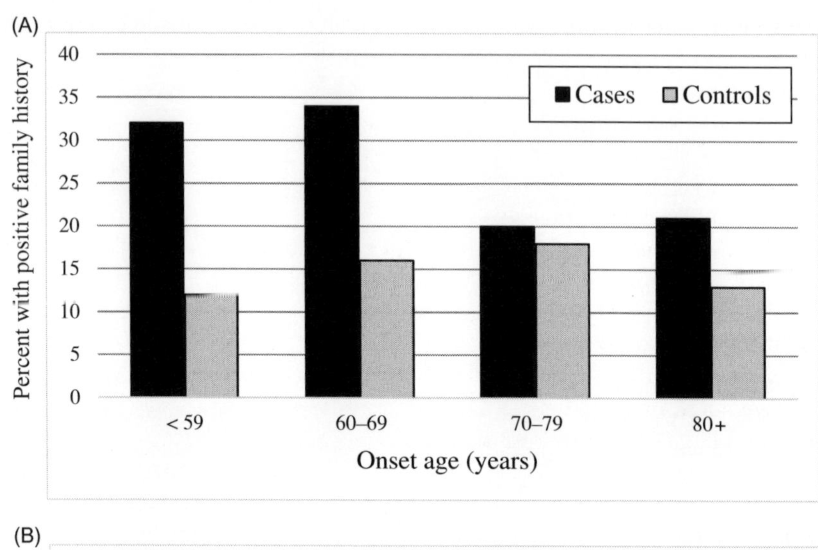

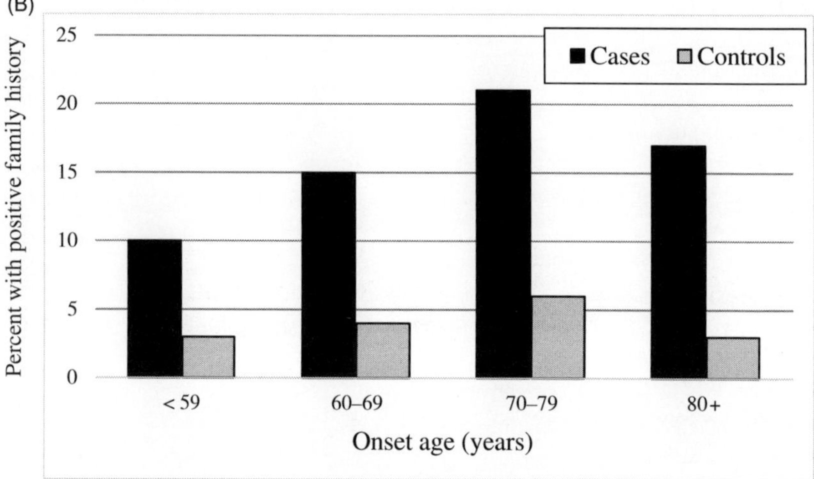

FIGURE 10.2 (A) Percent of AD cases and controls with a positive family history of dementia in the parents. (B) Percent of AD cases and controls with a positive family history of dementia in the siblings. *Adapted from van Duijn, Stijnen, and Hofman (1991).*

difference was apparent at all ages when dementia in siblings was considered (Figure 10.2B). Heston and others have reported that age at onset tends to be similar across affected first-degree blood relatives within a family. Therefore, parents of late-onset cases may not have survived to express dementia, whereas those of early-onset cases, because their age at onset was lower, had a greater opportunity to survive to develop this condition. Because of this bias and given the secular increase in life expectancy, it is likely that dementia in siblings is a better indicator of the genetic risk than dementia in parents.

COHORT STUDIES AND FAMILY HISTORY OF DEMENTIA

In comparison with case–control studies, relatively few cohort studies have reported on the association between family history of dementia and risk of incident AD. The main reason for this is the discovery of a major susceptibility allele for AD, the apolipoprotein E gene (APOE)-ε4 allele (Corder et al., 1993), which largely replaced family history in reports of potential genetic associations (even though it does not account for all of the genetic variation).

Findings from cohort studies on the association of family history of dementia have raised important epidemiologic issues regarding the way data are collected on risk factors for dementia. The Canadian Study of Health and Aging (CSHA) found family history to be a strong risk factor for AD in the prevalence phase of this study (1994), but not in the incidence phase (Lindsay et al., 2002). The relevant data are shown in Table 10.3. In the prevalence phase of this study, 258 cases of probable AD were compared with 535 cognitively normal controls. Analysis of data from this sample led to an odds ratio of 2.62 for family history of dementia. However, 5 years later when 194 incident cases of AD were compared with 3,894 participants who remained cognitively normal, the odds ratio for family history of dementia was only 1.02. A similar phenomenon occurred with head trauma. By contrast, both arthritis and taking

TABLE 10.3 Canadian Study of Health and Aging

Risk Factor		Odds Ratio (95% CI)	95% CI
Family history of dementia	Prevalence phase	2.62	1.53–4.51
	Incidence phase	1.02	0.59–1.77
Head injury	Prevalence phase	1.66	0.97–2.84
	Incidence phase	0.87	0.56–1.36
History of arthritis	Prevalence phase	0.54	0.36–0.81
	Incidence phase	0.61	0.43–0.87
Use of any nonsteroidal anti-inflammatory drugs	Prevalence phase	0.55	0.37–0.82
	Incidence phase	0.65	0.44–0.95

Source: Adapted from The Canadian Study of Health and Aging: risk factors for Alzheimer's disease in Canada (1994).
Risk factor associations found in the prevalence and incidence phases of the study.

any nonsteroidal anti-inflammatory drug at baseline were similarly protective in both phases of the study. Why might this occur? The data on exposures in the prevalence risk factor analysis came from informants or proxies for both cases and controls. At that time, the nondemented controls themselves also reported their own exposures. It is this self-reported set of exposures that formed the basis for the incident risk factor study. A plausible explanation for the loss of association with family history of dementia is that the participants who reported their own risk factors at baseline and went on to develop AD forgot to report many secondary cases of dementia in their families. Using a similar argument, the strong decline in risk due to head trauma could have been due to people developing dementia neglecting to report some of their own head traumas. We do know that AD is preceded by a period of time during which there is substantial memory loss (MCI), so there is an explanation for selective forgetting of past exposures by those who would later go on to AD. It is of interest that exposures related to *current* status (vs history), such as arthritis and the use of nonsteroidal anti-inflammatory drugs (NSAIDs), did not show this difference.

Because of the dependence on the memory of someone who is soon to develop AD, it is possible that cohort studies may work best for objective measures, such as blood levels or genes, and for current conditions that participants are experiencing, and may not be as valid for historical exposure information. However, if the exposure data are collected from participants many years and preferably decades prior to onset of cognitive impairment, prospective cohort studies are preferred to case–control studies because they provide a real measure of the speed of developing new disease, and we can make valid conclusions about the temporal sequence between the exposure(s) of interest and the outcome(s).

HOW GENETIC IS ALZHEIMER'S DISEASE?

While family and case–control studies suggest that a family history of dementia significantly increases the risk for Alzheimer's, this question is best addressed by twin studies in which concordance rates in monozygotic and dizygotic twins can be compared. Because siblings share both genes (on average one-half) and early-life environment, it is difficult to tease apart the effects of shared genes from shared environment. However, this is not a problem in studies that compare monozygotic or identical twins to dizygotic or fraternal twins, where the same early-life environment is shared in both types of twins, but in the case of identical twins, all rather than half of the genes are shared. If a disease is caused by genes inherited from one's parents, identical twins will both have the same risk, while fraternal twins will have a lower risk. Therefore, comparison of the concordance rates of disease in identical and fraternal twins provides a measure called heritability, reflecting how heritable or genetic a disease is. The detailed techniques and computations involved in determining heritability of AD are beyond the scope of this book.

In the largest population-based twin study of dementia, in which over 2,700 intact twin pairs over age 65 (1,083 MZ or identical twin pairs and 1,688 same-sex DZ or fraternal pairs) were clinically assessed for dementia, heritability for AD was estimated to be 79%, with a 95% confidence interval ranging from 67% to 88% (Gatz et al., 1997). While smaller studies also have suggested a major role for genetic inheritance in the causation of AD, the narrow confidence interval suggests that the vast majority of cases of this illness can be explained by genes inherited from parents.

FAMILIAL AD AND THE DISCOVERY OF GENETIC MUTATIONS

It has been known since the early 1950s that a small percentage of cases of AD (around 2–5%) show autosomal-dominant transmission in single families. Identifications of three genes in which mutations reliably produce AD in carriers were important milestones in our understanding of the pathogenesis of this illness. The first mutation to be found was in the gene for APP located on chromosome 21. This finding by a team led by Dr. John Hardy, was the result of 7 years of work showing that the amyloid accumulating in neuritic plaques was derived from a large precursor protein called APP, the gene for which was located on chromosome 21 (Goate et al., 1991). The first gene mutation in APP was identified in two unrelated families. Subsequently, 30 different mutations in this gene causing Alzheimer's were identified (www.alzgene.org). Onset age in the patients carrying these mutations has generally been in the 40s and 50s (Hardy, 2006).

With the realization that the APP gene accounted for only a minority of cases of autosomal-dominant Alzheimer's disease, the race was on to find other gene(s) that might lead to this form of the disease. The next discovery came within 4 years when a mutation in a gene located on chromosome 14 was shown to cause autosomal-dominant transmission of the disease in families (Sherrington et al., 1995). The protein encoded by this gene was called presenilin 1 (PSEN1). Mutations in this gene account for about half of all early-onset AD in families (Sherrington et al., 1996), making it the most important mutation for early-onset disease. People with mutations in PSEN1 develop AD at early ages, ranging from 29 to 62, with an average age of about 44 years. Families with a particular PSEN1 mutation tend to develop Alzheimer's at around the same age (Fox et al., 1997). To date, almost 200 different mutations in this gene have been identified that lead to early-onset AD. PSEN1 is known to be involved in processing of APP, most likely as a component of gamma secretase, an enzyme critical to cutting the larger protein to produce the β-amyloid fragment that accumulates in Alzheimer plaques.

The final gene leading to early-onset AD was named presenilin 2 (PSEN2). It is a very rare cause of familial AD found predominantly in a relatively small group of German families from Russia, the so-called Volga Germans. Age at onset in these families varies widely from 40 to 84, but the majority of cases have onset in their 50s (Bird et al., 1989). To date, seven mutations have been identified in this gene that cause AD. Like PSEN1, the protein encoded by this gene is known to be involved in splicing APP to produce Aβ, the main component of Alzheimer plaques.

Together, mutations in the three genes identified for dominantly transmitted AD account for <5% of the total cases of this disease. Their utility resides predominantly in genetic screening for the early-onset form of this illness and for the insight they give us into the pathogenesis of AD. It is unclear whether additional mutations will be found or whether these three constitute the basis for most cases of early-onset disease. It has now been over 16 years since the discovery of the presenilin mutations, and no additional genes have been identified by genetic linkage analysis in families with autosomally dominant transmitted disease.

The dominant role played by genes evident from the high heritability coefficient suggests that additional genes are likely responsible for a large percentage of AD cases and that genetic variants or common polymorphisms are likely involved rather than mutations. The discovery of the gene for APOE on chromosome 19 as the major susceptibility gene for AD in 1993 by Strittmatter et al. (1993) and Corder et al. (1993) provided an explanation for the high heritability of this disease. There are three principal alleles for APOE, the most common or ε3 allele, occurring with a frequency of 75–85%, the second most common or ε4 allele occurring with a frequency of 10–16%, and the least common or ε2 allele occurring with a frequency of 5–7% in most European Caucasian populations. Figure 10.3 shows the effect of higher doses of the ε4 allele, which produces earlier onset in individuals with two ε4s (ε4 homozygotes, 4/4) than in people with one ε4 (ε4 heterozygotes, 3/4) or no ε4s. Although the effect of ε4 is exaggerated in this paper because families with late-onset disease with multiple cases were studied, studies of representative populations like the Cache County Study shown in Figure 10.4 (Breitner et al., 1999), demonstrate similar differences in age at onset by allelic distribution in APOE genes. In the latter study, women carrying one or two ε4 alleles had higher risks than men, but the peak age of prevalent AD for each APOE genotype did not differ by sex.

The relative frequency of the principal alleles for APOE varies greatly between populations, with the ε4 allele occurring at a lower frequency in Chinese (Borenstein et al., 2010) and Asian populations (Borenstein et al., 2014) and at a higher frequency in African, African-American (Borenstein et al., 2006), and certain Caucasian subgroups, mostly from Northern Europe. The population rates of AD appear to reflect these variations in frequency, with lower incidence of AD in Asian populations and higher incidence in African-Americans, for example.

While there is some variability from study to study, the results of a meta-analysis of 42 case–control studies of AD (Rubinsztein & Easton, 1999) demonstrated an increased risk for cases over 65 to carry one of more ε4 alleles

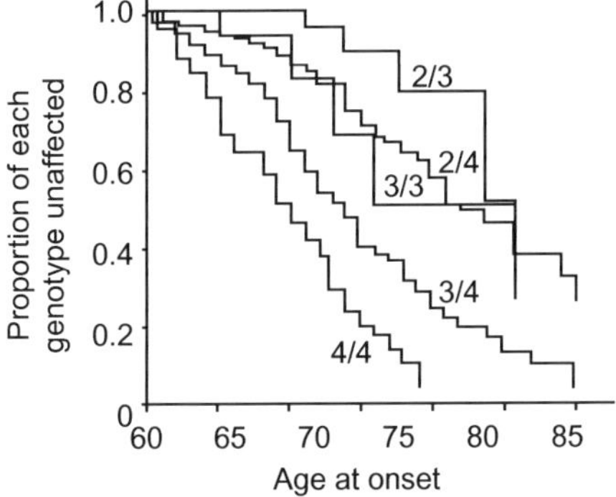

FIGURE 10.3. The dosage effect of the ε4 allele of the apolipoprotein E gene on age at onset of Alzheimer's disease. *Reprinted from Corder et al. (1993).*

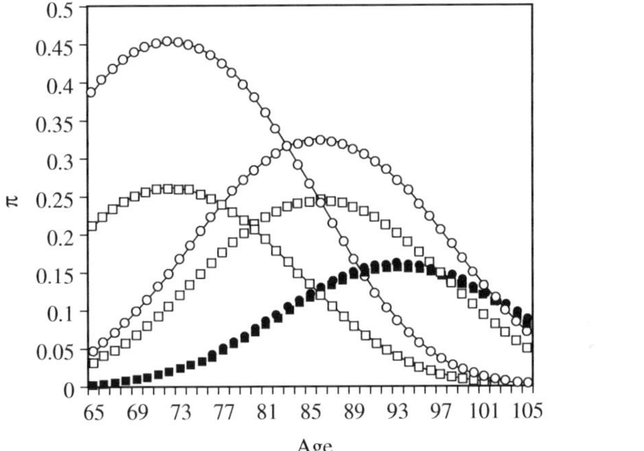

FIGURE 10.4. Probability of prevalent AD by age and apolipoprotein E ε4 dose in the Cache County Study. Squares: men; Circles: women. Black symbols (men and women)—no e4 alleles (peaks at 95 years old), Gray symbols—one e4 allele (peaks at 86 years old), Open symbols—two e4 alleles (peaks at 73 years old). *Reprinted from Breitner et al. (1999).*

(pooled OR = 3.18; 95% CI = 2.93–3.45) and a reduction in risk for those carrying ε2 alleles (pooled OR = 0.67; 95% CI = 0.58–0.79) in comparison to those with two ε3 alleles. From this meta-analysis, the population attributable fraction (PAF) or proportion of AD cases attributable to the APOE genotype was estimated to be 60% (95% CI = 48–68%). Another meta-analysis (Farrer et al., 1997) reported a pooled OR of about 3.0 for ε4 heterozygotes and 13.0 for ε4 homozygotes. Comparison of African-Americans, Hispanics, Japanese, and Caucasians revealed major differences in the association of the ε4 allele with AD. African-Americans and Hispanics showed much smaller odds ratios than Caucasians, while Japanese had higher odds ratios. The PAFs were approximately 12% among African-Americans, 25% among Hispanics, and 63% among Japanese. Because the frequency of ε4 genotypes varies considerably in different populations and the relative risks vary as well, it is difficult to put a confident estimate on the PAF associated with the APOE genotype. From the meta-analyses, it appears that among Caucasians the PAF is likely to be around 50%. It is important to note that the meta-analyses likely undersample patients with AD above age 80, in whom the risk attributable to this gene might be considerably lower.

The Nun Study included participants from 75 to 102 years of age at entry and followed those participants to death. Mean age of death was around 90 years old in this sample. In this study, the etiologic fraction, which is interpreted similarly to the PAF, was 37.8% for one or more ε4 alleles, lower than that observed in the meta-analyses that included younger cases. However, the PAF for fulfilling neuropathologic criteria for AD at death in the Nun Study was 60.5%, suggesting that ε4 alleles account for more than 60% of neuropathologic AD.

OTHER SUSCEPTIBLITY GENETIC VARIANTS

In 2007, using a candidate gene approach, the neuronal sortilin-related receptor, SORL1, was found to be genetically associated with AD (Rogaeva et al., 2007). This receptor is involved in APP trafficking and when it is underexpressed, production of β-amyloid is increased.

The era of GWAS has led to the identification of many genetic variants in addition to APOE and SORL1 associated with AD. In addition, several candidate genes have shown significant associations in large meta-analyses. Although none of these variants explains as high a percentage of cases as APOE, their combination may well explain considerable genetic variance. Genes associated with AD include those coding proteins in pathways involved in inflammation, movement of proteins within cells, lipid transport, and APP processing. Lists of genes associated with AD are updated regularly in AlzGene (www.alzgene.org). Understanding the interaction of these genes with each other and APOE will be very important in interpreting their significance in the pathogenesis of AD. Because clinically expressed AD includes two set of risk factors, those for pathology and those for clinical expression, a clearer picture of genetic involvement in pathogenesis is likely to come from genetic studies of neuropathology from autopsied brains unselected for dementia.

As might be expected, genes for clinical AD can have different effects in different racial or ethnic groups. A GWAS to examine the genetics of late-onset AD among 1,968 African-American AD cases and 3,928 controls found that, in addition to APOE, a single-nucleotide polymorphism (SNP) called *ABCA7* (rs115550680) also located on chromosome 19 had an effect size similar to that of APOE in this group (Reitz et al., 2013). By contrast, among non-Hispanic whites, the *ABCA7* SNPs had much lower effect sizes (Naj et al., 2011). *ABCA7* plays a major role in lipid metabolism and may be related to the higher frequency of cardiovascular and cerebrovascular frequencies in African-Americans as compared to Caucasians. In this respect, it may be affecting clinical expression rather than affecting amyloid processing.

It is clear that expression of genes plays a major role in their influence over the lifespan. Understanding the role of methylation and environmental triggers for turning genes off and on will likely be important for AD (Bennett et al., 2015). Epigenetic changes, whether protective, benign, or harmful, may help explain, for example, why one twin or sibling develops the disease and another does not, or why onset can be separated by a number of years.

In summary, there is abundant evidence that genes play a major role in AD and that most of the risk of this condition can be attributed to common genetic polymorphisms. To date, only one major gene responsible for about half of the disease (APOE) has been identified. The remainder of the heritability is likely explained by small effects from many other genes with a few exceptions in specific racial and ethnic groups.

DOWN SYNDROME

For many decades, it has been recognized that individuals with DS are likely to develop dementia during middle age. In fact, as early as 1974, it was acknowledged that "In Down's syndrome, the reward for survival beyond age 40 is presenile dementia" (Ellis, McCulloch, & Corley, 1974). DS results from having three copies of a critical segment of chromosome 21, the same chromosome containing the gene for APP. Triplication of the genetic locus for APP has been shown to result in higher production of Aβ across the lifespan in Down patients (Englund et al., 2007) and it has been suggested that the increased production of this protein accelerates the neuropathology of AD. In 1998, Prasher showed that AD was absent in DS cases when the triplication of the chromosome did not involve the region coding for APP (Prasher et al., 1998).

Figure 10.5 shows increasing cumulative prevalence rates of dementia in four different studies of individuals with DS (Schupf & Sergievsky, 2002). The cumulative prevalence increases exponentially as seen in people without DS, but the curves appear to be shifted around 25 or 30 years earlier compared to individuals without DS, and the percent affected by age 60 is about twice as large as the percent affected at age 85 in individuals without DS. This observation is of considerable interest, since the triplication of chromosome 21 will increase the production of Aβ on average by 50%. If the onset of the disease is related to the rate at which Aβ is produced over the lifespan, an increased rate of 50% would correspond to 25–30 years.

A second connection between AD and DS is that they occur more frequently in the same families, suggesting a genetic association. The first epidemiologic evidence of such an association was published in 1981 from Heston's family study described earlier. Heston looked at the excess of DS cases in first-degree relatives of Alzheimer patients and noted that especially among cases of AD with

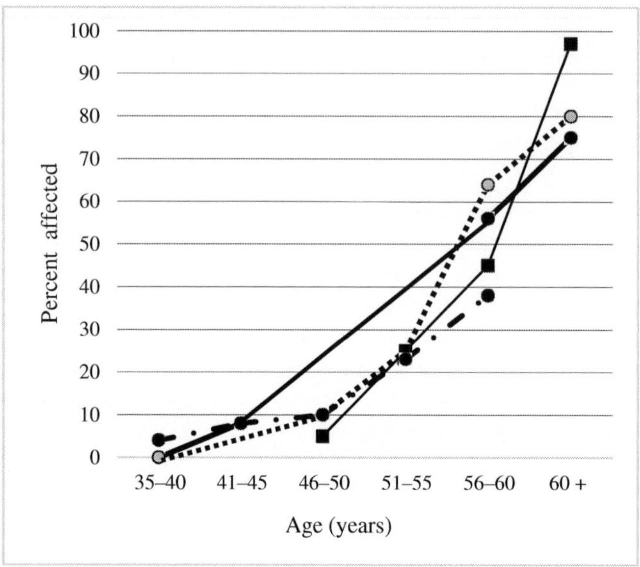

FIGURE 10.5. Cumulative prevalence of dementia in Down syndrome in four studies. *Adapted from Schupf and Sergievsky (2002).*

onset in their 50s, there was a marked increase in risk. This increase declined with age of the Alzheimer patient, with no additional risk of secondary DS cases for individuals with onset of AD after age 70. This association was reexamined in the pooled reanalysis of case–control studies (van Duijn, Clayton, et al., 1991). For early-onset disease (before age 65), the association was statistically significant (OR = 3.0, 95% CI = 1.1–7.5). For late-onset disease the odds ratio (2.6) was similar, though not statistically significant. It is of interest that the association of AD with family history of DS was much stronger in those with a family history of dementia (OR = 4.0, 95% CI = 1.3–12.5) than in those without such a history (OR = 1.9; 95% CI = 0.6–6.0), suggesting that there might be a genetically inherited susceptibility to DS that is shared with AD.

Because DS is a rare outcome, the statistical power to examine associations with AD is limited when one begins with AD and examines family history of this event. To get adequate power to examine this association, several hundred Alzheimer cases and controls must be studied as in the pooled analysis. An alternative and more efficient approach is to begin with DS patients and examine their family history for the more common event, AD. This approach was taken by Schupf, Kapell, Lee, Ottman, and Mayeux (1994). Beginning with 96 adults with DS and 80 with other forms of mental retardation, the risk for AD was assessed in the biologic mothers and fathers of these individuals. An increased risk for AD of around 2.5 was found in the mothers, but not the fathers of DS children. More importantly, when the mothers were 35 years of age or

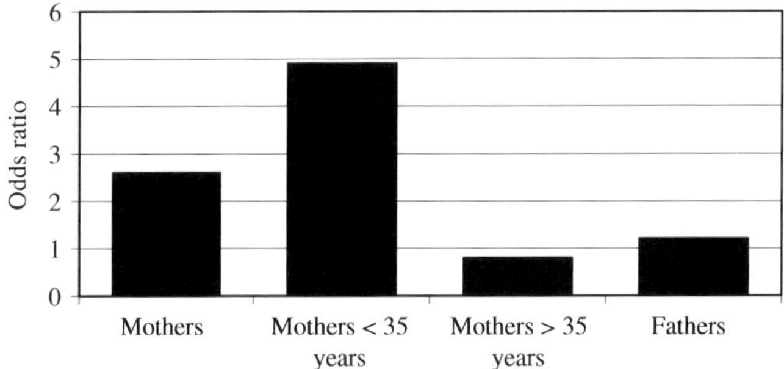

FIGURE 10.6. Odds ratios for dementia in all mothers of Down syndrome adults compared to mothers of other mentally retarded adults (Mothers), Mothers less than 35 years at the birth of the Down syndrome child (Mothers <35 years), Mothers greater than 35 years (Mothers >35 years) at birth, and Fathers. *Adapted from Schupf et al. (1994).*

older when they had their DS child, they had *no* increased risk for AD. However, there was a marked *increase* in risk in the more uncommon situation where a mother *under* the age of 35 had a DS child (Figure 10.6).

Heston noted that the risk for AD in blood relatives of DS patients declined with age at onset. However, when this issue was examined with greater power by Schupf and her colleagues, the risk for AD in mothers who had DS children continued through very old age (Figure 10.7). The findings that only mothers are affected is consistent with the observation that 95% of DS is associated with a nondisjunction event in chromosome 21 in the maternal gamete. This nondisjunction event might have two etiologies depending on the mother's age, a genetic predisposition to nondisjunction in young mothers and a nongenetic predisposition in older mothers.

Why might such an event be associated with AD? The gene for APP is located on chromosome 21, for which an extra copy in all or most cells leads to DS. Three copies of this gene would lead to increased production of β-amyloid and consequently increased Alzheimer neuropathology. Studies have shown a greater frequency of aneuploidy, particularly, trisomy 21 in neurons and other cells in Alzheimer patients compared to controls (Granic, Padmanabhan, Norden, & Potter, 2010). In addition, APP triplications have been described in families with a variant of AD (Rovelet-Lecrux et al., 2006). Therefore, a possible explanation for the genetic association between AD and DS is a shared genetic defect leading to increased chromosomal nondisjunction and trisomy of some cells, including gametes (leading to DS in children) and brain cells promoting increased accumulation of beta-amyloid and eventually AD. In this view, an unknown proportion of AD cases might represent a genetic mosaicism with trisomy 21 expressed in some, but not all brain cells (Geller & Potter, 1999).

While many individuals with DS develop dementia relatively early in life, many do not. The fact that age at onset and frequency of dementia vary widely

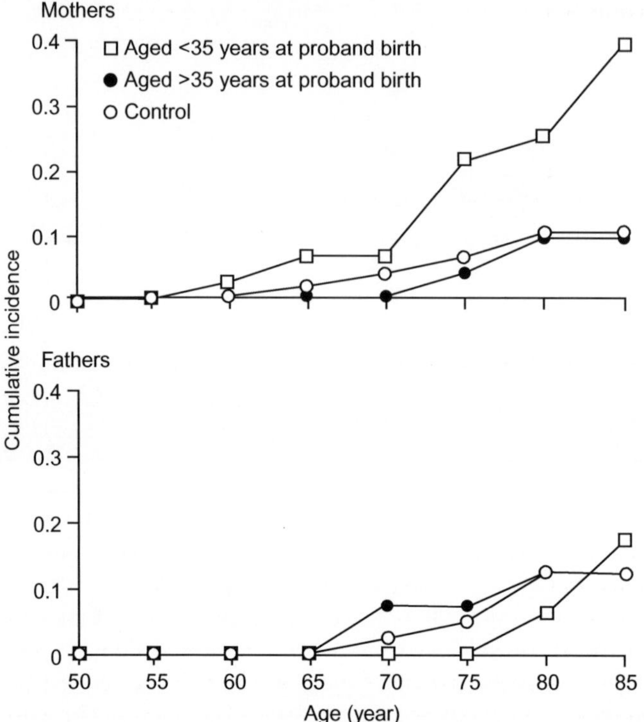

FIGURE 10.7. Cumulative incidence of dementia in parents of adults with Down's syndrome by age of the mother at birth and of adults with other forms of mental retardation (controls). *Reprinted from Schupf et al. (1994).*

in DS suggests the existence of risk factors for dementia in DS. It is likely that some of these risk factors might be similar to those identified in AD. Schupf examined the cumulative incidence of dementia in adults with DS and found that as in individuals without this condition, the age at onset was significantly earlier in carriers of the APOE-ε4 allele (Schupf & Sergievsky, 2002). Other genetic variants conferring susceptibility to AD in both DS as well as in people without DS include SORL1, BACE1, RUNX1 and ALDH18A1 (Patel et al., 2011). Regardless of the modifying effect of AD susceptibility genes, the curves for age-specific incidence of dementia appear to be shifted on average 25–30 years earlier in those with DS, likely due to a higher production of beta-amyloid across the life course.

Chapter 11

Early-Life Factors

THE LIFE COURSE APPROACH

We can use the threshold model discussed in Chapter 5 to frame the role of early-life factors in the causation of dementia and Alzhemier's disease (AD). Under this model, individuals who start adult life with less reserve can lose brain tissue at the same rate as people who start adulthood with more reserve, but will attain the clinical dementia threshold sooner given a fixed amount of pathology. Conversely, building reserve or preventing its loss across the life span could result in delaying the onset of cognitive decline to older ages. Life course epidemiology attempts to weave together the effects of genes and pre- and postnatal development, with childhood and adult exposures that influence the incidence of disease in mid- to late-life (Kuh, Ben-Shlomo, Lynch, Hallqvist, & Power, 2003; Lynch & Smith, 2005). Central to this approach is the timing of exposures, their interactions, and the manner in which they increase the risk of disease over time. Three theoretical models that have been used to understand this process are the *critical period model*, the *accumulation of risk model*, and the *chains of risk model* (Lynch & Smith, 2005).

The *critical period model* refers to an exposure at a particular time in life that produces an adverse outcome that would not have occurred if the same exposure had been experienced at a different time. Examples include fetal exposure to diethylstilbestrol, which is known to produce various adverse outcomes if exposure occurs before week 11 of gestation (Reed & Fenton, 2013), and toxicologic exposures such as lead in childhood that have lifelong health consequences (Dietert et al., 2000). Barker and his team in the United Kingdom (Barker, 2004) made key observations in this area, showing that prenatal and postnatal growth and its determinants could have lasting effects on human health in adulthood. According to Barker's fetal origins hypothesis, these associations can be explained by plasticity of the body's organs and systems at critically sensitive times when the environment determines how that system will develop. Most of this developmental plasticity occurs *in utero*, and much of it is determined by the mothers' own exposures, including her exposures during pregnancy, her own growth, and lifetime nutritional status, which in turn affect her ability to nourish the fetus (Barker, 2004). An example of a critical time

Alzheimer's Disease. DOI: http://dx.doi.org/10.1016/B978-0-12-804538-1.00011-0

period phenomenon called "programming" is that of the adaptation to environmental heat and the development of sweat glands. "In the early years of this century Japanese military expansion took their soldiers and settlers into unfamiliar climates. They found that there were wide differences in people's abilities to adapt to hot climates. Physiological studies showed that this was related to the number of functioning sweat glands. People with more functioning sweat glands cooled down faster. Rather than attributing the differences in sweat gland numbers to 'genetic effects,' Japanese physiologists explored the early development of the glands. They found that at birth all humans have similar numbers of sweat glands, but none of them function. In the first 3 years after birth a proportion of the glands become functional depending on the temperatures to which the child is exposed. The hotter the conditions the greater the number of sweat glands that are programmed to function. After 3 years the programming is complete and the number of sweat glands is fixed. The development of sweat glands encapsulates the essence of programming – a critical period when the system is plastic and sensitive to the environment, followed by loss of plasticity and a fixed functional capacity" (Barker, 1998).

Barker's fetal origins hypothesis in its early days encountered its share of criticisms (Paneth & Susser, 1995), including possible selection bias, confounding effects of exposures between early- and mid-life, and overinterpretation of inductive causal reasoning (Rich-Edwards & Gillman, 1997). However, data in the last 20 years support the hypothesis and it is now generally accepted that fetal growth is associated with a range of chronic conditions and aging-related outcomes, including coronary heart disease, breast cancer, stroke, diabetes, hypertension, and mortality (Barker & Thornburg, 2013; Delisle, 2002; Lynch & Smith, 2005).

The specific application of critical exposure periods to *in utero* exposures is difficult in life course research, because it requires data that have been collected on a cohort across the life span from gestation to mid- and to late-life. Birth cohort studies are extremely expensive and resource-intense, and as a result, are few in number. The investigation of critical exposure periods would also require knowledge of exposures during the induction period between the initial exposure and outcome, and repeated measures are rarely available at those specific times, even in birth cohort studies. In countries that have excellent medical registries, for example, Sweden, these types of studies may be more feasible than in countries that do not have organized registries.

In AD epidemiology, an example of a critical period finding is the use of hormone replacement therapy (HRT). In 2003 and 2004, the Women's Health Initiative Memory Study published results from a clinical trial that showed that HRT (both estrogen alone and estrogen plus progestin) increased the risk for dementia (Shumaker et al., 2004, 2003). This led to major national news stories and caused women of all ages to ask their doctors to take them off these medications. As we shall see in more detail in Chapter 19, observational studies suggest that rather than increasing the risk of dementia, estrogen may be *inversely* related with this outcome, exerting most of its neuroprotective benefits around the time of menopause or in the period immediately following it (Whitmer, Quesenberry, Zhou, & Yaffe, 2011).

The *accumulation of risk model* posits that exposures across the life course have a cumulative effect when there is excessive damage to a system and/or when the system becomes vulnerable or weakened in keeping up with the accumulated damage (Kuh et al., 2003). In AD, this model could be interpreted in terms of the loss of functioning brain tissue across the life course resulting from exposures to genetic and environmental risk factors. Those with faster rates of loss secondary to these exposures would experience earlier onset of cognitive impairment assuming they had similar amounts of brain reserve at the beginning of adult life.

The accumulation of risk model raises the question whether or not risk factors act independently or interactively (additively or multiplicatively) across the life course. Because no one study can provide the longitudinal data necessary to assess all relevant exposures occurring in fetal life, childhood, and adult life, the answers to this question are usually limited to measures obtained in single studies. For questions related to interactions, most studies have studied genes, in particular apolipoprotein E (APOE), in the modulation of exposure effects, such as vascular disease (Borenstein, Wu, & Larson, 2005) or head circumference (HC) (Graves et al., 2001). One can also examine how variables related to reserve interact with one another (Barker et al., 2012). Analysis of these interactions is enabled by the fact that genes and some childhood and adult measures, e.g., HC and attained education, change little after their maximum values have been attained. The possibly more interesting issue of interaction of exposures that change over the life course is more difficult to assess.

The application of the accumulation of risk model to chronic diseases is not unique to AD. In 1972, Kannel and Dawber, leaders of the Framingham Heart Study, remarked, "There is a growing conviction that the only way to substantially reduce the toll from atherosclerotic disease is to attack its constitutional and environmental precursors long before overt symptoms occur. Epidemiologic and pathologic studies suggest that only early intervention is likely to have a major impact on the evolution of the disease. The pathologic changes which lead to atherosclerosis begin in infancy and progress during childhood. Consideration of the possible value of prophylaxis beginning in childhood is therefore in order" (Kannel, 1972). Preventive measures suggested by Kannel and Dawber (1972) included the reduction of obesity and cigarette smoking, as well as improved diet and exercise. The idea that adoption of a healthy lifestyle early in life could delay the pathology of atherosclerosis and the eventual occurrence of a cardiac event was also put forth in this seminal paper. These ideas are slowly gaining favor in the study of the causes of AD, where the situation could be very similar.

Although it is well accepted that AD begins at least two decades before clinical onset with the accumulation of insoluble amyloid-ß (Aß) deposits (neuritic plaques), cerebral amyloid angiopathy, and aggregated tau in neurofibrillary tangles (Jack & Holtzman, 2013), researchers are investigating the possible causal roles of other forms of amyloid, including soluble ones (Lesne et al., 2013; Mucke & Selkoe, 2012), that may produce neurotoxicity over a *much longer* time period. Neurofibrillary tangles, which are better correlated with cognition in older age than neuritic plaques (Bennett, Schneider, Wilson, Bienias, & Arnold, 2004), are known to be present as early as the 20s (Braak et al., 1997). Therefore, it is biologically plausible that AD pathology begins early in life and accumulates over a very long time period before clinical symptoms become manifest. It also is plausible that genes and environmental exposures behave independently and cumulatively, to reduce reserve below the clinical threshold of dementia, and that this trajectory is reflected in individual risk profiles across the life course.

The third model, known as the *chains of risk* model, describes exposures that are linked, with one exposure's consequences leading to the next exposure (either protective or increasing risk) (Kuh et al., 2003). Under this model, exposures may have independent effects on disease risk in addition to being mediated by earlier exposures. When exposures increase or decrease the risk cumulatively, this is called an "additive effect" and is a special case of the accumulation model (Kuh et al., 2003). Some diseases have a final triggering event that is determined from earlier events that are the primary causes of disease onset. In AD epidemiology, early-life exposures may be linked through the chains of risk model as well as through the accumulation of risk model. For example, parental resources and cultural parental attitudes toward formal education determine to some extent the level of completion of education of the offspring, which determines the extent to which that individual engages in cognitively stimulating activities throughout their lives, which in turn may increase reserve, acting to delay the onset of clinical dementia in older age.

Most epidemiologic studies use the "one exposure-one outcome" approach. Therefore, epidemiologists must piece together bits of information about how different exposures interact and contribute to the outcome. In AD, cohort sample sizes may be insufficient to address multiple interactions in a single model (particularly higher-order interactions).

You may be wondering how many studies exist that cover up to a 100-year exposure period, and your intuitive answer is correct: none. The Framingham Study (of over 5,000 individuals started in 1948) is the longest running cohort study in the United States, and in Japan, the Adult Health Study (of about 20,000 subjects begun in 1958) is still ongoing. The British Birth Cohort studies, namely the National Survey of Health & Development and the National Child Development Study, began in 1946 and 1958, respectively, have been instrumental in the development of life course epidemiology in the United Kingdom. Another set of studies from Scotland, the Lothian birth cohort (LBC) studies, begun in 1921 (LBC1921) and 1936 (LBC1936), have contributed important information to our understanding of life course epidemiology of AD. In the LBC1936 study, of 3,686 people living in this area, 1,091 were successfully tracked to the mid-2000s and were interviewed and neuropsychologically tested (about 30% participation) (Deary et al., 2007). One of the problems with this study design and other studies that have long lag periods between "visits" is the lack of information about the interceding period, and the reliance on late-life recall, which may result in measurement error and recall bias (Lynch & Smith, 2005).

Other studies, primarily in Europe, the United States, Australia, the UK, and Scandinavia were initiated in the early 1970s to the late 1990s to evaluate the early-life origins of cardiovascular disease (Magnussen, Smith, & Juonala, 2014). These studies link early-life with adult-life vascular outcomes. Additional studies initiated in the same time period link cardiovascular and cerebrovascular disease in adult-life with late-life outcomes, including dementia.

It is important to acknowledge that genetics sets the stage for lifetime risk (see Chapter 10), so that in a sense AD risk begins at conception. In this chapter, we consider factors that can build reserve during the first 25 years of life. Early-life risk factors are grouped into six categories: (i) prenatal environment, (ii) early-life brain development, (iii) early-life body growth, (iv) early-life socioeconomic conditions, (v) education and intelligence, and (vi) linguistic ability. It is important to recognize that these risk factors are related both to genes and to environmental exposures *in utero* and early life. It also is important to acknowledge the possible role played by the environment in regulating our genes ("epigenetic" effects). In addition, the fetal and early-life origins of adult hypertension, diabetes, hyperlipidemia and obesity suggest that these vascular risk factors which contribute to the expression of dementia, have a very early start as well. (This association is discussed in more detail in Chapter 14.)

The Prenatal Environment

The Intrauterine Environment

There are no studies linking fetal exposures directly with AD for the reasons we discussed above. The fetal origins hypothesis has spurred research showing that the gestational environment influences the development of the fetus in critical periods, which affects homeostatic regulatory mechanisms. Such environmental programming can have far-reaching effects, including changes in the structure, physiology and function of body organs and processes, as well as epigenetic effects (Ross et al., 2007; Veeraswamy, Vijayam, Gupta, & Kapur, 2012). There is now extensive evidence that intrauterine growth restriction is linked to an increased risk for Type II diabetes mellitus, obesity, hypertension, dyslipidemia, and insulin resistance (known in combination as the metabolic syndrome) (Chernausek, 2012). Together these conditions lead to increased risk for cardiovascular and cerebrovascular diseases (Barker, Winter, Osmond, Margetts, & Simmonds, 1989), which in turn are associated with increased risk for AD (Qiu, 2011) (see Chapter 14). While the mechanisms of such effects are not completely understood, epigenetic effects appear to play a role in programming activities *in utero*. In particular, fetuses that are deprived of nutrition can have a paradoxical response in which the child develops obesity, hypertension, and glucose intolerance in adulthood (Ross et al., 2007). In the Helsinki Birth Cohort of more than 13,000 individuals born during the period 1934–1944 (Barker et al., 2012), the incidence of sudden cardiac death was related to the thinness of the placenta at birth ($p = 0.006$), and there was a qualitative ($p < 0.10$) interaction with lower birth weight. Women in that study who were born of mothers with a larger placental surface area were at increased risk for sudden cardiac death, which was explained as a compensatory mechanism for a thin surface (the placenta grows a larger surface area to compensate for its thinness). Sudden cardiac death was also related to lower paternal socioeconomic status (SES) and to lower SES and education of the subject herself, consistent with a combination of an accumulation of risk model with a chains of risk model.

In a study of 25,283 people in the Netherlands exposed to the "Dutch famine" of 1944–1947, it was reported that those exposed to the famine during *early* gestation had a higher risk for mortality (HR = 1.12, 95% CI = 1.01–1.24), but those who were exposed in *late* gestation did not (HR = 1.04, 95% CI = 0.96–1.13), demonstrating a critical period effect (Ekamper, van Poppel, Stein, & Lumey, 2013). In that study, socioeconomic life conditions had independent effects from early-life exposure to famine. Related to the same exposure, another analysis examining cognition at age 59 compared individuals exposed to famine to those not exposed as well as to same-sex siblings born outside of the famine period (February 1, 1945–March 31, 1946) (de Groot et al., 2011). Weight and BMI at age 59 were significantly higher among individuals exposed to the famine during gestation ($p = 0.01$ for weight and $p < 0.001$ for BMI). While not statistically significant, there was a strong trend for performance on a Z-scored general cognitive index to be lower at age 59 among individuals exposed in the first 10 weeks of gestation (mean difference = −4.37, 95% CI = −9.04 to 0.67) compared with later weeks of gestation ($p = 0.08$). However, no associations were observed for overall exposure to famine and cognitive scores at age 59.

In another analysis of 737 individuals from the Dutch Famine Birth Cohort (de Rooij, Wouters, Yonker, Painter, & Roseboom, 2010), associations with cognitive function measures including the Alice Heim test of general IQ (AH4), a memory task (paragraph recall), a perceptual motor-learning task (mirror drawing), and a selective attention task (a Stroop-like color-word test) were examined. Those exposed to famine, regardless of which trimester, had smaller adult head circumferences (HC) compared with those not exposed to famine. Prenatally famine-exposed subjects performed worse on a sex-adjusted score on a Stroop-like task compared with unexposed subjects ($p = 0.047$), with a stronger effect among those exposed in early gestation ($p = 0.009$). Response times on the Stroop-like tests also were slower in the exposed group, and a more pronounced effect was again seen in those exposed to famine in the earlier part of gestation (first and second trimesters) ($p = 0.002$). None of the other tests showed associations with the famine-exposed group, including the intelligence and memory tests. The authors interpreted these findings as suggesting that the poorer performance in attention in famine-exposed participants was due to more rapid aging in this group. Vascular changes, specifically white matter lesions in the brain, could be mediating the association, since the authors published another paper showing that famine-exposed individuals, particularly those exposed in early gestation, had a more atherogenic lipid profile and higher risk of coronary heart disease (Roseboom, de Rooij, & Painter, 2006).

The causal pathways between gestational exposures and late-life AD could possibly behave as a chains of risk model with triggering events. Such a causal mechanism was proposed by Lahiri and Maloney (2010). In their model (Latent Early-Life Association Regulation (LEARn)), a "two-hit" model was described for "sporadic" AD, in which the first hit might occur during gestation or in early-life, primarily affecting epigenetic changes such as methylation; and the second hit would occur later in life, with adult exposures such as poor nutrition or head injury. According to this model, early-life influences, including exposure in gestation to toxins, inadequate nutrition, and other stressors, may alter expression levels of AD genes. These latent changes are proposed to be retained by epigenetic markers in the promoter sequences of these genes, by DNA methylation, DNA oxidation, and chromatin organization (Lahiri & Maloney, 2010). In adulthood, genes that have been altered in these ways, if they are exposed to additional hits, would express themselves in pathologic ways to cause disease. This model assumes that the epigenetic changes precede the pathology of the disease. However, there is no evidence about when during the lifetime these changes occur. As we pointed out in Chapter 10 (Genetics), the heritability of sporadic AD is high (Gatz, Reynolds, et al., 2006). Therefore, much of sporadic as well as familial disease may be explained by Mendelian genetics. This does not imply that the "two-hit" model is wrong, but rather that it should be considered hypothetical until more evidence is developed.

Because the study of the gestational period and early life is so novel, the effects of this critical period of development on the brain are just beginning to be recognized (Faa et al., 2014). During this time, neuronal cell, and neuronal and glial cell connections are being made that will be modified further during development. Environmental factors acting during gestation, including maternal nutrition, maternal hypertension and gestational diabetes mellitus may critically impact the developing brain, but little data are available at present to address this issue.

BIRTH ORDER AND SIBSHIP SIZE

There is some evidence to suggest that the uterine environment is an important determinant of birth outcomes, including birth weight (Gibbons, Cedars, & Ness, 2011). Whether multiparity (having multiple offspring) is associated with maternal fetal outcomes is still under debate. Although older studies suggested this association, more recent ones do not support it. Some of the positive findings may be attributed to the definition of parity, to confounding by maternal age (also linked to AD, see Chapter 10) and SES, to access to prenatal care, and to methodological differences in study design (Aliyu, Jolly, Ehiri, & Salihu, 2005). The definition of what constitutes a "very high" parity where there is an increased risk of adverse birth outcomes is not uniform across studies. Another problem plaguing these early-life studies is the rarity of "great grand multipara"—women having more than 10 pregnancies—and the small absolute risk of adverse birth outcomes, resulting in insufficient sample size in many studies. Despite these reservations, high parity appears to be a risk factor for specific medical conditions, such as diabetes and certain placental problems (Aliyu et al., 2005).

There are a few studies of AD that have examined birth order, and the results have shown no association. In a case–control study of 133 AD cases from Canada who were compared with six control groups from a population registry, there was no effect of birth order (De Braekeleer, Froda, Gautrin, Tetreault, & Gauvreau, 1988). In another case–control study derived from Group Health Cooperative (GHC), a health maintenance organization in Seattle, WA (Moceri, Kukull, Emanuel, van Belle & Larson, 2000), 393 prevalent cases and 377 controls selected at random from the enrollment lists were frequency- matched by age ±2 years and sex, and analyses were based on data from proxy informants for both groups. For each unit increase in birth order, the OR for probable AD by NINCDS-ADRDA criteria was 1.04 (95% CI = 0.96–1.12), missing statistical significance. However, there was an association with the number of siblings in this study. The OR per additional sibling was 1.08 (95% CI = 1.02–1.15), and there was an increasing risk with sibship group size (OR = 1.0 for < 5 siblings; OR = 1.07 (95% CI = 0.68–1.68) for 5–6 siblings; OR = 1.72 (95% CI = 1.01–2.43) for 7–9 siblings and OR = 2.66 (95% CI = 0.92–7.99) for 10+ siblings ($p = 0.008$)). These findings are consistent with "resource dilution" where a greater number of siblings leads to fewer resources, and suggest that relative deprivation during the first few years of life rather than in utero exposures may be related to increased risk for AD. It is known that both lower SES and higher maternal age are strong confounders of the association between sibship size and later life outcomes. The necessary studies to disentangle birth order from sibship size from other confounding variables have not yet been done.

In another paper (Moceri et al., 2001), researchers used 239 incident AD cases and 245 controls selected at random from the enrollment lists of GHC in Seattle, WA, frequency-matched by age and sex. This analysis did not rely on proxy informant interviews, but instead gathered data from the US Census and the birth certificates of cases and controls. There was no clear effect of birth order here either, but sibship size was nearly statistically significant with the OR = 1.39 (95% CI = 0.99–1.95) for five or more siblings compared with fewer than five.

Sibship size is well known to be associated with cognitive performance as well as with final educational achievement. The resource dilution hypothesis maintains that since parental resources are limited, the access children have to such resources becomes diluted with each additional sibling (Downey, 2001). Therefore, children with no or few siblings have greater access to increased educational opportunities compared with children with many siblings. Possible early-life advantages of larger sibships, including increased environmental stimulation and developing better social interaction styles, may offset the resource dilution hypothesis to some degree, but there exists considerable evidence to support it (Jaeger, 2009). For example, when sibship size was examined in relation to adult intelligence, memory, and executive function, an association was seen for executive function and working memory, but not for intelligence (Holmgren, Molander, & Nilsson, 2006).

BIRTH WEIGHT

Undernourishment in gestation and other maternal risk factors may cause the brain to not develop to its full potential during gestation. *In utero*, the brain grows to about one quarter of its adult weight. At birth, the rate of growth is highest, and by age 1 the brain weighs 75% of its adult weight (Chase, 1973). In the last trimester of gestation, a growth spurt occurs in which glial cells rapidly develop, axons grow, dendritic branches expand, and synapses form (Ross et al., 2007). Therefore, insults sustained by the fetus during the last trimester have an important impact on final brain size (Muller et al., 2014a; Muller 2014b). In animal studies, brain and body weight are permanently stunted by gestational and infant undernutrition. In addition, when rapid postnatal catch-up growth occurs in infants, the risk of central obesity and development of insulin resistance is higher (Bieswal et al., 2006).

Low birth weight can negatively impact brain development in very early life, which can have a permanent effect on the number of neurons and their interconnections (Clark, Zamenhof, Van Mathens, Grauel, & Kruger, 1973; Martyn, Gale, Sayer, & Fall, 1996). Lower brain weight is well correlated with smaller HC, as we shall see in a later section of this chapter. The goal to build the maximum amount of brain reserve gestationally and in the first few years of life is met when conditions actively promote optimal brain development and the attainment of the largest size of the brain within that individual's genetic potential. Early-life brain growth, whether it meets an individual's full genetic potential or not, will form the baseline complement of neurons and their interconnections, represented by the intercept in figure 5.2. With regard to dementia, an individual starting life with a smaller brain may be more likely to reach the clinical threshold for clinical dementia earlier than a person starting life with a larger brain.

In a review of life course epidemiology as it pertains to dementing illnesses, Whalley, Dick, and McNeill (2006) postulate that genes, the intrauterine environment, placental insufficiency, maternal malnutrition, and perhaps other influences, such as inadequate prenatal care and socioeconomic conditions during gestation, lead to low birth weight. Through a chains of risk model, low birth weight, coupled with socioeconomic conditions in early life, result in lower childhood intelligence. In turn, lower intelligence is associated with lower educational and occupational opportunities, as well as adverse lifestyle factors, such as smoking, poor nutrition, and sedentary lifestyle that can lead to lower social and mental stimulation throughout adulthood. These risk factors, coupled with vascular diseases (diabetes, hypertension, obesity) raise the risk for dementia, accelerating the onset of clinically detectable cognitive symptoms through a reduction of reserve, which occurs throughout the life course.

Little evidence exists to support direct relationships between birth weight and late-life cognition, but data covering only part of the life course can be considered in this regard. In a national birth cohort study in the United Kingdom, higher birth weight was associated with higher educational attainment at age 26 (OR for an increase in five birth weight categories = 1.12, 95% CI = 1.04–1.20) (Richards, Hardy, Kuh, & Wadsworth, 2001). Birth weight in this study also was associated with cognitive function at age 8 and age 26. However, a word-list learning task administered at age 43 (different from the tests administered at earlier ages) was not associated with birth weight. The authors concluded that the lack of association seen with the measure given at age 43 could be due to the use of different tests at the different ages. In another paper based on the same cohort, among individuals born between 1920 and 1943, a measure of cognitive decline was derived using the difference observed between a measure of fluid intelligence (the AH4 test) and a measure of crystallized intelligence (the Mill Hill vocabulary test) (Martyn et al., 1996). The authors found no association between birth weight and cognitive function at age 61, but acknowledge that their cohort was still highly functioning at this age. One problem with using standardized measures to assess cognitive function in individuals who are functioning well above the clinical threshold is their lack of sensitivity. Although the AH4 test requires greater manipulation of information than the Mill Hill Vocabulary Test, it is still basically an IQ test and lacks the sensitivity to detect subtle deficits in nondemented people.

The fetal origins hypothesis, with determinants of birth weight at the center of the puzzle, is a burgeoning area of interest in the etiology of neurodegenerative diseases such as AD and Parkinson's disease (Faa et al., 2014). A paper presented at the 2014 Alzheimer's Association International Conference using archived records in Reikjavik, Iceland reported an additive effect of low birth weight in relation to height (ponderal index), and adult hypertension on brain volumes in late-life. Compared with individuals with high ponderal index scores at birth and no hypertension in midlife, individuals with low ponderal index scores at birth and midlife hypertension had a 5.9 mL (95% CI = 0.2–11.9) smaller total brain volume, and a 3.8 mL (95% CI = 0.7–7.0) smaller white matter volume in late life (Muller, 2014a).

EARLY-LIFE BRAIN DEVELOPMENT

We have discussed the importance of brain development during gestation and the problems accompanying suboptimal growth, resulting in low birth weight. During the first 2 years of life, the brain undergoes rapid growth in overall size, reaching 80–90% of its adult volume (Knickmeyer et al., 2008), accompanied by a burst of new synapses and overall gray matter volume. A study of 98 healthy children and mothers in North Carolina who were recruited during their second trimester of pregnancy and followed until the child was 2 years old showed that total brain volume increased 101% in the first year and 15% in the second. The authors suggest that, while lasting damage can occur in this critical period of brain growth, this is also the time when preventive measures can alleviate such damage (Knickmeyer et al., 2008). For example, babies subjected to extreme deprivation in orphanages who are placed in foster care before age 2 show much better improvements in cognitive development than those placed in such care after this age (Nelson et al., 2007).

Because most of the final size of the brain is determined in the first few years of life, we can use adult measurements of intracranial brain volume to make inferences about early brain growth. In 1988, Katzman and colleagues identified a group of 137 nursing home subjects who had been clinically tested during life and also had neuropathologic examinations for AD. Among this group, the investigators found a group of 10 individuals who, on autopsy, had "definite histologic changes of the Alzheimer type" (Katzman et al., 1988), but whose cognition and function were comparable to age-matched controls with no histologic evidence of AD. The finding that differentiated this group was that they had a greater number of large neurons in the frontal, parietal, and temporal cortices than other groups that were either not demented with no brain lesions, demented with AD pathology, or demented with no AD lesions. Their brain weights were also higher than any of the other groups. The authors concluded that this group of 10 individuals either had less atrophy of the brain, or that they "started with more neurons and a larger brain, and thus had a greater reserve," implying that they "had incipient Alzheimer's disease but did not show it clinically because of this greater reserve" (Katzman et al., 1988).

Maximal attained brain size in adulthood can be determined from the volume of the skull (intracranial volume) using structural MRI. A related measurement given the approximately spherical shape of the head is HC, which is more easily obtained in epidemiologic studies. In adulthood, the correlation between HC and intracranial volume ranges between 0.50 (in 24–43 year olds) (Tramo et al., 1998) and 0.70 (in a sample of 75–85 year olds) (Wolf et al., 2003). HC remains fairly constant throughout the life course, permitting estimates of brain size in earlier life from adult measurements. Because the correlation between HC and intracranial volume is only moderate, utilization of HC in place of intracranial volume as a measure of maximal attained brain size should result in nondifferential misclassification leading to reduction in the strengths of association between brain size and cognitive outcomes in comparison with the more accurate measure of intracranial volume. Although both measures (intracranial volume and HC) are appropriate for estimating maximal attained brain volume, use of the more accessible measure (HC) likely reduces the statistical power to see associations (Wolf et al., 2003).

The paper by Katzman et al. (1988) triggered research to examine the association between premorbid brain size (measured by intracranial measurements on imaging and/or HC) and dementia. In 1995, Schofield et al. measured cross-sectional intracranial areas from computed tomography (CT) scans of 28 women with probable AD as a surrogate for brain volume and reported a correlation of 0.48 ($p = 0.009$) between age at first AD symptom and intracranial area. For each increase of 1 cm^2 in cross-sectional intracranial area, the age at first symptom was delayed by 4 months (Schofield, Mosesson, Stern, & Mayeux, 1995). When education, height, and ethnic group were additionally adjusted, this correlation increased to 0.64 ($p = 0.01$). In 1997, Schofield et al. published a second population-based finding, in which HC was analyzed in relation to prevalent dementia (Schofield, Logroscino, Andrews, Albert, & Stern, 1997). In this study, women in the lowest quintile of HC had the highest frequency of AD (22%), and a significant dose–response was observed, with only about 7% of those with the largest quintile of HC having AD ($p = 0.001$). However, there was no significant dose–response among men ($p = 0.18$), which may have been due to the smaller number of men in the sample. The OR for AD associated with the lowest quintile of HC (<53.5 cm) for women was 2.9 (95% CI = 1.4–6.1), and for men (<55.5 cm), 2.3 (95% CI = 0.6–9.8).

In 1991, when we began the *Kame* Project, we measured HC on all 1985 participants. In 1996, we published the first population-based study in which the association between HC and cognitive ability was addressed (Graves et al., 1996). Each unit increase in the measure of HC was associated with a 3.8 (95% CI = 2.3–5.3, $p = 0.0000$) points higher score on a global measure of cognitive function, the Cognitive Abilities Screening Instrument (CASI) after adjusting for age, sex, and education. The HC measure did not independently predict prevalent probable AD in our baseline sample. However, when we stratified the finding among AD cases and those who were cognitively normal in the baseline cohort, we found that smaller HC was associated with lower CASI scores only among the AD cases and not among controls, indicating that HC predicted the *severity* of cognitive impairment in Alzheimer patients. These findings suggested that initial brain size is likely not relevant for people without a predisposition to AD. However, among people who have this disease, reserve measured by HC modifies the clinical presentation.

In a study of 181 AD, VaD, and MCI patients referred to a Memory Disorders Clinic in Sweden and 85 age-matched controls, Wolf, Julin, Gertz, Winblad, and Wahlund (2004) reported that smaller intracranial volume increased the risk for cognitive impairment (MCI or dementia), with greater severity of cognitive impairment among people with dementia, similar to our initial findings from the *Kame* Project. In addition, they reported that the association between intracranial volume and severity of cognitive impairment was not modified by hippocampal atrophy. Because hippocampal atrophy is an important marker of the AD neuropathologic process, absence of modification by hippocampal volume of the association between intracranial volume and cognitive impairment points to the existence of two types of risk factors: one (hippocampal volume) associated primarily with Alzheimer's pathology, and the other (intracranial volume) that determines the degree to which Alzheimer pathology influences cognition (reserve).

An important question is whether one should adjust for height when investigating the association between HC and AD. We know that on average taller people have larger heads and that brain volume matures to its adult size in the first decade of life, while adult height is attained in the second decade. Thus, we are looking at two processes that, while they share some variance, may have independent determinants. Height was not a major confounder in our analyses, nor of those by Schofield et al. However, if the critical variable is the size of the brain (intracranial volume), height adjustment is unlikely to be necessary.

The early studies of maximum brain volume using HC spurred other investigators to examine the role of maximal brain size on the risk for cognitive decline and AD and most supported the initial findings. In the MoVIES cohort (Reynolds, Johnston, Dodge, DeKosky, & Ganguli, 1999), among 825 individuals aged around 78, each 1 cm increase in HC was cross-sectionally associated with a decreased risk of a low score on the Mini Mental State Examination (OR = 0.83, 95% CI = 0.69–0.99), similar in men and women. In Korea (Kim et al., 2008), among 916 community-dwelling participants, each standard deviation (3 cm) decrease in HC was associated with an increased risk of prevalent AD (OR = 1.66, 95% CI = 1.3–2.1). By contrast to these findings in cohorts, two case–control studies in which brain volume was compared between a group of cases coming to a clinic and control volunteers failed to show differences. Among 692 people recruited from the memory disorder clinic at the University of Kentucky, mean HC was similar among cases and controls, and increased risk for conversion to AD with smaller HC was not seen among 459 persons who were initially free of AD and who were followed over time (Espinosa et al., 2006). When cases derived from the Mayo Clinic's Alzheimer's Disease Patient Registry and Alzheimer's Disease Research Center were compared with controls from the surrounding community, no difference in total intracranial volume was found (Edland, Rocca, Petersen, Cha, & Kokmen, 2002). Studies that use dementia referral clinics to identify cases may be biased because higher-educated individuals are more likely to find their way to these specialty clinics, and these people may have larger HCs. HC has been associated with education level in many studies, which is known to be associated with health-seeking behaviors. If the controls come from a different population, comparisons may be invalid. In the case of the Mayo Clinic study, cases coming from around the world to see neurologists at Mayo Clinic would likely be more highly advantaged throughout their lives in comparison to local residents of Olmsted County who are representative of the local population and constituted the majority of controls in the Mayo Clinic study. Violation of the study base principle, which maintains that cases and controls must come from the same underlying population (Wacholder, McLaughlin, Silverman, & Mandel, 1992), may have biased the results toward the null value. A multisite study using registries and specialty memory clinics, MIRAGE (Perneczky et al., 2010), also did not find an association between HC and performance on the MMSE per se, but did find that brain atrophy in those with larger HC had less of an impact on cognitive performance than in those with smaller HC, thus supporting the brain reserve hypothesis.

In a small study of 85 AD cases, 22 of whom had familial AD and 52 healthy controls, Jenkins, Fox, Rossor, Harvey, and Rossor (2000) was unable to replicate Schofield's age at onset-intracranial volume study. However, they did find that familial AD cases had smaller total intracranial volumes (TIV) (1359.5 cm^3) than controls (1407.1 cm^3) or sporadic cases (1419.5 cm^3). It is important to note that their sample size was small, they used a matched design without a matched analysis, there were differences in education level between cases and controls, and the control group consisted of volunteers, violating the study base principle.

Another interesting study is that by Staff, Murray, Deary, and Whalley (2004). The authors set out to test how well different measures of reserve (education, occupational attainment, and head size) predict late-life cognition. They used data on 92 subjects who participated in the 1932 Scottish Mental Survey of 11-year olds, when they were given a test of intelligence. They also measured neuropsychological performance on reasoning, intelligence, and memory at age 79, as well as total intracranial volumes (TIV) on MRI. They found effects on late-life cognition from education and occupational attainment but not from TIV. However, it is noteworthy that their model was adjusted for childhood intelligence. If lower HC is a cause of lower late-life cognitive performance, it may act through lower IQ in childhood, which is well known to be correlated with brain volume (Reiss, Abrams, Singer, Ross, & Denckla, 1996). Thus, lower IQ in childhood may be a mediating, rather than a confounding, variable. Adjustment for IQ in childhood may have nullified the HC-late-life cognition association (Figure 11.1). The authors did not test the association between childhood intelligence and TIV, the critical element in the causal pathway. If the authors had examined that part of the pathway, they may have reached a different conclusion.

The largest cross-sectional study that addressed the association between HC and dementia was conducted by the 10/66 Dementia Research Group (DRG), which conducted population-based cross-sectional studies of dementia at 17 sites in 12 low- and middle-income countries (Prince et al., 2011). For each country, the target sample size was between 2,000 and 3,000. A total of 14,960 individuals completed the assessments, with response rates between 72 and

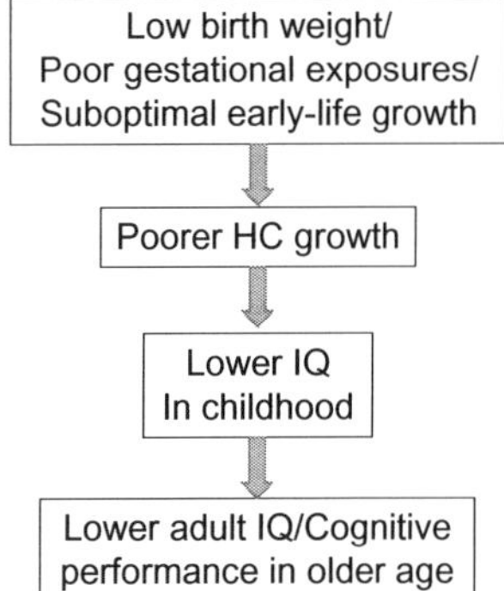

FIGURE 11.1 Simplified causal pathway of adverse early-life exposures to lower cognitive performance in older age.

98%. In Cuba and Peru (rural samples), HC was statistically inversely associated with the prevalence of dementia, adjusting for age, sex, education, and family history of dementia. The association was inverse in 7 of the 11 sites, with some sites just missing statistical significance. The authors conducted a pooled meta-analysis of the data, which showed an adjusted prevalence ratio (PR) of 0.75 (95% CI = 0.63–0.89). One problem with this point estimate is that the analysis was performed comparing the lowest quartile of HC to the highest (presumably leaving out the middle two quartiles). This omission of data can bias the point estimate away from the null, thus overstating the results. The 10/66 authors examined effect-modification of the HC-dementia association by education level, and found an inverse trend, with the PR's upper confidence interval missing statistical significance (PR = 0.96, 95% CI = 0.91–1.01). In the Nun Study, this interaction was both statistically and clinically important for the clinical expression of dementia or AD (Mortimer, Snowdon, & Markesbery, 2003).

Cross-sectional studies are vulnerable to survival bias, the idea that the study findings might be distorted if the exposure interacts with the outcome to cause removal from the cohort (through illness, death, or other dropout). Because AD patients with smaller HCs have more severe cognitive impairment (Graves, Mortimer, et al., 1996) and those with dementia and larger HC have somewhat better survival (HR = 0.86, 95% CI = 0.69–1.06) (Jotheeswaran, Williams, Stewart, & Prince, 2011), it is possible that the association of HC with AD is underestimated in cross-sectional studies.

Epidemiologists and scientists in general should never simply "count" the number of positive and the number of null studies. Making a table that shows which studies were null and which found an association is meaningless without detailed critique of each paper and a deep appreciation of methodological difficulties that can distort study findings. In the case of HC and AD, the association is best studied in large, population-based cohort studies in which there is a good distribution of the exposure variable and in which the study base is known for the comparison groups. Such studies have generally supported an association between HC and cognitive impairment or dementia.

In the few cohort studies in which HC was measured, it was not directly associated with incident AD, but could be seen clearly interacting with other variables to increase risk for the disease. In the *Kame* Project, we followed 1869 nondemented Japanese-American residents of King County, WA for 10 years. HC was measured at baseline (1992–1994) and incident probable AD was defined by NINCDS/ADRDA criteria. HC did not differ significantly between incident cases and those who did not become demented. For the lowest tertile of HC compared with the upper two tertiles, the HR for AD was 2.26 ($p = 0.16$), suggestive of an association. However, when APOE status was analyzed as an effect-modifier, those with HC in the lowest tertile who had one or two APOE-ε4 alleles had a 12-fold increased risk for AD (95% CI = 2.76–52.64, $p = 0.0009$), which did not change when adjusting for height or body-mass index. This finding suggests that individuals with smaller brain volumes early in life who are at higher genetic risk for AD represent a particularly vulnerable subgroup (Graves et al., 2001).

In an analysis from the Nun Study (Mortimer et al., 2003), participants were stratified into those with less than 16 years of education (low education) and those with 16 or more years of education (high education). HC was stratified into tertiles and interactions with education examined with regard to risk for dementia. Among nuns with HC in the low or middle tertiles, the odds for having dementia were significantly higher if education was low (adjusted OR for dementia = 4.1, 95% CI = 1.7–9.9; 68.4% had dementia) than if education was high (OR = 1.0, 95% CI = 0.6–1.8, 33.5% had dementia). Again, there was no effect of low HC by itself. The strong increased risk could only be seen when the association was examined among those with low education. Importantly, in this study, autopsy data available for 60 of the 294 participants in this analysis showed that both educational attainment and HC were unrelated to the fulfillment of the neuropathologic criteria for AD, consistent with independence of brain reserve from Alzheimer pathology.

In 2008, a second finding was published from the Nun Study showing that among nuns carrying an APOE-ε4 allele, small HC was associated with lower educational attainment (OR = 6.27, 95% CI = 1.21–32.48) (Mortimer, Snowdon, & Markesbery, 2008). We also found the same association of small HC with lower educational attainment among those with incident dementia (OR = 3.23, 95% CI = 1.27–8.21) and with neuropathologic AD at autopsy (OR = 5.03, 95% CI= 1.29–19.66). By contrast, in those without an ε4 allele there was no association between small HC and education (OR = 1.4, 95% CI = 0.63–3.12). This also applied to participants without dementia (OR = 0.53, 95% CI = 0.11–2.47) or neuropathologic AD (OR = 1.04, 95% CI = 0.17–6.26). Therefore, individuals with small HC are likely to receive less education if they are at greater risk for AD neuropathology as reflected by their

APOE-ε4 status, dementia outcomes or AD neuropathology. The findings also were not explained by a birth cohort effect (with earlier birth cohorts having smaller HCs). This study suggests that among those predisposed to AD pathology, educational attainment, which is largely determined by young adulthood, is already limited by this time in those with smaller brains and less brain reserve. Conversely, in those not at high risk for AD, brain size does not seem to have an important influence on educational attainment. Other studies have shown that individuals who carry an ε4 allele leave school earlier than those without such an allele (Codemo, Corti, Mazzetto, et al., 2000; Winnock et al., 2002). In these studies, the critical decision to leave school was determined on average around age 12, indicating an effect of this AD susceptibility gene on brain or cognitive reserve at a very young age.

EARLY-LIFE BODY GROWTH

While HC is almost fully developed by age 6, a person's full height is not attained until the end of the second decade of life (a little longer in males). Again, genes determine to a great extent how tall a person will be, but in populations deprived of adequate nutrition, individuals can fail to reach their full height potential.

Adult height has been positively associated with increased birth weight and birth length. In a study that examined men between the ages 18 and 20 and linked data to the Danish Medical Birth Register (Sorensen et al., 1999), mean adult height was 175.7 cm for birth weights of ≤2,500 g and 184.3 for those with birth weights of >4,501 g, with a consistent dose–response effect for the middle six categories. This trend remained after adjusting for gestational age, birth order, maternal age, and marital and employment status of the mother. A study from Israel found that babies born small-for-gestational-age had an increased risk of being shorter by the late teen years (Paz et al., 1993). Interestingly, the association between adult height and socioeconomic conditions is inconsistent and unreliable, and adult height is considered to be a function more of genetics and net nutrition in early childhood (the difference between intake of food and losses to activities and disease, e.g., diarrheal diseases in developing countries) (Deaton, 2007), although there may be intrinsic confounding in lower income countries between SES and nutritional status.

Some longitudinal studies that investigated height, but not HC, as a measure of early-life growth, found increased risks for poor cognitive performance, and/or AD associated with shorter stature. The Honolulu-Asia Aging Study examined height among 3,733 Japanese-American men living on Oahu, Hawaii and their cognitive performance on the Cognitive Abilities Screening Instrument (CASI). After age adjustment, the prevalence of poor performance on the CASI declined in a dose–response fashion with increasing height ($p < 0.001$). Among men who were under 5′1″, 25% performed poorly, compared with only 9% among those who were taller than 5′8″. This association remained after removing men who had dementia or stroke (Abbott et al., 1998). In Israel, about

10,000 men initially identified in 1963 at the age of 40–65 were followed to 1999, screened with the Modified Telephone Interview for Cognitive Status (N = 2,040) and evaluated with standard criteria for dementia and AD (Beeri et al., 2005). Body height was measured in 1963 to the nearest centimeter and stratified into quartiles. The tallest group had the highest SES, a consistent finding in the literature. Relative to the shortest quartile, the prevalence of dementia and AD decreased with increasing height. For AD, by comparison with the first quartile, the ORs were, for quartile 2: 0.81 (95% CI = 0.56–1.2); quartile 3: 0.46 (95% CI = 0.31–0.70) and quartile 4: 0.57 (95% CI = 0.38–0.85), controlling for age, SES, and geographic location of birth. A similar dose–response trend was found for VaD. The findings are likely underestimated because nonsurvivors (who died prior to the current study) and refusers had more risk factors for cognitive impairment and were shorter than those included in this analysis.

Knee height, leg length, and arm span have been used to estimate height. Leg length is a better measure of attained height in adulthood, since it remains more stable than height over the life course, due to reduction of trunk length associated with osteoporosis and vertebral collapse (Bannerman, Reilly, MacLennan, Kirk, & Pender, 1997; Mak, Kim, & Stewart, 2006). One study by Kim et al. (Kim et al., 2011; Kim, Stewart, Shin, & Yoon, 2003) found cross-sectional associations between arm span and leg length and dementia prevalence, but this was only present among women. The finding was consistent for both AD and VaD diagnoses. A prospective examination in an American cohort (Huang et al., 2008), the Cardiovascular Health Study (CHS), found that women with greater knee heights and arm spans had a reduced incidence of dementia and AD, but not VaD (HR for AD per inch increase in knee height = 0.78 (95% CI = 0.65–0.93), HR for AD per inch increase in arm span = 0.90 (95% CI = 0.85–0.96)). Among men, only arm span was inversely associated with AD (HR = 0.92, 95% CI = 0.84–1.00). The reason that women show stronger associations compared with men might be that we see the effects of reserve in a more pronounced way in individuals with lower levels of reserve, and women are shorter than men and have smaller head sizes in absolute terms.

In the large 10/66 study of seven countries, the meta-analyzed result for leg length and prevalence of dementia comparing the longest to the shortest quartile was 0.82 (95% CI = 0.68–0.98), adjusted for age, sex, education, and family history of dementia (Prince et al., 2011). The potential longitudinal role of leg length for cognitive decline was examined in 290 African Caribbeans living in the community in south London who were recruited from primary care practices, 216 of whom were seen at baseline and three years later (Mak et al., 2006). Cognition was ascertained from a composite score on the MMSE and other standard neuropsychological tests. Cognitive decline was defined as performing in the bottom 20% of a factor score calculated from a principal components analysis. Leg length was analyzed in relation to the baseline score and the change in score over 3 years. The OR for cognitive impairment at baseline associated with the lowest quartile of leg length was 2.1 (95% CI = 1.0–4.4), but no association was found for leg length quartiles and cognitive decline. This is consistent with the threshold model presented in Chapter 5 in which low reserve is represented by the intercept but not the *slope* of change. Low reserve operates by lowering the intercept, which is associated with the maximum amount of functioning brain tissue throughout the life course.

An important question that remains is whether HC may explain the body stature findings. In one study (Prince et al., 2011), the main effect of leg length moved from statistical significance to marginal nonsignificance when HC was added to the model (0.82, 95% CI = 0.68–0.98 to 0.84, 95% CI = 0.70–1.01). The similarity of the point estimates suggests that leg length likely had independent effects from HC. In the *Kame* Project (Graves et al., 2001), the interactions between HC and APOE-ε4 were not impacted by the addition of height into the model. However, in that study height was itself not a significant predictor of AD (HR = 1.06, 95% CI = 0.90–1.25). The relationships between small head size, short limb length and height, and cognition in older age may all be mediated by poor gestational and childhood nutrition related to both brain and body development.

EARLY-LIFE SOCIOECONOMIC CONDITIONS

The SES of the family of origin can be measured by parental education and occupation, living conditions, and number of siblings. Early-life SES is associated with intellectual or mental stimulation at home, access to education and patterns of socialization. These variables also are associated with intrauterine growth and development, gestational through early-life nutrition, and other factors that we have discussed. No study exists that has included all of these variables, but more evidence is accumulating to suggest that childhood SES may have independent effects from adult-life SES on cognition in old age and on the incidence of dementia and AD. In this section, we focus on early-life SES, but will also discuss adult- and late-life SES.

One of the first reports of an association between early-life SES and risk for AD was from a population-based case–control study of 122 cases of AD and 297 normal controls matched for age and sex identified from an age- and sex-stratified random sample of 1887 persons aged 70 and over living in the Saguenay-Lac-Saint-Jean region of Quebec (Mortimer, Fortier, Rajaram, & Gauvreau, 1998). Data on family history of dementia, educational attainment, and childhood SES were obtained from informants for both cases and controls. Thirty-seven percent of cases and 11% of controls had a positive family history of dementia defined as dementia in one or more siblings. SES in childhood was defined by a question, "What was his/her financial situation when s/he was a child?" Possible answers included: no difficulty, better than most families, about the same as most families, worse than most families, and very difficult. Those reported as having a family financial situation worse than most or very difficult were considered as having low SES in childhood. Adjusting for age, sex, and educational attainment, low childhood SES was associated with a 10-fold increased risk for AD (OR = 10.8, 95% CI = 1.2–94.6) among those with a positive family history of dementia, but no association was found among those with a negative family history of dementia (OR = 1.4, 95% CI = 0.7–2.6). The powerful modifying effect of a positive family history of dementia on the association between low SES in early life and AD suggests that among those with a genetic predisposition to the disease, early-life social disadvantage can play an important role in increasing the risk of the clinical disease at older ages.

As discussed earlier, the risk for dementia increases with increasing number of siblings (Moceri et al., 2000, 2001), consistent with the resource dilution effect that would likely be enhanced in families with lower SES. Moceri et al. also reported that suburban residence was inversely associated with prevalent AD (OR = 0.36, 95% CI = 0.2–0.7). Suburban residence could represent higher SES in the family, given that during the period when subjects would have lived in the suburbs, they were considerably more affluent than those who lived in urban or rural areas.

In the second study, Moceri et al. attempted to reconstruct the early-life environment of these subjects, obtaining birth certificates and census records for 82% of the cases and 87% of the controls (Moceri et al., 2001). Three variables indicative of early-life SES in the model together were predictive of AD: father's occupation (manual vs nonmanual): OR = 2.0 (95% CI = 1.2–3.3); household size 7+ versus <7: OR = 1.5 (95% CI = 0.9–2.4) (not significant); and high school graduate or less versus more education (OR = 1.7, 95% CI = 1.1–2.6). When subjects with no risk factors were compared with those who were APOE-ε4 positive, had 7+ siblings, and had a father whose occupational status was manual, the OR for AD was 14.8 (95% CI = 4.9–46). This is quite remarkable, and shows that the strength of the associations are larger when variables are combined, which is usually difficult to do in a study with limited sample size (292 cases and 282 controls). This also is consistent with our findings for the interaction between HC and APOE-ε4, where we found a combined risk for AD of 12.1 (95% CI = 2.8–53) (Borenstein Graves et al., 2001). The presence of adverse early-life conditions may be particularly important for people who carry genetic risk for AD, a similar finding to that of the Quebec study cited above.

In the *Kame* Project, we used two variables to index childhood SES, small HC (HC ≤ 54.35 cm), and number of children in the home when the subject was age 2–3 (Borenstein, Wu, & Larson,, 2005). Among participants carrying an APOE-ε4 allele, both of these variables were significant predictors of probable AD (HR for HC: 2.56, 95% CI = 1.04–6.34; HR for >4 children in the home at age 2–3: 3.27, 95% CI = 1.17–9.17). This population-based cohort study replicates the findings of increased risk for AD with increased numbers of siblings seen in the earlier Moceri case–control study. Moreover, it extends the earlier findings in Caucasians to a different ethnic group, Japanese-Americans. These findings in combination with those from the Nun Study discussed above point to a number of low reserve-related variables acting in concert to increase the risk for AD among people who are particularly vulnerable because of their genetics or early-life environment.

In the Chicago Health and Aging Project (CHAP), participants' county of birth and 1920 US Census data were used to calculate county-specific literacy rates, percent of children in school, and mean household socioeconomic position for 4,268 participants (Wilson et al., 2005). The exposures were summarized in a composite measure of birth county SES as a *Z*-score ranging from −3.81 to 1.31 with higher scores representing higher SES. Education and occupation were used as measures of adult SES. Childhood household SES was additionally measured using parental levels of education, paternal lifetime occupation, and by asking subjects to rate their family of origin's financial situation when they were a child. Cognitive function was measured by four tests (immediate and delayed episodic memory, perceptual speed, and the MMSE). County and household SES were both related to level of cognitive function measured around age 74, but were not associated with decline in such function, again showing the effect on the intercept, but not the slope of decline. In addition, adult SES partially mediated but did not eliminate the association between county SES and cognition in older age. When adult SES was included in the same model as household SES, the latter was no longer statistically significant.

An important question that addresses the temporal sequence of the life course model is whether SES measured in different time periods affects AD risk equally, or whether a critical time period exists. One of the methodological problems in addressing this question has to do with the use of different measures to measure SES in childhood versus early and late adulthood. For example, the Finnish Kuopio Ischemic Heart Disease Risk Factor Study of 496 men aged 58–64 (Kaplan et al., 2001) measured early-life SES using four variables (mother's and father's education and occupation), while adult SES was measured using the subject's own education only. Of these variables, maternal education was the most important predictor of subjects' cognitive function in midlife. This association remained after adjustment for the subject's own education level, meaning that early-life SES remained important to cognition in mid- to late-adulthood and the effect did not appear to be mediated through adult education.

In a study conducted in Eastern Europe (Horvat et al., 2014), almost 29,000 people age 45–69 were recruited in 2002–2005 from population registers in six towns in Czechoslovakia, Novosibirsk in Russia, Krakow in Poland, and Kaunas in Lithuania. Three measures of cognition were used, a 10-word memory list recall, verbal fluency, and a speeded measure of concentration. Maternal education and access to basic household amenities at the age of 10 (cold and hot tap water, radio, refrigerator, household own kitchen, own toilet) were used as indicators of childhood SES. Adult SES was measured as subject's education (in three strata) and household assets owned (range of 0–11). Structural equation modeling (SEM) was used for the analysis with a latent variable of cognitive function as the outcome. This type of modeling (SEM) is superior to logistic regression-type analyses, since this model can simultaneously take into account both direct and indirect effects. The results showed a significant but weak direct path from the mother's education to cognition in mid- to late-adulthood (ß = 0.21), and a stronger association of the subject's own education with cognition (ß = 1.01). However, the mother's education strongly influenced the subject's own education (ß = 0.50).

The association between deprivation and risk of cognitive impairment in old age may be more pronounced among those who are very deprived. One study that focused on this association was the Chinese Longitudinal Healthy Longevity Survey (CLHLS) (Zhang, Gu, & Hayward, 2008). This study's baseline examination was conducted in 1998 with several follow-up waves. For this analysis, only data from 1998 and 2000 were used. There were over 8,800 subjects aged 80–105 in 1998 recruited from name lists that are commonly available to researchers in China; 4,691 were reinterviewed in 2000. The sample was representative of the oldest old living in 22 provinces in China. The Chinese version of the MMSE was used as the measure of incident cognitive impairment (defined as the change from a score of 18 or greater to a score of less than 18 over the 2-year follow-up). Early-life SES (birth to age 14) was measured by place of birth (urban/rural), going to bed hungry, and education. Education was considered a childhood SES variable because in this period of time, schools were private and only families who had sufficient monetary resources could send their children to school (Zhang et al., 2008). Adult SES was quantified using the participant's primary occupation before age 60 and their current residence (urban/rural). Occupation was dichotomized into two groups (professional/administrative versus lower status jobs). Baseline MMSE score was entered into the model to control for initial level of performance. The analysis showed that a model including childhood SES *but not adult* SES was significantly associated with the odds for incident late-life cognitive impairment. When adult SES was added to this model, higher childhood SES continued to robustly predict a reduced OR for incident cognitive impairment in old age. Among men, adult measures of SES (occupation and urban residence in adulthood) were not associated with cognitive impairment. Among women, adult urban residence reduced the risk for cognitive impairment in old age by 19% ($p < 0.01$) and increased childhood SES continued to show trends or significant inverse associations with the probability of incident cognitive impairment in old age. Men who had the highest SES (born in urban areas, were not hungry, had some schooling, and had a better job) had an OR of 0.24 for being cognitively impaired at baseline compared with men who had all the risk factors. For women, the OR was similar (OR = 0.32).

The studies reviewed above suggest that early-life SES has a persistent influence on cognition in later life, and while some of this effect appears to be the result of higher adult SES among those raised in more affluent circumstances, the early effects of childhood SES remain an important influence on later cognitive outcomes independent of adult SES.

New research shows significant associations between parental SES (education and income in particular) and brain structure in childhood and adolescence. In a cross-sectional study of 1,099 volunteer parents and their children (average age 11.9 (sd = 4.9)) called the Pediatric Imaging, Neurocognition and Genetics (PING) Study (Noble et al., 2015), total cortical surface area among children was positively correlated with parental education and these associations were even stronger for family income ($p = 0.03$ and $p = 0.004$, respectively). Interestingly, the association also was stronger at the lower end of the income distribution, implying that among more socioeconomically deprived children, even a modest increase in family income resulted in a bigger increase in surface area (whereas a smaller increase in surface area resulted from gains in the high income strata). When both parental education and family income were in the model together, only income predicted surface area. In this study, family income was also marginally associated with greater cortical thickness ($p = 0.054$), but parental education was not. Parental education was correlated with children's left, but not right, hippocampal volume. Income was unassociated with either left or right hippocampal volumes. Finally, this study showed that surface area partially mediated the significant effects of family income on performance on four cognitive tests. Building a larger cortical surface area in early life likely leads to more reserve, potentially resulting in a better ability to stave off cognitive dysfunction in late life.

Finally, there are two important studies that have examined the associations between childhood SES and brain imaging features that are commonly seen in dementia and AD. Both of these analyses are from the Scottish Mental Survey of 1947. In the first, the authors examined SES in childhood (age 11) (Staff et al., 2012). In this analysis, 934 of 2,620 participants in Aberdeen were traced in 1998, and 235 had complete data from an MRI sub-study in 2004–2005. Childhood SES data were obtained from the participants when they were 64 years old and an MMSE score <24/30 was used as a screen for a clinical assessment for dementia, which was completed by the study physician. Participants were asked to recall their father's occupation at age 11, the number of public rooms in the family home, and the number of residents expected to share the same bathroom. The subject's education and adult occupation, as well as local area deprivation based on the participant's home address at baseline (using an ecologic quantification) were used to index adult SES. A structural equation model was used to assess the effects of childhood and adult SES on right and left hippocampal volumes. The results showed a significant linear association between childhood SES and hippocampal volumes at age 68 ($p = 0.03$), but not between childhood SES and overall brain volume ($p = 0.53$). However, individuals with high childhood SES had larger brain sizes than those with lower childhood SES, likely reflecting a nonlinear association between these variables. In separate analyses, childhood SES had an important effect on education, which in turn, had a strong effect on adult SES. This study suggests that conditions in early life can have a long-lasting effect on the development of the brain that persists for over 50 years. Alternatively, it is possible that differential atrophy of the hippocampus may have occurred later in life among people with lower versus higher childhood SES.

In a second analysis from the same dataset (Murray, McNeil, Salarirad, Whalley, & Staff, 2014), paternal occupation at age 11 was used to measure childhood SES and the participant's occupation served as the measure of adult SES. Regional scores were derived for white matter, gray matter, periventricular and infratentorial hyperintensities on T2 and FLAIR MRI images. Lower childhood SES was strongly related to greater whole brain white matter hyperintensity burden adjusting for childhood intelligence, education, adult hypertension, and adult SES. Interestingly, this analysis found no association between adult SES and the volume of white matter hyperintensities or other vascular lesions visible on MRI.

The importance of early-life deprivation has been highlighted by the studies reviewed in this section. Most studies of ethnic and racial disparities in adult outcomes do not focus on childhood exposures, but rather on adult conditions and contextual effects in the adult environment, such as adult poverty, access to good nutrition/grocery stores, access to parks, and neighborhood safety. The need to consider the early-life origins of late-life diseases is underscored by the strong associations between childhood SES and outcomes like cognitive impairment or dementia that occur many decades later.

EDUCATION AND INTELLIGENCE

That there is a strong association between educational attainment and performance on mental status and other neuropsychogical tests has been clear for over 50 years (Mortimer & Graves, 1993). Although diagnostic assessment was not performed, Weissman et al. (1985) reported that in a random sample of elderly living in New Haven, CT, the rate of severe cognitive impairment was highly correlated with educational attainment, ranging from 0.2% for those with 16 or more years of education to 6.1% for those with 8 or fewer years. In 1988, we proposed that individuals with more years of formal education are likely to have a reduced risk of dementia or Alzheimer's disease by virtue of having more "intellectual reserve" (Mortimer, 1988). The first large epidemiologic study to consider education as a risk factor for dementia and Alzheimer's disease was a prevalence survey carried out in Shanghai, China (Zhang, Katzman, Salmon, et al., 1990). In that study, individuals with no education had a significantly higher prevalence of dementia than those with formal education. Since then, numerous case–control and cohort studies have considered the association between educational attainment and AD or dementia risk. Several reviews (Katzman, 1993; McDowell, Xi, Lindsay, & Tierney, 2007; Mortimer, 1993; Sharp & Gatz, 2011) of this relationship have been published in addition to four meta-analyses (Beydoun et al., 2014; Caamano-Isorna, Corral, Montes-Martinez, & Takkouche, 2006; Meng & D'Arcy, 2012; Valenzuela & Sachdev,

2006). All of these concluded that low education is an important risk factor for Alzheimer's disease. Three of the four meta-analyses reported pooled risk ratios for low education in incidence studies of dementia of 1.59 (95% CI = 1.43–2.27) (Caamano-Isorna et al., 2006), 1.89 (95% CI = 1.61–2.22) (Valenzuela & Sachdev, 2006), and 1.88 (95% CI = 1.51–2.34) (Meng & D'Arcy, 2012). When Alzheimer's disease was considered as the outcome in place of dementia, the pooled estimates of risk associated with low education were generally somewhat higher: 1.80 (versus 1.59 for dementia) (Caamano-Isorna et al., 2006) and 1.99 (95% CI = 1.30–3.04) (Beydoun et al., 2014).

In addition to the studies demonstrating a lower risk for AD or dementia with high education, a few studies did not find a significant association. However, examination of these studies generally showed RRs less than one, consistent with a protective effect of greater education. Those that did not show a significantly decreased risk with greater education either failed to control for age (Elias et al., 2000); adjusted for variables strongly associated with education, such as occupation, cognitive activity or IQ (Valenzuela & Sachdev, 2006); suffered from a potential selection bias of cases or controls (Beard, Kokmen, Offord, & Kurland, 1992; Munoz, Ganapathy, Eliasziw, & Hachinski, 2000) or lacked statistical power. One of the first null studies was that of Beard et al. (1992), which was based on 241 cases of AD and 241 controls identified by the Rochester Epidemiology Project. Because education was obtained from medical records, the results were based on only 60% of the cases and controls, leaving open the possibility that missing data on education may be related to case–control status.

Given that low education appears to be a strong risk factor for dementia, it is of interest to ask why this may be the case. McDowell and his colleagues (2007) suggested several hypotheses for this association. We list these below with some additions and modifications.

Hypothesis 1. The association between low education and dementia is not real, but is due to bias.

Several authors have pointed to the importance of "test bias" leading to the finding of a higher risk of dementia diagnosis with less education (Kittner, 1986). Community-based epidemiologic studies generally identify potential cases of AD through a screening procedure, such as the Mini Mental State Examination (MMSE). Because scores on mental status examinations are known to be strongly correlated with education (McDowell et al., 2007), well-educated individuals may score high enough on the screening test to evade detection as potential cases. Although this is a possible explanation of the low education-dementia association, examination of those who screened negative in cohort studies suggests that the number of such individuals is too small in most studies to have an appreciable effect on the association (McDowell et al., 2007).

A second way of spuriously producing an association between low education and dementia would be for selection of subjects in case–control studies to be related differentially to education (selection bias). This could happen if, for example, cases identified in a clinic were matched to volunteers in the surrounding community. If more well-educated individuals volunteered, this would induce a selection bias, resulting in the finding that controls were more well educated than cases. It is impossible to determine to what extent this is true. In cohort studies it is usually found that less-educated participants are more likely to die or drop out. Ascertainment of the clinical status of such individuals suggests that many of them become demented after leaving the study. Therefore, differential dropout by education is more likely to result in an *underestimation* of the number of cases with low versus high education and a reduction in the strength of the association between low education and dementia. This is often the case in epidemiologic studies. We are more at risk of making a Type II than a Type I error. However, we must guard against both.

Hypothesis 2. The association between low education and AD is related to the more rapid accumulation of Alzheimer pathology in those with less education.

If low education were a risk factor for more rapid accumulation of Alzheimer pathology, it would be a risk factor for the disease by virtue of this association. However, large autopsy studies have shown no association between educational attainment and quantitative measures of Alzheimer lesions (Bennett et al., 2003; Mortimer, Borenstein, Gosche, & Snowdon, 2005; White, 2009).

Hypothesis 3. The association of low education with dementia is related to risk factors associated with lower SES.

Low SES is known to be related to many adult risk factors for dementia, including poorer cardiovascular and cerebrovascular health. In addition, low SES is a risk factor for infectious diseases and accidents, as well as chronic conditions, including cancer and obstructive pulmonary disease. Adult risk factors for the above conditions, including hypertension, obesity, poor nutrition, smoking, and alcohol abuse, also occur more frequently in persons of lower SES. Therefore, there are numerous pathways through which low education can be associated with dementia. It is remarkable therefore that adjustment for these diseases and risk factors has been shown to have little effect on the association between low education and dementia (McDowell et al., 2007).

Hypothesis 4. Education may be a surrogate for cognitive ability, in particular IQ, which is an important factor influencing dementia risk.

In many cultures, higher educational attainment is related to higher IQ or cognitive ability (Graves et al., 2001; Pavlik, Doody, Massman, & Chan, 2006). In their review of the relationship between education and dementia, Sharp and Gatz (2011) noted that "It appeared that a more consistent relationship with dementia occurred when years of education reflected cognitive capacity." Systematic studies of the association between IQ and dementia risk were undertaken by Schmand, Smit, Geerlings, and Lindeboom (1997), who found that a strong relationship between education and incident dementia in a population-based sample of 1,063 older subjects became nonsignificant when a measure of IQ was added to the model. Education did not have a reciprocal effect, that is, IQ was still significantly associated with dementia (OR = 0.61 (95%

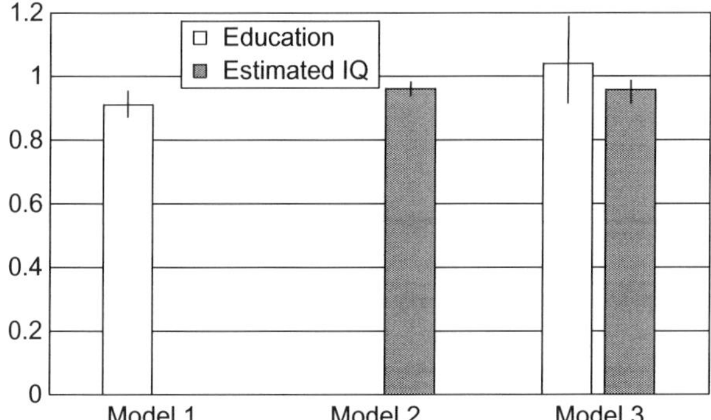

FIGURE 11.2 Hazard ratios for incident dementia, The *Kame* Project. Model 1: Education, adjusted for age; Model 2: Estimated NART verbal IQ (VIQ) adjusted for age; Model 3: Education and VIQ, adjusted for age. Unpublished data.

CI = 0.41–0.91)) in the same model. Similar findings have been obtained in Alzheimer patients where an association between education and decline in cognitive performance was evident without IQ in the model, but was no longer significant when IQ was added (Pavlik et al., 2006). When analyses were carried out using the data from the *Kame* Project, we obtained similar results (Figure 11.2). The fact that addition of IQ to a model containing education eliminated the significant effect of this variable suggests that IQ mediates the association between education and risk of dementia or rate of decline. The published findings are consistent with the view that much of the education effect is likely to be explained by IQ or cognitive ability.

Hypothesis 5. Greater education leads to increased lifelong cognitive stimulation that influences brain growth.

It is important to emphasize that higher education facilitates entry into more cognitively challenging occupations and is likely to increase lifelong cognitive stimulation. Education is usually completed in young adulthood, leaving many decades before death during which cognitive activity can affect brain growth and intellectual development. As discussed in Chapter 17, this effect of education may also be important for decreasing the risk for dementia.

Finally, it is of interest to ask how important education is in accounting for cases of Alzheimer's disease in comparison to other established risk factors. Norton, Matthews, Barnes, Yaffe, and Brayne (2014) compared population attributable fractions for several potentially modifiable risk factors, including diabetes mellitus, midlife hypertension, midlife obesity, physical inactivity, depression, smoking, and low educational attainment. Of these variables, worldwide low educational attainment was associated with the highest PAF, 19.1%. This estimate was based on a meta-analysis of 13 cohort studies yielding a RR of 1.59 for low education (Barnes and Yaffe, 2011). The pooled risk estimate obtained by the same authors based on six case–control studies was higher

(1.89). Had this estimate been used instead, the estimate of the PAF would have been 24.2%. The latter PAF is similar to that for one of the strongest risk factors for AD, family history of dementia in first degree relatives (28.6%), based on the pooled reanalysis of seven case–control studies (van Duijn, Clayton, 1991), and considerably larger than that for another established risk factors, head trauma (3.7%), based on a pooled reanalysis of seven case–control studies (Mortimer et al., 1991).

IDEA DENSITY IN EARLY ADULTHOOD

Prospectively collected information on early-life characteristics is rarely available on cohorts that have been followed for development of AD many decades later. One of the few groups to preserve this type of information systematically are Catholic nuns. The discovery of a treasure trove of information on the nuns we were studying came serendipitously during a visit to one of the retirement convents of the School Sisters of Notre Dame by my principal colleague on the Nun Study, Dr David Snowdon. He happened upon a room that resembled a museum and met the archivist, who showed him a vault with numerous file cabinets containing "high school transcripts, photographs, … and other detailed records describing the sisters' lives from childhood to late adulthood" (Snowdon, 2001).

It would be some time until we began to analyze what would turn out to be the most important document in the archives, an autobiography written by each sister when she took her final vows, around age 22. While we certainly can't claim that the Nun Study began in the early part of the twentieth century and spanned almost 75 years (the actual study did not begin until 1992 when we enrolled surviving sisters who were 75 years or older), we couldn't have asked for better colleagues than the Catholic sister who left detailed instructions for writing autobiographies that were both sufficiently specific to guarantee uniformity and sufficiently long for linguistic analysis. Sisters taking their final vows in the 1930s were asked to: "Write a short sketch of your own life. This account should not contain more than two to three hundred words and should be written on a single sheet of paper. …Include place of birth, parentage, interesting and edifying events of your childhood, schools attended, influences that led to the convent, religious life, and its outstanding events" (Snowdon et al., 1996).

Given the association of lower IQ with higher risk of dementia and the knowledge that many IQ measures are based on vocabulary, we initially focused on the words used in the essays. We decided on two measures, the use of monosyllabic versus multisyllabic words, and the use of less common or rare words. In the analysis of monosyllabic versus multisyllabic words, we found that the sisters who developed dementia more frequently used monosyllabic words. The second measure was based on a database of usage of 10,000 English words prepared in 1921 by Edward Thorndike, a Columbia University researcher (Thorndike, 1921). Using this resource, we examined the vocabulary in the essays for the occurrence of less common or rare words, and again discovered that those who more frequently used rare words in their essays were less likely to become demented 60 years later.

Although the initial findings were encouraging, our findings were limited to the lexical (word) level of analysis. Language also involves grammatical structure or syntax, and content or semantics that might yield additional information that could be used in predicting risk for dementia. In collaboration with Dr. Susan Kemper, a psycholinguist from the University of Kansas, we added two other measures, grammatical complexity, which addresses the average complexity of sentence structure in the essays, and idea density, which measures the number of individual ideas expressed per ten words, a measure of semantic density or information per word of the essay. Analyses of these two measures in the essays we found in the archives were carried out completely blinded to the clinical and neuropsychological assessments. Of the syntactic and semantic measures, grammatical complexity adjusted for idea density was not associated with either dementia or neuropathologic AD 60 or more years later (unpublished data). However, idea density predicted *both* the existence of dementia and the severity of Alzheimer lesions at autopsy.

In our 1996 publication (Snowdon et al., 1996), of 25 sisters who were autopsied and had data on idea density, those whose essays scored in the lowest third of idea density were *59 times* more likely to develop Alzheimer's disease *defined by both neuropathology and clinical expression* more than 60 years later compared to those with idea density in the upper two-thirds of the distribution. However, there was a wide 95% CI (4.6–746.6). The magnitude of this association was unlike anything we had seen in our careers, and we suspected that we had found an early marker or sign of the disease. Given the appearance of neurofibrillary tangles in the brains of people without dementia who died in their 20s and the findings from PET scans of changes in brain glucose utilization around the same age, could it be that a subtle linguistic measure associated with semantic information processing was an early sign of a disease that would not be diagnosed until five or more decades later?

As commonly happens with small samples, the association between idea density and Alzheimer's disease was not as strong when a larger and more representative sample was analyzed. When analyses were carried out later on 164 nuns who were autopsied and had data on idea density, sisters who had the lowest third of idea density were found to be approximately six times as likely to have clinical and pathologic AD, adjusting for age of death and educational attainment compared to those with those whose idea density fell in the upper two-thirds of the distribution (OR = 6.2, 95% CI = 2.96–13.00), still a very strong and highly significant association. This OR, while much smaller, was contained within the original confidence interval. Additional analyses showed that idea density was associated with both clinical dementia (OR = 4.86; 95% CI = 2.44–9.66) and fulfillment of neuropathological criteria for Alzheimer's disease (OR = 3.98; 95% CI = 1.77–8.94). Idea density was also strongly associated with Braak neurofibrillary stage controlling for age of death ($t = 4.53$; $p < 0.0001$).

Although Catholic nuns provided a unique resource to study the association of linguistic measures early in life with neuropathological outcomes, other studies have examined this association with clinical and cognitive outcomes. In the Johns Hopkins Precursors Study, the association between idea density determined from essays written for admission to medical school and later clinical diagnosis of AD was examined in 54 applicants (Engelman, Agree, Meoni, & Klag, 2010). As in the Nun Study, higher idea density at an average age of 22 was associated with a lower risk for Alzheimer's disease. In case–control analyses matched on age and sex, the OR for AD associated with lower idea density was 6.25 (95% CI = 1.11–33.3), despite a small sample size. In another study Farias et al. (2012) followed 81 older adults for an average of 4.3 years. Idea density was derived from oral speech samples at baseline when the participants were already in the age range of risk for Alzheimer's. Lower idea density was associated with greater decline in global cognition, semantic memory, episodic memory, and spatial abilities, consistent with the cognitive decline expected to occur in Alzheimer's disease.

Given the early age at which the writing samples in the Nun Study and the Johns Hopkins Precursors Study were obtained, the critical exposure had to occur either at conception through inheritance of genes or in childhood. Medina et al. (2011) examined the association between idea density derived from autobiographical essays written by 35 nondemented adults at risk by way of familial AD mutations (mean age = 35) and APOE genotype. They found idea density to be related to the presence of one or more ε4 alleles ($p < 0.0001$) and proposed that the risk for AD in persons with low idea density seen in the Nun Study may be mediated by APOE genotype.

Recent analyses of the Nun Study data show that the presence of an APOE-ε4 allele is significantly associated with having low idea density (OR = 2.24; 95% CI = 1.12–4.45). However, adding the APOE-ε4 genotype to idea density in logistic models for dementia and neuropathologic AD outcomes had little effect on the associations of idea density with these outcomes (dementia: OR = 4.2 (95% CI = 2.1–8.8) without APOE-ε4 in the model versus OR = 3.8 (95% CI = 1.9–8.1) with APOE-ε4 in the model; neuropathologic AD: OR = 3.4 (95% CI = 1.3–8.8) without APOE-ε4 in the model versus OR = 3.0 (95% CI = 1.1–7.9) with APOE-ε4 in the model). If idea density *mediated* the association between APOE-ε4 and dementia or neuropathologic AD, we would expect the Odds Ratios with and without APOE-ε4 in the model to be substantially different. We also examined whether idea density predicted clinical and neuropathological outcomes in 150 individuals who did not carry an ε4 allele, and continued to observe a strong association between idea density and clinical (OR = 3.5, 95% CI = 1.5–8.2) and pathologic AD (OR= 4.2, 95% CI = 1.4–12.0) in this group. In ε4 carriers, the OR for clinical dementia was 10.0 (95% CI = 2.2–45.5). Because nearly all carriers of the ε4 allele fulfilled criteria for neuropathologic AD, there was insufficient power to calculate the OR for the idea density-AD association among ε4 carriers.

Although Catholic sisters with low idea density were more than twice as likely to carry an ε4 allele as those with high idea density, low idea density continues to be strongly associated with an increased risk for both dementia and neuropathologic AD in those not carrying an ε4 allele. The very strong association between idea density determined in early adulthood and neuropathologic AD late in life suggests that idea density may reflect genes associated with neuropathologic AD, including, but not restricted to APOE.

Finally, given the strong association between idea density and dementia in late life, it is of interest to ask whether other types of lesions may be involved in this association. Analyses of associations of idea density with both Alzheimer and cerebrovascular pathology at death showed that the association with Alzheimer neuropathology was strong, while no association was found between idea density and the presence or severity of cerebrovascular disease (Snowdon, Greiner, & Markesbery, 2000). Idea density appears to be one of the best early indicators of an Alzheimer neuropathologic process. Although it would be difficult to replicate this measure in other autopsy series because of the lack of systematically collected linguistic samples, oral or written samples of language collected for another purpose could be used to examine whether idea density is a strong predictor of dementia in late life.

Chapter 12

Traumatic Brain Injury

In 1928, Martland published a paper on the neurologic effects of traumatic brain injury (TBI), in which he noted slowed movement, gait disturbances, forgetfulness, and "slight mental confusion" in about 50% of prize fighters (Martland, 1928). Critchley proposed the term "traumatic encephalopathy" for this syndrome and observed that it was a progressive condition with a mean latent period of 16 years (range 6–40) between first exposures as a boxer and development of neurologic symptoms and signs (Critchley, 1957). In 1959, Corsellis and Brierley described the clinical history and neuropathology of dementia following a TBI in a healthy 50-year-old man who had been knocked unconscious for a few minutes in a car accident. Following this TBI, he became confused and gradually deteriorated over time until his death at age 55. On histopathologic examination, he had intense deposition of "typical senile plaques" in all cortical regions examined, especially in the outer cortex. He also had a large number of cortical neurofibrillary tangles. The authors concluded that it is unknown as to whether this was a typical case of AD in which the TBI occurred at the very start of the clinical onset or whether it represented a true "post-traumatic dementia" that arose as a direct result of the TBI (Corsellis & Brierley, 1959). In 1975, Corsellis described a case series of boxers who primarily had tangles in the hippocampus and medial temporal gray matter but very few plaques, and he proposed that chronic traumatic encephalopathy (CTE) and Alzheimer's disease have different pathologies (Corsellis, 1975). Following another case report in 1982 of a 22-year-old man who died 16 years later with typical neuropathologic AD (Rudelli, Strom, Welch, & Ambler, 1982), the findings of the first systematic case-control studies of head trauma and AD were published. These studies addressed two important questions: whether a single blow to the head could increase the risk for AD and whether mild TBIs contributed to its risk. A separate literature evolved for CTE that focused on repetitive TBI in the context of contact sports. In this chapter, we will focus on TBI as an etiologic factor for AD, but will make some comments about CTE in the conclusion.

From a public health standpoint, TBI is the leading cause of morbidity and mortality in the world for people younger than 45 (Sundman, Hall, & Chen, 2014). Globally, 10 million people have a TBI each year. In the United States in 2010,

Alzheimer's Disease. DOI: http://dx.doi.org/10.1016/B978-0-12-804538-1.00012-2

the CDC cites 2.5 million TBIs as an isolated injury or in combination with other injuries (www.cdc.gov/traumaticbraininjury/). In Europe, about one million TBI cases are hospitalized annually. Among civilians, TBI is most often caused by traffic accidents (60%), falls (20–30%), contact sports and work-related accidents (10%), and violence (10%). In athletes, repetitive TBI is common among those who play contact sports such as American football, boxing, ice hockey, wrestling, rugby, and soccer (Moretti et al., 2012). In addition, between 12% and 14% of combat casualties of the Vietnam War were due to TBI, but this has risen to 22% in the Afghanistan and Iraq wars, mostly due to increases in blast-related injuries (Institute of Medicine [IOM], 2009), making military injuries a major cause of TBI. Among older people, TBI incidence has been rising due to increased incidence of falls (61% of TBIs in people over age 65 are due to falls) and traffic accidents (pedestrian, driver, or passenger, 8%). Many TBIs result in life-long disabilities, with attention, memory, and executive function the most affected aspects of cognition (Moretti et al., 2012).

TBI can be defined as a "non-degenerative, non-congenital insult to the brain … from an external mechanical force (usually from acceleration/deceleration forces), possibly leading to permanent or temporary impairment of cognitive, physical and psychosocial functions, with an associated diminished or altered state of consciousness" (Dawodu, 2015). The Glasgow Coma Scale (GCS) is commonly used to measure the severity of TBI and includes items related to eye opening, motor and verbal response, and cognitive function. The Head Injury Interdisciplinary Special Interest Group of the American Congress of Rehabilitation Medicine defines a mild TBI, also called a concussion, as "a traumatically induced physiologic disruption of brain function as manifested by any period of loss of consciousness (LOC), any memory loss for events immediately before or after the accident, or focal neurologic deficits that may or may not be transient" (Mild Traumatic Brain Injury Committee of the Head Injury Interdisciplinary Special Interest Group of the American Congress of Rehabilitation Medicine, 1993). In addition, mild TBIs must have a GCS score of greater than 12, no abnormalities on CT scan, no operative lesions, and involve a hospital stay of less than 48 h. A moderate TBI is defined as a GCS score of 9–12, abnormal findings on CT scan, operative intracranial lesion, and a hospital stay of at least 48 h. A severe TBI is defined by a GCS score of 9 or below within 48 h of the injury.

In epidemiologic studies, when we do not have medical records available or the TBI was not otherwise documented, we must rely on recall for identification of the circumstances surrounding the event, the age(s) at which events occurred, whether there was anterograde or retrograde amnesia, if there was a loss of consciousness (LOC) and for how long, and whether and where the individual sought medical care for the injury. In case-control studies, informant recall of TBI is dependent on the relationship of the informant to the case or control as well as how long and how well they know one another. Recall may be different for informants of cases versus controls, so comparisons on the degree of agreement between controls and control informants may not necessarily be similar to those between cases and case informants were the cases able to answer for themselves. Additionally, we need to be alert to over- or under-reporting on the part of the case and control informants, because these differential errors between the groups will be reflected in the final ORs obtained. The degree of agreement between control and control informants on the presence or absence of TBI has been examined (Graves et al., 1990a). In our case-control study of 130 pairs matched on age, sex, and informant type, 24% of controls were interviewed to assess concordance between responses from control informants and controls. The kappa statistic for TBI was 0.5, indicating moderate agreement. Importantly, when discordant responses were analyzed, the lack of agreement was due to *underestimation* of the control's exposure by the control informant (false-negative reports). In our experience, it is more common for control informants to under-report exposures than for case informants to over-report, as we saw in Chapter 9. Control under-reporting can lead to a Type I error, since lower exposure rates in controls would translate into a higher and perhaps spurious OR for the exposure.

CASE-CONTROL STUDIES OF HEAD TRAUMA AND AD

During the late 1970s and 1980s, many of the first case-control studies included a question about head trauma on their questionnaires. Generally, this was one of many exposures being investigated in these early studies, so details about the head trauma were not sought. In 1983, we published an abstract from the first case-control study on this topic (Mortimer et al., 1983), which was followed by an article in 1985 (Mortimer, French, Hutton, & Schuman, 1985). In the study, 78 AD patients from the Veterans Administration Medical Center were compared with two sets of matched controls—a hospital-based and a neighborhood-based group. Cases and hospital controls were of similar mean age (73.2 and 73.6, respectively), but hospital controls were less educated than cases or neighborhood controls (9.3 vs 10.6 and 10.8 years, respectively). Informants were interviewed for both groups; and 25.6% of cases' versus 5.3% and 14.6% of hospital and neighborhood controls' respondents, respectively, reported head injuries with LOC and the year the event(s) occurred. Matched-pair analyses yielded ORs of 4.5 ($p<0.01$) and 2.8 (not statistically significant) comparing cases to hospital and neighborhood controls. Events among cases occurred between 4 and 62 years before the interview date, with a mean of 35 years; for controls the mean was 40 years. Analysis of false-negative reports was examined by a 10-question survey given to hospital controls, which identified only one false-negative report on the part of the hospital control informants. We took steps to reduce the likelihood of recall bias by masking the hypotheses of the study to the interviewers and subjects. We also argued that if recall bias were responsible for the findings, the head traumas would be concentrated in the years just before symptom onset; this did not occur.

The second case-control study to examine the association between head trauma and AD, by Heyman and colleagues at Duke University in North Carolina enrolled 40 AD cases who had onset of dementia before age 70 and matched them by age, sex, and race to 80 community-based controls (Heyman et al., 1984). Cases were more highly educated than controls. The matched OR was 5.31 ($p < 0.05$). In four of the six cases with TBI, the event occurred 30–40 years before the onset of dementia, and in another case it occurred 19 years earlier. In these five cases, the TBI was accompanied by LOC, retrograde amnesia, and multiple fractures. In the sixth case, the TBI occurred after the onset of the disease. Three controls had had a TBI. One was severe and occurred 40 years earlier; the other two were mild. None of these TBIs was associated with abnormal mental function following the incident. Although this study was based on very small numbers, it provided further support for a potential association.

A number of other case-control studies where head trauma was studied were conducted during the 1980s. In one of these, we obtained more detail about the TBI events than had been done previously (Graves et al., 1990a). We categorized head traumas into three groups: (1) those that led the subject to visit a physician for the injury, (2) those that led the subject to seek hospital care in the emergency room or as an inpatient, and (3) those that resulted in LOC, even for a few seconds. We all hit our heads once in a while, so it was important not to include head injuries that were likely biologically inconsequential. We also gathered data on the duration of LOC, the age at the time of the event, and the circumstances surrounding the event. One-hundred and thirty cases of probable AD from the University of Washington Geriatric and Family Services Clinic were enrolled and matched to 130 controls who were friends or relatives (not related by blood) of the case and case informant. Using friends as controls is appropriate when one is not interested in exposures that are at risk for being "overmatched," such as smoking or other lifestyle habits. For one or more episodes of head trauma with LOC the OR adjusted for age and family history of dementia was 2.9 (95% CI = 1.1–7.53), and for one or more episodes of head trauma without LOC, it was 5.5 (95% CI = 1.35–22.5). This latter OR could be at least in part attributed to recall bias, because control proxies may recall only more severe head injuries. The average duration from the latest head trauma to the reference year (the year before symptom onset as reported by the informant in the medical record) was 21.3 years for cases (range 1–64 years) and 32.5 for controls (range 1–51 years). The difference was not statistically significant ($p = 0.22$). An important observation was that the OR increased as the time since the last head trauma episode decreased ($p = 0.002$). Compared to those with no head trauma, the OR for ≥ 30 years was 1.5 (95% CI = 0.44–5.17), for 10–29 years, 5.0 (95% CI = 1.25–19.84), and for 1–9 years, 9.7 (95% CI = 1.12–83.34). This is of great interest, since we want to know whether head injuries more remotely in time or closer to the onset of dementia matter more. In our study, it appeared that those that occurred when the subject was older were more important. While the increasing ORs with decreasing time before the onset of AD could be explained by recall bias, sensitivity analyses excluding episodes occurring within 5 years of the reference year did not change the interpretation of the findings.

In 1990, we worked with a team of investigators at Erasmus University in the Netherlands on a reanalysis of raw data from 11 case-control studies published in the 1980s (EURODEM) (van Duijn, Stijnen, & Hofman, 1991), eight of which had included TBI as a risk factor (Mortimer et al., 1991). The three studies we have just reviewed were the only ones that had statistically significant findings. Others (Amaducci et al., 1986; Chandra, Philipose, Bell, Lazaroff, & Schoenberg, 1987; Ferini-Strambi, Smirne, Garancini, Pinto, & Franceschi, 1990; Shalat, Seltzer, Pidcock, & Baker, 1987) found elevated ORs (although two found ORs of 1.0 and 1.2), but the ORs were not statistically significant. We calculated the *post hoc* statistical power for these individual studies to detect an OR of 2.0 ($\alpha = 0.05, \beta = 0.80$) and found that it ranged from 12.7% to 40.5%. By contrast, the pooled analysis had a *post hoc* power of 97%. The pooled OR for AD associated with head trauma with LOC adjusted for education, family history of dementia, and alcohol consumption was 2.20 (95% CI = 1.14–4.22) with no evidence of heterogeneity. The higher power offered by the pooled analysis allowed several subgroup analyses. "Sporadic" cases (those without a family history of dementia) had a somewhat larger OR than "familial" cases (OR = 2.31, 95% CI = 1.17–4.84 and OR = 1.42, 95% CI = 0.76–2.71, respectively). There was effect-modification by sex, such that TBI was a risk factor for AD among men (OR = 2.67, 95% CI = 1.64–4.41), but not in women (OR = 0.85, 95% CI = 0.43–1.70). Age at onset of AD did not affect the risk. For subjects less than 70 years of age the OR was 1.95 (95% CI = 1.12–3.48), and for those age 70 and over it was 1.81 (95% CI = 1.03–3.25).

To replicate the study of Graves et al. (1990a), an analysis was run to examine the time from head trauma episode to disease onset ($\leq$10 years and >10 years). Head traumas that occurred within 10 years were associated with an OR for AD of 5.33 (95% CI = 1.55–18.3), while those more remote had an OR of 1.63, which while smaller was still statistically significant (95% CI = 1.04–2.57). This and the finding of Graves et al. (1990a) of increased risk for head traumas occurring closer in time to the onset of dementia have several possible explanations. First, they could be attributed to enhanced case informant recall of more recent events versus head injuries that occurred decades before. The fact that the mean number of years between the injury and disease onset/reference year was similar for cases and controls ($p = 0.21$) in the Graves et al. study makes this explanation unlikely. Second, recovery of the brain from more remote injuries could decrease the likelihood that such injuries would be risk factors for AD in comparison to more recent head injuries for which there would be less time to recover. A third explanation is that head trauma may be more likely to have an impact on triggering AD if it occurs in the presence of significant AD brain pathology. This would favor an association between head trauma occurring at a more advanced age and AD. It is also consistent with the enhanced risk experienced by carriers of the Apolipoprotein E (APOE)-e4 allele, in whom AD pathology would develop more rapidly over the life course, placing carriers at higher risk of triggering AD at younger ages. Lastly, the type of informant may have influenced the times of recall of head trauma events. However, in a separate analysis that retained only pairs that were matched on informant relationship, the pooled OR was higher than the overall pooled OR (2.13, 95% CI 1.37–3.12), indicating that differences in informant relationships did not explain the finding.

Another meta-analysis of case-control studies conducted after the Mortimer et al. paper did not pool the raw data, but analyzed existing publications of studies that followed the original case-control studies (Fleminger, Oliver, Lovestone, Rabe-Hesketh, & Giora, 2003). Inclusion criteria for the meta-analysis included TBIs with LOC, use of the NINCDS-ADRDA criteria for probable or possible AD or the DSM criteria for AD, an attempt to rule out controls who might be demented, symmetric data collection (use of proxies for both cases and controls), and exclusion of controls recruited from psychiatric departments. In addition, sensitivity analyses were conducted for studies that matched on proxy relationship (i.e., case's daughter vs control's daughter). The search procedure successfully retrieved the studies included in Mortimer et al.'s 1991 pooled reanalysis. Of 43 case-control studies eligible, 15 were conducted before 1991 and 21 were published after that date; and of these 15 met inclusion criteria. After stratifying on the eight studies in Mortimer et al.'s reanalysis, seven studies were meta-analyzed using a fixed-effects model. The pooled OR was 1.35 (95% CI = 0.94–1.94), with no significant heterogeneity. The association was again modified by sex, with men incurring a significant risk of 2.26 (95% CI = 1.13–4.53) and women no increased risk (OR = 0.92, 95% CI = 0.53–1.59). The sensitivity analysis that matched on proxy informant type yielded an OR of 1.42 (95% CI = 0.75–2.67). In the Mortimer et al. reanalysis, exclusion of studies that did not match on informant type increased the OR to 2.13 (95% CI = 1.37–1.42). Therefore, the issue of how informant type affects the point estimate remains unclear.

COHORT STUDIES OF HEAD TRAUMA AND AD

TBI has historically been treated as a relatively low-frequency event, with lifetime prevalence estimates around 5–10% for at least one TBI with LOC, but this frequency varies depending on the source of controls selected in a case-control study. For example, an ex-military population would likely have a higher frequency. Because of the relatively low frequency of head trauma, cohort studies of this exposure with risk for AD may be limited in their statistical power to detect a significant effect. For example, in 1,000 people being followed in a cohort study, only about 62 will have had a TBI, and of these, only about 1–2 will develop AD in 1 year. We must keep this in mind when we talk about TBI as a risk factor in prospective cohort studies.

Other methodological problems with cohort studies are related to the nature of AD and its long prodrome, as well as the fact that information on head injuries are obtained at baseline from all nondemented participants. The assumption that everyone who is not prevalently demented is "disease-free" may not accurately reflect the variable degrees of AD pathology in such individuals. The problematic issue here is that people who develop incident AD within the first few years of the study likely have substantial AD pathology and many of them may meet criteria for mild cognitive impairment (MCI). Such participants may be poor historians and omit reporting TBIs that occurred long before baseline. In cohort studies, proxy informants are typically not interviewed along with the "nondemented" individuals at baseline, since it is assumed that they could accurately report their own histories. One study in which both disease-free and proxy informants were interviewed was the Canadian Study of Health and Aging (CSHA), where the investigators were interested in conducting a case-control study as the first phase of a longitudinal study. In the CSHA, the analysis of head trauma as a risk factor for AD using proxy informants and prevalent cases at baseline yielded a suggestive OR of 1.66 (95% CI 0.97–2.84). However, in the same cohort using information from all nondemented participants at baseline, the OR for head trauma for incident cases was 0.87 (95% CI 0.56–1.36). These findings could be explained by the fact that individuals who would soon become demented may not have recalled some head injuries that occurred in the past, while their informants may have recalled such episodes.

Among the cohort studies that found no association with TBI and incident AD, some were from well-known studies such as Rotterdam (Mehta et al., 1999), ACT (Dams-O'Connor et al., 2013), the CSHA, EURODEM, the Mayo Clinic (D. B. Williams, Annegers, Kokmen, O'Brien, & Kurland, 1991), and an early cohort study by Dr Katzman and his colleagues in New York (Katzman et al., 1989). One problem in these studies leading to a null association could be their short follow-up (Launer et al., 1999; Mehta et al., 1999), resulting in under-reporting of TBI from "nondemented" cohort members who developed incident AD shortly after baseline. Another study examined TBI in 811,622 Swedish men who conscripted for military service between 1969 and 1986 (Nordstrom, Michaelsson, Gustafson, & Nordstrom, 2014). The mean age of TBI was in the mid- to late-30s, and the cohort was followed to a mean age of 52, after which 177 early-onset AD diagnoses were made. There was no statistically significant association with one mild TBI and AD (HR = 1.0, 95% CI = 0.5–2.0), at least two mild TBIs (HR = 2.5, 95% CI = 0.8–8.1), or one severe TBI (HR = 0.7, 95% CI = 0.1–5.2). However, the confidence intervals were very wide, indicating a lack of power. Despite the lack of association with AD, these authors did find statistically significant associations with other forms of dementia (vascular, alcohol, and dementia of unspecified type), another fairly consistent finding in the literature.

Conversely, some smaller cohort studies have reported a positive association with TBI. One early study recruited 271 people age 60 and over living in north Manhattan (the prequel of WHICAP) from nursing homes, home care agencies and other healthcare providers (Schofield, Tang, et al., 1997). Participants were followed over a mean of 20.5 months with 48 incident cases of dementia diagnosed. Nineteen head traumas with LOC were found, and the Cox model yielded an adjusted RR of 3.6 (95% CI = 1.2–11.2). This was modified by the duration of LOC (for ≥5 min, the RR for AD was 11.2 [95% CI = 2.3–59.8] and for <5 min, RR = 1.7 [95% CI = 0.4–7.5]). Additionally, people who had their head injury more than 30 years before did not have an elevated risk, whereas those whose head injury was <30 years before did (RR = 5.4, 95% CI = 1.5–19.5), again pointing to the association between more recent head trauma and AD.

Rather than relying on participants' or proxy informants' memories to document head injuries, the use of medical records would increase the validity of exposure ascertainment. An historical cohort study was conducted with Navy and Marine veterans of World War II who were hospitalized during their military service with a nonpenetrating TBI (exposed, n = 548) or pneumonia laceration, puncture or incision wounds (unexposed, n = 1,228) (Plassman et al., 2000). Dementia and AD were identified using a three-phase process, culminating in consensus diagnoses using DSM-III-R and NINCDS-ADRDA criteria. APOE genotypes were available from 46 of 54 incident dementia cases and from 356 nondemented participants. The age-adjusted HR for AD associated with a history of head injury was 2.01 (95% CI = 1.03–3.91) and was larger for other dementias (HR = 3.23, 95% CI = 1.33–7.82). Severity of the head injury was defined as mild (LOC or post-traumatic amnesia <30 min with no skull fracture), moderate (LOC or post-traumatic amnesia >30 min but <24 h and/or a skull fracture), and severe (LOC or post-traumatic amnesia >24 h). While a mild injury did not incur an increased risk for AD (HR = 1.33, 95% CI = 0.51–3.47), both a moderate and a severe head injury did (HR = 2.32, 95% CI = 1.04–5.17 and HR = 4.51, 95% CI = 1.77–11.47, respectively with $p_{\text{for trend}} = 0.0013$). Although there were too few subjects to show a statistical interaction with APOE-ε4, there was an increasing, albeit nonsignificant HR associated with head injuries among veterans carrying one or two ε4 alleles (OR for AD associated with head injury in those with no ε4 alleles, 0.62 [95% CI = 0.24–1.65]; OR for AD associated with head injury in those with one ε4 allele, 1.53 [95% CI = 0.33–7.15] and 4.50 [95% CI = 0.23–88.41] for those with two ε4 alleles). Men who had a head injury also had an earlier age at onset of AD by about 2 years (73.06 [n = 17] in those with a head injury vs 74.94 [n = 18] in those with no head injury), although this finding was not statistically significant. Given that these veterans had their head injuries 50 years before outcomes were ascertained, the authors conclude that their result is "consistent with the perspective that AD is a chronic disease that unfolds over many decades, with an extended latent phase as well as a prodromal stage and the stage of fully expressed dementia" (Plassman et al., 2000).

A more recent historical cohort study of 188,764 US veterans with a mean age of 68 examined ICD-9 codes for TBI and dementia in electronic medical records (Barnes, Kaup, et al., 2014). Because TBI in veterans is often accompanied by depression, post-traumatic stress disorder (PTSD), and cerebrovascular disease, one goal of this analysis was to examine these comorbidities as effect-modifiers of the TBI-dementia association. Data were obtained from the Veterans Health Administration National Patient Case Database and included a random sample of 200,000 veterans who were 55 years or older and had at least one inpatient or outpatient visit at baseline (2000–2003) and follow-up (2003–2012). Prevalent dementia subjects were excluded ($n = 11{,}236$). In this database, the date of the TBI was not available. Fine-Gray proportional hazards regression accounting for competing risks was used. HRs from the fully adjusted models (demographics, comorbidities and psychiatric conditions) were 2.13 (95% CI = 1.20–3.77) for AD, 2.41 (95% CI = 1.35–4.31) for VaD and 4.14 (95% CI = 1.32–13.01) for Lewy body dementia. No multiplicative effect-modification was found for depressive symptoms, PTSD, or cerebrovascular disease and TBI. Instead, these were found to act additively to increase risk for dementia. The age at onset of the dementia was found in this study to be 2 years earlier in those with TBI compared with those without TBI, similar to the study of Plassman et al. (2000).

A different approach to investigating the association between TBI and AD was taken by the Biologically Resilient Adults in Neurological Studies (BRAiNS) at the University of Kentucky's Alzheimer's Disease Center (Abner et al., 2014). The participants in this study were 649 volunteers who self-reported head injury with LOC, and the study examined the timing of the event and duration of LOC, which was dichotomized at <5 min and greater than 5 min. One important feature of this study was that a subset of 238 subjects died and had neuropathologic evaluations. The authors used a multistate Markov chain model that adjusted for competing risks to examine the effect of head injury on transitions between four transient states (normal cognition, aMCI based on neuropsychological testing, mixed MCI based on testing, and MCIcc based on clinical consensus), and three absorbing states (dementia, drop-out, and death). Over a mean of 10.4 annual examinations, the OR for a transition from normal cognition to any type of MCI for participants with a head injury was age-dependent. For a 1-year increase in age, the OR for this transition was 1.21 (95% CI = 1.15–3.56) and for a transition from MCIcc to dementia, it was 1.34 (95% CI = 1.11–1.61). The neuropathologic data revealed that men with a history of head trauma had higher mean diffuse plaque counts in the parietal and occipital regions, including the entorhinal cortex, and more neuritic plaques in all regions of the neocortex compared with men without such a history ($p < 0.05$). Women did not show this trend. The OR for having AD-positive pathology was significantly elevated for men with head injuries compared with those without (OR = 1.47, 95% CI = 1.03–2.09) but this was not observed in women (OR = 1.18, 95% CI = 0.86–1.68). Adjusting for

APOE-ε4, sex, age at death, and congophilic amyloid angiopathy, mean neurofibrillary tangles were not elevated in any region in men compared to men without head injury. An interesting explanation advanced by the authors for the disparity in findings between men and women is that male sex could be a proxy measure for the severity and frequency of TBIs, because in their study, men reported injuries that led to LOC in excess of 5 min more than women. Plassman et al. (2000) also found that risk for AD was elevated for moderate and severe, but not mild, injuries. The BRAiNS study reported that women who came to autopsy were more likely than men to have more than two events with LOC ($p = 0.03$) and were more likely to report a TBI after age 55 ($p = 0.03$). More work needs to be done to tease out the effects of severity of the head injuries, but as we have seen, this kind of information requires studies with very large numbers of participants. Historical cohort studies using medical records may not contain sufficient detail on each event, as we saw in the study of Barnes et al. (2014).

As noted above, case-control studies also have found an elevated risk for AD associated with head trauma in men, but not in women (O'Meara et al., 1997; Salib & Hillier, 1997; van Duijn et al., 1992). One study found this association only in women, although this could have been due to few men in the sample (Mayeux et al., 1993). Multiplicative effect-modification by APOE-ε4 has been seen only in one case-control study, where the OR for AD associated with head trauma and APOE-ε4 was 10.2 (95% CI = 1.2–8.9) (Mayeux et al., 1995; Tang et al., 1996a). Two other studies found the effects of TBI and APOE-ε4 to be additive (Luukinen et al., 2005; Sundstrom et al., 2007), as was suggested by Dr Katzman in 1996 (Katzman et al., 1996). One study (Guo et al., 2000) found an increased risk only among ε4 negatives, while another (O'Meara et al., 1997) found no effect-modification by APOE-ε4. Most studies that have looked at the timing of the injury found that head traumas within 5 or 10 years of AD onset incur the highest risk (Gilbert et al., 2014; Graves et al., 1990a; Mayeux et al., 1993; Schofield, Tang, et al., 1997; van Duijn et al., 1992).

In a Finnish study of 1,113 residents age 70 and over living in five rural communities (Luukinen et al., 2005), 325 individuals who scored 26 or higher on the MMSE were followed for 9 years and mild and moderate TBIs resulting from falls were recorded by a diary method and confirmed by hospital records. Over the follow-up, 23 head injuries occurred among 17 individuals who were treated at the Oulu University Hospital. Dementia was diagnosed by consensus according to DSM-IV criteria. Adjusting for age, sex, APOE, and low education the HR for incident dementia was 2.61 (95% CI = 1.25–5.46). The interaction term for TBI × APOE-ε4 was statistically significant (HR = 4.06, 95% CI = 1.96–8.41), with individual effects for TBI being 2.43 (95% CI = 0.70–8.43) and for APOE-ε4, 1.51 (95% CI = 0.70–3.24), implicating an additive model. However, exclusion of MMSE scores of 27 and 28 resulted in an interaction implicating a multiplicative model. Because this study actually followed subjects through time to document their head injuries using a diary method, the effect of recall bias was minimized.

MECHANISMS

As we have seen, studies have found that a TBI advances the age at onset of clinical AD by about 2 years. Among susceptible individuals, TBI may act as a "triggering" event, pushing people closer to the clinical threshold. This is supported by one study conducted at Mayo Clinic in Rochester, MN, in which medical records were searched between 1935 and 1984 for TBI, and AD was documented using records until 1988 (Nemetz et al., 1999). Among 1,283 TBIs, 31 individuals developed AD and the standardized incidence ratio (another measure of the relative risk) was found to be 1.2 (95% CI = 0.8–1.7). Even though there was no overall effect of TBI on incident AD (the numerator was also quite small), this study did find that the time to AD from the TBI was 8 years earlier compared with individuals who did not have a TBI ($p = 0.015$).

If genetic predisposition is required for TBI to be a risk factor for AD, one would expect that TBIs would not be associated with AD neuropathology in cognitively normal individuals, but would be in those who are on their way to or already have dementia. This was seen in the Mayo Clinic Study of Aging (MCSA; Mielke et al., 2014). In this analysis, 448 cognitively healthy controls and 141 individuals diagnosed with MCI had a Pittsburgh compound B-Positron Emission Tomography (PET) to detect amyloid in living brain, a fluorodeoxyglucose-PET (FDG-PET), and an MRI to measure hippocampal volume. MCIs and controls did not differ by the frequency of self-reported head trauma ($p = 0.74$) or the age at first self-reported head trauma (58 for controls and 56 for MCIs, $p = 0.70$). The main finding was that among cognitively normal controls, a history of head trauma was not associated with amyloid load, hippocampal volume or FDG-PET hypometabolism. Conversely, in those with MCI, persons with head trauma had about an 18% higher global amyloid load ($p = 0.002$), which translated into an OR of 4.95 (95% CI = 1.69–18.29) of elevated amyloid accumulation in TBI subjects compared with non-TBI subjects. In addition, the mean difference in adjusted hippocampal volume, controlling for age and sex between individuals with and without a history of head trauma reached a p-value of 0.07, close to significance. No association was present for FDG-PET. These findings imply that among people who are vulnerable to MCI and dementia, head trauma may enable the neuropathology or cause the cognitive disorder to clinically manifest, but may have less consequence for people who are not inherently susceptible to the disease.

That the AD neuropathologic cascade could be triggered by overexpression of β-amyloid precursor protein (APP) following a TBI was suggested as early as 1991 by Roberts and his colleagues (Roberts, Gentleman, Lynch, & Graham, 1991) and confirmed repeatedly since that time (Ikonomovic et al., 2004; Roberts et al., 1994). These studies reported that severe TBI caused cortical Aβ deposition in 30% of individuals with such injuries. They also noted that the presence of Aβ increased more with increasing age in TBI patients compared with controls (Roberts et al., 1994). TBI patients who fell into the 30% with cortical deposition of Aβ were more likely to be APOE-ε4 carriers (Nicoll, Roberts, & Graham, 1995). In addition, ε4 carriers were found in a meta-analysis to have poorer outcomes post-TBI than noncarriers at 6 months (RR = 1.36, 95% CI = 1.04–1.78) (Zhou et al., 2008). Finally, it has been shown that $A\beta_{42}$ (vs $A\beta_{40}$) is the more common form of the amyloid β-protein produced after a fatal TBI (DeKosky et al., 2007; Johnson 2010, 2012), consistent with the generation of amyloid plaques.

In the hours following a TBI, microstructural white matter injuries occur (called diffuse axonal injuries, DAIs) as a result of shearing of fragile axons by acceleration/deceleration forces (Blennow, Hardy, & Zetterberg, 2012), which lead to swelling and damage to the axonal cytoskeleton. This impairs axonal transport and promotes abnormal production and accumulation of toxic proteins and peptides. In AD, the most affected protein is APP. Other proteins appear to be predominantly involved in other neurodegenerative processes, such as α-synuclein in Lewy body dementia. The increased production of APP leads to the release of excess amounts of Aβ that aggregate to form Aβ plaques. In animal experiments, the extent of disruption of axonal transport is proportional to the severity of the injury. DAI studies in humans and experimental animals also show that axons continue to degenerate and swell for lengthy periods of time and that Aβ continues to accumulate in the swollen axonal bulbs, leading to further abnormal APP metabolism (Blennow et al., 2012). Impairment in this system occurs as a normal part of aging, but DAIs cause an acceleration of this process, advancing the age at onset of an underlying neurodegenerative pathology (Sundman et al., 2014).

As suggested in our early papers on head trauma, a TBI also can result in transient opening of the blood–brain barrier, allowing in materials normally excluded from the brain (Mortimer et al., 1985, 1991). In recent work, it was demonstrated that TBI results in focal microbleeds and breakdown of the blood–brain barrier in the white matter. These areas then become foci of inflammation, which results in degeneration of the white matter (Glushakova, Johnson, & Hayes, 2014). Within minutes after the TBI, microglia aggregate around the site of injury and proinflammatory cytokines and chemokines are released that persist for at least a year (Giunta et al., 2012) and up to 17 years (Ramlackhansingh et al., 2011). Natural flavonoids (see Chapter 15) have been proposed as a potential treatment to reduce the risk for AD after TBI (Diamond et al., 2000; Giunta et al., 2012) by modulating microglial activation and neuronal damage induced by inflammatory pathways initiated by TBI. The chronic neuroinflammation seen after TBI is now the subject of intense research (Faden & Loane, 2014; Johnson et al., 2013; C. Smith, 2013). The blood–brain barrier in the hippocampus has been shown to fail progressively with age in older cognitively healthy individuals and this finding is more pronounced in MCI (Montagne et al., 2015). Thus, changes in the integrity of the vasculature may be an early event that facilitates neuropathologic processes in AD.

TBI leads to progressive white- and gray-matter atrophy, as well as atrophy of the anterior hippocampi, regardless of the location of the injury (Ariza et al.,

2006). While some view TBIs as potentially decreasing neuronal reserve leading to an earlier manifestation of clinical dementia (Lye & Shores, 2000), others have shown that the TBI-AD association is modified by reserve, such that, for example, people with higher education can recover functionally (E. B. Schneider et al., 2014) and cognitively (Sumowski, Chiaravalloti, Krch, Paxton, & Deluca, 2013) more quickly from a TBI compared with lower-educated people. It is clear from the wealth of experimental and pathologic data available that head trauma or TBI is a risk factor for the pathology of AD. However, the bulk of the data suggests that TBI does not "cause" AD on its own, but operates in concert with ongoing neurodegenerative mechanisms that together accelerate neuropathologic processes already in play. This view is consistent with the earlier age at onset of AD following a head trauma, the higher susceptibility to AD pathology following a severe head trauma in people carrying the ε4 allele, and the general finding that head injuries occurring later in life nearer to the time of AD onset appear to have more impact on the incidence of this illness.

POPULATION ATTRIBUTABLE FRACTION FOR HEAD TRAUMA

The population attributable fraction for AD associated with head trauma or TBI using a prevalence in the population of 0.10 and a RR of 2.0, is 9.1%. This estimate will of course vary by sex, with men having a much higher PAF than women.

CHRONIC TRAUMATIC ENCEPHALOPATHY

We end this chapter with a few words about CTE, which shares one neuropathologic characteristic with AD that is attributable to TBI. Much of the work on CTE assumes that it occurs primarily as the result of repetitive, mild traumas as experienced by boxers and professional athletes of contact sports, but more recent work acknowledges that it can be caused by a single blow or episodic blows accompanied by acceleration/deceleration forces (Omalu, 2014). Much public attention is now being focused on American football. Findings from autopsies of National Football League (NFL) players have found neuropathologic changes similar to those found in professional boxers in the twentieth century (Omalu et al., 2005).

CTE is one of the major reasons that TBI was investigated as a risk factor for AD. However, it has a very different clinical and neuropathologic picture than AD. Neuropathologically, very little or no Aβ is seen (except perhaps when CTE and AD overlap in a single person). Hyperphosphorylated tau deposits and neurofibrillary tangles represent the hallmarks of this illness (McKee et al., 2009; Omalu et al., 2005). Clinically, CTE patients show irritability, impulsivity, aggression, depression, short-term memory loss, and an increased risk for suicide. Over decades these symptoms may progress to other cognitive deficits and eventually to dementia (Stein, Alvarez, & McKee, 2014). Among professional

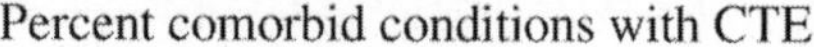

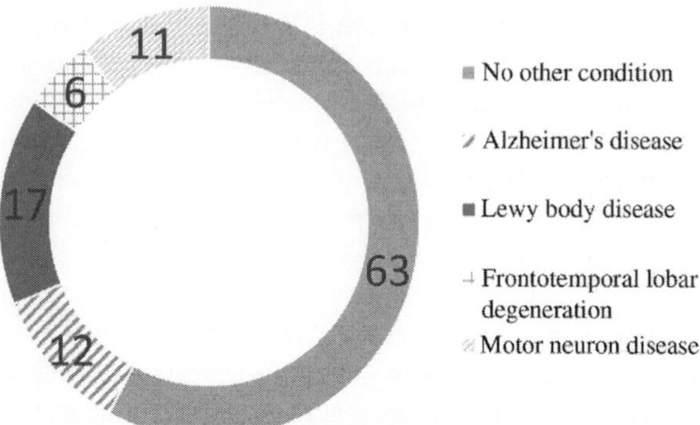

FIGURE 12.1 Percent of CTE cases with other neurodegenerative comorbidities. *Adapted from Stein et al. (2014).*

football players, it has been noted that the severity of CTE is associated with the number of years playing football and the number of years postretirement (McKee et al., 2013), as well as the age at which the individual began playing (Stamm et al., 2015). Among 68 autopsies of persons who had been diagnosed with CTE (all men, aged 17–98 [mean of 59.5] including 64 athletes, 21 military veterans [86% who were also athletes], and one person who engaged in self-injury of the head), 12% had comorbid AD, 17% had concomitant Lewy body disease, 11% had comorbid motor neuron disease and 6% had frontotemporal lobar degeneration (Stein et al., 2014) (see Figure 12.1). Among CTE cases in this series, there was no Aβ deposition. Sparse diffuse and neuritic plaques were observed in about 13%. Marked global atrophy of the brain and decreased brain weight also typically were seen, in addition to severe atrophy of the frontal and temporal lobes, medial temporal lobe, and anterior thalamus. There was also marked atrophy of the white matter.

The distribution of neurofibrillary tangles in CTE is different from AD with extensive tangles found in the more superficial neocortical layers, whereas in AD the distribution is in deeper layers of the cortex. Interestingly, Hof et al. reported that two other presumably environmentally triggered tauopathies, postencephalitic Parkinson's disease (PD) and the amyotrophic lateral sclerosis (ALS)-parkinsonism dementia complex of Guam, also show more superficial distributions of NFTs. In addition, they observed that NFTs in CTE are larger than those found in AD (Hof et al., 1992). Others have shown that phosphorylated tau in CTE tends to be perivascular and distributed irregularly compared with AD (Geddes, Vowles, Nicoll, & Revesz, 1999). Among boxers, APOE-ε4 carriers who were "high-exposure" (had 12 or more professional bouts), had higher clinical ratings on the Chronic Brain Injury Scale than ε4 noncarriers (mean [SD] = 3.9 [2.3] vs 1.8 [1.2], $p = 0.04$) (Jordan et al., 1997). This might imply, that like in AD, if a neuropathologic process is occurring, having an ε4 allele acts as an accelerator, or it could indicate the presence of comorbid AD with CTE.

Because autopsy samples are highly biased, particularly among those case series we have been discussing, the prevalence and incidence rates for CTE in representative samples of NFL players, boxers, military personnel, and other special groups with unique TBI exposures are unknown. One study examined neurodegenerative causes of death, in particular AD, PD and ALS, in relation to having been a professional NFL player (Lehman, Hein, Baron, & Gersic, 2012). They acquired underlying- and multiple- cause-of-death rate files and stratified NFL players who had at least five pension-credited playing seasons from 1959 to 1988 into speed players (all players except linemen and punters/kickers) and nonspeed players (linemen). Standardized mortality ratios (SMRs) were calculated using the US population. As expected, overall mortality among players was reduced (SMR = 0.53, 95% CI = 0.48–0.59) compared with the general population (a good example of the "healthy worker effect"). Neurodegenerative mortality was increased among speed players only (SMR = 4.74, 95% CI = 2.59–7.95). For AD, the SMR for speed players was 6.02 (95% CI = 2.21–13.1); for ALS it was 6.24 (95% CI = 2.29–13.6). No significant findings were observed among nonspeed players or for PD. Others have shown that speed players suffer more concussions than nonspeed players.

In general, the findings regarding CTE suggest that as originally proposed by Corsellis (1975), it likely represents a separate neuropathologic process from AD. However, in those genetically susceptible to AD, particularly at more advanced ages, both pathologic processes can coexist in the same individuals. The inclusion of head injury as a potential risk factor in the early case-control studies was largely motivated by the "punch drunk" CTE presentation in boxers. These studies have led to numerous investigations that suggest that TBI may accelerate existing AD pathologic processes through mechanisms based on production of excess amounts of $A\beta_{42}$, the form of Aβ with the highest potential to give rise to neuritic plaques.

Chapter 13

Cigarette Smoking and Alcohol Consumption

One of the advantages of studying Catholic nuns is that they have fairly similar lifestyle habits, so the confounding effects of variables such as smoking cigarettes and drinking alcohol are minimized. The disadvantage of conducting research in homogeneous populations like these is that these types of lifestyle exposures cannot be studied. Outside the convent, modifiable exposures such as tobacco and excessive alcohol consumption are important public health hazards. In the 1980s when the first case-control studies of Alzheimer's disease (AD) were being conducted, these exposures were included in "fishing expeditions," explorations of many different exposures that might be associated with case-control status.

CIGARETTE SMOKING

The results of the first case-control studies that investigated smoking cigarettes were quite surprising. Most of the associations discovered were inverse. In a pooled reanalysis of raw data from eight case-control studies (Graves et al., 1991), we observed a statistically significant pooled odds ratio (OR) of 0.78 (95% CI = 0.62–0.98), with a strong p-value for dose-response ($p = 0.0003$) for pack-years of smoking (ORs = 0.73, 95% CI = 0.50–1.09 for <15.5 pack-years; 0.63, 95% CI = 0.42–0.95 for 15.5–37 pack-years; and 0.50, 95% CI = 0.31–0.80 for >37 pack-years). Further analyses stratified by the presence of a family history of dementia in first-degree relatives showed ORs that were more protective among those with a family history of dementia compared with those with a negative family history, but this difference did not achieve statistical significance. These studies were matched for age and sex, and the findings remained after adjusting for education level of the participants.

At the time of these studies, strong evidence also was emerging demonstrating an inverse association between smoking and Parkinson's disease (nicely summarized in Wirdefeldt, Adami, Cole, Trichopoulos, & Mandel, 2011). Because Parkinson's and Alzheimer's are both neurologic diseases and some overlap of the two conditions was known to occur (Lewy body variant of AD), the "argument by analogy" was deemed valid at the time. In addition, the inverse

Alzheimer's Disease. DOI: http://dx.doi.org/10.1016/B978-0-12-804538-1.00013-4

association of smoking with AD was consistent with a well-known biologic mechanism. For decades, beneficial short-term effects of nicotine on various domains of cognition were thought to exist (Heishman, Kleykamp, & Singleton, 2010), including working memory and short-term episodic memory. Nicotine is known to bind to presynaptic nicotinic acetylcholine receptors, resulting in increased release of a number of neurotransmitters, including acetylcholine (reduced in Parkinson's disesae (PD)) and dopamine (reduced in PD). Nicotine introduced experimentally is known to increase the number of nicotinic cholinergic receptors in the cerebral cortex and to stimulate the release of acetylcholine (Graves et al., 1991; Perry et al., 1987). Additionally, nicotine improves attention and memory in animal models, effects that are thought to be related to increased activation of the prefrontal cortex, parietal cortex, thalamus, and hippocampus (Heishman, Kleykamp, & Singleton, 2010).

Early on, we and others (Graves and Mortimer, 1994; Riggs, 1992) raised a methodological concern regarding these inverse associations between cigarette smoking and PD and AD. For PD, there were other explanations, for example, the propensity to smoke may be decreased for people who may have a lower complement of dopamine throughout the life course and are destined to develop PD in late-life. For AD, if smokers who develop AD are more likely to die than nonsmokers who develop AD, smoking-AD cases will be differentially under-ascertained in case-control studies (using either prevalent or incident cases), and smoking will appear to be inversely associated with AD. For example, it has been reported that 5-year mortality is greater in demented smokers (HR = 3.5, 95% CI = 1.4–8.8) than in nondemented smokers (HR = 0.8, 95% CI = 0.5–1.2; $p_{\text{for interaction}} = 0.04$) (Wang, Fratiglioni, Frisoni, Viitanen, & Winblad, 1999).

In addition to a survival bias potentially explaining the inverse association between smoking and AD in case-control studies, other methodological problems may be even more important. For example, early case-control studies, in an effort to focus on pure AD, excluded cases with a history of cerebrovascular disease. This exclusion was not applied to controls, who were often identified from other hospital patients who were more likely to have smoking-related diseases. The combination of selecting patients without smoking-related conditions like stroke with the selection of controls who were likely to have smoking-related diseases could easily lead to inverse associations with smoking and smoking intensity. In the case of smoking, a variable that one would think is relatively easy to measure, methodological concerns make this exposure a relatively complex one to study in AD.

The prospective cohort studies would provide further evidence of the role of smoking in the etiology of AD. However, as we shall see, the association would be positive rather than inverse. Because these studies enumerated incident cases of all-cause dementia and clinical subtypes that allowed for "possible" AD diagnoses involving processes other than "pure" AD, vascular risk factors, including smoking, began to emerge as potential causes of this disease. We know that smoking is a major risk factor for all stroke types (Shah & Cole, 2010), so it is not surprising that smoking is associated with vascular dementia (VaD) and vascular cognitive impairment (VCI). Smoking increases the risk for VaD independently of stroke status. Therefore, smoking may impact risk for VaD through mechanisms other than completed strokes (Beydoun et al., 2014). The association between smoking and increased risk for incident AD could be explained by smoking-related oxidative stress and inflammation in addition to its effect on cerebrovascular disease, which increases the risk of clinical expression of AD.

One of the early prospective studies to examine smoking as a risk factor for AD was the Rotterdam Study (Ott et al., 1998). Over an average of 2.1 years of follow-up, 105 incident cases of AD were identified in a population of almost 7,000 people age 55 and over. Current smokers had a 2.2-fold (95% CI = 1.3–3.6) increased risk for AD compared with never-smokers. This association was more pronounced in men (RR = 5.8, 95% CI = 1.6–20.9) than in women (RR = 2.0, 95% CI = 1.0–3.7). Risks were not statistically elevated for all former smokers, but were for former male smokers (RR = 3.9, 95% CI = 1.1–13.5). A second paper from the same study (Reitz, den Heijer, van Duijn, Hofman, & Breteler, 2007) published 8 years later after a mean follow-up of 7 years found an attenuated risk estimate for AD (HR = 1.56, 95% CI = 1.2–2.0) when the cohort was older.

In 1999, a pooled reanalysis of data from four population-based cohort studies in Europe (the Odense study from Denmark, the PAQUID study from France, the Rotterdam Study from The Netherlands, and the MRC-ALPHA Study from the United Kingdom) (Launer et al., 1999) reported an overall RR for AD of 1.74 (95% CI = 1.21–2.50) for current smoking versus never-smoking, and a RR for AD of 1.19 (95% CI = 0.80–1.51) for former smoking. Again, estimated risks were higher among men who were current smokers (RR = 3.17, 95% CI = 1.42–7.07) compared with women (RR = 1.50, 95% CI = 0.94–2.40, $p_{\text{for interaction}} = 0.16$). Interestingly, the association was only present among people without a family history of dementia (RR = 2.28, 95% CI = 1.49–3.50); there was no association of smoking in people with a family history. A similar finding was found in the Rotterdam Study with regard to Apolipoprotein E (APOE)-ε4 (Ott et al., 1998). Smokers who did not carry an APOE-ε4 allele had a pronounced increased risk (RR = 4.6, 95% CI = 1.5–14.2), compared with the RR for AD among smokers who were APOE-ε4 positive (RR = 0.6, 95% CI = 0.1–4.8). In the study of Launer et al., the Rotterdam Study contributed 34% of the total sample to the pooled analysis, so it is likely that some of this finding was to some extent driven by that study.

In the WHICAP cohort in New York, current smoking was found to increase risk for AD among 142 incident cases, with an adjusted RR = 1.7 (95% CI = 1.1–2.8) (Merchant et al., 1999); former smoking incurred no increased risk (RR = 0.7, 95% CI = 0.5–1.1). The main effect of smoking was examined for interaction with a composite vascular disease variable, and some evidence was found for additive, but not multiplicative, interaction. Stratification also was performed by APOE-ε4 status, and the authors reported that the association was present only among ε4 noncarriers (RR = 2.1, 95% CI = 1.2–3.7), as shown in other studies.

Some studies have produced null findings. For example, the Kungsholmen Study found no effect of smoking over a 3-year follow-up period (HR for incident AD for ever smoking = 1.1, 95% CI = 0.5–2.4). This cohort was older than that in many studies, which may have reduced the risk due to smoking-related mortality. Because there could be a differential bias by mortality among prospective studies (e.g., with ε4 carriers who smoke having a higher mortality before and during a prospective study), it would be more informative to examine this association using smoking in midlife as the exposure.

Midlife exposure was studied in the Cardiovascular Risk Factors, Aging and Dementia (CAIDE) study (Rusanen et al., 2010). Participants were selected from four population-based samples that formed different studies starting in 1972. At baseline, the participants were on average almost 51 years old. Follow-up about 21 years later was conducted with a random sample of 1,449 survivors age 65–79 in 1998. In this study, smoking in midlife increased the risk for AD 6.6-fold (95% CI = 1.80–23.94) among APOE-ε4 carriers (the opposite from findings from earlier studies showing the association only among ε4 noncarriers), and an inverse, but nonstatistically significant (RR = 0.56, 95% CI = 0.11–2.88) risk was observed among ε4 noncarriers. The risk in the overall sample (regardless of APOE status) was 2.17 (95% CI = 0.87–5.36). Imputing the status of nonparticipants who were somewhat older, less educated and less healthy on vascular variables such as blood pressure and cholesterol in a sensitivity analysis, the RR was 0.86 (95% CI = 0.49–1.52). This study is important in that smoking was measured in midlife and the follow-up was very long. Overall, the findings paint a mixed picture, with midlife smoking a risk factor for incident AD only in certain subgroups.

Hernan, Alonso, and Logroscino (2008) examined 12 prospective cohort studies published between 1989 and 2007. They reported a weighted average RR of 1.71 for AD among smokers compared with nonsmokers for studies for which the minimum age category at baseline was 55–64 (two studies), an RR of 1.17 for those that used a minimum age stratum of 65–74 (seven studies), and an RR of 0.52 for those using a minimum age stratum of 75 years (three studies). In cohort studies, Hernan et al. postulate that most smokers who are susceptible to AD already develop the disease by age 75. Therefore, the cohort studies including only older age groups are already depleted of susceptible smokers, leading to an apparent inverse association between smoking and incident AD (Hernan et al., 2008). The authors also noted that other risk factors that we will explore later, such as hypertension and obesity, also have their adverse effects in midlife, and in very old people, such risk factors may be protective.

Rusanen, Kivipelto, Quesenberry, Zhou, and Whitmer (2011) used medical records from the Kaiser Permanente Medical Care Program of Northern California to examine the midlife effects of smoking by number of cigarettes smoked. If there is a dose-response association between the exposure and the disease, that is, the higher the exposure, the higher the risk for disease (or with an inverse association, the higher the exposure, the lower the risk for disease), our confidence would be increased in concluding that the exposure is causally associated with the disease. Dose-response is only one of the causal criteria that we use in epidemiologic causal inference, but it does give us biologic support for the association. In this study, the authors electronically traced the medical records of participants in this health maintenance organization among those who participated in the Multiphasic Health Checkup in San Francisco and Oakland in 1978–1982 when they were on average 58 years old. Follow-up was 23.1 years, and among 21,123 people in this analysis, there were 1,136 AD cases, 416 VaD cases, and dementia diagnoses in 5,367 people. Former smoking (quitting by age 58) again was not associated with any outcome (dementia, AD, or VaD by ICD-9 codes). The results are shown in Figure 13.1. While there was a slightly increasing risk with increasing strata of pack-years, the increasing risk was not linear, and the elevated risk was most evident in those smoking two packs of cigarettes or more per day at midlife. An editorial about this paper

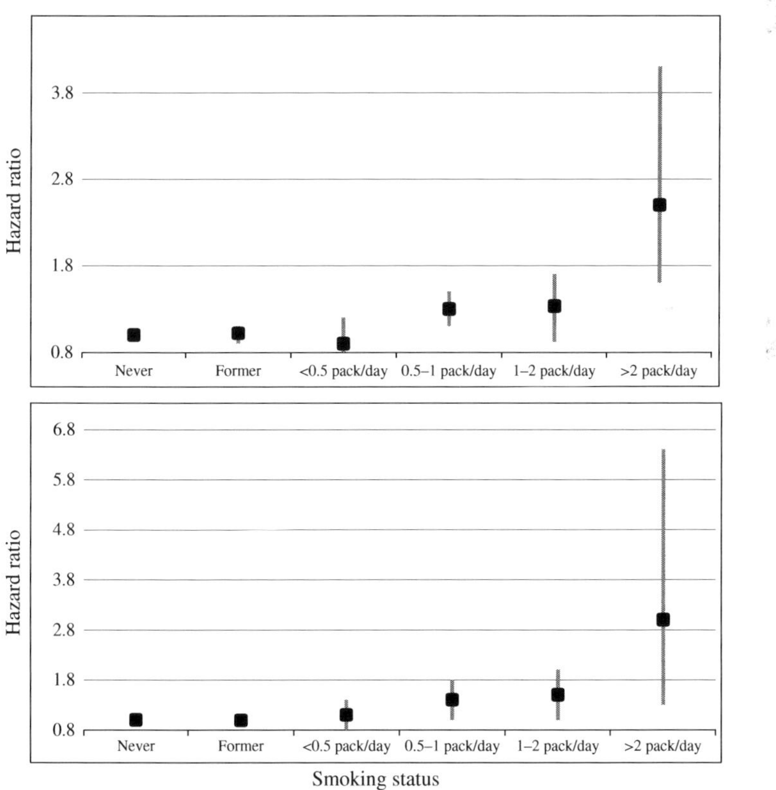

FIGURE 13.1 Hazard ratios for AD (upper panel) and VaD (lower panel) with 95% CI according to smoking amount in midlife. Values from Cox proportional hazards models adjusted for age, sex, education, race, marital status, hypertension, high cholesterol, BMI, diabetes, heart disease, stroke, and alcohol drinking. *Adapted from Rusanen et al. (2011).*

called attention to the fact that chronic smoking is associated with global brain atrophy (Pines, 2011).

Two papers that have meta-analyzed the smoking-AD association also bear discussing. In the first (Anstey, von Sanden, Salim, & O'Kearney, 2007), researchers from Australia conducted a meta-analysis limited to studies that were prospective, and reported outcomes for dementia and its subtypes and for cognitive decline. Incidence waves had to be at least 12 months apart. Data on smoking at baseline were required, and any study with a sample size of less than 50 was excluded. The final sample included 19 papers, 10 of which measured the association of smoking with AD (rather than dementia). For current versus never-smoking, four studies were included in the analysis for AD, and the pooled measure of association was 1.79 (95% CI = 1.43–2.23). The pooled estimates for former versus never and ever versus never-smoking were not statistically significant. Only two studies met inclusion criteria for the outcome of VaD, and the pooled estimate here for current versus never-smoking was similar to that for AD (RR = 1.78, 95% CI = 1.28–2.47). For the analysis of annual cognitive change (using the MMSE), three studies were included and the effect size was –0.13 MMSE points per year (95% CI = −0.18 to −0.08) comparing current smokers to nonsmokers. In this meta-analysis, all of the included studies utilized elderly cohorts. Therefore, the effect size may be smaller than in the population at large if one were able to include people who smoked and developed AD but who died before they could participate in a study. The included studies also adjusted for different confounders, so residual confounding cannot be ruled out.

In a second meta-analysis, Peters, Poulter, et al. (2008) searched the literature between 1996 and 2007. Twenty-three studies, including mostly cohort studies were selected. Of these, six found no association between current smoking and dementia or cognitive decline, five found an association between current smoking and incident dementia, and seven found an elevated risk between smoking and risk of cognitive decline. No studies found an association between former smoking and incident dementia or cognitive decline. The pooled analyses compared current versus former and never-smokers. The RR for AD was similar to the study of Anstey et al. (2007) (RR = 1.59; 95% CI = 1.15–2.20). For VaD, the RR was nonsignificant (RR = 1.35, 95% CI = 0.90–2.02), and this was also true for cognitive decline, 1.20 (95% CI = 0.90–1.59). For analyses of former smokers compared with never-smokers, none of the point estimates was statistically significant. This meta-analysis used somewhat different databases and search terms, yielding divergent results from the Anstey et al. paper. Both papers caution the reader about the results for former smokers, as nondifferential misclassification may have obscured the findings. Neither meta-analysis investigated the existence of a dose-response association using more detailed measures of exposure to tobacco smoking, such as pack-years.

On the basis of the Peters et al. meta-analysis, Barnes and Yaffe (2011) estimated a population attributable fraction of almost 14% (4.7 million) of AD cases globally (11% in the United States) could be prevented if smoking could be eliminated (using a prevalence of smoking of 27.4% globally and 20.6% in the United States). Furthermore, if smoking could not be totally eliminated, but reduced by only 25%, this would prevent one million of existing cases today globally and 130,000 in the United States.

Mechanisms

In the last 15 years or so, much research has been done on the molecular mechanisms that are impacted by smoking. Whereas early studies focused primarily on the vascular and pulmonary systems, more recent work has focused on neurobiologic and neurocognitive sequelae of smoking (Durazzo, Mattsson, & Weiner, 2014). In their comprehensive review, Durazzo et al. suggest that smoking is linked to biologic functions that can impact mild cognitive impairment (MCI) and AD. Chronic exposure to cigarette smoke and nicotine causes a state of chronic oxidative stress, which upregulates activity in the pathways that propagate Aß isoforms ($Aß_{1-40}$ and $Aß_{1-42}$) and abnormal phosphorylation of tau. These authors have also shown that current smokers demonstrate a higher 2-year rate of global brain atrophy compared with never-smokers in anterior frontal, temporal, posterior cingulate, and posterior parietal regions (Durazzo, Meyerhoff, & Nixon, 2010).

In the same paper (Durazzo et al., 2014), the authors conducted an analysis from the Alzheimer Disease Neuroimaging Initiative (ADNI). ADNI investigates the use of biomarkers, including blood-based, cerebrospinal fluid, magnetic resonance imaging (MRI), and Positron Emission Tomography (PET) imaging in over 1,000 cognitively normal individuals, MCI, and AD from 55 research centers in the United States (for more information, see www.adni.org). They compared 109 cognitively normal people age 65 and over who had ever smoked for 1 year or longer (12 current and 97 former smokers) to 154 similar people who had never smoked. All subjects received Florbetapir F-18 PET scans that show binding to fibrillar Aß deposits in neuritic plaques. Although the data were not given, the groups were said to be similar by sex, APOE-ε4 status, vascular and Chronic Obstructive Pulmonary Disease (COPD) medications, lipid profiles, modified Hachinski scores (measuring cerebrovascular risk), and white matter hyperintensity volumes on MRI. However, smokers were more likely to have had a history of alcohol abuse. The composite gray matter florbetapir retention cut-off of ≥ 1.11 was considered amyloid-positive in this study. Current and former smokers were more likely to be amyloid-positive compared with never-smokers in the cingulate, temporal, parietal areas and for composite gray matter (p-values around 0.02 or less). When former smokers were considered separately from current smokers, results were similar to the analyses in which former and current smokers were treated together (89% of smokers were former smokers). However, there was no association with florbetapir retention for any smoking dose variable (pack-years, lifetime years or years since smoking cessation). The authors state that the lack of dose-response associations might be due to confounding by other variables ("premorbid or comorbid factors") or that the amyloid deposition in their cohort may have been stable for many years (Durazzo et al., 2014).

About 30% of cognitively normal people age 65 and over have a positive florbetapir retention level, overlapping with people who have MCI or AD, though these results vary, likely due to methodological differences between studies (Chetelat et al., 2013). Interestingly, this 30% is in agreement with the proportion of cognitively normal individuals found in community-based studies who meet neuropathologic criteria for AD at death (Bennett, Schneider, Arvanitakis, et al., 2006; Snowdon et al., 1996). In the study of Durazzo et al. (2014), the proportion of smokers that had amyloid-positive PET scans was 40%, compared with 25% for never-smokers. They conclude that this elevated proportion among smokers is 10% higher than expected for this age group of cognitively normal persons. However, the crucial analysis, comparing current smoking to never-smoking was not done, likely due to small sample size ($n = 12$). Most studies of AD do not observe former smoking to be a risk factor for AD, and in fact, former smoking also is known not to be associated with the risk for stroke (Wolf, D'Agostino, Kannel, Bonita, & Belanger, 1988), one of the primary mechanisms by which the increased risk for AD or dementia may occur.

Finally, lifetime smoking is associated with other poor lifestyle habits, such as excessive alcohol consumption, poor dietary and physical activity patterns, depression and increased risks for cardiovascular and cerebrovascular diseases. Smoking also is associated with lower education and socioeconomic levels (Clare et al., 2013). Lower SES sets the stage for increased vascular disease, which in turn increases the risk for AD. The life course chains of risk and accumulation models likely apply here with regard to risks that act as intermediates and as interactions over the decades. While further work is necessary to determine what direct effects smoking may have on the pathogenesis of AD, it most likely reduces adult brain reserve through its cerebrovascular effects, facilitating clinical expression of the disease.

ALCOHOL CONSUMPTION

Individuals who abuse alcohol may develop cognitive dysfunction that is characterized by deficits in multiple domains, rather than a more typical amnestic syndrome that is the hallmark of AD. Binge-drinkers include alcoholics and problem drinkers. Problem drinkers are not addicted to alcohol but can become disinhibited in public places or on the road. In the United States, about 7% of adults and 19% of adolescents are alcoholics or have a drinking problem, and alcohol consumption is responsible for over 100,000 deaths per year, accounting for 5% of total mortality in the country (Brust, 2010). Wernicke encephalopathy and Korsakoff syndrome are caused by a deficiency in thiamine (vitamin B_1), which is commonly seen in alcoholics. Wernicke encephalopathy damages the thalamus and hypothalamus, while Korsakoff syndrome occurs when there is permanent damage to the hippocampus. Wernicke-Korsakoff syndromes are relatively rare (0–2% internationally) and both diseases have been recognized since the late 1880s (even before Alzheimer's disease).

"Alcoholic dementia" can be present without Wernicke syndrome or even without thiamine deficiency. On CT scanning, ventricular and sulcal enlargements coupled with whole brain volume atrophy are seen. This atrophy can reverse upon cessation of drinking. Women show greater susceptibility to the effects of alcohol, but also a greater ability to recover (Mann et al., 2005). Proposed mechanisms for alcohol's neurotoxicity include glutamate excitotoxicity, oxidative stress (in some cases aggravated by thiamine deficiency), hyperhomocysteinemia resulting from folate deficiency, as well as reduction of brain-derived neurotrophic factor (BDNF) and nerve growth factor (Miller, King, Heaton, & Walker, 2002).

How much is too much? The National Institute on Alcohol Abuse and Alcoholism defines "at-risk" or "heavy" drinking as more than four drinks on any day or 14 drinks per week for men and more than three drinks on any day or seven drinks per week for women. Men over age 65 are advised to reduce their alcohol consumption to the recommended amounts for women, due to interactions with medications and presence of comorbid conditions.

The inverse association between light-to-moderate drinking and cardiovascular disease outcomes and all-cause mortality is well-known. Ronksley, Brien, Turner, Mukamal, and Ghali (2011) conducted a meta-analysis of 84 prospective cohort studies comparing alcohol drinkers at baseline (defined as "active alcohol" consumption) to lifetime nondrinkers ("teetotalers") for overall mortality, mortality from cardiovascular disease and coronary heart disease, incident coronary heart disease, incident stroke, and stroke mortality. Mean follow-up time in these studies was 11 years, and on average six confounding factors were adjusted (range 0–18). Pooled RRs and 95% CIs were, for overall mortality, RR = 0.87 (95% CI = 0.83–0.92); for cardiovascular disease mortality, RR = 0.75 (95% CI = 0.70–0.80); for coronary heart disease mortality, RR = 0.75, (95% CI = 0.68–0.91); for incident coronary heart disease RR = 0.71 (95% CI = 0.66–0.77); for incident stroke, RR = 0.98 (95% CI = 0.91–1.06); and for stroke mortality, RR = 1.06 (95% CI = 0.91–1.23). Analyses to examine dose-response (in grams of alcohol/day) revealed protective RRs for cardiovascular/coronary heart disease outcomes at levels of 2.5–14.9 g alcohol per day (≤1 drink). In addition, for stroke incidence and mortality, and for cardiovascular disease mortality, the dose-response data were consistent with U or J-shaped curves (example in Figure 13.2), indicating higher risks with heavier drinking. The RR for incident stroke associated with >60 g/day (over 4 drinks per day) was 1.62 (95% CI = 1.32–1.98). The lack of a significant association for "active" drinking versus teetotalers on stroke could be due to the canceling effect of the two parts of the J-shaped curve. A meta-analysis in 2003 showed that while drinking more than 60 g of alcohol per day increased the risk for total stroke (RR = 1.64, 95% CI = 1.39–1.93), drinking less than 12 g per day

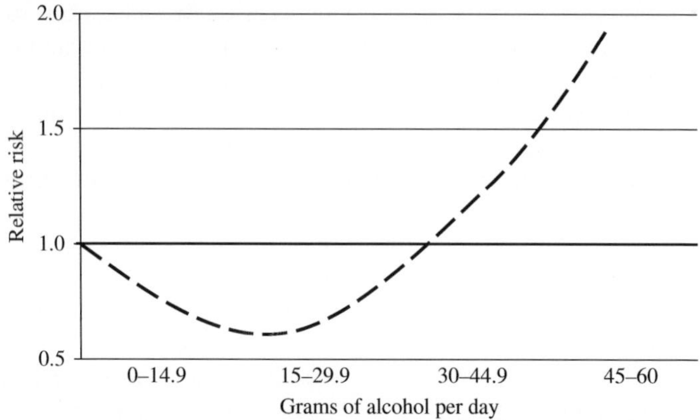

FIGURE 13.2 J-shaped curve for the relationship between alcohol consumption and cardiovascular and cerebrovascular outcomes.

reduced this risk (RR = 0.83, 95% CI = 0.75–0.91). Similar risks were seen for both ischemic and hemorrhagic stroke (Reynolds et al., 2003). This is relevant, because overt and clinical strokes are the major determinants for VaD and cerebrovascular disease greatly increases the expression of AD. These associations are discussed in more detail in the following chapter.

There are several published meta-analyses of alcohol and cognitive outcomes. The earliest was a pooled reanalysis of case-control studies of AD that we conducted with the EURODEM Risk Factors group (Graves et al., 1991) that showed no effect. In a later meta-analysis of published studies (Peters, Peters, Warner, Beckett, & Bulpitt, 2008), 26 papers based on prospective cohort studies were included, with most studies having five or more years of follow-up. Most studies were from North America and Europe. A methodological problem with such a meta-analysis is that exposure definitions were nonuniform, varying from number of daily or weekly drinks, to examining only wine consumption, stratifying drinks by sex, or classifying "frequent" and "infrequent" drinkers. These nonstandardized definitions plague the field and result in difficulties in comparing studies and thus in drawing firm conclusions from the data. If we look at the overall direction of the RRs from these studies, a trend is evident. Of 27 point estimates given, only five were 1.0 or higher, with the remaining estimates being less than 1 (52% were inversely statistically significant). The pooled RR was 0.63 (95% CI = 0.53–0.75) for all incident dementias. Looking specifically at AD as the outcome, 13 point estimates resulted in a pooled RR of 0.57 (95% CI = 0.44–0.74). Five point estimates were used in the analysis for VaD; the pooled RR was 0.82 (95% CI = 0.50–1.35). No significant finding emerged when the authors considered cognitive decline as the outcome. The authors discuss these findings in light of varying methodologies among the studies, different periods of follow-up, various definitions of exposures (which the authors collapsed to obtain their pooled estimates), and definition of the term, "low-to-moderate alcohol levels," which varies significantly by country. In addition, the extent to which studies obtained information about past alcohol consumption habits versus only current drinking varied.

In a second meta-analysis, 15 prospective studies with follow-ups ranging from 2 to 8 years estimated pooled RRs for incident dementia or AD (9 studies), VaD (5 studies), MCI, cognitive impairment, or cognitive decline (18 studies) (Cummings et al., 2013). Most studies compared drinkers in strata of use (ranging from very light to moderate or heavy, or zero drinks versus number of drinks per day or week). The definition of "light and moderate consumption" was not modified from the original studies for this analysis. Sufficient data were present to compare light and moderate drinkers to teetotalers, and heavy drinking versus teetotalers for AD, VaD, and any dementia. Data were not sufficiently comparable for the outcomes of cognitive impairment or cognitive decline. For light-to-moderate drinkers versus teetotalers, the pooled RR for AD was 0.72 (95% CI = 0.61–0.86) with significant heterogeneity ($p = 0.04$); for VaD, 0.75 (95% CI = 0.57–0.98) and for any dementia, 0.74 (95% CI = 0.61–0.91). Effect estimates were somewhat stronger among men [light-to-moderate drinkers had an RR = 0.58 for AD (95% CI 0.45–0.75) with women light-to-moderate drinkers having an RR = 0.83 (95% CI = 0.81–0.85)]. Interestingly, no significant increased risk estimates were found comparing heavy/excessive drinkers to teetotalers. It is possible that older age cohorts have healthier participants, and that heavy drinkers are excluded from these studies due to comorbidity or death. Unfortunately, neither meta-analysis was able to analyze data by beverage type or look at interactions with other variables, such as APOE genotype.

In a study restricted to women, the Women's Health Initiative Memory Study (WHIMS; Espeland et al., 2005), the potential protective effect of alcohol on cross-sectional performance of cognition and on incidence of MCI and probable dementia was examined. This study was considered the "definitive" study of postmenopausal hormone replacement therapy and its alleged protective role on cognition, MCI, and dementia/AD, which we will examine further in Chapter 19. The WHIMS followed 4,461 community-dwelling women aged 65–79 for about 4.2 years and examined cognitive decline on the Modified Mini-Mental State Examination (3MSE) as well as clinical incidence of MCI and dementia at 39 academic centers around the United States between 1996 and 2002. For less than 1 drink per day versus 0 drinks per day, the OR for a decline in 3MSE score (possible score range 0–100) of 8 points or more was 0.69 (95% CI = 0.49–0.97) in the crude model and 0.53 (95% CI = 0.28–0.99) in the fully adjusted model. Covariate adjustment included age, number of years since menopause, education, ethnicity, family income, smoking status, body mass index (BMI), presence of hypertension, prior cardiovascular disease, prior hormone treatment, and use of statins and aspirin. The fully adjusted model showed a HR for incident probable dementia (by DSM-IV criteria) of 0.81 (95% CI = 0.56–1.16) for <1 drink per day, and 0.57 (95% CI = 0.31–1.09) for ≥1 drink per day.

The Italian Longitudinal Study on Aging is a prospective study investigating 5,632 participants aged 65–84 years old living in eight Italian communities (Solfrizzi et al., 2007). Alcohol consumption data were obtained in 1992, and the incidence rate of MCI and the transition rate from MCI to dementia were investigated with Cox proportional hazards regression. Alcohol intake was measured as a continuous number of drinks per day and as a categorical variable [none (reference value), ≤1 drink/day, 1 to ≤2 drinks/day, and >2 drinks/day]. During 15,341 person-years, 105 participants developed MCI. For incident MCI, there were no significant associations with alcohol consumption. However, there was an inverse association (not statistically significant) for those drinking ≤1 drink per day. For MCI to dementia transitions, there was a highly statistically inverse association for drinking ≤1 drink per day (HR = 0.15, 95% CI = 0.03–0.78) for all types of alcohol and the same magnitude for consumption of wine only (HR = 0.15, 95% CI = 0.03–0.77). Drinking more than one glass of alcohol per day was associated with inverse point estimates, but none of these was statistically significant. The authors did not adjust for APOE, nor did they look at effect-modification by this susceptibility gene.

Adjustment for confounding in studies examining the association between alcohol consumption and cognitive status requires the control of many characteristics that are related to drinking and cognitive outcomes. Drinkers tend to more commonly be current or former smokers. They have higher socioeconomic status, are more likely to live with others, to be men, to have no history of vascular disease, to be white, to be younger, and to have lower BMI. Women drinkers are more likely that nondrinkers to be hormone replacement users (Peters, Poulter, et al., 2008). Point estimates that are close to the null are more likely due to bias, and confounding bias may be one explanation for the inverse results. However, some studies found very strong point estimates, which are less susceptible to bias. Another methodological explanation for an inverse association is healthy-person bias. People who are healthier and have a higher socioeconomic status and a better risk factor behavior profile (including diet, physical activity, and social interaction) may be more likely to drink moderately. It may be the characteristics of these healthy people, which are difficult to adjust statistically, rather than alcohol intake itself, that are inversely related to AD and cognitive outcomes. A study in Denmark showed that wine drinkers ate more fruits and vegetables, fish, and olive oil than beer or liquor drinkers (Tjonneland et al., 1998).

In studies of older cohorts, we also have to consider reverse causation as an explanation of inverse results. Individuals who are starting to decline cognitively (but do not yet meet research criteria for any clinical outcome) may begin to limit alcohol intake. In epidemiologic studies, this would appear as an inverse association. Studies that document exposures in midlife are needed to resolve this question.

Effect-Modification

Individual studies have investigated effect-modification by several variables. In the Rotterdam Study, light-to-moderate alcohol consumption (1–3 drinks per day) was inversely associated with the risk for all dementia subtypes (HR = 0.58, 95% CI = 0.38–0.90), but this was present only among men. For VaD in both sexes, the HR = 0.30 (95% CI = 0.10–0.92), but sex-specific estimates were not significant. Hazard Ratios for AD were in the inverse direction for both sexes, but none of the estimates was statistically significant. For APOE-ε4 status, dose-response analyses showed that among ε4 carriers only, drinking between one drink per week and less than one drink per day was associated with a reduction in risk (HR for AD = 0.46, 95% CI = 0.23–0.94). No differences in risk estimates were found by the type of alcohol consumed (wine, beer vs liquor), but all effect estimates were nonstatistically significant, likely due to loss of power upon stratification (Ruitenberg et al., 2002).

In the Cardiovascular Health Study (Mukamal et al., 2003), a nested case-control analysis of 373 cases of incident dementia (258 with AD, 44 with VaD, and 54 with both) and 373 controls revealed a J-shaped curve for all dementias, AD, and VaD, with significant *p*-values for quadratic trend for all dementias and AD. In that study, drinking 1–6 alcoholic drinks per week was the most protective (OR = 0.46, 95% CI = 0.27–0.77) in a fully adjusted model compared to teetotalers. This amount of drinking was inversely associated with outcomes among both men and women in this study. A significant association was present only among people *without* an ε4 allele. However, this may have been due to reduced power to see such an association among carriers of this allele. No clear trends were evident for different types of alcohol in this study, although the consumption of liquor appeared, based on the point estimates for number of drinks per week, to have the weakest associations.

The CAIDE study, which included 1,464 men and women aged 65–79 who were followed over an average of 23 years, measured alcohol drinking in their 1972 and 1977 questionnaires and related this to MCI and dementia outcomes in 1998 (Anttila et al., 2004). In this cohort, about one-third of the cohort were teetotalers, 40% drank "infrequently" (less than once per month) and the remaining third drank "frequently" (several times per month). Adjusting for age, sex, education level, follow-up time, BMI, and measures of cardio- and cerebrovascular diseases, and using "non-ε4 carrier nondrinkers" as the reference group, no association was found for dementia, but when stratified by ε4 status, there was a strong effect present among ε4 carriers. Infrequent drinking incurred a risk of 4.08 (95% CI = 0.98–16.91) and frequent drinking was associated with a risk of 7.07 (95% CI = 1.37–36.6) compared to nondrinkers, while risks of infrequent and frequent drinking were not elevated for noncarriers. For MCI, teetotalers were found to have more than a twofold increased risk (OR = 2.15, 95% CI = 1.01–4.59) and frequent drinkers had an OR = 2.57 (95% CI = 1.19–5.52), but these estimates were not modified by APOE-ε4 status. Additionally, no interactions with sex were found.

Another example of effect-modification by APOE and type of alcohol was in an analysis conducted by the WHICAP investigators in New York City (Luchsinger, Tang, Siddiqui, Shea, & Mayeux, 2004). In this cohort study, 980 participants living in the community were followed for 4 years and 199 developed AD. Alcohol consumption was measured by means of a food frequency questionnaire (FFQ), and separate questions were asked for different types of alcohol. Participants were stratified according to their frequency of drinking [nondrinkers; light drinkers (1 drink per month to 6 drinks per week), moderate drinkers (1–3 drinks per day) or heavy drinkers (>3 drinks per day)]. Covariates included sex, race/ethnicity, education, self-reported history of heart disease, and APOE. Other vascular variables were not included because they did not improve the fit of the statistical model. No association was seen with VaD for any alcoholic beverage, although the point estimate was in the inverse direction. Only wine showed an inverse association with AD, where the HR was 0.55 (95% CI = 0.26–0.89) (Figure 13.3). In addition, this study found an interaction between alcohol intake and APOE in that noncarriers showed the association, while carriers did not. The authors proposed that the protective effect of wine may not be present among people who carry a genetic risk for AD, but that among those who do not, the biologic effects of wine may be sufficient to protect people from the disease.

More studies are needed to examine the roles of midlife versus late-life alcohol intake and how binge-drinking in midlife may affect AD risk. Studies like CAIDE where drinking was evaluated in midlife get us closer to a situation in which differential mortality by alcohol intake, APOE, and sex is less of a concern. The CAIDE results demonstrate that both infrequent and frequent drinkers who are ε4 carriers have an *increased* risk for dementia. The authors suggest that ε4 carriers may have impaired abilities for neural repair, which would make them more vulnerable to alcohol's damaging effects.

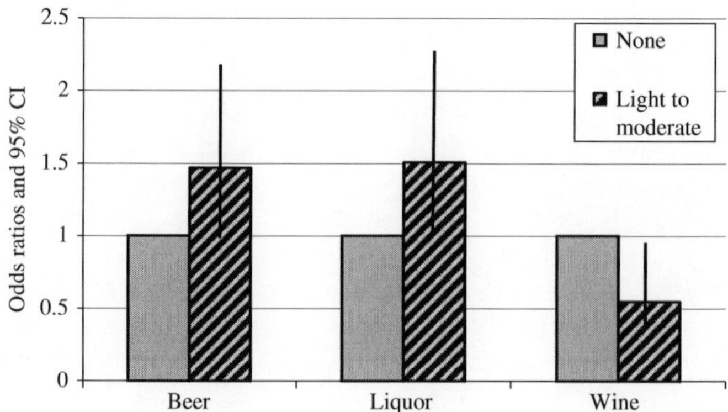

FIGURE 13.3 OR and 95% confidence intervals for Alzheimer's disease by amount and type of alcohol. *Adapted from Luchsinger et al. (2004).*

Mechanisms

Low-to-moderate drinkers have shown increases in the size of ventricles and increased sulci width, with a linear dose-response effect with amount of alcohol consumed (Ding et al., 2004). Increases in white matter volume and decreases in gray matter volume in frontal and parietal regions as well as generalized brain atrophy have been observed in long-term low-to-moderate drinkers (de Bruin et al., 2005). Other studies have found less white matter damage in low-to-moderate drinkers compared with teetotalers (Kim et al., 2012). Decreases in white and gray matter volumes may occur differentially among older men compared with women, because estrogen is protective against glutamate toxicity. In one study, elderly low-to-moderate drinkers showed reduced white matter hyperintensities and increased gray matter volumes, while women showed no benefit (Anstey et al., 2006).

Multiple biologic pathways have been proposed to explain alcohol's neuroprotective effects. The most commonly cited are its cardiovascular benefits, which have been linked to lower death rates from vascular diseases, as we discussed earlier. High-density lipoprotein level is increased with alcohol, and fibrinogen and other thrombotic promoters are reduced. Inhibition of platelet aggregation also is thought to occur with moderate alcohol intake (Mukamal & Rimm, 2001). Inflammatory markers, such as Il-6 and C-reactive protein, are reduced with exposure to alcohol, and in some studies such markers are associated with cognitive decline. Low-to-moderate alcohol intake also is known to protect against stroke (Reynolds et al., 2003) by delaying neuronal death, degeneration of neurons and dendrites, oxidative damage to DNA, activation of glial cells, and neutrophil infiltration (Kim et al., 2012). In addition, alcohol has polyphenols, among them resveratrol in red wine. Polyphenols are nonvitamin antioxidants that are 50–100 times more potent than conventional antioxidants (such as Vitamins E and C) (Dai, Borenstein, Wu, Jackson, & Larson, 2006) and also have strong anti-inflammatory effects. This topic will be discussed in Chapter 15.

Wine Consumption and AD

The first paper that looked specifically at wine intake and risk for AD was the PAQUID study of 3,777 community-dwellling individuals age 65 and over living in the Bordeaux area of France (Orgogozo et al., 1997). By virtue of the study being conducted in France (and particularly in Bordeaux), 95% of the alcohol consumed in the sample was wine. Drinkers were classified as nondrinkers (44% of the sample), mild (1–2 drinks per day, 41%), moderate (3–4 drinks per day, 12%), and heavy (more than 5 drinks per day, 3%). Dementia and AD were assessed using DSM-III-R and NINCDS-ADRDA criteria and 66 AD incident cases were found. Compared with nondrinkers, mild drinkers had almost half the risk for AD over a 3-year follow-up (adjusted OR = 0.55, 95%

CI = 0.31–0.99) and moderate drinkers had a third of the risk (OR = 0.28, 95% CI = 0.08–0.99). There was an insufficient number of heavy drinkers in the sample to provide a good estimate of the risk for AD in this group. There is some concern of reverse causality in this paper, since the follow-up was relatively short.

In Denmark, a study of 1,709 people aged 65 and over living in central Copenhagen who had participated in a study in 1976–1978 were included in a nested case-base analysis of alcohol and dementia prevalence identified in 1991–1994 (Truelsen, Thudium, & Gronbaek, 2002) (83 cases, 1626 controls). Drinking wine in the late 1970s was inversely associated with dementia in multivariate models. Using never/hardly ever as the reference group, monthly intake of wine reduced the risk for dementia. The OR for monthly wine intake, adjusted for age, sex, years of education, history of stroke, cohabitation status, income, systolic blood pressure, and current smoking, was 0.43 (95% CI = 0.23–0.82). Weekly intake had an OR of 0.33 (95% CI = 0.13–0.86) and daily intake an OR of 0.57 (95% CI = 0.15–2.11). In this study, monthly drinking of beer was associated with an elevated risk for dementia (OR = 2.28, 95% CI = 1.13–4.60), which curiously declined with increasing amounts of beer consumption (OR for weekly intake = 2.15, 95% CI = 0.98–4.78 and for daily intake = 1.73, 95% CI = 0.75–3.99). Similar findings for AD were reported, but only 40 AD cases were included in the analysis and data were not shown. Liquor drinking was not associated with dementia risk. Some of these estimates are based on very small numbers of cases, and the findings must be viewed in this context. The results for beer were unexpected and without biologic explanation. Drinking patterns likely differ for different types of alcohol, with wine intake occurring largely during meals and beer and liquor intake occurring more often in binge sessions. The inverse association with wine was attributed to flavonoid content, a type of polyphenol (see Chapter 15).

In the Canadian Study of Health and Aging, a nested case-control analysis using 194 incident AD cases examined "at least weekly consumption" of wine, beer, and liquor (Lindsay et al., 2002). Combining all alcohol types, a marginally significant inverse association was found with incident AD (OR = 0.68, 95% CI = 0.47–1.0). Although ORs for both beer and liquor were less than one, they were not statistically significant. Only the OR for wine was statistically significant (OR = 0.49, 95% CI = 0.28–0.88).

If wine consumption is inversely associated with the risk for AD, what is this potential biologic mechanism? In a study of transgenic mice (Tg2576) with human genes to produce AD, animals were randomized to three groups: those receiving Cabernet Sauvignon-extracted polyphenols, ethanol, or water for 7 months. Alcoholic beverages were diluted with water to produce a 6% concentration of ethanol equal to about one 5-oz glass for women and two 5-oz glasses for men (Wang et al., 2006). Wild-type mice matched for age and sex were subjected to the same treatment. At 11 months of age, spatial memory functions were assessed using a maze test and the animals were sacrificed and submitted to morphologic studies of the hippocampus, cingulate, and parietal neocortex. Over 7 months, the results showed that the polyphenol-treated mice had a slower decline in spatial memory, but no differences were found for the mice treated with plain ethanol or water. Additionally, polyphenol-treated wild-type animals (without the ability to produce AD neuropathology) were unaffected, suggesting that the polyphenol treatment among transgenic mice may work by modulating AD amyloid. This was indeed seen upon neuropathologic examination. The polyphenol-treated transgenic mice had lower $Aß_{1–40}$ and $Aß_{1–42}$ in the neocortex and hippocampus ($p < 0.05$). In the ethanol arm, there was a trend for reduction in $Aß_{1–40}$ and $Aß_{1–42}$ peptides, but this was not statistically significant. The Cabernet Sauvignon polyphenol treatment also promoted the production of nonamyloidogenic processing of APP in the brain with an accompanying increase in α-secretase activity, but not ß- or ɣ-secretase activity, and the extracted polyphenols were shown to prevent Aß peptide generation. Thus, the polyphenolic compounds in wine may have a beneficial effect on AD pathologic processes. Unfortunately, the authors did not look at a group of mice that received the wine-derived polyphenols and the ethanol together, mimicking the content of red wine. They also did not examine vascular mechanisms. Little is known about whether polyphenols have an effect on delaying the presentation of dementia through vascular effects in addition to modulating the underlying neuropathology.

New lines of evidence are emerging to favor a true role of wine in the etiology of AD. In WHICAP, high-resolution structural MRIs were obtained from 589 participants and total brain volume, white matter hyperintensity volume, and the presence of infarcts were cross-sectionally analyzed in conjunction with alcohol data derived from a FFQ. Fully adjusted models (including age, sex, education, race/ethnicity, APOE status, smoking, caloric intake, vascular disease history, and BMI) showed that total light-to-moderate alcohol intake was marginally associated with larger total brain volume ($p = 0.08$). In a model adjusted for some, but not all (vascular) variables, a modest effect ($p = 0.05$) was present for wine, but not beer or liquor consumption when all types of alcohol were in the model together (Gu et al., 2014). In the model adjusting for vascular confounders, this p-value increased to 0.09. In the model unadjusted for vascular variables, beer intake was marginally associated with white matter hyperintensity volume ($p = 0.06$), whereas wine and liquor were not ($p = 0.65$ and 0.68). Other studies have found inconsistent results for white matter hyperintensity volumes and alcohol consumption.

If alcohol consumption is inversely associated with AD, it may represent a true cause, or it could reflect a number of biases. Some of the biases we have considered in this chapter include survival, the “healthy-person” effect, reverse causation and confounding. Since light to moderate drinking has been shown to reduce mortality rates (Letenneur, 2004), differential mortality is unlikely to explain the finding. The healthy-person bias and related confounding should be controlled as tightly as possible, but there may be intrinsic confounding that is statistically difficult to adjust. It is likely, as we shall see in Chapter 15, that alcohol drinking in moderation in combination with other dietary patterns over a long time period work together to delay the risk for onset of AD by reducing amyloidogenic processes and increasing brain reserve perhaps through upregulation of BDNF pathways and reduction of cardiovascular damage.

Chapter 14

Vascular Disease

"What's good for your heart is good for your head" (Alzheimer's Association web page). This motto has found its way into the popular press, as well as appearing on the American Heart Association/American Stroke Association, WebMD, Alzheimer's Association, and other websites. The discovery that control of cardiac risk factors may benefit brain function emerged from prospective epidemiologic studies that found that vascular risk factors (VRFs) increase the risk for AD. In the previous chapter, we reviewed smoking and alcohol consumption, frequently considered to be "VRFs." A healthy diet, physical activity, and social and mental engagement are considered to have vascular as well as cognitive benefits. We will cover these protective factors in separate chapters because of the potential importance each of them has individually in the prevention of AD. In this chapter, we will focus on four VRFs for AD, diabetes, blood pressure, cholesterol, and obesity. Reviews of these and other risk factors, including homocysteine and systemic atherosclerosis can be found in Williams, Plassman, Burke, Holsinger, and Benjamin (2010) and Meng, Yu, Wang, Tan, and Wang (2014), and Qiu (2011).

We have seen earlier that vascular pathology by itself rarely causes dementia, but its presence increases the probability that a person with AD pathology will present with dementia (Snowdon et al., 1997). As we discussed in Chapter 4, there is strong evidence that vascular and Alzheimer pathologies occur independently of each other. The model we will use, which we refer to as "the man on the man" (Figure 14.1) posits that vascular and other pathologies in combination with AD neurodegenerative pathology stand on one another's shoulders to reach the clinical threshold for dementia, and attainment of the threshold will not occur if subclinical amounts of AD pathology or vascular or other pathologies are present alone (Bars B and C). However, AD pathology alone may be sufficient to cross the threshold (Bar A).

Recognizing that vascular and AD pathologies frequently co-occur and that vascular disease can facilitate the clinical expression of AD raises the question whether the two factors together behave in an additive or a multiplicative manner to produce cognitive impairment. It is also important to recognize that there is likely to be substantial misclassification of clinical dementia subtypes, such

Alzheimer's Disease. DOI: http://dx.doi.org/10.1016/B978-0-12-804538-1.00014-6

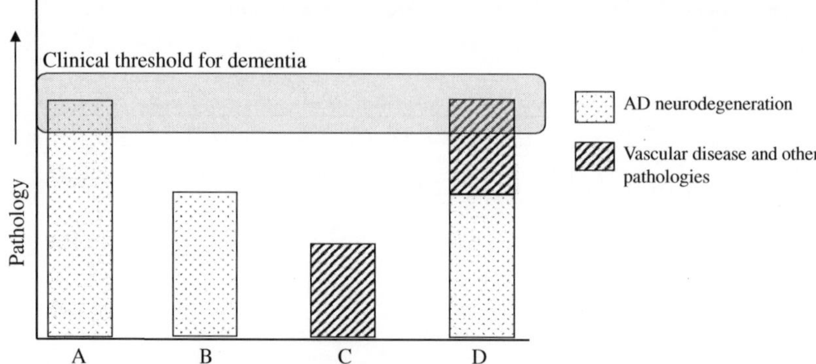

FIGURE 14.1 Additive model for mixed neuropathologies in achieving the clinical threshold for dementia. Bar A: Sufficient AD neurodegeneration alone; Bar B: Insufficient AD neurodegeneration alone; Bar C: Insufficient vascular/other pathologies alone; and Bar D: Combined pathologies achieves threshold.

that diagnoses of "Alzheimer's disease" often include vascular pathology, muddying the waters in interpretation of results on VRFs across studies. In 2002, Launer observed, with regard to the first studies showing that subclinical atherosclerosis increased the risk for prevalent dementia (Hofman et al., 1997) and higher blood pressure over 15 years predicted AD (Skoog et al., 1996), that "the critical question…is whether vascular disease is a *part of the AD pathology*, or is *independent of this pathology*" (Launer, 2002). It is our view that these two types of pathology are largely independent of one another. However, some overlap is inevitable from the presence of congophilic amyloid angiopathy, in which breakdown in the walls of small vessels caused by aggregation of $A\beta_{1-40}$ occurs in some cases of AD. It is important to recognize that this vascular lesion occurs independently of other vascular lesions and is part of an Alzheimer pathologic process, not a vascular pathologic process.

The discovery of apolipoprotein E (APOE)-ε4 as a major susceptibility gene for AD in 1993 was one of the first clues that vascular disease may be involved in AD. APOE is a cholesterol-carrying protein associated with very low-density lipoproteins (LDLs) and its job is to remove excess cholesterol from the blood and transport it for processing in the liver. It is thought that people with the APOE-ε4 allele are unable to clear amyloid from the brain as efficiently as those with the ε3 alleles; while those with ε2 alleles are considered to remove amyloid more efficiently (Jiang et al., 2008).

Researchers have proposed that the brain's vascular system is designed to prevent damage to the neurovascular unit. Such protection involves maintenance of adequate blood flow and integrity of the blood–brain barrier (Kalaria, Akinyemi, & Ihara, 2012). It also has been suggested that cerebrovascular disease can reduce cerebral blood flow and that reduced cerebral blood flow can lead to a progressive cerebrovascular insufficiency that over time destabilizes

	Autopsy	No autopsy
Demented during life	a	b
Not demented during life	c	d

FIGURE 14.2 Selection bias in dementia studies by autopsy status. In the population, dementia cases are more likely to be autopsied compared with nondementia cases. Thus, cells "c" and "d" are not properly enumerated. Only studies that seek autopsy on all participants regardless of dementia status can claim no selection bias.

neurons, synapses, neurotransmission, and eventually evolves into a neurodegenerative process involving an AD cascade (de la Torre, 2013). These observations are supported by studies in animals. In one study, clamping the carotid artery to deprive the brain of blood in transgenic mice was shown to accelerate ß-amyloid deposition (Kitaguchi et al., 2009). Another study in rhesus monkeys showed that dystrophic axons labeled for ß-amyloid cleaving enzyme 1 (BACE1) were in close proximity to cortical blood vessels (Cai et al., 2010). These studies led to speculation that vascular damage may *cause* or accelerate the formation of AD neuropathologic lesions. If vascular lesions cause AD pathology, one would expect that individuals with more vascular pathology would have more AD pathology. However, as we have reviewed in Chapter 4, autopsy studies provide very strong evidence that vascular and AD lesions occur independently of each other. It is conceivable that extreme ischemic events such as major strokes could increase the frequency of AD pathology in the immediate surrounding area, but it does not appear that subclinical cerebrovascular disease affects the frequency of AD lesions, a prerequisite for the existence of a causal pathway from vascular to Alzheimer pathology.

Because of the common co-occurrence of vascular and AD pathology, autopsy studies that are mostly restricted to demented subjects can induce an association between vascular disease and AD. As shown in Figure 14.2, in such autopsy studies, demented individuals are more likely than nondemented individuals to have an autopsy (cell "a" will be proportionately larger than cell "c"). If vascular lesions disclose the presence of underlying AD pathology only in those who become demented, autopsy studies largely restricted to such demented cases will produce the finding that vascular pathology is more likely to occur in those with AD pathology. On the other hand, an autopsy study that includes participants regardless of dementia status prior to death will not suffer from this disclosure bias and will give an accurate picture of the independence of Alzheimer and vascular pathologies.

The first study in which autopsies were obtained regardless of cognitive status prior to death was the Nun Study. Since one of the inclusion criteria for this study was the donation of the brain upon death, virtually all sisters who died had neuropathologic examinations regardless of their cognitive status during life. As reviewed in Chapter 4, this study as well as two others that obtained autopsies independent of clinical status at death, the Religious Orders Study (ROS) and the HAAS, found no association between the severity of Alzheimer and vascular lesions, suggesting that these pathologies occurred independently of one another. To illustrate this point, we can look at correlations from the Nun Study between vascular and AD neuropathologies. Table 14.1 shows such correlations, partialling out the variance due to age at death. The correlations between Alzheimer and vascular variables ranged between −0.008 and 0.09, with *no correlation achieving statistical significance*. If vascular pathologies *caused* AD pathologies and/or vice versa, correlations among these variables would be evident.

The ROS was conducted in a population of Catholic nuns, priests, and brothers (Bennett, Schneider, Arvanitakis, & Wilson, 2012). Participants who were not demented were followed annually and ultimately to brain donation. From January 1994 through October 2011, the study enrolled 1,162 participants, of whom 69% were women and 88% were non-Hispanic white with a mean age of 76 years and a mean education of 18 years. By 2013, the study had identified 387 incident mild cognitive impairment (MCI) cases (132 amnestic MCI (aMCI)) and 287 incident dementia cases, 273 with incident AD. The ROS reported that cerebral infarcts were associated with dementia risk. As in the Nun Study, AD pathology and cerebral infarcts were additively related to the odds of dementia (Schneider, Wilson, Bienias, Evans, & Bennett, 2004). The investigators also considered whether there might be a multiplicative interaction between subcortical and cortical infarctions, but found no effect beyond an additive one on the probability of expressing dementia. In addition, there was no correlation between AD pathology and the presence of infarctions ($r = 0.04$, $p = 0.56$). These results thus agree with the "man-on-the-man" mechanism of crossing the threshold of cognitive impairment by means of multiple additive brain pathologies.

The Rush Memory and Aging Project (MAP), which began in 1997 (Bennett, Schneider, Buchman, et al., 2012), also required brain donation of its participants. To increase representation among lower SES individuals, the investigators recruited from subsidized housing facilities, local churches, and social service agencies. This study claimed to reduce the "healthy person effect," because participants were seen at home and the only exclusion criterion was the inability to sign the Anatomical Gift Act for organ donation at death. Because participants often died in a nursing facility, the researchers were able to work with facility staff to make sure the autopsy was performed. From November of 1997 through November 2011, 1,556 participants agreed to participate, with the cohort being 73% women and 88% non-Hispanic white, and a little older (80) and with somewhat lower mean education (14.4 years) than the ROS. Three-hundred and forty-three incident aMCI cases and 250 incident dementia cases

TABLE 14.1 Correlations and *p*-Values Between AD Neuropathologic Measures (Neurofibrillary Tangles, Neuritic Plaques, and Braak Stage) and Vascular Pathologic Measures (Lacunar Infarcts, Big Infarcts, Microinfarcts, and Atherosclerosis Rating in the Circle of Willis) Adjusted for Age at Death, The Nun Study, N = 326 (Mean Age at Death = 90.7)

	Neurofibrillary Tangles	Neuritic Plaques	Braak Stage	Lacunar Infarcts	Big Infarcts	Microinfarcts	Atherosclerosis Rating in the Circle of Willis
Neurofibrillary tangles	1.0	0.50 (<0.0001)	0.74 (<0.0001)	−0.008 (0.89)	−0.025 (0.65)	0.03 (0.58)	−0.03 (0.60)
Neuritic plaques		1.0	0.53 (<0.0001)	−0.04 (0.43)	−0.05 (0.36)	−0.05 (0.39)	−0.06 (0.27)
Braak stage			1.0	−0.0008 (0.99)	0.05 (0.38)	0.09 (0.11)	0.004 (0.94)
Lacunar infarcts				1.0	0.34 (<0.0001)	0.34 (<0.0001)	0.19 (0.0006)
Big infarcts					1.0	0.16 (0.004)	0.17 (0.02)
Microinfarcts						1.0	0.05 (0.34)
Atherosclerosis in the Circle of Willis							1.0

(238 AD, mixed or not) were identified in this cohort. Examining the joint effects of AD pathology and cerebral infarcts yielded no interaction beyond additivity on the odds for dementia. The authors concluded that cerebrovascular and other pathologies (such as Lewy bodies) "reduce the ability of the brain to tolerate any given amount of AD pathology making it more likely that it will lead to cognitive impairment and dementia. Thus, the prevention of cerebrovascular and Lewy body disease will reduce the numbers of persons meeting clinical criteria for AD" (Bennett, Schneider, Buchman, et al., 2012).

In addition to large vascular lesions leading to clinical outcomes, subclinical vascular lesions are increasingly being recognized for the important role they play in cognition in older age (DeCarli, 2013). Subclinical vascular lesions visible on MRI include lacunar infarcts and white matter hyperintensities (WMH). The latter are seen on T2-weighted MRI in the white matter and likely reflect a number of characteristics and consequences of small vessel disease, including microinfarcts, microhemorrhages, cerebral amyloid angiopathy (CAA), demyelination, and subsequent loss of axons (Shim et al., 2015). The most consistent predictor of WMH is advanced age. Risk factors for WMH that have been identified include hypertension, diabetes, smoking, hyperlipidemia, and cardiovascular disease (CVD), consistent with their vascular origin (Jeerakathil et al., 2004). Associations with AD pathology, in particular with neurofibrillary tangle density (Shim et al., 2015), have been observed and have led some to suggest that some WMH may also reflect Wallerian degeneration secondary to neuronal death in AD. Evidence in favor of this view is provided by the spatial location of WMH. WMHs in the parietal lobe, for example, were specifically associated with incident AD in the WHICAP study, while more anterior WMHs were associated with mortality (Brickman et al., 2014). However, in dementia patients as well as subjects with normal cognition, WMHs occurred independently of APOE genotype, suggesting that AD pathology may play a role in their formation in only a minority of older individuals (Hirono, Yasuda, Tanimukai, Kitagaki, & Mori, 2000; Paternoster, Chen, & Sudlow, 2009).

In a systematic review and meta-analysis of the role of WMH on dementia occurrence, longitudinal human studies were included if WMH were measured by MRI (not by computed tomography), had an MRI at baseline, and included more than 50 people (Debette & Markus, 2010). For incident dementia, 14 studies were included, three of which were population-based, the Framingham Study, the Three-City Dijon Study, and the CHS-Cognition Study. In these three studies, the pooled HR for dementia comparing the highest category of WMH to the lowest was 2.9 (95% CI = 1.3–6.3). Among the nonpopulation-based studies (mostly selected cohorts of MCI patients), the HR was 1.4 (95% CI = 0.9–2.3). In this review, WMHs were also associated with an increased rate of mortality (HR = 2.0, 95% CI = 1.6–2.7). Among current smokers, the risk for WMH progression in the Atherosclerosis Risk in Communities Study was higher (OR = 1.57, 95% CI = 1.05–2.36) compared to nonsmokers (OR = 0.91, 95% CI = 0.62–1.33) (Power et al., 2014).

In the 1970s and 1980s, it was believed that repeated strokes alone caused "multi-infarct dementia" (now called "vascular dementia"). In addition, "silent" vascular damage was believed to be part of normal aging. As more is understood about the vascular system, the role of microinfarcts in contributing to impairments in cognition is emerging. Microinfarcts in the brain are defined as "sharply delimited microscopic regions of cellular death or tissue necrosis, sometimes with cavitation (a central fluid-filled cavity)" (Smith, Schneider, Wardlaw, & Greenberg, 2012) and visible only by light microscopy. They are common (present in about one-third of people over age 65, though estimates vary among studies), but the unique contribution to dementia from microinfarcts is complicated by the copresence of other vascular pathologies (macroinfarcts and white matter lesions). The cognitive consequences of microinfarcts likely depend on their location. For example, cortical but not subcortical microinfarcts have been found to be associated with poorer cognition (Smith et al., 2012).

The Honolulu-Asia Aging Study (HAAS) is a longitudinal study of 3,733 Japanese American men begun in the early 1990s. The cohort from which this study was derived were originally enrolled in 1965 in the Honolulu Heart Program, a study of cardiovascular and cerebrovascular disease. When the HAAS began, it included a significant autopsy component. The autopsy study differed from the last three studies discussed, since brain donation was not an inclusion criterion of the study. In a substudy of 439 men autopsied between 1992 and 2001 (Launer, Petrovitch, Ross, Markesbery, & White, 2008), the average age at death was 85. In this sample, 99% of the cohort had some AD pathology and 78% had vascular lesions. No association was present for AD pathology with vascular pathology of any type, including microinfarcts. The authors concluded that Alzheimer and vascular lesions are independent of one another, supporting an additive effect of these lesions on cognitive dysfunction.

The Adult Changes in Thought (ACT) Study, conducted within Group Health Cooperative of a primarily Caucasian population representative of the Caucasian population in Seattle, WA, is methodologically standardized with The *Kame* Project, HAAS and the Adult Health Study in Hiroshima, Japan. In this study too there was no association between pathologic morbidities; thus different neuropathologies were observed to be independent of one another and to act additively to produce dementia (Sonnen, Larson, Haneuse, et al., 2009).

The additive effect of Alzheimer and vascular lesions is especially evident for microinfarcts. In both HAAS and ACT the burden of microinfarcts in the brain was related to cognitive performance independently of Alzheimer lesions. In HAAS, investigators entered all cerebrovascular variables together into a regression and found that only microinfarct number predicted scores on the CASI global cognitive function test. In ACT, the only vascular measure that predicted dementia status was the presence of three or more cerebral microinfarcts (adjusted RR = 4.80, 95% CI = 1.81–10.26). Along with this variable, the two pathologic variables predictive of dementia status in ACT were Braak neurofibrillary tangle stage (V/VI, RR = 5.89, 95% CI = 1.62–17.6) and a combination of Braak stage and Lewy bodies in the neocortex (RR = 5.08, 95% CI = 1.37–18.96). The corresponding adjusted population attributable fractions (PAFs) were 33% for microinfarcts, 45% for Braak stage, and 10% for cortical Lewy bodies (Sonnen et al., 2007).

Another recently recognized type of vascular damage that can have cognitive sequalae is cerebral microbleeds. These can be seen on MRI and their prevalence is thought to range from 10% to 25% in community-dwelling older people (Greenberg et al., 2009). Microbleeds in a lobar cortico-subcortical distribution are associated with APOE-ε4 status and thought to be due to CAA. In the Australian Imaging, Biomarkers, and Lifestyle Study of Ageing (Yates et al., 2014), when high global Aß burden and APOE were in a model together, Aß burden but not APOE-ε4 was associated with incident lobar microbleeds, as might be expected given their association with CAA. In a cross-sectional analysis from the AGES-Reykjavik Study in Iceland (Qiu et al., 2010), 3,906 individuals with a mean age of 76 had MRI scans and digital retinal images from which cerebral microbleeds and retinal microvascular features were measured. Outcomes in this study included a composite *Z*-score of memory, processing speed, and executive function tests. Prevalent dementia diagnoses and their subtypes were made using standard clinical criteria. Participants with multiple cerebral microbleeds (2 or more) had lower *Z*-scores on tests of processing speed and executive function. The OR for VaD was 2.32 (95% CI = 1.02–5.25) for multiple cerebral microbleeds and 1.95 (95% CI = 1.04–3.62) for retinal microvascular disease. The associations were particularly pronounced in deep hemispheric or infratentorial regions, which could result from hypertensive vasculopathy, and the authors suggested that cerebral microbleeds may be part of the pathogenesis linking hypertension to vascular cognitive impairment and dementia.

In the Amsterdam Dementia Cohort, WMH, number of microbleeds (>3 and 0–2), number of lacunes and medial temporal atrophy were examined among 334 individuals whose average age was 62 (47% women) to predict the progression of subjective memory impairment (self-rating of memory problems) to MCI or to all-cause dementia (Benedictus et al., 2014). Over an average follow-up period of 5 years, mild WMH increased the risk for transitioning from subjective memory impairment (SMI) to MCI or dementia (HR = 2.8, 95% CI = 1.2–6.3) and severe WMH increased this risk by 4.2-fold (95% CI = 1.2–13.8). In this cohort, lacunes and microbleeds did not predict progression from SMI to MCI or dementia.

DIABETES

While secular trends for AD forecast a decline in incidence rates with better brain development and increasing educational attainment, the increasing incidence rate of Type 2 diabetes (T2D) could lead to a large increase in the burden of AD and dementia in developed and developing countries in the future. In

2013, the prevalence of T2D was about 10% in the United States, about 7% in Europe (Norton, Matthews, Barnes, Yaffe, & Brayne, 2014), highest in the Middle East and North Africa (11%), and lowest in the rest of Africa (about 6%). In the United States, the rates of T2D were highest in Native Americans (15.9%) and lowest in non-Hispanic whites (7.6%). Rates for non-Hispanic blacks and Hispanics were about the same (13%), and for Asian Americans, 9% had diabetes. In 2010, diabetes was the seventh leading cause of death in the United States (N = 69,071) and was listed as a cause of death for 234,051 people. Diabetes often occurs in combination with other vascular conditions, such as hypertension, dyslipidemia, and stroke. The cost for caring for diabetics in the United States exceeds that of AD. In 2012 alone, the annual cost was $245 billion. Until about 1995, the rate of diabetes remained fairly stable at around 3%. Since then, the rates have been climbing steadily.

Cohort Studies

The question of whether and how T2D is involved in AD etiology has been the subject of intense investigation over the past 20 years. Earlier case–control studies were subject to multiple methodological shortcomings, including the problem of restricting attention to "pure" AD cases. The initial population-based association of diabetes and AD was reported from the cross-sectional phase of the Rotterdam cohort study (Ott et al., 1996). This study reported a nonstatistically significant effect for AD (OR = 1.3, 95% CI = 0.9–1.9), with a more pronounced effect among insulin-treated participants (OR = 2.8, 95% CI = 1.0–8.0). The OR for VaD was elevated (2.1, 95% CI = 1.1–4.0 for all diabetics; and 5.4, 95% CI = 1.2–23.8 for insulin-treated diabetics). Shortly after this study was published, Leibson et al. (1997) published the first incidence data from an historical cohort study from the Mayo Clinic in which incident T2D cases were identified between 1945 and 1989. In a model adjusted for the nonlinear effects of age and calendar year, the RR for AD was statistically elevated for T2D among men (RR = 2.27, 95% CI = 1.55–3.31) but not among women (RR = 1.37, 95% CI = 0.94–2.01). When the authors excluded 18 cases diagnosed with AD that also fulfilled criteria for other types of dementia from the diabetes cohort, the RR was attenuated (1.22, 95% CI 0.93–1.57). In 1999, Ott and colleagues followed their 1996 paper with an incidence analysis, and found that the RR for AD associated with T2D was 1.9 (95% CI = 1.2–3.1). The magnitude of the association was higher in AD cases with concomitant cerebrovascular disease (RR = 3.0, 95% CI = 1.0–9.3), but even in those with no cerebrovascular disease, the RR was elevated (RR = 1.8, 95% CI = 1.1–3.0). The authors also replicated their cross-sectional finding that the risk was more pronounced among those who had been treated with insulin (RR for dementia in this group was about four times higher among both men and women, with only the RR for women being statistically significant). Those on oral medications were at about a twofold higher risk, again significant only for women.

Another study that included neuropathologic data was the HAAS (Peila, Rodriguez, & Launer, 2002). In an analysis of 2,574 men, 1,674 of whom did not have T2D and 900 of whom did, the adjusted RR for incident AD was 1.8 (95% CI = 1.1–2.9) and 1.6 (95% CI = 0.9–3.0) for AD without accompanying CVD. The RR was highest for VaD (RR = 2.3, 95% CI = 1.1–5.0). When interaction between APOE-ε4 and diabetic status was investigated, the RR for AD without CVD for both factors combined was 5.5 (95% CI = 2.2–13.7). When diabetes and APOE-ε4 status were analyzed for their associations with vascular and neurodegenerative pathologies, diabetes by itself was statistically significantly associated only with large infarcts, but not with Alzheimer neuropathology; while the presence of both diabetes and ε4 were significantly associated only with neurodegenerative but *not* vascular pathologies.

In the past 12 years, a number of high-quality prospective population-based studies on the association between T2D and AD have been published. A meta-analysis of this association from 15 studies yielded a summary RR of 1.57 (95% CI = 1.41–1.75) (Vagelatos & Eslick, 2013). There was moderate heterogeneity ($p = 0.07$) and no publication bias was detected ($p = 0.22$). An interesting finding from this meta-analysis was a *lower* pooled RR associated with studies that used blood glucose measurements (RR = 1.46, 95% CI = 1.30–1.64) compared with those that used self-reported T2D (RR = 1.98, 95% CI = 1.64–2.40). Those who had blood glucose measurements may represent a biased subpopulation, since obtaining fasting glucose tests in community-based studies is expensive and logistically challenging, and not all subjects may have participated in this aspect of a study. On the other hand, self-reports of diagnosed diabetes also may involve error. About 30% of T2D is undiagnosed in the community based on NHANES data (Cowie et al., 2006). If this occurred equally among AD and unaffected cohort members, the RRs associated with T2D could be underestimated. However, if incipient AD cases are more or less likely to be misclassified by diabetes status, the RRs could be over- or underestimated. A second interesting finding was that adjustment for cardiovascular risk factors changed the RR very modestly (RR = 1.51, 95% CI = 1.34–1.70 adjusting for age and sex alone; RR = 1.66, 95% CI = 1.31–2.10 adjusting additionally for CVD factors), implying that the association for diabetes is likely independent of other VRFs. The PAF for AD associated with diabetes was estimated from this review to be about 8% in the United States (implying the elimination of almost half a million cases out of 5.4 million prevalent cases if diabetes could be eliminated) and 6% overall in the world (about 1,440,000 cases).

Since the HAAS findings were published, only a few studies have examined the interaction between diabetes and APOE-ε4 with the risk of incident AD. One might expect that these risk factors interact, since there may be shared pathways between T2D and AD, including those related to cholesterol transport, which may be related to APOE. For example, Aß clearance from the brain may involve the lipidation status of APOE, with highly lipidated APOE increasing exit of Aß from the brain, and poorly lipidated APOE slowing down such clearance (Craft,

2009). Vagelatos and colleagues meta-analyzed epidemiologic data from five studies obtaining a pooled RR of 2.29 (95% CI = 1.12–4.67) for the interaction of diabetes with APOE-ε4 (Vagelatos & Eslick, 2013), but with a highly significant *p*-value for heterogeneity ($I^2 = 74.85\%$, $p = 0.003$). The studies included HAAS, the Kungsholmen Study, the *Kame* Project, the CHS-Cognition Study, and the Framingham Study. Only HAAS and the CHS-Cognition Study found a statistically significant multiplicative interaction (RRs ranged from 4.4 to 5.0). In the *Kame* Project, we found a nonstatistically significant inverse HR for AD among ε4 carrier diabetics (HR = 0.51, $p = 0.38$), while non-ε4 carriers with diabetes had an elevated HR for AD (HR = 2.98, 95% CI 1.30–6.83) (Borenstein, Wu, & Larson, 2005). Some investigators believe that there are different pathways to AD, one being driven by APOE-ε4 and its related neurodegenerative factors and another pathway being mediated by insulin resistance (Suzanne Craft, webinar 10/29/2009, http://vimeo.com/98659146). If this were true, our findings would support this hypothesis.

A synergistic modifying role of APOE-ε4 on the association between T2D and AD might be suspected because presence of an APOE-ε4 allele increases oxidative stress and damage, resulting in reduced ability for neurons to remodel (Axelsen, Komatsu, & Murray, 2011). The role of insulin has been studied extensively for its role in the brain in experimental studies, and we now know many of its functions. Synapses of astrocytes and neurons have insulin receptors, which are primarily present in the olfactory bulb, cerebral cortex, hippocampus, hypothalamus, amygdala, and septum. In these areas, insulin signaling contributes to the generation of new synapses as well as their remodeling (Cholerton, Baker, & Craft, 2013). In T2D, chronic metabolic stress conditions and proinflammatory signaling result in less efficient insulin signaling and a decreased responsiveness of the insulin receptors, which like APOE-ε4 would reduce the ability of neurons to remodel and grow new synapses.

Mechanisms

Over the past 10–15 years, the causative role of ß-amyloid plaques in AD pathogenesis has been called into question. It has been known for some time that the density of amyloid plaques in the brain do not correlate well with cognition, while NFTs and loss of synapses (also seen in brain atrophy) correlate better (Bennett, Schneider, Wilson, Bienias, & Arnold, 2004; De Felice, Lourenco, & Ferreira, 2014). Although plaques are thought to be neurotoxic, the idea that *soluble* bioactive Aβ oligomers (AβOs) might be the real culprits in the ß-amyloid cascade has been put forth by several AD researchers (Lesne et al., 2013; Mucke & Selkoe, 2012). There are multiple lines of evidence supporting the notion that AßOs disrupt normal brain insulin signaling pathways by increasing inflammation (De Felice, Lourenco, & Ferreira, 2014). It is possible that throughout the life course, individuals who generate more soluble Aß may increase their risk for AD in part due to disruption of insulin-signaling pathways. Insulin is known to reduce the phosphorylation of amyloid precursor protein and to increase the level of proteins that are antiamyloidogenic, such as insulin-degrading enzyme. Insulin also helps to traffick $Aß_{1–40}$ and $Aß_{1–42}$ to the cell membrane and out to the extracellular space. Therefore, a lack of insulin signaling as occurs in insulin resistance can slow down the process of clearing Aß from neurons. Interestingly, insulin also reduces oligomer formation (Cholerton et al., 2013). While it is beyond the scope of this chapter to review all of insulin's neuroprotective roles, these are eloquently reviewed in several articles (Cholerton et al., 2013; Correia et al., 2012; Nelson et al., 2009). The interaction of insulin and Aß would suggest T2D and AβOs may interact multiplicatively.

Autopsy studies provide additional information on the effects of T2D on Alzheimer and vascular lesions. In the ACT cohort, 196 autopsied participants were analyzed in four groups: those who had neither dementia nor diabetes, those who had one and not the other, and those who had both (Sonnen, Larson, Brickell, et al., 2009). In the nondiabetic dementia group, participants had more AD neuropathologic outcomes (Aβ load and free radical damage), while the diabetic dementia group had more vascular markers and neuroinflammation. In addition, treated diabetics had more deep microvascular infarcts than nontreated diabetics. The authors concluded that patients with T2D and dementia die with a lower Aß burden compared with those who have dementia and are not diabetic.

A study examining the genetic determinants of diabetes found no association with late-onset AD, and concluded that the observed epidemiologic associations between T2D and AD could result from "secondary disease processes, pleiotropic mechanisms and/or common environmental risk factors" (Proitsi, Lupton, Velayudhan, et al., 2014). On the other hand, the ACT Study found that the risk for incident dementia (not specifically AD) was elevated in a dose-response fashion even among nondiabetics with higher glucose levels (for levels above 100 mg/dL, the HR ranged 1.10–1.18 for each increase in 5 mg/dL, p-value for trend = 0.01). Conversely, for diabetics, the risk for dementia was 1.15 (95% CI = 0.98–1.34) at 180 mg/dL glucose and 1.40 (95% CI = 1.12–1.76) at 190 mg/dL (p-value for trend = 0.002) (Crane et al., 2013; Expert Panel on Detection, 2001). Consistent with these findings, we had previously reported an elevated risk for dementia (Mortimer et al., 2010) versus aMCI for fasting blood glucose in the *normal* range (≤110 mg/dL or 6.1 mmol/L) (OR = 7.75, 95% CI = 1.10–55.56) adjusting for age, sex, education, modified Hachinski Ischemic score, hippocampal and total brain volume (TBV), WMH volume, body mass index (BMI), and stroke identified by MRI, suggesting that prediabetic pathology may play a role in the causation of dementia.

Treatment Studies

Another strong piece of evidence for or against insulin resistance and diabetes as a direct player in AD pathogenesis would be whether treatment of VRFs, including diabetes, lowered the risk for AD. So far, the findings are mixed.

In an historical cohort study of 301 AD patients without CVD seen at a memory clinic at the University of Lille in France with a mean MMSE score of around 22 and mean age around 71, 93% had at least one VRF, including hypertension, dyslipidemia, T2D, smoking, and atherosclerotic disease (Deschaintre, Richard, Leys, & Pasquier, 2009). At baseline, VRFs were treated with antihypertensives, statins, or fibrates for dyslipidemia, oral antihyperglycemics or insulin for T2D, and smoking cessation. Patients were followed for about 2 years. Participants were included if they had MMSE tests done at least twice, 6 months apart. Patients were stratified into three groups: 72 with no VRFs treated, 119 with some VRFs treated, and 89 with all VRFs treated. In adjusted mixed random effects regression models, decline in MMSE score over 2 years was slower in the group that had all VRFs treated compared with the group with no VRFs treated ($p = 0.002$). The group with some VRFs treated did not differ from the group with no VRFs treated. The authors then analyzed each VRF separately and found that the effect was limited to treated patients with dyslipidemia treatment and atherosclerosis. Although no effect was found for T2D, hypertension, or smoking treatments, untreated diabetic patients had a marginally faster decline on MMSE than those without diabetes ($p = 0.06$), and treated diabetic patients had a decline similar to nondiabetics ($p = 0.79$). Only 36 patients had T2D, so the authors caution that the absence of significant findings could be due to low power. This study was not a randomized trial, and used only the MMSE as the outcome.

A randomized controlled trial (RCT) focusing on intensive glucose lowering in Type 2 diabetics (ACCORD-Memory in Diabetes Study) examined change in the Digit Symbol Substitution Test (DSST) score and TBV over a 40-month period (Launer, Miller, et al., 2011). This was a double 2 × 2 factorial, parallel group randomized trial of 2,977 individuals aged 55–80 (mean age 62) with hemoglobin A_{1c} (HbA_{1c}) concentrations of >7.5%. The DSST was measured at baseline, and at 20 and 40 months. A subsample of 632 participants also received MRIs to measure TBV. The goal of the intensive glycemic-lowering treatment group was to decrease HbA_{1c} levels to <6%; a second group, the standard glycemic-lowering treatment, was studied to reduce levels to 7.0–7.9%. Each participant received customized interventions, including diabetes education, glucose-monitoring equipment, and antidiabetic medications. Intensive therapy included increasing doses or adding new medications monthly if HbA_{1c} levels were ≥6% or if >50% of premeal or postmeal glucose readings exceeded 5.6 mmol/L. The standard treatment group received more intensive therapy when HbA_{1c} levels exceeded 8% or >50% of their glucose levels exceeded 7.8 mmol/L. The intensive therapy group was stopped at the beginning of 2008 because the mortality rate in this group was elevated (HR = 1.27, 95% CI 0.83–1.93), with 47 deaths in this arm versus 39 in the standard arm. Nevertheless, most participants were able to complete at least 34 months of therapy. The findings showed no benefit on DSST (or other cognitive tests including the Rey Auditory Verbal Learning Test, Stroop test and MMSE). However, TBV loss was smaller in the intensive compared with the standard treatment group (difference in means = 4.6 (95% CI = 2.0–7.3), $p = 0.0007$). This translated into an annualized decline in TBV of 3.9 cm^3, which was 26% lower than that in the standard treatment group (5.3 cm^3). We know that cognitively healthy individuals with a mean age of 76 lose about 0.4% volume per year; in MCI or dementia cases, this decline is approximately double (Jack et al., 2004). From this study, the comparative annual declines were 0.42% in the intensive treatment group and 0.57% in the standard treatment group. The authors pointed out that we would expect structural brain measures (such as TBV) to change before cognitive measures do. They suggested that if the cohort was followed for long enough, cognitive differences may be observed. The authors used younger participants in this trial because they considered this the critical period in which brain disease processes begin to manifest, leading to the increased risk for dementia or AD associated with T2D. It is possible that this cohort was too young to observe significant differences in cognition. Although it is necessary to begin modifying such risk factors as early as possible, studies also need statistical power to detect their primary outcomes.

A more promising set of results from randomized clinical trials for AD and T2D is that for intranasal insulin (Freiherr et al., 2013). Because insulin administered into the body can lead to hypoglycemia, a safer method is to spray insulin into the nose. The nasal cavity provides a direct pathway into the brain, bypassing the blood–brain barrier. Concentrations of insulin are detectable in the cerebrospinal fluid 30–40 min after administration, and biologically important levels do not alter levels of insulin or glucose in the peripheral tissues. In an early (nonrandomized) study conducted by Dr Suzanne Craft and her group at the University of Washington (Reger et al., 2006), intranasal insulin administration increased verbal memory recall in 13 early AD and 13 aMCI cases relative to 35 healthy controls, but the effects were significant only in those not carrying an APOE-ε4 allele receiving 40 IU of insulin ($p = 0.0005$), while the ε4 carriers unexpectedly showed reduced performance in the 40 IU scenario ($p = 0.004$).

In the first clinical trial of intranasal insulin also by Craft and her colleagues (2012), 64 aMCI and 40 mild-to-moderate AD patients were randomized to receive placebo, 20 IU of insulin or 40 IU of insulin for 4 months intranasally. The dose of 20 IU statistically significantly increased scores on delayed memory (story recall), and both doses improved general cognition (ADAS-cog score) among younger subjects. CSF biomarkers for AD were not altered, but function rated by caregivers and cerebral glucose metabolism improved. Larger randomized clinical trials of intranasal insulin are in progress at the time of writing this book, which may reveal additional findings.

Diabetes and Brain Atrophy

Another way in which T2D might affect the risk of AD would be through accelerated brain atrophy leading to loss of volume in critical brain regions.

A cross-sectional MRI comparison of 350 individuals with T2D with a mean age of 68 and 363 individuals without T2D with a mean age of 72 showed significantly greater atrophy in those with T2D (Moran et al., 2013). This was particularly evident for gray matter volumes in regions that are affected early in AD including the hippocampus, medial temporal lobe, anterior cingulate, and medial frontal lobe. These findings are also consistent with another study of 372 normal middle-aged participants, which showed that the degree of insulin resistance was associated with medial temporal lobe atrophy as well as the rate of progressive atrophy over 4 years (Willette et al., 2013). Both sets of findings suggest that glucose dysregulation may contribute to the pathophysiology of AD through increased atrophy in critical brain regions.

Population Attributable Fraction for Diabetes

As we have seen in previous chapters, the PAF is the measure of the proportion of a disease that can be attributed to or caused by an exposure. The PAF is a useful indicator of the potential primary prevention that a risk factor might offer. Calculation of the PAF for one risk factor at a time assumes that risk factors are independent of one another; thus it is desirable to take shared variance into account. In one such study, adjusted PAFs were calculated for seven risk factors (Norton et al., 2014) that had been previously published as independent PAFs (Barnes and Yaffe, 2011). To account for collinearity between risk factors, a novel method was devised, which weighted the PAF for each risk factor. The "adjusted" PAF ranged between 1.9% and 4.5% for T2D. The calculation of the PAF takes into account the prevalence of the exposure. Because T2D is relatively rare in the population (5–11%), the PAF for T2D also is relatively low. Further study on diabetes and insulin resistance is necessary to elucidate the exact role of this condition and insulin in the etiology of AD.

HYPERTENSION

About 70% of diabetics also have hypertension, and the OR for diabetes associated with hypertension is approximately 2 (Lago, Singh, & Nesto, 2007). Today, hypertension affects about a quarter of the adult population and it is estimated that half of all hypertensive patients are insulin resistant (Craft, 2009). Among people age 70 and over, the prevalence of hypertension is about 50% (Skoog & Gustafson, 2002). By 2025, it is expected that almost 1.6 billion adults will be hypertense. Comorbid diabetes and hypertension place an individual at risk for chronic kidney disease (Lago et al., 2007), which has been found in some studies to be related to cognitive function (Yaffe et al., 2010) but not in others (Helmer et al., 2011). Both conditions together also raise the risk for coronary artery disease and stroke (Willey et al., 2014). Hypertension is considered to be a major risk factor for vascular cognitive impairment and vascular dementia (Gorelick, 2004).

Hypertension is diagnosed if systolic blood pressure (SBP) exceeds 140–160 mm Hg or diastolic pressure exceeds 90 mm Hg. Population-based epidemiologic studies of AD have defined hypertension in a number of ways: (i) by measuring actual blood pressures, (ii) by classifying as positive a person who reported that a physician diagnosed them with hypertension, and (iii) by the subject taking medication for hypertension. A few studies have been able to examine blood pressure data from midlife. These studies are most useful because older populations may be biased by survival and because AD is associated with a drop in blood pressure, as we shall describe.

Cohort Studies

In the Longitudinal Population Study in Göteborg, Sweden (the H70 study), 973 of 1,148 70-year olds were enrolled from a population census (Skoog et al., 1996). Of these, 382 nondemented subjects were selected randomly for a psychiatric evaluation. At age 85, these participants had an evaluation for dementia. Despite a very small number of incident AD cases in this study (n = 10), subjects with high diastolic blood pressure at age 70 had a higher risk for developing AD at ages 79–85. Over the 15-year follow-up of this study, incident AD cases had a larger decline in SBP and diastolic blood pressure (DBP) compared with people who did not develop AD. This general trend has been seen throughout the literature, starting with cross-sectional studies that reported an inverse association between SBP and DBP and prevalent AD (Guo, Viitanen, Fratiglioni, & Winblad, 1996). In a follow-up to the Göteborg study, Skoog and his colleagues described declining blood pressure in the years immediately preceding and following AD onset (Skoog, Andreasson, Landahl, & Lernfelt, 1998).

Some studies have found increased risks for poorer cognition associated with higher SBPs, including the Atherosclerosis Risk in Communities study and the Framingham Study (Elias, Wolf, D'Agostino, Cobb, & White, 1993), but even these have mixed results (Qiu, Winblad, & Fratiglioni, 2005). Because longitudinal, population-based studies provide the most information about the temporal sequence of the association between hypertension and AD, we will focus on these. Those that examined midlife blood pressure and cognition were fairly consistent in finding that midlife high systolic blood pressure (HSBP) has harmful effects on cognition in later life.

For the outcome of dementia and its subtypes, some studies have found that hypertension (usually self-reported when the cohort was nondemented) or history of hypertension is associated with incident VaD, but not necessarily AD. For example, in the Hisayama Study, a prospective population-based study in Japan, among 828 participants followed over 7 years, blood pressures exceeding 160/95 mm Hg were not associated with AD, but were associated with VaD (OR for increase of one standard deviation in SBP = 1.6, 95% CI 1.2–2.2) (Yoshitake et al., 1995). Similarly, in the WHICAP cohort, history of hypertension was related with incident VaD (RR = 1.8, 95% CI = 1.0–3.2) but not with

AD (RR = 0.9, 95% CI = 0.7–1.3) (Posner et al., 2002). In the *Kame* Project, we measured blood pressure at baseline and incident AD over a 6-year follow-up. While the univariate analysis showed that blood pressure ≥140 mm Hg at baseline was marginally associated with increased risk for AD ($p = 0.05$), this association was absent upon multivariate analysis (Borenstein et al., 2005). In these studies, cohorts were age 65 and over and had relatively short follow-ups (<10 years, usually in the range of 5–8 years). It is not surprising that high blood pressure would be a risk factor for VaD. Hypertension is the major risk factor for stroke, and stroke is the main determinant (with silent strokes and white matter disease) of VaD. That hypertension is generally unrelated to AD from these studies also is not surprising, given the observation that blood pressure begins to drop with increasing age, particularly in those at risk for AD. There are several methodological artifacts that may contribute to a null or inverse association of hypertension with AD. Because studies often limit enrollment to people over age 65, those with severe hypertension or stroke before this age may not participate because of prior stroke history, limiting the severity of hypertension of enrollees and therefore reducing the strength of the association. The relatively brief follow-up time between enrollment and incidence of AD also could lead to findings of lower blood pressures in those at risk for AD given the drop in blood pressure prior to AD onset. Underadjustment or overadjustment for potential confounders may also result in reduction of the strength of the hypertension-AD association. In addition, the decision to use only probable AD incident cases by NINCDS-ADRDA criteria as the outcome would result in the exclusion of possible AD cases in which VRFs may play a more important role. Finally, the exposure based on self-report may be misclassified, most frequently by underreporting of hypertension.

When a meta-analysis of studies with relatively brief follow-ups was performed of the association between a history of hypertension obtained from baseline interviews with nondemented cohort participants and incident AD, the pooled estimate was RR = 0.97 (95% CI 0.80–1.16) (Power et al., 2011). For a 10 mm Hg increase in SBP, the association with AD was RR = 0.95 (95% CI 0.91–1.00) and for a 10 mm Hg increase in DBP, it was RR = 0.94 (95% CI 0.85–1.04) (Power et al., 2011). Although several explanations can be given for these findings, it is likely that predisease onset drops in blood pressure are responsible for the inverse association with SBP.

What does stand out in the literature is the consistency of results among the few studies that were able to measure blood pressure in midlife and follow cohorts over several decades for late-life dementia outcomes and neuropathology. The HAAS measured blood pressures three times five minutes apart beginning in 1968–1970 (Launer, Masaki, Petrovitch, Foley, & Havlik, 1995; Launer et al., 2000). In 1995, they reported that high SBP levels in midlife were associated with the risk for cognitive impairment (CASI score <82/100) when the HAAS men were about 78 years old. By contrast, midlife DBP was not associated with late-life cognitive impairment (Launer et al., 1995). A few years later, this group published their results with clinical outcomes (Launer et al., 2000). Blood pressures were stratified into four categories: for SBP, <100 mm Hg (low); 100–139 (normal); 140–159 (borderline); and 160+ (high); and for DBP, <80 mm Hg (low); 80–89 (normal); 90–94 (borderline); and 95+ (high). Hypertension was said to be present when it was outside of the normal limits in two out of three assessments. For this study, blood pressures were measured *an average of 27 years* before dementia outcomes were ascertained (DSM-III-R and NINCDS-ADRDA criteria for AD). The analyses were adjusted for age, education, APOE-ε4, smoking, alcohol consumption, prevalent cerebrovascular accident, prevalent coronary heart disease, and subclinical atherosclerosis. The men were about 53 years old in 1965–1968 (over 60% were 45–55 years old) and were assessed for dementia for the first time in 1991–1993. About 57% of the sample had never been treated for their high blood pressure; therefore the results were stratified by treatment status. For prevalent dementia among men who were never treated, the OR associated with an SBP of 160 mm Hg or higher compared with an SBP in the normal range was 4.85 (95% CI = 1.99–11.83). For DBP of 90–94 mm Hg versus normal blood pressure, the OR for dementia among those never treated was 3.78 (95% CI = 1.59–8.95). For those with DBP over 95 mm Hg, the OR was 4.00 (95% CI = 1.56–10.25). Interestingly, no associations were found in men treated for their hypertension. For AD, none of the adjusted ORs was significant for SBP, but for untreated high SBP, the adjusted OR for VaD was 11.80 (95% CI = 3.52–39.5). Conversely, for untreated DBP, the OR for AD was 4.47 (95% CI = 1.45–13.1) (not significant for VaD) and for untreated low DBP, it was similarly elevated for AD (OR = 1.86, 95% CI = 1.01–3.46) (not significant for VaD). This was the first study that measured blood pressure in midlife that found a strong association between DBP and AD.

In 2000, the HAAS group published a second paper that examined midlife hypertension in relation to the presence of neurofibrillary tangles, neuritic plaques and low brain weight in 243 cohort members who came to autopsy (Petrovitch et al., 2000). SBP ≥160 mm Hg in midlife was associated with lower brain weight and a higher number of neuritic plaques in the neocortex and the hippocampus, while DBP ≥95 mm Hg was associated with a higher number of neurofibrillary tangles in the hippocampus. These results suggest that there may be a direct relationship between elevated blood pressure and AD neuropathology. An alternative explanation is that among individuals with extensive AD lesions, those with higher BP may have survived longer, leading to greater progression of the underlying disease. Although not from a representative autopsy study, Sparks et al. (1995) reported that individuals with a history of hypertension had higher densities of senile plaques and neurofibrillary tangles than did a similarly aged group of individuals without cardiac disease. Unfortunately, the latter group was not characterized by the presence or absence of hypertension, so the findings do not necessarily show that hypertension increases Alzheimer lesions. Outside of the presence or absence of heart disease, little information was provided on confounders such as sex and other AD risk factors that could influence AD pathology.

Other studies support the additive joint effects of hypertension and AD biomarkers. For example, in a cross-sectional study of 115 cognitively healthy volunteers (Glodzik et al., 2012), MRI and cerebrospinal fluid tests were obtained. Hypertension was defined based on whether the subjects were currently on antihypertensive treatment or had SBP $\geq$ 140 mm Hg or DBP $\geq$ 90 mm Hg. CSF AD biomarkers were defined as high if t-tau > 350 pg/mL, p-tau$_{231}$ > 18 pg/mL, and Aß$_{42}$/Aß$_{40}$ < 0.11, which are standard cut-scores. For other biomarkers (p-tau$_{231}$/Aß$_{42}$, t-tau/Aß$_{42}$) the medians were used since no standard cut-scores existed. The hypertensive and nonhypertensive groups were similar for AD biomarkers after adjusting for age and sex, but white matter lesion (WMH) scores were higher in hypertensive subjects ($p < 0.001$). Hypertensive subjects had more gray matter atrophy in the cerebellum, occipital, and frontal regions. Although elevated CSF AD biomarkers and hypertension were both related to more gray matter atrophy, no multiplicative interactions were found, and the authors concluded that among asymptomatic individuals, AD pathology and hypertension act additively with regard to damage to the gray matter.

In 2001, a Finnish research group reported their findings for midlife VRFs and AD in later life based on a longitudinal population-based study that began in 1972 (North Karelia project and FINMONICA) (Kivipelto et al., 2001). Those who were aged 65–79 in 1997 were worked up for dementia and AD. There were 1,449 participants from an original population of 2,293 people. Midlife blood pressure was classified as normal if SBP < 140 mm Hg, borderline if SBP fell in the range of 140–159 mm Hg, and high if it exceeded 160 mm Hg; for DBP, the cut-scores were < 90, 90–94, and $\geq$ 95 mm Hg. The examination in 1998 was the first time the cohort had been evaluated for cognition and dementia. Therefore, prevalent AD (n = 48 vs 1352 nondemented participants) was the outcome used. Dementia, AD, and VaD were defined using standard research criteria (DSM-IV for dementia, NINCDS-ADRDA for AD). At exposure assessment, the cohort was on average 50 years old. At outcome ascertainment, they were on average 71 years old, with 60% of the study population being women (as opposed to HAAS, which included only men). The odds ratios for AD, adjusted for age, education, BMI, history of myocardial infarction and cerebrovascular symptoms, smoking, and alcohol consumption increased with increasing SBP compared to normal SBP (OR = 2.1, 95% CI = 0.8–5.0) for borderline SBP and OR = 2.8 (95% CI 1.1–7.2) for high SBP). No significant findings were identified for DBP. While the study design was similar to that of HAAS, the studies differed in that HAAS showed an association with high DBP whereas this exposure was not related to the outcome in the Finnish study. The Finnish group did not stratify on treatment status, nor were there autopsy data, as in HAAS. Besides the different population and ethnic group, the authors of the Finnish study cite nonresponse bias as possibly influencing their findings. SBP was higher in midlife among nonparticipants, and if cognition in later life was lower in nonparticipants, their results would be underestimated (for both SBP and DBP). The prevalence of dementia in this cohort also may be underestimated, since cognitive screening in the first phase of the diagnostic process did not include screening of any subjects with MMSE scores ≥24/30. Therefore, some hypertensives may have escaped detection as being demented.

A third study published in 2005 used a different approach (Whitmer, Sidney, Selby, Johnston, & Yaffe, 2005). Employing electronic medical records from Kaiser Permanente Medical Care Program of Northern California from January 1994 to April 2003, Whitmer and colleagues defined hypertension if subjects met one of the following criteria: they had a self-reported history of physician-diagnosed hypertension, they used antihypertensive medication, or they had a measured SBP ≥140 mm Hg or a DBP of ≥90 mm Hg. Dementia diagnoses were also obtained from the database, using five ICD codes. The population was younger at exposure assessment than in the HAAS and Finnish studies (42 years old), and they were about 68.4 (nondementias) and 69.3 (dementia cases) in 1994. In Cox proportional hazards regression models, the presence of hypertension increased the risk for incident AD by 24% (HR = 1.24, 95% CI = 1.04–1.48), adjusted for age at midlife exam, age at baseline of the dementia study, sex, race, education, presence of diabetes, high cholesterol, and smoking. Interestingly, when the four cardiovascular measures (hypertension, diabetes, high cholesterol, and smoking) were in the model together, each was independently statistically associated with the risk for dementia (HRs varying between 1.24 and 1.46), and when the number of cardiovascular risk factors were summed, the risks for dementia increased in a dose-response manner from 1.27 (95% CI = 1.02–1.58) for one risk factor to 2.37 (95% CI = 1.10–5.10) for four. Because outcomes were ascertained from ICD codes, no attempt was made to determine the subtype of dementia.

In the ACT cohort in Seattle, WA, hypertension was measured among participants age 65 and over from 1994 onward (Li et al., 2007). This study had a 52% refusal rate, enrolling 2,581 of 5,422 members of the HMO. It was argued that the high refusal rate did not impact the results, because refusals were similar to participants by demographic characteristics (although a detailed medical record analysis of this issue was not conducted). SBP and DBP were measured at baseline and at four incidence waves of the cohort and clinical outcomes (dementia and AD) were ascertained using standard criteria for those who scored less than 86/100 on the CASI. At the end of 2004, there were 380 new dementia cases and 1,289 nondemented subjects. Two blood pressure measurements were taken 5 min apart and averaged; 2,342 had a valid measurement from baseline and at least one follow-up visit. SBP and DBP were stratified similarly to other studies, with SBP ≥160 mm Hg, borderline 140–159, and normal <140 mm Hg; DBP was high if DBP ≥90 mm Hg, borderline at 80–89 mm Hg, and normal at <80 mm Hg. Cox proportional hazards regression models were adjusted for sex, education (years), race (white/nonwhite), APOE-ε4 presence, history of coronary heart disease, cerebrovascular disease, and T2D, as well as use of antihypertensive medications. Although only baseline SBP and DBP were used in the main analyses, the authors also investigated whether BP declined more in demented than in nondemented subjects in the years prior to dementia onset.

They also stratified their analyses into three age groups (65–74, 75–84, and ≥85) to investigate whether there was effect-modification by age, hypothesizing that the association would be positive for younger participants and null or inverse for older participants.

High SBP (≥160 mm Hg) was associated with incident dementia (HR = 1.60, 95% CI = 1.01–2.55), but only in the youngest age stratum. Only borderline DBP increased dementia risk (HR = 1.59, 95% CI 1.07–2.35), again in the lowest age stratum; high DBP (≥90 mm Hg) was inverse (0.69) and not statistically significant. The same trends were evident with risk for incident probable AD, but none of the HRs was statistically significant. The authors found no differences between the dementia and nondementia groups in terms of the number of years prior to outcome when the blood pressures were measured. SBP and DBP declined similarly in both groups over time.

While different studies have somewhat different findings regarding SBP and DBP, hypertension appears to be a risk factor for AD if it occurs in mid-adulthood (40s–60s). The null or inverse associations found for older individuals may be an artifact of design (incipient dementia cases may forget their hypertension history even when they are "nondemented") or may be spurious due to characteristics of older cohorts (reverse causality or survival bias). Additionally, some studies suggest that among subjects older than 70, low DBP (<70 mm Hg) may be associated with increased risk for dementia and AD (Fournier et al., 2009). This finding was reported in HAAS, the Kungsholmen Study, and in the East Boston study as well as others (Dickstein et al., 2010). While the mechanism for this risk factor is unclear, a lack of perfusion to the brain could be one explanation or the low DBP could be a consequence of neuropathology. This finding is important because it implies that the risk for AD with regard to blood pressure may vary considerably with age. While midlife hypertension is likely to be a risk factor for late-life dementia, hypotension in old age may be a marker for incipient AD.

Treatment Studies

Given the association between midlife hypertension and AD, an important question is whether antihypertensive treatment slows down cognitive decline or reduces the risk for AD. According to some observational studies (Nagai, Hoshide, & Kario, 2010), antihypertensive treatment is associated with reduced cognitive decline or a lower incidence of dementia. For example, in the Cache County study in Utah, among 3,227 individuals age 65 and over who were permanent residents of the county in 1995, the use of any antihypertensive medication at baseline predicted a reduced risk for AD (HR = 0.64, 95% CI = 0.41–0.98); with the lowest HR being associated with potassium-sparing diuretics (HR = 0.26, 95% CI 0.08–0.64) (Khachaturian et al., 2006). Other studies such as the Rotterdam Study (in't Veld, Ruitenberg, Hofman, Stricker, & Breteler, 2001), the Kungsholmen study (Guo et al., 1999), and the Indianapolis study (Murray et al., 2002) have reported similar findings for cognitive performance and dementia. In an autopsy study of 291 brains from the Mt. Sinai School of Medicine in New York City (Hoffman et al., 2009), there was less AD pathology among hypertensive subjects who had been treated than among subjects who had normal blood pressure levels in midlife (ascertained from medical records). Antihypertensive medications may have a beneficial effect on AD neuropathology, perhaps even in excess of their effect on blood pressure.

A more definitive answer to the question regarding the efficacy of antihypertensive medications requires data from RCTs. In 2014, a trial of almost 3,000 T2D patients using intensive blood pressure and lipid-lowering interventions over 40 months failed to show differences in cognitive function at the end of the trial (Williamson et al., 2014). In this trial, the group with intensive blood pressure control actually showed a *reduction* in TBV compared to the group receiving standard therapy.

RCTs of blood pressure medications to reduce cognitive impairment and AD have been reviewed by Nagai and colleagues (2010). In this paper, the authors reviewed eight trials that were conducted prior to 2010. Although the sample sizes were very large in these trials (ranging from 2,418 to 9,297 subjects), inclusion and exclusion criteria, treatments, choice of neuropsychological tests, and clinical outcomes and periods of follow-up (2.2–4.5 years) varied. In general, these studies showed that the treatments did reduce blood pressures and that there was a trend toward better neuropsychological performance and lower incidence rates of dementia among those treated. However, few trials achieved statistical significance (Nagai et al., 2010). In a meta-analysis, Peters, Beckett, et al. (2008) combined results from four placebo-controlled trials that assessed whether antihypertensive medications reduced the incidence of dementia. They show a combined HR of 0.87 (95% CI 0.76–1.0). A second meta-analysis (McGuinness, Todd, Passmore, & Bullock, 2009) also combined four trials (including three that were included in the first meta-analysis) of hypertensive subjects without a prior history of cerebrovascular disease, and reported a similar point estimate (OR = 0.89, 95% CI 0.74–1.07) that was not statistically significant for the outcome of incident dementia. These meta-analyses suggest that antihypertensive medications might lead to small to moderate reductions in incident dementia. In the meta-analysis by McGuinness and colleagues, an analysis of cognitive change from baseline including three of the four studies demonstrated that MMSE scores benefited from the treatment (mean difference 0.42 (95% CI = 0.30–0.53). In all studies, blood pressure values (diastolic: −4.28 (95% CI = −4.58 to −3.98) and systolic: −10.22 (95% CI = −10.78 to −9.66)) were significantly reduced by the treatments.

The most promising RCT of antihypertensive treatment in the secondary prevention of dementia was the Systolic Hypertension in Europe (Syst-Eur) Study (Forette et al., 2002). In this study, nondemented participants with SBPs of 160–219 mm Hg and DBP less than 95 mm Hg were randomized to the active treatment dihydropyridine calcium channel blocker nitrendipine (10–40 mg/day). This drug could be supplemented with or substituted with enalapril maleate (5–20 mg/day), hydrochlorothiazide (12.5–25 mg/day) or both together. The placebo group was treated the same way with matching pills. The goal for blood pressure was to reduce SBP by at least 20 mm Hg to a level below 150 mm Hg. Participants were screened for dementia at baseline using cognitive screening criteria and were administered the MMSE annually. If the MMSE score fell below 23, the participant was worked up for dementia using DSM-III-R criteria (standard in 1988 when the trial began). Stroke was the primary outcome. Nineteen European countries and 106 centers participated in the trial, which enrolled 3,228 individuals. In the trial, 1,485 people with a median age of 68 were randomized to treatment and 1,417 to placebo and followed for 3.9 years. Sixty-four incident dementia cases occurred with an overall incidence rate of dementia of 5.2/1000 person-years. The adjusted HR for dementia associated with treatment was 0.38 (95% CI = 0.23–0.64). For each 1,000 person-years of treatment, the authors estimated that 20 cases of dementia (95% CI = 7–33) could be prevented. The results were also applicable to AD, for which there were 12 new AD cases in the treated group and 29 in the placebo group.

The issue of whether specific drug classes are more effective than others has been examined by Fournier et al. (2009). These investigators have proposed that dihydropyridine calcium channel blockers and angiotensin-AT1 receptor blockers have greater neuroprotective effects than other classes of antihypertensives, such as diuretics and angiotensin-converting enzyme inhibitors. Potassium-sparing diuretics have been shown to reduce incident AD only in prospective cohort studies, but not in randomized clinical trials. In the Syst-Eur trial (Forette et al., 2002), the authors cited impaired regulation of intracellular calcium in aging as a possible mechanism of action of calcium channel blockers, which lead to other cell abnormalities and to neuronal death. Calcium homeostasis also is affected by aging and by AD pathology, and among people with dementia, ß-amyloid may increase levels of intraneuronal free calcium, exposing the brain to oxidative and inflammatory stress (Fournier et al., 2009).

Further studies to answer the question regarding which antihypertensives are most effective in preventing AD are difficult because of ethical decisions about randomizing people to certain medications that may not work best to reduce their hypertension. All of the studies included in the meta-analyses had cardiovascular or cerebrovascular diseases as their primary outcome. For example, the Syst-Eur trial had to be stopped because a clear benefit was evident for incident stroke outcomes. It is likely that clinical trials are needed to fully investigate the effects of antihypertensive drugs on dementia occurrence. McGuinness, Todd, Passmore, and Bullock (2009) point out that it would be most useful to follow people in trials from midlife onward, but this is neither ethical nor feasible.

Mechanisms

The term, "arteriosclerotic brain disease" was an early term used for vascular dementia, and in the evolution of our knowledge of AD, the term "senility" was often used in conjunction with the term, "hardening of the arteries." While these definitions have been rejected, some of these concepts have come full circle. Aging is accompanied by increasing stiffness of the large and small arteries, which leads to increases in SBP; and in turn, SBP increases arterial stiffness. Elevated SBP also affects atherosclerotic processes and changes in the autoregulation of blood flow to the brain.

Elevated SBP also has been associated with increased brain atrophy, as well as white and gray matter injury, including WMH and asymptomatic infarcts (Maillard et al., 2012). In a study of 579 of over 4,000 participants in the third-generation Framingham Study who had MRIs (Maillard et al., 2012), diffusion tensor imaging was used to measure fractional anisotropy and mean diffusivity. These measures of white matter integrity are more sensitive than WMH. This cross-sectional analysis of young people who were on average 39 years old, with a mean SBP of 115 and DBP of 74 (60% women) found a linear association between SBP and decreased regional fractional anisotropy and increased mean diffusivity, as well as with lower gray matter volumes, implying that subtle vascular impairments to the brain may occur in response to high SBP even in young middle age (Maillard et al., 2012).

Population Attributable Fraction for Hypertension in Midlife

The global PAF for AD associated with midlife hypertension has been estimated at 5.1% (95% CI 1.4–9.9) (Barnes and Yaffe, 2011), assuming an RR of 1.61 (95% CI 1.16–2.24) and a prevalence of 8.9%. In the United States, this estimate would be higher (8.0%, 95% CI = 2.2–15.1), based on a higher prevalence of hypertension in midlife (14.3%) (Norton et al., 2014). In a systematic review (Kloppenborg, van den Berg, Kappelle, & Biessels, 2008), the PAF for dementia (not AD alone) associated with hypertension was estimated to be 30% based on an OR for dementia of 2.3 and an estimated prevalence of hypertension of 30–40%. Because hypertension is considerably more prevalent than T2D, from a public health viewpoint, it has a greater impact on the frequency of dementia and AD.

CHOLESTEROL

In 1994, Sparks and his colleagues described an experiment in rabbits fed either a high cholesterol diet or a placebo diet for 4, 6, and 8 weeks (Sparks et al., 1994). Neuropathologic analyses revealed that the high cholesterol diet led to increased accumulation of intracellular immunolabeled ß-amyloid in the brain that was higher the longer the diet was continued.

Elevated cholesterol levels, particularly low-LDL cholesterol, increase the risk for death from CVD (Eichner et al., 2002), and cholesterol levels, like blood pressure, drop with increasing age (Chui, Zheng, Reed, Vinters, & Mack, 2012). Therefore, in any cohort study of cholesterol and AD, midlife cholesterol will be a better target than late-life cholesterol. Indeed, a similar situation that we have discussed regarding hypertension applies to the epidemiologic investigation of cholesterol levels and risk for AD. We also need to consider the amount of follow-up time in cohort studies. For late-life assessment of serum cholesterol levels and AD, studies either show null results, as in the Framingham Study (Tan et al., 2003) or inverse associations, as in the WHICAP cohort (Reitz et al., 2010a) and in the H70 Göteborg study (Mielke et al., 2005).

Cohort Studies

Four studies assessed midlife cholesterol levels, three of which looked at AD outcomes specifically. The first study (Notkola et al., 1998) examined 444 men age 70–89 years old who were survivors of a large cohort called the Seven Countries Study, a study initiated in 1959 when the men were 40–59 years old. They related serum cholesterol levels, defining "high" as ≥6.5 mmol/L, to the prevalence of AD and reported an OR of 3.1 (95% CI = 1.2–8.5), adjusting for age and APOE-ε4. This early study also found that prior to AD onset, cholesterol levels began to decline.

The second study (Kivipelto et al., 2002) measured serum total cholesterol concentrations in 1972–1977 and 1982–1987, with 48 cases of probable and possible AD diagnosed according to standard criteria and 82 cases of prevalent MCI diagnosed by Mayo criteria (Petersen et al., 1995). APOE-ε4 carriers had slightly higher cholesterol levels in mid- and late-life compared with noncarriers, but were similar with respect to BMI, blood pressure, and other cardiovascular and cerebrovascular characteristics. Adjusting for age, sex, education, APOE, smoking, and alcohol consumption, the OR for AD associated with high cholesterol was 2.8 (95% CI = 1.2–6.7). Importantly, adjustments for APOE status did not change the estimates. High midlife SBP also was an independent predictor of prevalent AD in this sample, as was a history of myocardial infarction. The authors concluded that the association between APOE-ε4 and AD was not mediated by lipid levels. When the OR was calculated for combined risk factors (APOE-ε4, high midlife cholesterol and high midlife SBP) by scoring each individual as a 0, 1, 2 or 3, the OR for AD comparing all three risk factors to no risk factors was 8.4 (95% CI = 2.0–36.0) adjusting for age, sex, education, smoking, and alcohol. This OR is consistent with an additive interaction of these risk factors.

The third study that examined total cholesterol at midlife was the HAAS (Kalmijn et al., 2000). The adjusted OR for prevalent dementia associated with one standard deviation of higher cholesterol at the average age of 53 was 1.10 (95% CI 0.95–1.26). For AD, the point estimate was not elevated (OR = 1.00, 95% CI = 0.94–1.05) but that for VaD was (OR = 1.11, 95% CI 1.05–1.18). The authors proposed that these are underestimates of the effect of cholesterol due to survival bias with carriers of high cholesterol dying before dementia would occur.

Investigators of the Kaiser Permanente Multiphasic Health Checkups (MHC) study (Solomon, Kivipelto, Wolozin, Zhou, & Whitmer, 2009) also examined midlife lipid levels with regard to dementia risk. In an historical cohort analysis of 9,844 members spanning three decades, dementia was diagnosed by ICD-9 codes. There were 469 incident cases of AD between 1994 and 2007. At baseline, the cohort was about 42 years old. Adjusting for age, sex, education, race/ethnicity, midlife BMI, diabetes, hypertension, and late-life stroke, the HRs for AD were 1.23 (95% CI = 0.97–1.55) for borderline cholesterol levels (200–239 mg/dL) and 1.57 (95% CI 1.23–2.01) for high cholesterol levels (≥240 mg/dL). In this study, the HR for VaD was statistically significant only for borderline cholesterol levels and not for high levels, which may have reflected lower statistical power in this stratum. Further analyses revealed that a threshold of > 220 mg/dL defined a cut-off whereby risk for AD began to increase. Although LDL cholesterol levels are considered the most proatherogenic, in 1964–1973 when the level of total cholesterol was determined, these measures were not available. The main shortcoming of this study was the inability to standardize the diagnosis and subtypes of dementia. Specifically, there was no allowance for mixed dementias by ICD-9 codes. However, this study represents the largest sample size and longest follow-up to determine the importance of high cholesterol concentrations in midlife for the risk for AD. The more modest effects of high cholesterol in the US studies compared to the Finnish studies may be related to the higher stroke risk among Finns.

With regard to LDL specifically, Yaffe and her colleagues followed over 1,000 postmenopausal women with coronary heart disease for 4 years who were enrolled in a clinical trial of estrogen/progestin (the HERS trial) (Yaffe, Barrett-Connor, Lin, & Grady, 2002) with lipoprotein measurements before and after follow-up. Prevalent cognitive impairment was defined as a Modified Mini-Mental Examination Score (3MS) of <84 of 100. They found that high LDL as well as high total cholesterol levels were associated with prevalent cognitive impairment.

Kloppenborg et al. (2008) included eight studies on dyslipidemia in their systematic review. Of these, most obtained serum cholesterol levels, while others also included triglycerides and specific lipoproteins (high-density and low-density). Of four studies that examined AD as an outcome, two found statistically significant associations. No studies examining triglycerides found any association with AD or VaD.

Mechanisms

A number of mechanisms increase the biologic plausibility of a relation between higher cholesterol levels and risk for AD. Cholesterol has been shown to increase the activity of the ß- or γ-secretase enzymes that drive Aß production from APP, with a lower amount of APP metabolized through the nonamyloidogenic α-secretase pathway (Shepardson, Shankar, & Selkoe, 2011a). Other mechanisms through which high cholesterol could act include increased inflammation and phosphorylated tau. The idea that cholesterol could affect aggregation of Aß also has been proposed.

It is known that optimal cholesterol concentrations are important to maintain the health of neurons. These observations have led to the question of whether treatment by statins, drugs to reduce cholesterol levels, has led to a concomitant reduction in AD incidence. Preclinical studies (conducted in cell culture or in experimental animals) suggest that statins have the potential to reduce Aß production (Shepardson et al., 2011a). Several observational studies also suggest that statins reduce AD risk. In a case–control study from the UK clinical practices that donate data to the UK-based General Practice Research Database (Jick, Zornberg, Jick, Seshadri, & Drachman, 2000), 284 dementia cases were compared with 1,080 controls, all of whom had hyperlipidemia. The OR was not statistically significant for any comparison for untreated hyperlipidemia or non-statin lipid-lowering medications, but for statins, the OR was 0.29 (95% CI = 0.13–0.63). An analysis from the Cache County Study (Zandi et al., 2005) found an inverse association between statin use and prevalent dementia (OR = 0.44, 95% CI = 0.14–0.86), but no association with incident dementia (HR = 1.19, 95% CI = 0.53–2.34) or AD (HR = 1.19, 95% CI = 0.35–2.96). It is risky to use a cross-sectional design to examine this question, since prevalent dementia or AD cases may be less likely to be prescribed a statin (Hofman et al., 1997). They also may be more likely to go off treatment when AD symptoms develop. In addition, the use of statins may be more prevalent among people with healthy lifestyles (i.e., controls). Cross-sectionally, these kinds of problems can lead to the appearance of an inverse association between statins and AD.

Randomized Clinical Trials

RCTs of statins in AD have yielded inconsistent results. Shepardson and colleagues (Shepardson, Shankar, & Selkoe, 2011b) summarized the findings of five trials with four different lipid-lowering agents (atorvastatin, lovastatin, simvastatin and pravastatin). The only trial that was deemed effective had only 94 participants, a 12-week follow-up, and the outcome was reduction of serum Aß levels (Friedhoff, Cullen, Geoghagen, & Buxbaum, 2001). Others showed null results for incidence of AD, or no change in cognition in AD patients. A major limitation of the RCTs was their relatively brief duration (about 1–2 years). Studies starting in midlife aimed at reducing cholesterol in asymptomatic individuals at risk for AD are needed to better determine the effectiveness of statins in reducing incidence of AD. However, trials of such long duration are not practical.

APOE Interaction

APOE-ε4 has also been shown to interact with total cholesterol levels on AD risk, but in an unexpected way. In the Indianapolis study of 2,212 African

Americans, AD prevalence was associated with higher total cholesterol levels among ε4 noncarriers, but among carriers, there was no association between total cholesterol and AD risk (Evans et al., 2000). This is similar to our findings from the *Kame* Project, where VRFs (diabetes and transient ischemic attack or TIA) were associated with incident AD among ε4 noncarriers, but not among ε4 carriers (Borenstein et al., 2005). Other studies, as we have reviewed in the section on diabetes, have found the opposite association, that is, significant associations among carriers versus noncarriers.

Population Attributable Fraction for Cholesterol in Midlife

For midlife cholesterol, Kloppenborg et al. calculated an estimated PAF for high cholesterol in midlife of 18–22%, based on an OR for dementia of 2.1 and an estimated prevalence of 20–25%. In late-life, the estimated PAF was 0. It is likely that like blood pressure, the association of high cholesterol with AD may differ depending on when it is measured. In midlife, high cholesterol likely increases the risk for late-life AD through increased vascular damage, whereas in late-life, high cholesterol is unrelated to this risk.

OBESITY

That we are in the midst of a global obesity epidemic has been extensively covered in the media. What might be less well known is the number of health conditions that are affected by obesity. Among older people, obesity is associated with at least 10 forms of cancer, diabetes, hypertension, cardiovascular and cerebrovascular diseases, metabolic syndrome (MetS), obstructive sleep apnea, osteoarthritis, depression, disability, and quality of life (Salihu, Bonnema, & Alio, 2009; Solomon & Manson, 1997). Obesity also is associated with higher mortality risk, although the adiposity measure that is most harmful is still disputed (Solomon & Manson, 1997). Central obesity (using waist circumference or waist-to-hip ratio) appears to be particularly harmful (the "apple" shape). According to the most updated data from the World Health Organization (apps.who.int/bmi/index.jsp) the countries with more than 30% of obese adults (BMI $\geq$30) include Egypt, French Polynesia and several other small islands in the South Pacific, Panama, Saudi Arabia, the United Arab Emirates, and the United States. However, there are no data for a number of countries, including the Russian Federation. The worldwide prevalence of obesity is increasing and by 2030, it is predicted that 20% of the global population will be obese, with the prevalence in women exceeding that of men (Finkelstein et al., 2012). What is more alarming still is that increasing proportions of children and adolescents are meeting the definitions of overweight and obese (Ogden et al., 2006), meaning that higher adiposity may contribute to increasing incidence rates of disease, including AD, in the future.

The most common method of ascertaining adiposity in epidemiologic studies is to measure BMI, which is the ratio of weight (kg) to height (m) squared (weight in kg/(height in m)^2). In pounds, this is calculated as (lbs/in^2) $\times$ 703.

The World Health Organization traditionally classifies overweight and obesity into four strata: underweight (BMI <18.5), normal weight (18.5–24.9), overweight (25–29.9), and obese (≥30). Others have used percentile groups from the distribution of BMI (e.g., quantiles). Additional measures used to assess obesity include waist circumference by itself, waist-to-hip ratio, skinfold thickness, and others that are not used in population-based studies, such as bioelectrical impedance. Methods used to validate adiposity measures such as MRI or dual energy X-ray absorptiometry also exist. BMI as a measure of adiposity is considered indirect and imperfect, as body fat cannot be distinguished from lean body mass and body composition. Definitions of BMI strata may vary in different populations. For example in some Asian populations, the cut-off used for "overweight" is 23 instead of 25. BMI itself has good specificity but poor sensitivity for adiposity (sensitivities of 36% in men and 49% in women using NHANES-III data) (Romero-Corral et al., 2008). As one might expect, there is a tendency for self-reported weight to be underestimated, and height to be overestimated in both men and women, resulting in lower BMIs, likely underestimating the RRs for outcomes associated with BMI. In the Nurses' Health Study, Pearson correlations were similar for men and women, and were about 0.84–0.88 for self-reported hip measurements compared with two technician-measured measurements, and around 0.70 for waist-to-hip ratios (Rimm et al., 1990). Importantly, BMI underrepresents body fatness in older populations because older people lose muscle mass and generally have more fat than younger people (Gallagher et al., 1996; Kuczmarski, 1989).

There are problems interpreting the effect of BMI in persons of advanced age. For example, there is evidence that greater BMI is associated with increased all-cause mortality up to age 75, but that after this age, this association is lost (Stevens et al., 1998). In one study (Dahl et al., 2013), greater BMI was inversely associated with mortality in older age groups (RR = 0.80, $p = 0.01$) controlling for weight change and multiple morbidities. Furthermore, either a loss or a gain of BMI (defined here as 5% change over 18 years relative to stable BMI) was associated with increased mortality risk (RR = 1.65, 95% CI = 1.34–2.04 for loss and RR = 1.53, 95% CI = 1.18–1.99 for gain) (Dahl et al., 2013). This might be explained by confounding by smoking or other unmeasured covariates that are associated with BMI and reduced survival. Another explanation is that studies that adjust for intermediate variables in the causal pathway (such as diabetes, hypertension, and dyslipidemia) may erroneously reduce the association between obesity and mortality. Other data, such as a study in over 8,000 Seventh-Day Adventists who have strict dietary guidelines and generally do not smoke (Lindsted, Tonstad, & Kuzma, 1991) found that, with regard to mortality, men with BMIs below 22.3 (in the lowest quintile in that population) had the lowest rates of all-cause mortality. The question of how adiposity is related to mortality is not yet settled.

Obesity provides a common denominator for the other adverse vascular outcomes we have reviewed in this chapter. It is estimated that 80% of obese individuals are insulin resistant (Craft, 2009). The ORs associated with increasing strata of BMI (overweight, obese Class 2 and obese Class 3) increase for diabetes, hypertension, and hyperlipidemia. For example, for diabetes the ORs are 1.59 (95% CI = 1.46–1.73), 3.44 (95% CI = 3.17–3.74), and 7.37 (95% CI = 6.39–8.50) for the three BMI strata, respectively, compared with normal weight based on data from over 195,000 US adults age 18 and over who participated in the 2001 Behavioral Risk Factor Surveillance System (Mokdad et al., 2003). The ORs are similar for hypertension, but are lower for the association between hyperlipidemia (total cholesterol) and BMI strata (ORs = 1.5–1.9, all highly significant). In early old age, the co-occurrence of these morbidities is stronger, but likely decreases in the 80s and 90s when the prevalence of vascular morbidities begins to decline.

Insulin resistance exerts adverse effects on the vasculature. For example, insulin impacts capillary recruitment, vasodilation, and regional blood flow, and this results in a positive feedback system that worsens insulin resistance, further impairing the neurovascular unit (Craft, 2009). Adipose tissue produces adipokines, such as adiponectin, leptin, resistin, and cytokines, including Tumor Necrosis Factor-α and Interleukin-6, which may themselves be related to AD or may only be associated with AD through vascular conditions (Luchsinger & Gustafson, 2009). Leptin is an important player in the obesity story, since it is potentially neuroprotective (Anstey, Cherbuin, Budge, & Young, 2011).

There are a number of systematic reviews (Emmerzaal, Kiliaan, & Gustafson, 2014; Luchsinger & Gustafson, 2009) and meta-analyses (Anstey et al., 2011; Beydoun, Beydoun, & Wang, 2008) of the associations between body composition and AD, and it is not our purpose to review all of the studies. We will discuss some of the overall findings as well as controversies. In addition to body composition measured in mid- and late-life and AD measured in late-life, there are different findings depending on whether we are considering overweight or obesity as the exposure, or whether we look at the trajectory of weight loss over time. The question as to weight loss before and following AD onset is also pertinent. Each of these topics will be considered below.

Methodological difficulties involved in the investigation of adiposity aside from its measurement are similar to the other VRFs. Measurement time is critical as there is compelling evidence that the association with AD differs by whether adiposity is measured in mid- or late-life. Despite the relatively simple ways in which weight and height can be obtained, use of self-reported data will likely distort the effect measure toward the null for reasons given above. In addition, studies frequently use different cut-off scores for defining obesity, limiting the validity of comparisons. Another problem in comparing results between studies is the different variables used to adjust the RR for AD and dementia. We will consider only prospective cohort studies in our discussion.

Midlife Overweight and Obesity

In a systematic review and meta-analysis (Beydoun et al., 2008), four studies were considered that examined the association between obesity and dementia.

The overall RR for incident AD associated with obesity in this analysis was 1.8 (95% CI = 1.0–3.3). No effect-modification was reported by sex. For studies that assessed adiposity before the age of 60, the RR for AD was 3.10 (95% CI = 2.19–4.38), whereas for those assessing exposures later, it was 1.38 (95% CI = 0.94–1.66). When studies were limited to obesity assessed in midlife in another meta-analysis (Anstey et al., 2011), the pooled RR (using fixed effects) was 2.04 (95% CI = 1.59–2.62). In a third meta-analysis (Kloppenborg et al., 2008) the OR for dementia (not AD) was 2.0 based on three studies for obesity at midlife (age 45–65). However, not all studies have found this association. In a more recent systematic review (Emmerzaal et al., 2014), although six studies showed that midlife overweight and obesity increased the risk for dementia, three others did not, and one demonstrated significant risk only for obese subjects. In this review, the risk was stronger among obese women compared with obese men, although the findings from the individual studies were mixed.

In the largest study published to date (Qizilbash et al., 2015) the authors examined historical records from almost two million people aged 40 and higher from the Clinical Practice Research Datalink (CPRD), the routine primary care database in the United Kingdom and related BMI to incident dementia. A previous study had found that only 48% of cases identified as dementia or AD in the CPRD were deemed to meet stricter NINCDS-ADRDA criteria (Seshadri et al., 2001). For the BMI measurement, of over 6 million individuals in the database, only 32% had nonmissing data and had more than 12 months of historical data (from 1992 to 2007). The authors excluded prevalent cases of dementia by excluding dementia in the records if they were present within 12 months of the first BMI measurement. The follow-up for incident dementia cases occurred over a 9.1-year period. After adjustments for age, sex, smoking, alcohol status, diabetes, previous myocardial infarction, statin use, antihypertensive use, and the J-shaped effect of BMI on mortality, the authors found that underweight individuals (with a BMI <20) were 1.39 times more likely to develop incident dementia (95% CI = 1.36–1.42) compared with those of a healthy weight, and that with increasing BMI category, the risk for incident dementia decreased in a dose-response fashion. This trend was present even when the measurement of BMI occurred 15 years before dementia onset. Because the age distribution of the population was very broad, a large proportion of the sample was over age 65 at first BMI measurement, and in these people, weight loss is likely to precede dementia onset. The authors stated that further analyses would examine weight loss as a possible explanation for their findings. In addition, no adjustment was made for socioeconomic conditions across the life span. If SES is inversely associated with BMI in the United Kingdom, and SES is inversely associated with incident dementia, this could serve to attenuate the results. Stratifying the results by height might be another way to examine whether the association between BMI and incident dementia varies by a proxy measure of nutritional status across the life course. While this study (with over 45,000 dementia events) is certainly impressive with regard to its very large size, there are methodological questions regarding outcome and exposure ascertainment, selection bias, and confounding that cast some doubt on the findings.

Several studies with exceptionally long follow-ups are worthy of a closer look. In the Kaiser cohort (Whitmer, Gunderson, Barrett-Connor, Quesenberry, & Yaffe, 2005), 10,276 men and women were seen from 1964 to 1973 when they were ages 40–45 and those who were still members in 1994–2003 were evaluated for dementia. The authors included demographics, smoking, alcohol use, and cardio- and cerebrovascular diseases as covariates in Cox proportional hazards regression models. Obese subjects (BMI ≥30) had a HR for dementia (not specifically AD) of 1.74 (95% CI = 1.34–2.26), while overweight subjects had a HR of 1.35 (95% CI = 1.14–1.60) compared with normal weight individuals. Subscapular and triceps skinfold measurements also showed that those in the highest quintile incurred a HR of 1.72 (95% CI = 1.36–2.18) and 1.59 (95% CI = 1.24–2.04) respectively. This study is one of the first that had almost a 30-year follow-up period, a large sample size (713 dementia cases) in a representative population and adjusted for relevant confounders. In fact, adjustments for comorbid vascular conditions increased the HRs.

In the CAIDE study, 1,449 participants aged 65–79 years old were examined for dementia and AD (Kivipelto et al., 2005) and followed for 21 years. In this study, despite a statistically elevated OR for prevalent dementia when the model was adjusted only for demographic variables, when vascular variables related to obesity were sequentially adjusted, the OR became nonstatistically significant (OR = 1.88, 95% CI 0.76–4.63). In this study, being overweight in midlife was not associated with dementia risk (OR = 0.99, 95% CI = 0.47–2.15).

In HAAS, 1,890 men age 77–98 were monitored for incident dementia (Stewart et al., 2005) until 1999. Weight was measured in 1965 at the baseline of the Honolulu Heart Study and twice before 1999. Among 112 incident cases, baseline weight from mid- to late-life was similar to unaffecteds. In the Framingham Offspring Study, obesity assessed by BMI and waist-to-hip ratio in 1988–1990 in the age range 40–69 predicted poorer cognitive performance in executive function and visuomotor skills assessed in 1999–2002 (Wolf et al., 2007).

Another important study (Whitmer et al., 2008) attempted to examine specifically whether central obesity incurred more risk that total body obesity. Abdominal fat is more highly associated with T2D, insulin resistance, coronary artery disease, stroke, and mortality than total body fat. In the Kaiser Permanente Medical Care Program of Northern California cohort that participated in the Multiphasic Health Checkups study (MHC), sagittal abdominal diameter (SAD) was obtained to measure central obesity and sagittal thigh diameter to measure peripheral obesity; BMI also was measured. Sex-specific quintiles were calculated. Interestingly, while quintile of thigh diameter did not predict risk for dementia in any quintile (HRs range from 0.99 to 1.01, nonsignificant), there was a clear dose-response effect between SAD and dementia risk (Figure 14.3). What is even more compelling is that, while a Cox proportional

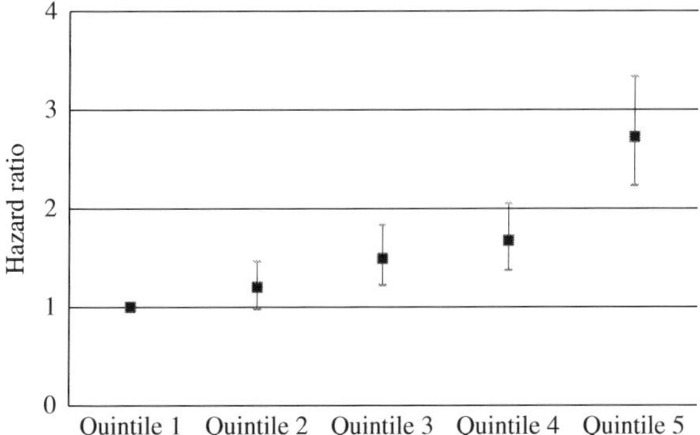

FIGURE 14.3 Hazard ratios for dementia by quintiles of sagittal abdominal diameter, Kaiser Permanente. *Adapted from Whitmer et al. (2008).*

hazards regression model adjusted for age, sex, race, education, marital status, medical care utilization, diabetes, hyperlipidemia, hypertension, ischemic heart disease, and stroke produced results similar to those in Figure 14.3, when the model was additionally adjusted for BMI, it was attenuated, but still showed the same shape, especially the increased risk in the highest quartile, suggesting that central adiposity predicts dementia independently from overall BMI. The authors also showed that, while overweight/obese adults without central adiposity had a RR of 1.8 for dementia, those who were both overweight and obese who also had central obesity had a RR for dementia of 2.34 and 3.60, respectively. This study had a follow-up time of 36 years and a large sample size, increasing the validity of the findings.

Late-Life Overweight and Obesity

The first investigation of the association between BMI and AD was in the Göteborg Study in Sweden (Gustafson, Rothenberg, Blennow, Steen, & Skoog, 2003). Over an 18-year follow-up of the population age 70 in Göteborg, BMI at age 70, 75, and 79 significantly predicted the risk for AD (range of HRs 1.23–1.36) but did not increase risk for VaD. However, it turns out that their study result was an outlier. All other studies that started with an older sample (≥65) found *inverse* associations between overweight or obesity measured in late-life and risk for AD, but not all were statistically significant. Emmerzaal et al. (2014) summarized studies of BMI and dementia or AD from 2003 to 2013 where BMI was measured in older populations but purposefully did not calculate pooled estimates because of the difficulty in pooling studies in which exposures and outcomes were measured in different ways and varying adjustments for confounders were made. The studies summarized for overweight and obesity measured late in life clearly showed an inverse risk present for AD and dementia.

In the CHS, a change was seen in the RR from a positive association for midlife measurement of BMI to a negative association with late-life measurement. At age 50, CHS participants self-reported their weight, and at baseline of the CHS-Cognition Study in 1992–3, participants were weighed and had their height measured (Fitzpatrick et al., 2009). For the midlife measurement, a statistically significant HR for dementia (not AD) was reported for obesity (RR = 1.39, 95% CI = 1.03–1.87 adjusting for demographic and VRFs). For the late-life measurement, an inverse association was found, in which each increased unit of BMI was associated with an HR of 0.95 (95% CI = 0.92–0.98) in the fully-adjusted model.

While adjusting for other VRFs is important to test the hypothesis that adiposity predicts dementia or AD independently, the analyses should also attempt to tease out the extent to which the other VRFs mediate the association between adiposity and cognitive outcomes. This has not been done systematically to date.

Weight Reduction and Underweight in Late-Life

In the *Kame* Project, we measured height and weight at baseline when the cohort was almost 72 years old. Over a follow-up period from 1992 to 1994 through 2001, higher baseline BMI was associated with a reduced risk for dementia (HR = 0.37, 95% CI = 0.14–0.98) (Hughes, Borenstein, Schofield, Wu, & Larson, 2009). We found additionally that those participants with a slower rate of decline in BMI had a lower risk for dementia. This was particularly evident among individuals who were initially overweight or obese (HR = 0.18, 95% CI = 0.05–0.58) (Hughes et al., 2009). Therefore, those who experienced a faster decline in BMI in their later years were at a higher risk for AD than those who lost weight less rapidly.

A similar finding was obtained in HAAS with a much longer follow-up period. During the first 26 years of follow-up, there were no differences in changes in weight in the incident dementia group and the unaffected group (Stewart et al., 2005). However, in the last 6 years of follow-up, men with incident dementia had an annual weight loss that exceeded that in men without dementia (−0.30 kg/year, 95% CI = −0.52 to −0.08). These and other data point to the now well-accepted prodrome of weight loss in individuals as they approach onset of AD. Weight loss continues throughout the course of the disease, accelerating during late disease stages. In the Japanese American populations studied in the *Kame* Project and in HAAS, frank obesity was rare, and the HAAS investigators point out that most of the weight loss in their sample occurred from a normal weight to underweight. The lack of obesity in this population may also be responsible for the null association between midlife obesity and risk for AD in HAAS. While it is known that underweight and obesity are associated with increased mortality, selective attrition of such individuals in these cohort studies would likely underestimate the HRs for dementia.

The CHS-Cognition Study reported that being underweight (defined as a BMI <20) was associated with an increased risk for dementia (HR = 1.62, 95%

CI = 1.02–2.64), while being overweight (BMI between 25 and 30) was not associated with dementia risk (HR = 0.90, 95% CI = 0.70–1.16). These results were similar for AD and VaD, except that the risks associated with underweight suggested a stronger association with VaD (Bennett, Schneider, Arvanitakis, et al., 2012; Fitzpatrick et al., 2009). Underweight is more difficult to study than overweight/obesity, because of small sample sizes of underweight participants who develop AD in longitudinal population-based studies.

Weight loss during AD is thought to be regulated through the hypothalamus, but there has been little systematic research into its mechanisms in preclinical AD (Stewart et al., 2005). In AD, cachexia (ill health that occurs with emaciation) often develops in mid- and late-stages, which can to some extent be attributed to changes in environment (e.g., moving to a nursing home from living independently), eating a different diet (potentially a poorer one), skipping meals, and behavioral problems. Cachexia is also known to be strongly related to the risk for death from AD (Evans et al., 1991).

If weight loss occurs as a prodromal sign before AD onset, how many years before can it occur? In one study from the Mayo Clinic, the Rochester Epidemiology Project, a matched case–control study was performed of 564 incident cases of dementia (1990–1994) (Knopman, Edland, Cha, Petersen, & Rocca, 2007). Weight was obtained cross-sectionally and at five previous time points. Cases and controls had similar weights 21 and 30 years before the study, but in the 9–10 years before the study, controls lost about 7.5 pounds, and dementia cases lost about 12 pounds. Among women, but not men, weight loss began 11–20 years before dementia onset. To explain these findings, the authors suggest that weight loss in women may be related to hormonal influences. In addition, reduced olfaction (ability to smell) may be partly responsible. Both loss of olfaction and increased depression have been shown to be markers of cognitive decline and AD, and these markers will be further discussed in Chapter 20.

Population Attributable Fraction for Obesity

We found three estimates of the PAF for AD attributable to obesity. Kloppenborg et al. (2008) estimated a PAF of 26–29% due to midlife obesity (ages 45–65, prevalence 35–40%) and zero for late-life obesity. Beydoun estimated a PAF of 21.1% (95% CI = 0–43%) for incident AD and 19.6% for VaD (95% CI = 21.5–64.2) using NHANES obesity prevalence rates from 1999 to 2002 (Beydoun et al., 2008). The lowest PAF comes from the analysis by Norton et al. (2014) based on midlife obesity. In this paper, the PAF was 7.3% (95% CI = 4.3–10.8) based on a prevalence of midlife obesity of 13.1% in the United States. The comparable PAF in Europe was 6.8% (95% CI = 1.9–13.0) based on a prevalence of 7.2%. For obesity globally, the PAF was estimated to be 2.0% (95% CI = 1.1–3.0) based on a prevalence of 3.4%. The latter prevalence is expected to continue to increase. Therefore, the global PAF estimate is likely conservative for future risk.

OTHER VASCULAR RISKS

We would like to close this chapter with a few words about stroke, coronary heart disease, the MetS, and other VRFs, including sleep-disordered breathing. Clinical and subclinical infarcts are important risk factors for VaD and VCI. We have discussed these at length. When vascular dysfunction combines with AD neuropathology, human studies have found an additive interaction. In population-based epidemiologic studies, clinical phenotypes can be misclassified. A case that is called "Alzheimer's disease" may in fact have a significant vascular contribution, but because of certain features and timing of cognitive dysfunction relative to silent or overt infarcts, may not meet criteria for VaD. Some Alzheimer epidemiologists have advocated for the investigation of causes for "dementia" rather than for AD and other subtypes due to this misclassification. The converse argument is that the risk factors for the subtypes are different, so we have to think about what we want to prevent. Prevention of AD neuropathology will likely require treatments that address this pathologic cascade. Clinical expression of MCI and dementia on the other hand, may be prevented through the reduction of modifiable risk factors, including those related to vascular disease. To prevent significant cognitive decline, we will need to monitor cognition over time, just as we monitor our PSA or our mammograms, and couple this with decreasing our risk for clinical expression through control of modifiable risk factors.

Very little research on the incidence of AD has been conducted in individuals with existing coronary heart disease. Because neither of these conditions is rare, they will obviously coexist frequently. Some studies have suggested that AD cases have more CVD (Breteler, 2000). For example, the CAIDE study has shown that atrial fibrillation in late-life increases the risk for AD 2.5-fold (95% CI = 1.04–6.16) and that this association is more pronounced in APOE-ε4 noncarriers (Rusanen et al., 2014). In the *Kame* Project, we found that having had a transient ischemic attack increased the risk for AD (HR = 5.12, 95% CI = 1.69–15.54), but only among APOE-ε4 noncarriers (Borenstein et al., 2005). In people who do not have the major susceptibility gene for AD (APOE-ε4), a lower level of AD neuropathology combined with vascular disease might be the enabling factor for the "man-on-the-man" that raises brain pathology over the threshold for clinical expression.

The MetS is characterized by the presence of three of the following vascular conditions: abdominal obesity, hypertriglyceridemia, low HDL, hypertension, and high fasting blood glucose (Expert Panel on Detection, 2001). In a cross-sectional study of 980 population-based subjects aged 65–74 in Finland, 43.6% met the criteria for MetS (Vanhanen et al., 2006). The OR for prevalent AD associated with MetS was 2.46 (95% CI = 1.27–4.78). When the analysis was limited to nondiabetics, the OR was even higher (3.26, 95% CI = 1.45–7.27). By contrast, in the Three-City (3C) cohort in France (Raffaitin et al., 2009), no association was found between MetS (diagnosed in 15.8% of over 7,087 population-based individuals aged 65 and over) and incident AD (HR = 0.81, 95% CI = 0.50–1.31) over a 4-year follow-up. In this study, there was a statistically elevated risk for VaD associated with MetS, (HR = 2.42, 95% CI = 1.24–4.73). However, the only MetS component that affected the risk for VaD was high triglycerides ($p = 0.02$) at baseline with low HDL cholesterol having a smaller effect ($p = 0.07$). More studies of the associations between dementia with the MetS are needed. Given that many cohort studies have obtained data on its components, this should be relatively easy to do using already collected data.

Sleep-disordered breathing can lead to hypoxia, limiting the delivery of oxygen to key regions of the brain. Two-hundred and ninety-eight women who had overnight polysomnography in a substudy of the Study of Osteoporotic Fractures were followed for a mean of 4.7 years for incident dementia (Yaffe et al., 2011). Compared to 193 women without sleep-disordered breathing, 105 women with sleep-disorder breathing had a higher risk for incident dementia adjusted for age, race, BMI, education, smoking status, diabetes, hypertension, antidepressant use, benzodiazepine use, and use of nonbenzodiazepine anxiolytics (OR = 2.04. 95% CI = 1.10–3.78).

It is of interest how combinations of VRFs predict dementia risk. In CAIDE, an analysis was conducted taking into account midlife obesity, high total cholesterol, and high systolic blood pressure (Kivipelto et al., 2005). When these risk factors were in a model together (BMI>30 vs <30; SBP>140 mm Hg vs <140 mm Hg; and total cholesterol >251 mg/dL vs <251 mg/dL), the ORs for dementia were: 2.09 (95% CI = 1.16–3.77), 1.97 (95% CI = 1.03–3.77), and 1.89 (95% CI = 1.02–3.49), respectively. The authors counted the number of these three risk factors for each subject. The OR for dementia associated with zero risk factors was treated as the reference value (1.0). The ORs for 1, 2, and 3 risk factors were: 1.37 (95% CI = 0.44–4.27), 3.03 (95% CI = 1.03–8.89), and 6.21 (95% CI = 1.94–19.92). This shows that the independent effects of VRFs sum in terms of their impact on dementia or AD risk.

When should we start to control our VRFs if we are interested in preventing AD? The answer to the question is probably the usual, "It's never too early." If we view the challenge of staying ahead of the curve as a balance between limiting damage to the vascular system and accumulation of AD pathology (plus other non-AD pathologies) versus building reserve through avoidance of modifiable risks by improving lifestyle behaviors, we can buy time, thus delaying the onset of cognitive impairment to later ages.

Chapter 15

Diet

Many changes in the diets of Americans have occurred over the past 50 years, according to a USDA report (Office of Communications, 2003). Between 1970 and 2000, e.g., the number of calories per capita increased by almost 25% (up 530 calories per day). This gain can be attributed to an almost 10% increase from refined grain products, 9% from increased fats and oils, and almost 5% from added sugars. The "food away from home" sector provided about one-third of total food energy consumption in the mid-1990s, an increase of 18% over the late 1970s. The USDA's Economic Research Service suggests that when eating away from home, people eat more food and/or eat higher calorie foods. With this trend has come reduced physical activity such that the equation "energy intake = energy expenditure" has been thrown severely off-balance. In a survey in 2002 about attitudes toward food and calories, only 18% of respondents said they were concerned about the nutritional content of their food, and of these, only 13% said calories was one of their concerns (Office of Communications, 2003). With regard to the latter, 49% were concerned about fat content and 18% about sugar content. The report ascribes changes in consumption of food in the United States to changes in prices, increases in disposable income, increases in food assistance for the poor, increases in "convenient" products (e.g., availability of prepackaged and prepared frozen foods and fast-food), more advertising, and food fortification programs. Social and economic drivers include smaller households, increases in two-income households, more ethnic diversity and an aging population. Other changes from 1950 to 2000 are increases in the consumption of red meat, poultry (and less of an increase in fish and seafood), and cheese, and decreases in the number of eggs and amount of milk consumed. Consumption of soft drinks has soared. On the positive side, the use of heart-healthy fats, such as olive and canola oils in salads and for cooking is on the rise, while the use of lard and butter has decreased. Fruit and vegetable consumption is rising, with a 20% increase in 2000 compared with the 1970s. However, grain consumption has increased by 45% from the 1970s to 2000, with wheat flour far in first place, and very low amounts of whole grains being consumed. Dietary changes have also been marked by quadrupling of portion sizes, according to

Alzheimer's Disease. DOI: http://dx.doi.org/10.1016/B978-0-12-804538-1.00015-8

the CDC (Young & Nestle, 2002). This increase in food consumption is accompanied by increasingly sedentary lifestyles (see Chapter 16).

Dietary recommendations from the US federal government have varied greatly over past decades. In 2011, "MyPlate" replaced the food pyramid, which was introduced to the United States in 1992 and updated in 2005. Today, MyPlate recommends that half the food on our plates consist of fruits and vegetables (60% vegetables, 40% fruit), and that grains and proteins together form the other half of the plate, with at least half of grains being whole grains, and proteins being lean (and including at least 8 oz per week of seafood) (http://www.choosemyplate.gov/food-groups/). Dairy products are recommended in small amounts. These suggestions will likely continue to change with the evolving science of nutrition.

MEASUREMENT OF DIET

Our diets are incredibly complex and difficult to measure. Obviously, we eat different things every day, and our diet changes over the course of our lives. Diets vary based on geography, racial/ethnic group, culture, income, season, and age. Dietary elements can be thought of in terms of continuous nutrient variables with everyone having a value. Other ways to measure diet are by individual foods, food groups, or food patterns. Dr Walter Willett, perhaps the most well-known nutritional epidemiologist, describes one advantage of describing diet in terms of nutrients as its ability to reflect biologic processes. In epidemiologic studies, calculation of the total intake of a nutrient across a person's diet provides the most powerful test of a hypothesis, particularly when many foods each contribute only a small amount to the total intake of the nutrient (Willett, 2013). For example, consider the nutrient, caffeine. Caffeine can be found in a number of foods, but the amount of caffeine in a person's diet cannot be readily combined using whole foods. Instead, the caffeine content of each food is documented in a nutrient database that accompanies a food frequency questionnaire (FFQ) and summed across each person's diet. The nutrient database is obtained from 24-h recall data from external data sources, such as the NHANES and the US Department of Agriculture's Continuing Survey of Food Intakes by Individuals and refined for the study population at hand (Signorello et al., 2009).

Willett also points to an advantage of studying specific foods or food groups when "we suspect that a particular food may be associated with risk but we have not proposed a hypothesis… associations between foods and food groups with disease risk is appropriate for exploring the data" (Willett, 2013). An example might be the examination of fruit and vegetable juices as proxies for increased polyphenolic content in the diet, which led to mechanistic work of how polyphenols may protect against AD (Dai, Borenstein, Wu, Jackson, & Larson, 2006; Williams & Spencer, 2012).

There are three common ways to measure diet. One is to keep a food diary for 1 day (24 h) or a few days (3–7). Sometimes the food diary is repeated in each season, since diet is affected by seasonal offerings. This is participant-intensive and requires training of subjects. Another method is to conduct 24-h dietary recalls. This is expensive, as it requires highly trained interviewers to obtain the data. FFQs are built on these techniques, but measure a person's "usual diet" in the last few weeks or over the past year. The validity of these methods have all been studied and are in acceptable ranges (Rothman, Greenland, & Lash, 2008).

It is common to conduct pilot testing in a new population or harmonize the food list to the culture and location of the study. For example, in *Kame*, we used an FFQ that was written and validated in Japanese American populations in Hawaii and Los Angeles (Kolonel et al., 2000). In our studies in China, we used a different FFQ that was based on the Shanghai Women's Health Study (Shu et al., 2004) but modified by 24-h recalls conducted every month for a year. FFQs are the most common method of measuring diet, due to their relatively low cost and ability to capture "usual" dietary patterns (DP) as well as to capture most of the diet (85–90%). It is difficult to use FFQs to question respondents about past eating habits, and when this is done, it is likely done with substantial error. Nevertheless, as Willett states, "A central feature of the dietary intake of free-living individuals is variation from day to day superimposed on an underlying consistent pattern. (If there were no element of consistency, and daily intake were a completely random event, there would be no hope of measuring the effects of nutrients epidemiologically.)" (Willett, 2013). Of course, when possible, it is ideal to measure diet repeatedly in prospective cohort studies. In the Nurses' Health Study of over 122,000 nurses in the United States, investigators began collecting FFQs in 1980 and every 4 years thereafter, resulting in one of the richest datasets available to explore associations between diet and disease outcomes.

FFQs can also gather data on portion size (usually small, medium, large). An average portion can be described in words, pictures, or using food models to give the respondent a reference point. However, such added detail (known as "semiquantitative" FFQs) only slightly improves the estimation of nutrients (Rothman et al., 2008).

OBSERVATIONAL STUDIES AND RANDOMIZED CLINICAL TRIALS

If a nutrient is beneficial, one would think that randomized clinical trials (RCTs) are best suited to test their effects in human populations. Do RCTs provide superior scientific evidence compared with cohort studies for the same questions? Nutrients are consumed at very low levels each day over the course of our lifetimes. Such low-"dose," long-term exposures are better studied with longitudinal observational designs in which diet is measured repeatedly and outcomes are assessed over long follow-ups. The effect on disease incidence of high-"dose," short-term nutrient supplementation is more conducive to RCTs. Nutrient interventions work against the backdrop of a lifetime of dietary exposures, and in AD or MCI, trials have historically taken place in populations 60 and over among people who already have some degree of neuropathology. Therefore, cohort studies offer answers to a *different question* than RCTs with regard to dietary exposures. For cohort studies, this question is what is the role of usual dietary intake on the evolution of slow-progressing disease processes? For RCTs, the question is what is the effect of supplementation of a nutrient(s) on short-term outcomes?

Although there are many limitations of observational studies, it is important to recognize that RCTs also have limitations. In RCTs of AD patients, there are several methodological issues that should be considered. For example, the age at which the RCT is initiated, as we have seen from Chapter 14 with regard to vascular variables, may have important effects on interventions. Other issues that affect RCTs include the lack of knowledge of the latent period between having adequate levels of the nutrient and its specific effect on disease, not knowing the amounts of nutrient required to produce the intended benefit, and not knowing how the nutrient interacts with all other nutrients to result in benefit. In addition, when a trial is long, there are problems with compliance, especially when the nutrient may become perceived by people as being beneficial such that the placebo group begins taking it on their own. The sample sizes required for such RCTs are usually very large since one is trying to detect a relatively small effect. RCTs can also suffer from substantial selection bias. Frequently, healthier people who have higher levels of the nutrient in question choose to participate, limiting applicability of information obtained in the trial. If only people who are deficient in the nutrient benefit, the absence of such people from the trial may result in a null finding. On the other hand, observational cohort studies reflect more longstanding intakes of nutrients and can better answer questions related to dietary habits and disease outcomes. For this reason, our discussions will be grouped by observational and RCT evidence for selected dietary variables.

There are a number of published books and articles that recommend an "Alzheimer's diet." The number of websites about this topic is staggering, and many offer advice that is not substantiated in the scientific literature. Clearly, diet is an important predictor of health. It is also one of the most modifiable risk factors and one that is under our individual control. In this chapter, we will generally limit our discussion to observational and interventional studies with Alzheimer's disease (AD) and mild cognitive impairment (MCI) as outcomes, although we will also discuss some studies that examined cognitive impairment or decline. In addition, in our review of observational studies, we will limit our discussion to cohort studies, because early case–control studies are affected by a number of methodological shortcomings, limiting their validity.

We will begin with vitamins C, E, β-carotene, B and D, and then move on to polyphenols, a class of antioxidants, and highlight particular types. We will specifically consider six nutrients: curcumin, epigallocatechin-gallate (EGCG), resveratrol, coffee, chocolate, and soy products thought to have effects on AD.

Consumption of different types of fat, including fish and fish oils is an important topic that will be treated separately. Lastly, we will discuss novel research into dietary patterns.

VITAMINS C, E, AND β-CAROTENE

The first cohort study suggesting a role for vitamins in AD was the CHAP study (Morris et al., 1998). Although there was no association found with multivitamins, there were some weak trends between the use of vitamin E and vitamin C supplements and risk for AD. Two years later, investigators from HAAS reported that vitamin E and C supplement use reduced the risk for VaD and was cross-sectionally associated with better cognitive performance (Masaki et al., 2000). However, no association was found for AD. In 2002, the Rotterdam Study reported that high intake of vitamins C and E from the diet predicted lower risk for AD (RR = 0.82, 95% CI = 0.68–0.99 per standard deviation of increase in intake in vitamin C and RR = 0.82, 95% CI = 0.66–1.0 per standard deviation of increase in vitamin E) (Engelhart et al., 2002b). This study also reported an inverse association between intake of β-carotene and AD (RR = 0.54, 95% CI = 0.31–0.96). In 2002, Morris and colleagues published a second study from CHAP among 815 community-based residents age 65 and older who were followed for almost 4 years and reported that among noncarriers of the APOE-ε4 allele, successive quintiles of dietary intake of vitamin E decreased the risk for AD, with a $p_{\text{for trend}}$ of 0.05 (Morris et al., 2002). However, no association was found for vitamin C, nor was there an association for vitamin C or E from supplements.

Subsequent cohort studies produced variable findings. For example, in WHICAP, no associations were found with incident AD for vitamins C or E, either from the diet or from supplements (Luchsinger, Tang, Shea, & Mayeux, 2003). The Nurses' Health Study reported a modest inverse association (in the context of a large sample size, N = 14,968) between the use of vitamin E supplements and better neuropsychological performance. However, vitamin C had no association (Grodstein, Chen, & Willett, 2003). In the Cache County Study (Zandi et al., 2004), only individuals who took vitamin E and C supplements in combination were at reduced risk for AD (adjusted HR = 0.36, 95% CI = 0.09–0.99); those who took one or the other were not. A later paper from HAAS (Laurin, Masaki, Foley, White, & Launer, 2004) found an *increased* risk for AD for vitamin E from food measured 30 years before (RR = 1.92, 95% CI = 1.16–3.18 for Quartile 2; RR = 1.35, 95% CI = 0.78–2.31 for Quartile 3; and RR = 1.78, 95% CI = 1.06–2.98 for Quartile 4) all compared with the lowest quartile. The dose–response association was not statistically significant and the result was not adjusted for tofu/soy intake, which may have increased the risk (see "Soy Consumption" section).

Two cross-sectional studies, both conducted in 2005, examined plasma concentrations of antioxidant vitamins on the presence of prevalent dementia. In the InCHIANTI cohort, the lowest tertile of vitamin E plasma level was associated with an OR for dementia of 2.6 (95% CI = 1.0–7.1) compared with the highest tertile (Cherubini et al., 2005). The Rotterdam Study found no effect for plasma vitamin E or other antioxidants on the risk of prevalent AD (Engelhart et al., 2005).

Three clinical trials also are worthy of mention. The first, conducted in 1997, randomized 341 patients with moderate AD to selegiline, vitamin E supplements (2,000 IU/day), both, or neither for 2 years (Sano et al., 1997). The primary outcome was time to the occurrence of institutionalization or loss of the ability to perform basic ADLs or a CDR of 3 or higher, indicating severe dementia. Individuals treated with vitamin E took a longer time to achieve the primary outcome ($p = 0.001$), while those on both agents were also likely to delay the primary outcome ($p = 0.049$). However, treatment with vitamin E was not associated with changes in cognitive outcomes in this trial. The second trial enrolled 769 MCI patients (Petersen et al., 2005) treated with donepezil (Aricept) or vitamin E (2,000 IU/day) for 3 years. The primary outcome was progression from MCI to AD. Although donepezil showed a benefit throughout the follow-up, vitamin E did not, either in the whole sample or among ε4-positive patients. In 2014, another trial compared the Alzheimer's Disease Cooperative Study Activities of Daily Living score (range 0–78) (Galasko et al., 1997) in participants with mild-to-moderate AD randomized to 2,000 IU/day of vitamin E (α-tocopherol) and memantine, an NMDA-receptor antagonist treatment for AD (Dysken et al., 2014). Vitamin E treatment led to a 19% delay in clinical progression compared with placebo, equal to a delay of 6 months.

Experimental data provide evidence that chronic accumulation of reaction oxygen species in the brain caused by several types of free radicals is associated with neuronal dysfunction (Dai et al., 2006). Increased deposition of Aß in the AD process leads to greater oxidative stress (Markesbery, 1997) and may be mediated by hydrogen peroxide. Antioxidants such as vitamins C and E could therefore be neuroprotective. There are methodological difficulties in cohort studies of diet and use of supplements that can lead to Type II errors (usually resulting in underestimated measures of effect) that must be considered before making overall recommendations about the utility of vitamins to prevent or delay the onset of AD. First is the error in the measurement of dietary exposures and accompanying nutrients. If these do not depend on the measurement of outcome (which in cohort studies is usually the case), nondifferential misclassification may occur, resulting in attenuated measures of effect. On the outcome side, the development of AD occurs over decades. Examining diet and supplement use at age 65 and over does not adequately represent lifelong patterns, and intervention studies lasting 2–3 years may be insufficient in length to expect a reasonably strong effect on cognition or on the incidence of MCI or AD. The size of the sample also is important, in that we will need more statistical power if we want to detect incidence of clinical outcomes compared to changes in cognition. Type I errors can occur if we interview "nondemented" subjects who will present with incipient MCI or AD in the following years. These participants may underrecall dietary exposures relative to truly nondemented subjects, resulting in a measure of effect that is falsely inverse. Finally, there are concerns in nutritional epidemiology about the manner in which single dietary elements interact with other elements in the human body. Therefore, supplementation in observational or interventional investigations may not reflect the overall effect of a group of elements (e.g., antioxidants). These limitations have led to the analysis of *patterns* of intake of whole foods, food groups, and overall dietary patterns (Luchsinger & Mayeux, 2004), which are considered later in this chapter.

Despite the lack of evidence supporting vitamin C as protective for AD, a meta-analysis of studies (Li, Shen, & Ji, 2012) reported an overall effect from observational cohort studies of 0.83 (95% CI = 0.72–0.94) with little heterogeneity for "moderate or high intake" of dietary vitamin C. Since daily vitamin C supplements of moderate dose are not harmful, this analysis suggests some possible benefit of increasing vitamin C intake.

More evidence exists to support a neuroprotective role of dietary vitamin E in preventing AD. However, existing trials have not assessed primary prevention using supplementation of this vitamin in people who do not have symptoms. Meta-analysis of data from observational studies led to a pooled RR for vitamin E of 0.76 (95% CI = 0.67–0.84) (Li et al., 2012), a somewhat stronger effect than for vitamin C, with little to moderate heterogeneity. Vitamin E is lipid-soluble and is a fairly potent antioxidant. The importance of ingesting γ-tocopherols (the most abundant form of vitamin E in the diet) instead of α-tocopherols (the most biologically active form of vitamin E) has been emphasized. In fact, consumption of all eight forms of tocopherol decreases oxidative stress and inflammation better than α-tocopherol alone (Morris, 2009). Doses of vitamin E of < 400 IU/day are generally safe, but some evidence demonstrates that taking 400 IU/day or more for many years may increase the risk for heart failure among people with existing vascular disease or diabetes as well as increase all-cause mortality (Boothby & Doering, 2005). Foods containing vitamin E include vegetable oils, green leafy vegetables, fortified foods, eggs, and nuts. Eating a healthy diet is likely the best way to ensure adequate intake of vitamin E.

ß-carotene is the red-orange pigment present in plants and fruits, such as carrots, pumpkins, and sweet potatoes. It is the precursor for vitamin A. Absorption is enhanced when ß-carotene is ingested with fats. The meta-analysis by Li reported a pooled RR of 0.88 (95% CI = 0.73–1.03) for "moderate or high" dietary intake of ß-carotene from five studies (Li et al., 2012).

B VITAMINS, FOLATE, AND PLASMA HOMOCYSTEINE

The B vitamins refer to eight vitamins (B_1, B_2, B_3, B_5, B_6, B_7, B_9, and B_{12}) that together are referred to as the vitamin B complex and are important in cell metabolism. Most of the work on B vitamins and AD has focused on B_6 (which plays a role as cofactor in many enzyme reactions, including amino acid metabolism and biosynthesis of neurotransmitters), B_9 (folate, which plays a role in metabolism of nucleic acids and amino acids and also in the production of red blood cells), and B_{12}, which serves to metabolize carbohydrates, proteins and lipids as well as increase myelination. Good dietary sources of B vitamins include meats, fish, beans, whole grains, potatoes, bananas, and brewer's yeast. Although beer is a source of B vitamins, drinking alcohol has a negative impact on their absorption. Folate is naturally occurring in food, while folic acid is the synthetic form of folate used in supplements and fortification of foods.

Folate protects against increases in homocysteine, a sulfur-containing amino acid that can lead to vascular disease (Selhub et al., 1995; Ueland & Refsum, 1989) with consequences for the clinical expression of AD. High homocysteine levels have been shown to increase the risk for dementia (RR = 1.8, 95% CI = 1.3–2.5 in the Framingham Study) (Seshadri et al., 2002). In another population-based study of 816 subjects from Italy, hyperhomocysteinemia, defined as plasma tHcy > 15 μmol/L, led to a HR for AD of 2.11 (95% CI = 1.32–3.76) (Ravaglia et al., 2005). In that study, low folate concentrations (≤11.8 nmol/L) also increased the risk for AD (HR = 1.98, 95% CI = 1.15–3.40). Folate may be useful in preventing or delaying dementia through its effect in reducing levels of homocysteine or through other mechanisms including its effect in combination with vitamin B_{12} on brain growth (Ordonez, 1979).

In the Kungsholmen Project, people with low levels of B_{12} and folate had a twofold higher risk for developing AD compared with people with normal levels of both vitamins (Wang et al., 2001). In the Women's Health Initiative Memory Study, among 7,030 MCI- and dementia-free women at baseline, dietary folate intake below the Recommended Daily Allowance (<400 μg/day) increased the risk for incident MCI and probable dementia twofold (95% CI = 1.3–2.9), but no associations were found for dietary intakes of B_6 or B_{12} (Agnew-Blais et al., 2014). A similar effect was found in WHICAP (Luchsinger, Tang, Miller, Green, & Mayeux, 2007). In the Nun Study, low-serum folate levels were associated with cortical brain atrophy (Snowdon, Tully, Smith, Riley, & Markesbery, 2000), an important risk factor for AD and dementia. Other studies of folate on dementia risk have found null or even adverse cognitive effects, but most of these studies were case–control in design (inappropriate for this question if plasma vitamin B levels are compared in cases and controls, since vitamin B levels can be affected by prevalent disease).

Randomized controlled trials have demonstrated inconsistent findings with regard to B vitamins. The ADCS conducted an 18-month study of high-dose B vitamins (5 mg folic acid, 1 mg vitamin B_{12}, and 25 mg B6 vs placebo) among mild-to-moderate AD patients (Aisen et al., 2008). While the investigators were successful in reducing tHcy levels, there was no evidence of benefit for any outcome measure, including change on the cognitive subscale of the ADAS-cog, change in MMSE, CDR-sum of boxes, or ADCS-ADL scores.

In 2010, University of Oxford investigators published the results from VITACOG, a randomized controlled trial to reduce homocysteine levels with high-dose B vitamins (Smith, Smith, et al., 2010). The study included 271 volunteers aged 70 and over with a diagnosis of aMCI or naMCI by Petersen criteria randomized to 0.8 mg folic acid + 0.5 mg B_{12} + 20 mg B_6 versus placebo for 24 months. One-hundred and ten participants randomized to treatment and 113 randomized to placebo completed the trial. Final tHcy levels declined by almost 32% in the B vitamin treatment group with no safety issues. Brain atrophy per year was almost 30% lower in the treatment group compared with the placebo group (0.76%, 95% CI = 0.63–0.90 vs 1.08%, 95% CI = 0.94–1.22, $p = 0.001$). The effect was strongest in those with a high baseline tHcy level, where the atrophy rate declined by 53%. The main finding was present among those who increased either their vitamin B_{12} status or their folate status. Therefore, the authors were unable to state which change in B vitamins was responsible for the results. Other studies have found specific effects of B_{12} (de Jager, 2014), while others were inconsistent. For example, one study found protective effects among those with the highest plasma folate and lowest vitamin B_{12} levels (OR = 0.22, 95% CI = 0.05–0.92) (Doets et al., 2014). In VITACOG, the higher brain atrophy rate was associated with lower final scores on the MMSE. A follow-up paper published in 2011 from VITACOG showed that the active treatment improved scores in global cognition (measured by the MMSE) ($p < 0.001$), episodic memory (using the Hopkins Verbal Learning Test-delayed recall, $p = 0.001$), and semantic memory (using category fluency, $p = 0.037$) (de Jager, Oulhaj, Jacoby, Refsum, & Smith, 2012).

In 2014, a multicenter trial was reported from the Netherlands, which examined 2,919 people age 65 and over with high tHcy levels (12–50 μmol/L, <10 is ideal) who were cognitively normal (van der Zwaluw et al., 2014). Participants took a tablet of 400 μg folic acid and 500 μg of vitamin B_{12} or a placebo for 2 years. MMSE and episodic memory test scores were available for about 2,500 participants, and other measures (attention and working memory, information processing speed, and executive function) were available for about one-third of the total sample. The treatment was sufficient to lower tHcy levels (1.3 μmol/L in the placebo and 5 μmol/L in the vitamin group), but all comparisons between the two groups for cognitive outcomes were null. The authors and others not associated with the study commented on Alzforum.org (www.alzforum.org/news/research-news/older-adults-get-no-cognitive-boost-b-vitamins) that 2 years may not be long enough to give the B vitamins the chance to have an effect on cognition, even in such a large study.

A number of systematic reviews and meta-analyses have been published. In the most recent of these (Clarke et al., 2014), 11 large trials including 22,000 normal elderly were analyzed. While the meta-analysis supported the ability of folate and B_{12} to lower tHcy levels, the authors concluded that a 25% reduction in tHcy levels was equivalent to only 0.02 of a year in cognitive aging per year with no significant effect in either global cognition or domain-specific neuropsychological performance and no effect-modification by the presence of vascular disease.

Reviewing the success and failures of RCTs of B vitamins, de Jager (2014) adopted a causal pathway proposed by Douaud et al. (2013), which posited that

B vitamin treatment leads to a 32% decrease in plasma homocysteine, cutting brain atrophy by half, and which in turn leads to a decrease in the CDR-Sum of Boxes rating. De Jager also showed from VITACOG that only those with a high atrophy rate may be aided by the B vitamins, and because of this, she proposed that there appears to be a critical level of brain atrophy and an opportune period of time in which to intervene and have a beneficial effect on atrophy (de Jager, 2014). Because people with all levels of brain atrophy were included in the failed trials, we may be missing the signal. Many failed trials of drugs for AD also have taught us the lesson that early intervention is better than later intervention. It will likely be important to calculate a risk index for each individual, which for the case of B vitamins, would include measures of existing concentrations of B_6, folic acid, and B_{12}, and of brain atrophy to determine whether a response should occur, and also to design interventions with a longer follow-up than 2 years.

Proposed mechanisms for the effect of B vitamins and cognition include reductions in homocysteine or increases in brain growth, as noted above. Increased homocysteine could lead to increased white matter hyperintensities and cerebral infarcts (Tangney, Aggarwal, et al., 2011). Other potential pathways could exist through reduction of oxidative stress and neuronal DNA damage (Agnew-Blais et al., 2014; Malouf & Grimley Evans, 2008).

VITAMIN D

Globally, 1 billion people have low-serum levels of 25-hydroxyvitamin D (25OHD) (<30 ng/mL) (Annweiler et al., 2014). In particular, half of all adults aged 65 and over and 70–90% of individuals with abnormal cognition have hypovitaminosis D. In addition to vitamin D's known benefits on bone health, a burgeoning new direction in research has shown that vitamin D acts as a "neurosteroid hormone" through its effect on the vitamin D receptor, which is present in neurons and glial cells. Vitamin D is also known to be involved in the reduction of amyloid-induced cytotoxicity and the inflammation secondary to AD and cerebrovascular pathology. The presence of prevalent AD may affect 25OHD levels, since moderate-to-severe AD patients are likely to experience less exposure to the sun and also may have lower intake of foods rich in vitamin D. However, some have argued that differences in vitamin D concentrations between cases and controls can be seen in MCI as well as mild AD (Annweiler et al., 2012). The Osteoporotic Fractures in Men Study examined 25OHD levels at baseline with regard to performance on the 3MS and the Trail-Making Test Part B, as well as incident cognitive decline 4.6 years later. Some trends were evident in the direction postulated, but none achieved statistical significance either cross-sectionally or longitudinally (Slinin et al., 2010). In this study, crude associations that were statistically significant were attenuated in adjusted analyses, especially by race and education. Probably the best current evidence for an association between vitamin D and the risk for AD comes from the Cardiovascular Health Study (Littlejohns et al., 2014), in which serum 25OHD levels were measured from samples taken in 1992–1993 and 102 incident AD cases occurred over an average of 5.6 years. Levels <25 nmol/L were considered severely 25OHD-deficient, and levels from 25 to <50 nmol/L were considered deficient, compared with sufficient levels (≥50 nmol/L). Adjusted HRs followed a dose–response gradient, with participants with deficient levels incurring a HR for AD of 1.69 (95% CI = 1.06–2.69) and those with severely deficient levels a HR of 2.22 (95% CI = 1.02–4.83). Although the question of whether reverse causation may account partially or fully for the findings remains, the authors excluded incident cases developing within the first year of follow-up, arguing that this is not a likely explanation. However, without a much longer follow-up and perhaps 25OHD levels measured from midlife and at different points in time, the question of a potential association between low vitamin D and higher risk for AD remains open. Nonrandomized trials and small randomized trials with low-dose vitamin D supplementation have yielded null results (Annweiler & Beauchet, 2011). Larger trials in vitamin D-deficient participants need to be conducted.

POLYPHENOLS, FRUITS, AND VEGETABLES

Polyphenols are a class of nonvitamin chemicals present in a multitude of plants that have much more potent antioxidant capacity than do traditional vitamins, such as C and E. About 5,000–8,000 forms of polyphenols exist, and many coexist in single foods. Moreover, they produce metabolites that far outnumber the number of types of polyphenols and are subject to individual bioavailability and other host characteristics that affect the way they are processed. Investigation of health effects from these compounds is a great challenge to medicine and epidemiology.

Common food sources of polyphenols include fruits and vegetables, juices, tea, selected herbs, red wine, curcumin, coffee, chocolate, olives and olive oil, nuts, algae, soybeans, and cereals. Polyphenols were originally recognized as providing the plant's defense against ultraviolent radiation from the sun, pathogens, and physical damage (Sun, Wang, Simonyi, & Sun, 2008). To combat these threats, the majority of a plant's polyphenols are present in the outer sections of fruits and vegetables, giving them their deep color (such as berries and green, leafy vegetables). Importantly, the mode of food preparation can deplete polyphenolic content, and FFQs typically do not ask how foods are prepared. Because of this, it is difficult to measure dietary quantities of polyphenol intake (Dai et al., 2006). Much of the existing work in the health effects of polyphenols has been done in animals. Randomized controlled clinical trials in people are rare, because these trials are expensive, these compounds exist in commonly eaten foods and in supplements, and there is no monetary benefit to pharmaceutical companies. *Absence of evidence*, rather than an *evidence of absence* is what underlies statements such as, "Many purported health claims for specific polyphenol-enriched foods remain unproven" (http://en.wikipedia.org/wiki/Polyphenol#Potential_health_effects). Despite this, some epidemiologic evidence exists to support the role of polyphenols in reducing the risk of cognitive decline and AD.

In AD, it is believed that the long-term and chronic accumulation of reactive oxygen species (free radicals) and reactive nitrogen species may exhaust antioxidant mechanisms leading to neurodegeneration. Oxidative damage has been shown to occur before the formation of AD senile plaques (Petersen et al., 2007). It also occurs during normal aging. In addition to their antioxidant effects, polyphenols have anti-inflammatory properties, which is important since inflammation also plays an important role in AD pathogenesis (Kim, Lee, & Lee, 2010).

Measures of types of polyphenolic chemicals in various foods are provided in an excellent review of the potential role of the bioavailability and metabolism of polyphenols (Singh, Arseneault, Sanderson, Murthy, & Ramassamy, 2008). The basic classification of polyphenols can be broken down into flavonoids and nonflavonoids. Subclassifications of flavonoids include anthocyanins (pelargodinin in berries, red and purple grapes, red wine, cherries, rhubarb), flavonols (such as quercetin in red cabbage, yellow onion, cherries, tomatoes, broccoli, apples, teas), flavones (such as apigenin in parsley, celery, thyme, and hot pepper), flavanones, (such as naringenin in citrus fruits and juices), isoflavones (such as genistein in soybeans and legumes), monomeric and polymeric flavonols (such as epicatechin in tea, chocolate, grapes, berries, and apples), and proanthocyanidins (in chocolate, apples, berries, red wine). On the nonflavonoid side are hydrobenzoic acids, present in berries and black currants; hydoxycinnamic acids, present in blueberries, kiwi, cherries, plums, apples, pears, peaches, artichoke, potato, and coffee; lignans, present in flaxseed, lentils, garlic, asparagus, carrots, pears, and prunes; and finally stilbenes, such as resveratrol in grapes, pomegranate, and groundnuts. Actual levels of polyphenols in these foods vary by geography. In the United States, the consumption of total anthocyanins is 10 times higher than the intake of vitamin C and 100-fold higher than that of vitamin E. In the US diet, quercetin is the main flavonol consumed, with a mean intake of 16 mg/day. Lignans are also considered phytoestrogens, since they exert a pro-estrogenic effect. Flavonoids make up about two-thirds of our total phenol intake, while nonflavonoids comprise the remaining third (Kim et al., 2010; Singh et al., 2008). Table 15.1 shows 25 foods with the highest antioxidant content per serving (Halvorsen et al., 2002; Singh et al., 2008).

In the first half of the 2000s, three important studies specifically addressed the possible role of flavonoids in the etiology of AD. The first was in the PAQUID Study in France (Commenges et al., 2000). Over a 5-year follow-up, among 1,367 participants age 65 and over, the RR for dementia (not AD) decreased with increasing dietary flavonoids, but only the middle category was statistically significant (multivariate RR = 0.45, 95% CI = 0.22–0.92). Another

TABLE 15.1 Twenty-Five Foods with the Highest Antioxidant Content per Serving

Food	Antioxidant Content (mm/100 g)	Food	Antioxidant Content (mmol/100 g)	Food	Antioxidant Content (mmol/100 g)
Cloves, ground	125.5	Pecans	9.7	Chocolate, dark	4.2
Oregano leaf, dried	40.3	Unsweetened baking chocolate	8.9	Blackberries	4.0
Ginger, ground	21.6	Paprika	8.6	Whole-grain cereal	3.4
Cinnamon, ground	17.7	Chili powder	8.4	Cranberries	3.3
Turmeric powder	15.7	Parsley, dried	7.4	Pudding mix, chocolate	3.2
Walnuts	13.1	Molasses, dark	4.9	Raspberries, strawberries, blueberries	2.1–2.3
Basil leaf	12.3	Pepper, black	4.4	Wine, red	2.1
Curry powder	10.0	Artichokes, prepared	4.3	Milk chocolate candy	1.5
				Pistachios	1.4

Source: Modified from Halvorsen et al. (2002) and Singh et al. (2008).

interesting finding from this study was an attenuation of the RR for dementia for wine consumption when flavonoid intake was included in the model, (RR = 0.98, $p = 0.98$), indicating a mediating effect of flavonoids on the inverse effect from wine on incident dementia.

In HAAS, flavonoid intake was measured primarily by tea intake. Wine intake was considered, but is known to be low in the Japanese American population (Laurin et al., 2004). The estimated median intake in HAAS was 4.1 mg/day, much lower than the estimated 13 mg/day in the United States (Singh et al., 2008). As we saw earlier in our discussion of vitamins C and E, HAAS is the only study that found that antioxidants (but not flavonoids) increased the risk for AD. For flavonoids, there was no association. This result reflects the longest follow-up in the literature, flavonoid intake having been measured in 1965–1968 and outcomes assessed in 1991–1999. However, only a single exposure measurement was used.

In the Three-City cohort conducted in Bordeaux, Dijon and Montpellier, France, 8,085 nondemented individuals were followed for 4 years and 183 incident cases of AD were identified (Barberger-Gateau et al., 2007). For individuals eating raw or cooked fruits and vegetables every day, the HR for all-cause dementia adjusting for demographic variables, APOE-ε4, BMI, and diabetes, was 0.72 (95% CI = 0.53–0.97). For AD, the HR was statistically significant when adjusted for demographic variables, but lost significance when adjusted for all variables ($p = 0.09$, in a model with N = 7369). Among other foods analyzed (including butter, goose or duck fat, olive oil, omega-3 rich oil, and sunflower or grape seed oil), frequent fruit and vegetable intake was the only variable that approached statistical significance.

In the Nurses' Health Study, 121,700 nurses aged 30–55 in 1976 living in 11 states were followed every 4 years and were administered FFQs for the first time in 1980. In 2001, 22,213 nurses aged 70 and over who were stroke-free were administered a cognitive assessment by telephone. This consisted first of the Telephone Interview for Cognitive Status (TICS) and later, tests of memory and executive function were added. In an analysis of fruit and vegetable intake, for which dietary and cognitive data were available on 13,000+ nurses, intake of cruciferous vegetables in the highest quintile was associated with better performance on all cognitive tests; and the results were pronounced for episodic memory, the best indicator of AD. Intake of green leafy vegetables also impacted the rate of decline, analogous to a difference of 1–2 years in age. In this study, no effect from consumption of fruits was found (Kang, Ascherio, & Grodstein, 2005).

In CHAP, findings were generally similar to those of the Nurses' Health Study (Morris, Evans, Tangney, Bienias, & Wilson, 2006). These authors calculated a random effects model including 3,718 individuals who had cognitive testing over three time points (6 years). Cognitive function was measured by Z-scores on four tests. Considering quintiles of daily fruit and vegetable servings, the *p*-value for trend in the multivariable-adjusted difference in annual change was 0.04 for vegetables and 0.55 for fruits (Morris, Evans, Tangney,

Bienias, & Wilson, 2006). All vegetables, except for legumes, had significant inverse associations with the outcome, among them zucchini, summer squash, eggplant, broccoli, lettuce, and other greens, kale, and collards. The authors calculated that the decrease in the rate of cognitive decline over 6 years in this study was equivalent to 5 years of age younger in those who consumed more than two vegetable servings per day. In addition, the high content of vitamin E in vegetables and the use of salad dressings and other fats that can increase the absorption of vitamin E and other fat-soluble flavonoids could mediate the observed association. When the authors included vitamin E in the model, the association between vegetable intake and cognitive change was attenuated and was not statistically significant. The lack of an association with fruit intake was unexpected, and the authors recommended further study of this topic.

In the Swedish Twin Study, an abbreviated FFQ was administered in 1967 to 5,692 mono- and same-sex dizygotic twins. In the HARMONY substudy of dementia and AD, 3,424 nondemented participants and 355 demented (240 with AD) were used in the analysis of fruit and vegetable intake. Co-twin analyses included 81 twin pairs who were discordant for dementia. The assessment of fruit and vegetable intake was crude, ascertained by a single question about whether fruit and vegetable intake formed a "great, medium, small or no part" of the diet. For this analysis, we collapsed the first two and the latter two categories to form a dichotomous variable (Hughes et al., 2010). The adjusted OR for AD associated with the high intake of fruits and vegetables was 0.60 (95% CI = 0.41–0.86), and this association was present for women but not men (OR = 0.47, 95% CI = 0.31–0.73 in women vs 1.15, 95% CI = 0.60–2.20 in men). In the matched co-twin analyses, the risk for AD associated with high intake of fruits and vegetables was in the same direction (OR = 0.47) but was not statistically significant (95% CI = 0.08–2.71), likely due to a much reduced sample size.

In a later study using the PAQUID cohort, researchers examined quartiles of flavonoid intake and cognitive decline over 10 years (Letenneur, Proust-Lima, Le Gouge, Dartigues, & Barberger-Gateau, 2007) using scores on the MMSE as the outcome. Adjusting for demographic variables, baseline performance on the MMSE was better among those with higher flavonoid intake, and there was a significant test for trend in performance over time. At the end of 10 years, those with the lowest flavonoid intake had lost a mean of 2.1 points (of 30) on the MMSE, and those in the highest quartile had lost about half that. When smoking and BMI were included in the model, the p-value became nonsignificant but was still close ($p = 0.06$) for flavonoid quartiles.

A systematic review of cohort studies on fruits and vegetables and the prevention of cognitive decline or dementia included nine studies that met inclusion criteria (Loef & Walach, 2012). The authors concluded that the weight of the evidence favored a high vegetable intake (defined in this paper as at least three servings or more than 200 g/day) as being inversely associated with AD risk, but that evidence for high fruit intake was still lacking. Perhaps the carbohydrate/glycemic load of fruits offsets the benefits for AD.

In the *Kame* Project, we used fruit and vegetable juice consumption to indirectly assess the role of polyphenols in the prevention of AD. Juices are known to contain a high content of antioxidant polyphenols. Purple grape juice has the highest polyphenolic content (and the highest number of individual polyphenols, including flavan-3-ols, anthocyanins and hydroxycinnamates), while white grape, pineapple, and tomato juices have the lowest polyphenol content (Singh et al., 2008). When juice is mechanically extracted under high pressure, high concentrations of peel and pulp components enter into the product. This is where most polyphenols reside. In addition, the number of whole fruits or vegetables ingested in one glass of juice is much higher than those ingested by consuming a single piece of fruit, such as an apple or orange. Finally, because juices are not cooked, the polyphenol content is maintained. In the *Kame* Project, we administered an FFQ to all baseline (1992–1994) participants, which included a question about intake of fruit and vegetable juices and the frequency of such intake. Of 1,836 nondemented participants at baseline, FFQ data were available for 1,589 individuals. We used Cox models to calculate the HR for probable AD by NINCDS-ADRDA criteria through 2001, adjusting for age, education, sex, regular physical activity, BMI, baseline CASI score, olfaction diagnostic group, total energy intake, intake of saturated fatty acids, monounsaturated fatty acids (MUFAs), and polyunsaturated fatty acids (PUFAs), APOE, smoking, alcohol intake, vitamin C, E and multivitamin supplementation, tea drinking, as well as dietary intake of vitamins C, E, and β-carotene (Dai et al., 2006). For intake of fruit and vegetable juices 1–2 times per week, the adjusted HR was 0.84 (95% CI = 0.31–2.29), and for 3 times a week or more, the adjusted HR was 0.24 (95% CI = 0.09–0.61) ($p_{\text{for trend}} < 0.01$), with the associations being more pronounced among those with an ε4 allele ($p = 0.02$) and those who were not physically active ($p < 0.01$). Because our FFQ only asked about "fruit and vegetable juices" we could not determine what kind of juices need to be consumed to reduce the risk for AD. In addition, our results need to be replicated in other cohort studies.

There is evidence that polyphenols from apples and citrus, such as quercetin, cross the blood–brain barrier and protect against hydrogen peroxide oxidation. In our study, as well as others (Laurin et al., 2004) no benefit was found from tea intake. Other studies have shown that catechin, the major polyphenol from tea, is not protective against hydrogen peroxide toxicity (Ishige, Schubert, & Sagara, 2001). Polyphenols in juices also have powerful anti-inflammatory properties and have been shown to reduce plasma concentrations of F2-isoprostanes (a marker of oxidative stress), while vitamin E has little effect (Meagher, Barry, Lawson, Rokach, & FitzGerald, 2001). In a study of transgenic AD mice, pomegranate juice, which contains very high concentrations of polyphenols, was randomly assigned to mice aged 6–12.5 months of age, with sugar water as the placebo treatment (Hartman et al., 2006). The pomegranate-supplemented mice not only learned cognitive maze tasks more quickly and swam more quickly than the placebo-supplemented mice, but also accumulated only half of the soluble $A\beta_{42}$ and hippocampal amyloid deposition. These results support further studies to study the role of fruit and vegetables juice supplementation for prevention of AD in human populations.

Before we leave the polyphenols, we would like to say a few words about other selected foods with high polyphenol concentrations that are inconclusive as of yet but are being studied in relation to AD: curcumin, EGCG, resveratrol, coffee, and chocolate. While we cannot review all the molecular and animal studies in these areas, we will discuss briefly human studies that have been conducted, and any trials that may hold promise for the future of prevention of AD in humans.

Curcumin

Curcumin is the polyphenol that gives the spice turmeric its coloring. The systematic review by Brondino et al (2014) attributes the beginning of this growing area of inquiry to the results of the study of Ganguli and Chandra et al. in India, in which low frequencies of AD were found compared with a rural community in Pennsylvania (Chandra et al., 2001). It was postulated that the lower frequency of disease in India could be due to the widespread use of curry (containing turmeric) in the Indian diet. However, as we saw in Chapters 6 and 7, there are other differences between the two sites that could have led to the disparate findings. A cross-sectional population-based study from Singapore of 1,010 nondemented participants age 60–93 showed that curry consumption "occasionally" (about once a month to once every 6 months) had an adjusted OR for an MMSE score of $\leq$23 of 0.62 (95% CI = 0.38–1.03), and more frequent consumption (once a month or more) was associated with an adjusted OR of 0.51 (95% CI = 0.21–0.90). Confounding and reverse causality are problems in this study, but it provides preliminary epidemiologic evidence of an association (Ng et al., 2006). *In vitro* studies have found that curcumin can inhibit Aβ aggregation and Aβ-induced inflammation. In animals, curcumin has effects on β-secretase, Aβ oligomerization, and tau phosphorylation, as well as behavioral improvement (Cole, Teter, & Frautschy, 2007; Hamaguchi, Ono, & Yamada, 2010). Aβ generates oxidative stress through metal ions such as copper and zinc, and curcumin and other polyphenols have the ability to chelate metal ions, which may constitute part of their anti-AD effects (Smid, Maag, & Musgrave, 2012). To date, clinical trials with curcumin have yielded null results. However, RCTs with curcumin have enrolled very small samples (n ~ 35), used low doses, were carried out in AD cases instead of MCI or asymptomatic at-risk individuals, were brief in duration, and did not utilize pure curcumin (Gupta, Patchva, & Aggarwal, 2013).

Several better designed trials to assess the effect of curcumin are ongoing. Use of curcumin in the short-term studies has been deemed safe, and the pharmacodynamics properties of curcumin make it more conducive to acting as a neuroprotective factor than as an agent that can reverse existing pathology. Therefore, long-term supplementation with this agent over many years may be warranted (Brondino et al., 2014).

Epigallocatechin-Gallate (EGCG)

Green tea catechins, in particular (−)EGCG, protect neurons in culture against Aβ toxicity by inhibiting β-amyloid fibrils from forming and by disruption of mature fibrils. In this regard, EGCG has a general activity against the β-sheet motif in Aβ proteins, as well as in other proteins, such as α-synuclein, the misfolded protein in Parkinson's disease. EGCG also mediates secretase activity, reducing APP proteolysis through a protein kinase c-dependent pathway. It has potent antioxidant and anti-inflammatory activity and can inhibit apoptosis (death of cells). It also activates neuronal differentiation synergistically with nerve growth factor (Smid et al., 2012). Most of the scientific support from this polyphenol's neuroprotective properties comes from cell culture or animal experiments. Epidemiologic studies examining tea consumption and cognition have generally shown no effects (Dai et al., 2006; Laurin et al., 2004) with some inverse findings (Arab et al., 2011). A protective effect has been described for stroke (Sato et al., 1989). Some limitations of epidemiologic studies of tea polyphenols include the lack of valid measurement and measurement too late in life (in cohorts who are over 65 who already experience high oxidative stress levels).

Resveratrol

Resveratrol is a nonflavonoid polyphenol found in grapes, red wine, and berries. We saw in Chapter 13 that wine consumption has been found to be inversely associated with incident AD. Resveratrol also has experimentally been shown to have antioxidant, anti-inflammatory, anticarcinogenic, and antimutagenic properties (Singh et al., 2008). This is another area that is promising for future intervention research in AD.

Coffee and Caffeine

That coffee may be inversely associated with AD would be good news to many of us. A great deal of work has been done on this topic, since it was recognized that caffeine has a protective role in attention (Nehlig, Daval, & Debry, 1992) but an adverse one in hypertension (Nurminen, Niittynen, Korpela, & Vapaatalo, 1999). Caffeine is the most common psychotropic substance used in the world, present in coffee, tea, and many soft drinks. Its main action is as an adenosine-receptor antagonist. Coffee's polyphenols are mostly chlorogenic acids, particularly 5-O-caffeoylquinic acid, which has been shown to be anticarcinogenic in animals. Other polyphenols in coffee, such as caffeic and ferulic acids reduce cholesterol levels and lower blood glucose. Animal studies show that caffeine, equivalent to five cups per day in humans, added to the drinking water of both young and old transgenic mice for 1–2 months not only reversed cognitive impairment but also decreased brain Aβ levels, reducing Aβ deposition in the hippocampus by 40% and in the entorhinal cortex by 46%. It is known that caffeine suppresses both β-secretase and γ-secretase, both required to generate Aβ (Arendash & Cao, 2010).

Among epidemiologic studies that have studied coffee consumption, the Three-City Study examined 4,197 women and 2,820 men and followed them for 4 years. Women who drank more than three cups of caffeine per day (limited here to tea and coffee) had less decline in verbal retrieval (OR = 0.67, 95% CI = 0.53–0.85), and a trend was observed for less decline in visuospatial memory (OR = 0.82, 95% CI = 0.65–1.03). The effect became more pronounced with increasing age. Among participants age 80 and over, the OR was 0.30 (95% CI = 0.14–0.63), but no effect was found among men, and caffeine was not protective for dementia incidence. The authors concluded that caffeine may be effective in delaying the onset of MCI among women (Ritchie et al., 2007). Similar findings restricted to women have been found in the CHS and in a study in Portugal (Arab et al., 2011; Santos, Lunet, et al., 2010). However, in Finland, a statistically significant inverse association between coffee consumption and change in MMSE score over 10 years was reported among men, with a significant linear dose–response (van Gelder et al., 2007). Finally, in a quantitative meta-analysis (Santos, Costa, Santos, Vaz-Carneiro, & Lunet, 2010) the pooled RR was 0.93 (95% CI 0.83–1.04) from cohort studies, with substantial heterogeneity. This RR became statistically significant when the most influential study was excluded (RR = 0.77, 95% CI 0.63–0.95), $I^2 = 34.7\%$). Further research is needed on the effect of coffee consumption on incident AD, including cohort studies and RCTs.

Chocolate

Dark chocolate has about the same amount of caffeine as coffee by weight, though an average bar of milk chocolate contains about the same amount of caffeine as a cup of decaffeinated coffee. In addition, the three types of chocolate contain flavan-3-ols (catechins) and flavonoids in the average amounts shown in Table 15.2.

TABLE 15.2 Total Phenolic and Flavonoid Content of Three Types of Chocolates

Type of Chocolate	Total Phenolics (mg/100g)	Flavonoids (mg/100g)
Dark	579	28
Milk	160	13
White	126	8

Source: http://en.wikipedia.org/wiki/Health_effects_of_chocolate#Polyphenol_content

Depending on its preparation, dark chocolate may have higher amounts of flavonoids per serving than teas and red wines (Ding, Hutfless, Ding, & Girotra, 2006). *In vitro*, an experiment using lavado cocoa, with a high epicatechin content showed reduced oligomer formation of both $A\beta_{40}$ and $A\beta_{42}$ (Wang, Varghese, et al., 2014). Another experiment conducted in a *Caenorhabditis elegans* model (roundworm) showed that a cocoa peptide called 13L was protective for oxidative stress and reduced deposition of Aβ (Martorell et al., 2013). Another pathway through which cocoa may induce benefits is through polyphenols' modulation of brain-derived neurotrophic factor (BDNF) signaling, which has effects on both Aβ plaque and on Aβ oligomer-treated cells (Cimini et al., 2013). In a large population-based cross-sectional study in Norway, the Hordaland Health Study, the authors measured chocolate, wine, and tea consumption from FFQs and described cognitive impairment as performance in the bottom decile of a variety of neuropsychological tests: the Kendrick Object Learning Test, the Trail-Making Test, part A, Digit Symbol Test, Block Design, the MMSE and the Controlled Word Association Test (Nurk et al., 2009). After adjustment for sex, education, smoking, vitamin supplement use, history of CVD, diabetes, and total energy intake, the scores on all six tests were better among wine drinkers. Among chocolate consumers, mean scores were higher on all tests except the Block Design test and tea drinkers had better scores in four of the six tests. The authors then classified participants on the basis of how many of the three foods (wine, chocolate, and tea) they consumed. Odds ratios for poor cognitive performance decreased in a dose–response fashion with increasing number of the three flavonoid-rich foods consumed, For example, on the episodic memory task, the OR decreased from 1.0 for no intake of the three foods to 0.77 (95% CI = 0.52–1.17) for one, 0.54 (95% CI = 0.35–0.83) for two, and 0.36 (95% CI = 0.19–0.67) for three. Similar dose–response trends were significant for the other tests. For chocolate consumption, the authors found that the maximum benefit was at a level of 10 g/day.

A double-blind, placebo-controlled trial of dark chocolate was conducted on 101 nondemented participants with mean age of 68, in which 37 g/day of dark chocolate was tested against an artificially sweetened cocoa beverage for 6 weeks. No benefit was found for neuropsychological performance. It is important to recognize that 6 weeks is a very short intervention period for a trial size of 100 subjects. It is likely that to be adequately powered, a much larger sample size with a much longer follow-up would be necessary (Crews, Harrison, & Wright, 2008). Furthermore, the high education levels of the participants (>15 years) with higher levels of reserve may have reduced the ability of the study to detect an effect.

Soy Consumption

Phytoestrogens in soy products are similar in structure to 17-β-estradiol, the most common circulating estrogen. They are bioactive, interact with estrogen receptors and impact estrogenic responses. Phytoestrogens can mimic endogenous estrogen but have less effect. When endogeneous estrogens are high, phytoestrogens act as estrogen-receptor antagonists, and when they are low, phytoestrogens act as estrogen-receptor agonists (Soni et al., 2014). There are a number of different phytoestrogen types, including isoflavones, lignans, coumestans, and stilbenes. In animal studies, soy-fed female rats performed better than a placebo group in short-term cognitive tasks, but by 8 weeks of feeding, these effects reversed.

Given the rapid increase in soy consumption in western countries and the pervasiveness of its consumption in Asia, it is important that we learn how these products are associated with cognitive outcomes in humans. The HAAS reported that participants eating two or more servings/week of tofu (vs less) in midlife not only had *poorer* CASI scores but also had increased ventricular volumes and lower brain weights at autopsy compared with nonconsumers (White et al., 2000). Similar findings were obtained in the *Kame* Project, where we found that both men and women who were high tofu consumers had significantly lower CASI scores than low or moderate consumers (Rice et al., 1999). In addition, high tofu intake has been shown to be related to poorer memory performance among Javanese and Sundanese elders (Hogervorst, Sadjimim, Yesufu, Kreager, & Rahardjo, 2008). Among 1,362 breast cancer survivors in Shanghai, we found higher soy protein intake from all sources to be associated with a decline in long-term memory over 18 months of follow-up ($p < 0.01$) (Dai, unpublished data). In another longitudinal study, late perimenopausal women and postmenopausal Asian women with high isoflavone consumption performed better than their low isoflavone counterparts on tests of processing speed, but in early perimenopause and postmenopause, those consuming high amounts performed worse on verbal memory (Greendale et al., 2012).

Short-term, double-blind clinical trials in which the effects of soy isoflavones were compared to placebo in postmenopausal women have resulted in mixed findings. As we have seen before, in comparison with clinical trials in which the exposure is time-limited, observational studies are more likely to reflect long-term dietary intake, including during the premenopausal period in women. The fact that most longitudinal studies have shown negative effects of soy on cognition and/or markers of brain atrophy likely reflect long-term exposures across the life course. *In vitro* studies suggest that soy isoflavones actively inhibit synthesis of estradiol and other steroid hormones (Adlercreutz & Mazur, 1997). Reduction in circulating estrogen over a long time course could result in brain atrophy, increasing the risk for cognitive impairment. Short-term stimulation of estrogen receptors in postmenopausal women, on the other hand, could result in transient improvement in some cognitive functions, given the absence of appreciable circulating estrogen. Given the effects of soy isoflavones on estrogen synthesis, it is likely that its effect will be modulated by both age and sex. This view is supported by animal studies that have shown opposite effects of soy phytoestrogens on spatial memory in male and female rats (Lee, Lee, & Sohn, 2005).

The longest and largest trial of soy products and cognitive outcomes was the WISH trial (Henderson et al., 2012), in which 313 healthy postmenopausal women aged 45–92 were randomized to receive 25 g/day of isoflavone-rich soy protein (including 52 mg of genistein, 36 mg of daidzein, and 3 mg glycitein) or milk protein-matched placebo for 2.5 years. Data were analyzed as intention-to-treat. Fourteen neuropsychological tests were administered and the primary cognitive outcome was change from baseline on global cognition. Secondary endpoints included changes in cognitive factors and in individual test scores. There was no association by group with regard to global cognition. The treatment group experienced an improvement on a visual memory factor, but there were no associations in the other 3 cognitive factors or on any of the 14 individual test scores. When a younger subgroup of women was analyzed, no associations were observed. Among women who had had a surgical menopause, the soy isoflavone group performed worse on global cognition ($p = 0.058$). Even though this trial was quite lengthy, we do not know whether null results would have been obtained with an even longer follow-up. Based on the observational data from several studies, we believe that the use of high levels of soy products should not be pursued in men or in premenopausal women for the prevention of dementia, given the importance of estrogen in maintaining brain tissue.

FATS

Probably the most studied component of the diet with regard to AD risk, fish and Omega-3 oils are regarded as healthy for the brain as well as the heart. In fact, dietary fats and the distribution of types of fats consumed are important predictors of a healthy diet and a healthy cholesterol profile (Morris & Tangney, 2014). Phospholipids comprise a quarter of the brain's dry weight (Uauy & Dangour, 2006). As we have already discussed, high cholesterol in midlife increases AD risk, and APOE-ε4 is involved in cholesterol transport. There are four major types of dietary fatty acids: *trans*, saturated, monounsaturated, and polyunsaturated. *Trans* fats, otherwise known as partially hydrogenated oils are consumed at a low level in the United States currently due to legislation in 2006 that required labeling of such fats on foods and a subsequent public health campaign to increase awareness and reduce consumption. *Trans* fats have been shown to increase APP forms that are amyloidogenic and decrease those that are nonamyloidogenic (Grimm et al., 2012). A 4-month study in mice of a western-type diet that included 40% saturated fat found greater Aβ concentrations compared with those on a soy-based diet (Morris & Tangney, 2014; Oksman et al., 2006). Besides amyloid, saturated and *trans* fatty acids have also been shown to impair function of the blood–brain barrier and to reduce glucose uptake in the hippocampus.

One of the earliest systematic studies of dietary fat intake and cognitive outcomes was the Rotterdam Study (Kalmijn et al., 1997). Over 2 years of follow-up, 58 of 5,386 participants became demented (42 with AD). Dietary intake of fats was measured with a 170-item semi-quantitative FFQ. Linoleic acid intake was used to measure n-6 PUFAs because it is the major source of PUFAs in the Western diet. Intake of n-3 eicosapentaenoic acid (EPA) and docosahexaenoic acid (DHA) was measured by intake of fish in the diet, the major source of these PUFAs. In this study, only total fats were statistically significant for all dementias (RR = 2.4, 95% CI = 1.1–5.2); other associations indicated a trend toward increasing risk with increasing saturated fat and cholesterol. No association of fats of any type was found for AD. In this early study, only demographic factors and total energy intake were adjusted. This would prove later to be a methodological flaw. Linoleic acid (g/day) also was not associated with any dementia or the two subtypes, while fish consumption was inversely associated with total dementia (RR = 0.4, 95% CI = 0.2–0.9) and with AD without CVD (RR = 0.3, 95% CI = 0.1–0.9), but not with VaD, adjusted for age, sex, education, and total energy intake. The results did not change when analyses were conducted that excluded individuals with cardiovascular diseases. *n*-3 PUFAs in fish, in addition to being a "good" fat, may decrease AD risk through its anti-inflammatory effects and through decreased cytokine production. In addition, *n*-3 PUFAs are involved in brain development and nerve cell regeneration (Kalmijn et al., 1997).

In a subsequent paper published from the same study, this association was again investigated after 6 years of follow-up of the cohort (Engelhart et al., 2002a). In this paper, high intake of total, saturated, and *trans* fats and cholesterol and low intake of, MUFAs, PUFAs, *n*-6 and *n*-3 PUFAs were not associated with dementia or any subtype. The authors explained their previous positive findings as due to a shorter follow-up period and a smaller number of incident dementia cases. While a Type I error in this direction is possible, it is less likely that studies with larger sample sizes and longer follow-up periods would result in such an error.

In 2003, investigators from CHAP used the revised Harvard FFQ from their baseline examination in 1993 and 131 incident cases of AD arising over 3.9 years of follow-up to examine the associations between saturated fat, *trans*-fat unsaturated fat, *n*-6 PUFA, MUFA, total fat, dietary cholesterol, and animal and vegetable fat. A novel aspect of their analysis that corrected the methodological flaw pointed out earlier was to adjust for the other fats when examining a particular type of fat. *Trans* fats had increasing ORs with increasing quintiles (from an OR of 3.4 (95% CI = 1.3–8.8) for the second compared to the first quintile to 5.2 (95% CI = 1.5–18.5) for the fifth compared to the first quintile, but the *p*-value for trend was not significant. Vegetable fats were associated with an inverse OR from 0.9 (95% CI = 0.4–2.0) for the second quintile to 0.2 (95% CI = 0.1–0.7) for the fifth quintile ($p_{\text{for trend}} = 0.002$). Other types of fat, particularly *n*-6 PUFA and MUFA, showed trends toward being significant after adjusting for other types of fat ($p_{\text{for trend}} = 0.10$). These were the first investigators to examine the ratio of PUFAs to saturated fats, for which a significant 70% reduction in the OR was observed for the highest versus the lowest quintile.

Other fats were found to be correlated with one another and also to be strong confounders of the associations, as were the presence of cardiovascular conditions and antioxidant nutrients. In addition, for *trans* fats, the effect was found to be more pronounced among people with low PUFA intake and less deleterious for those with high PUFA ($p = 0.04$ for interaction). *Trans* fats also were particularly harmful to black participants, and the inverse association between *n*-6 PUFA and AD was present only among women.

In WHICAP, no association with AD was found for carbohydrates, fats, or protein, based on a 61-item semiquantitative FFQ administered by telephone between the baseline and first incident wave (Luchsinger, Tang, Shea, & Mayeux, 2002). In a critique of the null studies, Morris and Tangney (2014) state that lack of control for all confounders, including cardiovascular disease and related fats would result in negative confounding. In CHAP, the analysis of MUFAs and incident AD had an OR of 0.8 without adjustment for other fatty acids and 0.2 with adjustment. If *trans* fats are negatively related to MUFAs and positively related to AD risk, this would indeed produce negative confounding. Furthermore, Morris describes statistical difficulties in adjusting for all fatty acids in a single model because of problems with multicollinearity of these variables. This results in an inflation of the standard errors of the estimates (thus widening the confidence intervals) and increases the threat of making a Type II error. This type of problem is exacerbated by small sample sizes. Finally, when all fats are included in the model together, there is an admixture of both inverse and adverse effects, resulting in a measure of effect of questionable meaning.

Besides CHAP, the only other cohort study that adjusted for other types of fats in their analyses of clinical cognitive outcomes was CAIDE (Eskelinen et al., 2008). The investigators examined incident MCI and neuropsychological function on a variety of tests. In this study, saturated fats were measured from intake of milk, sour milk, and spreads; and information about fats used for cooking and baking was obtained by asking about use of vegetable oil, margarine, and butter. After an average follow-up of 21 years, saturated fats from the sources studied increased the risk for incident MCI (OR = 2.36, 95% CI = 1.17–4.74), adjusting for demographic and vascular variables, APOE and other fats. In addition, high intake of PUFAs predicted better semantic memory scores and higher PUFA:saturated fat ratios were associated with higher psychomotor speed and better scores in executive function tests. Generally for saturated fat, increased RRs for global cognitive outcomes and MCI, as well as for cognitive decline have been found, as well as fairly consistent inverse associations for MUFAs and PUFAs, with some of the findings being "trendy" but not statistically significant (Morris & Tangney, 2014).

PUFAs in Fish

Omega-3 fatty acids are long-chain PUFAs, with fish being the primary source of these fats (EPA and DHA). Nuts, seeds, and vegetable oils that contain α-linolenic acid also provide PUFAs. The cardiovascular benefits of omega-3 fatty acids are numerous and include anti-inflammatory actions, as well as beneficial effects on triglyceride levels, blood pressure, blood clotting, stroke risk, risk of cardiovascular diseases, sudden cardiac death, and arrhythmias. Current recommendations from the American Heart Association are that individuals with coronary heart disease (CHD) take 1 g/day of combined DHA and EPA as a capsule or by eating fatty fish, and that individuals without CHD take at least 500 mg/day. The evidence for primary and secondary prevention of CHD associated with fish oil is elegantly summarized in Cao et al. (2014). However, there are conflicting data between the observational and interventional studies, similar to what is seen in AD research for certain medications (anti-inflammatory drugs, statins, hormone replacement therapy, see Chapters 14 and 19). For the omega-3 fatty acids, issues of bioavailability and trial design have been cited as part of the explanation for the divergent results (von Schacky, 2014).

PUFAs are critical parts of neuronal membranes, and they lower the proportion of total cholesterol, increasing the fluidity of membranes, which is essential to the infrastructure that supports learning, memory, and other aspects of cognition. Emerging evidence also demonstrates that DHA may be critical to the formation of new memories and to hippocampal neurogenesis in adult brain (Jicha & Markesbery, 2010). One of the possible mechanisms of action of PUFAs, particularly DHA from fish, is through increasing production of BDNF. DHA also has potent antioxidant activity (Cole, Ma, & Frautschy, 2009). DHA is called an "essential" PUFA because humans are unable to produce it. Although α-linoleic acid can be obtained from plants and can to some degree be converted to DHA, DHA itself and EPA are only available from consumption of marine animals. Thus, the important role of fish in the diet becomes clear. Jicha and Markesbery also point to the importance of the ratios of omega-6 to omega-3 PUFAs, where high ratios are proinflammatory and pro-oxidative.

Fish that have particularly high levels of these types of good fatty acids include salmon, lake trout, herring, sardines, and tuna. Many other types of seafood have smaller amounts of omega-3s.

In Tg2576 transgenic mice, researchers added 0.6% DHA to the chow of old animals (aged 17–19 months) and compared them to mice fed two low-DHA diets (0.09% DHA or 0%). The high-DHA diet was shown to reduce total Aβ by more than 70% compared with the low-DHA or control diets, more so for insoluble Aβ but to a lesser extent soluble Aβ as well. $A\beta_{42}$ levels were below those seen in the control chow diet, and amyloid plaques were reduced markedly in the hippocampus and parietal cortex. The authors concluded that DHA might have beneficial effects on β-amyloid production, accumulation and toxicity (Lim et al., 2005). Given that DHA is abundant in neurons and synaptic membranes, low levels of DHA can cause increases in *n*-6/*n*-3 ratios, producing inflammation that increases cytokines and oxidative stress, which drive increased Aβ production. Other experimental data *in vitro* and from transgenic animals show that omega-3 PUFAs may upregulate α-secretase to produce nontoxic peptides and prevent the formation of Aβ, downregulate cleavage with γ-secretase, and inhibit fibrillation and formation of toxic oligomeric Aβ (Jicha & Markesbery, 2010).

Prospective Cohort Studies of Fish Intake and AD

Several large epidemiologic studies provide compelling evidence in favor of the consumption of fish and *n*-3 fatty acids being inversely related to incident AD. The first study to observe this association was the PAQUID study (Barberger-Gateau et al., 2002). In 1991–1992, 1,674 community-dwelling participants were asked how often they ate meat and fish or seafood. Seven years later, 135 new AD cases had been diagnosed by standard criteria. The HR for AD associated with eating fish or seafood at least once per week was 0.66 (95% CI = 0.47–0.93) adjusted for age and sex. However, adjustment for education led to a similar, though nonsignificant association (HR = 0.69, 95% CI = 0.47–1.01). The next important study was by the CHAP investigators (Morris et al., 2003), which accrued 131 incident cases of AD over 3.9 years of follow-up. The RR for AD associated with eating fish once per week or more was 0.4 (95% CI 0.2–0.9) ($p_{\text{for trend}} = 0.07$). This association held for total *n*-3 fatty acids and for DHA, but not for EPA or α-linolenic acid. For total *n*-3 fatty acids the association was significant only among women. These models were adjusted for age, sex, race, education, total energy intake, APOE-ε4 and included a race × APOE-ε4 interaction term. Alpha-linolenic acid was statistically significant among people who were APOE-ε4 positive, whereas no association was present among those who were APOE-ε4 negative when adjusted for vitamin E intake and other types of fat.

In the Three-City cohort (Barberger-Gateau et al., 2007), an inverse association was also noted in the full model adjusted for age sex, education, city, income, marital status, APOE-ε4, BMI, and diabetes, but only the stratum of eating fish 2–3 times per week was statistically significant (HR = 0.59, 95% CI = 0.37–0.94). Interestingly in this study, intake of omega-6 oils that were not counterbalanced with omega-3s incurred an increased risk for dementia of 2.12 (95% CI = 1.3–3.46), but only among APOE-ε4 noncarriers (risk estimates for AD were not provided). In addition, there were 679 participants who had a poor diet (defined as infrequent intake of fish, fruits, and vegetables and no regular use of omega-3 oils) and 39 of these became demented during the follow-up. The risk for AD associated with this dietary pattern was 1.63 (95% CI = 1.04–2.56). Finally, it appeared that each of the three types of protective foods (fish, fruits and vegetables, and use of omega-3 oils) was independently related to a reduced risk for AD, although the analysis lacked power. In this study, individuals who dropped out of the study were in worse health than those who remained in the cohort. This is quite typical of cohort studies in the general population, and will usually result in underestimation of the exposure-outcome effects.

The CHS-Cognition Study examined fish intake from a 90-item FFQ among 2,233 participants aged 65 and over who had an MRI and resided in four US communities (Huang et al., 2005). Over an average of about 5 years, 190 AD cases developed. No benefit was observed for consumption of fried fish. There was a decreasing trend in risk for AD with increasing numbers of servings of tuna and other fish (including baked and broiled) adjusted for age, race, sex, APOE-ε4, energy intake, BMI, and region of the study, with the HR = 0.54 (95% CI = 0.31–0.95) for four or more servings of tuna and other fish per week. When this estimate was adjusted for education and income, the direction of the HR remained inverse, but was no longer statistically significant.

The issue of confounding by education has appeared several times in various studies. A concern in the investigation of fish consumption is the many other healthy habits that people who consume fish frequently also have. Many of these are inversely associated with AD. This "healthy-person" bias can result in spurious inverse associations, because *all* possible variables that might differ between exposed and unexposed participants are not included in the models. To address this issue, the French group undertook an analysis of characteristics that differ between fish-consumers and nonconsumers in the Three-City Study (Barberger-Gateau et al., 2005). Among 9,280 participants in this population-based study, people who ate fish regularly (at least once per week) were significantly more educated, had higher incomes, ate more pulses, fruits and vegetables, were more likely to drink alcohol, rated themselves to be in better health and less depressed, and scored higher on the MMSE. However, their objective health status was poorer than nonregular fish consumers, and they had a higher prevalence of hypertension and past stroke, despite having a lower BMI than nonfish consumers. In the same paper, the authors also examined which foods were more commonly eaten by fish-consumers. Fish eaters also were more likely to eat meat and eggs more than once a week. Other foods were not discussed, nor were other habits, such as physical activity (and types of physical activity) or other socioeconomic variables, or even the family-of-origin's socioeconomic background, or childhood diet, any of which could have had a substantial impact on the probability of being a regular fish-consumer in adult and late-adult life. The authors recommended that further study of the association between fish intake and AD be adjusted for the factors they identified.

We also must consider the problem of reverse causation, because it is likely that as symptoms of AD begin, the quality of the patient's diet may decline. As we shall see in our discussion of other modifiable risk factors, such as physical, mental, and social activity, this is a methodological dilemma that plagues observational cohort studies. Ideally, we would like to be able to look at midlife consumption of fish and other sources of omega-3 fatty acids in relation to cognitive impairment in late-life, but such studies are rare. The most remote diet measurement is from the CAIDE cohort, which examined 1,449 individuals aged 65–80 who had dietary assessments 21 years before. Frequent fish consumption (twice per week vs less often) was associated with better performance in late-life on a test of global cognition and on a test of semantic memory (Eskelinen et al., 2008). The Framingham Study found that DHA blood level in the top quartile measured about 10 years before cognitive testing was protective for dementia and AD (Schaefer et al., 2006).

RCTs and Fatty Acids

The study design that overcomes many of these problems is the randomized controlled trial. As we have seen, such trials, usually offering fairly high-dose interventions for a short period of time, are beset by their own methodological problems, such as inadequate sample size, compliance, and follow-up time. A number of smaller trials were conducted, and showed possible efficacy when participants were limited to those with very early disease. One example is the study of Chiu et al. (2008), in which the investigators randomized 23 MCI and 23 mild–moderate AD patients for 24 weeks to omega-3 PUFAs 1.8 g/day or placebo (olive oil). There was no effect on the cognitive scale of the Alzheimer's Disease Assessment Scale (ADAS-cog). In addition, higher concentrations of EPA on RBC membranes were associated with better cognitive outcomes ($p = 0.003$). Observational and intervention trials that were conducted until 2008 are summarized in Cole et al. (2009). At the time of this writing, 12 studies concerning omega-3 fatty acids and AD or cognition are ongoing (see Clinical Trials.gov). Hopefully these studies will provide larger sample sizes and longer follow-ups. Given that the Western diet is severely deficient in omega-3 fatty acids, with DHA levels of about 200 mg daily required for protection to the brain and intake closer to 80 mg daily (Cole, 2009), this is an important avenue to follow in future research.

Structural Brain Measures and Fatty Acids

A growing body of research exists to support the role of polyphenols and PUFAs on markers of brain plasticity (reserve), including enhanced expression of neurotrophic factors, synaptic function, and neurogenesis during adulthood (Murphy, Dias, & Thuret, 2014). In a study that we conducted in Shanghai, China (Mortimer et al., 2013) we obtained MRIs on 92 community-dwelling elders with a mean age of 74. Proxy informants for 32 demented, 28 MCI and 32 cognitively normal controls were interviewed regarding fish consumption and physical activity when the subjects were age 50. Among women, brain atrophy (percent of the cranium not occupied by gray or white matter) was associated with number of grams of fish consumed (divided at the median) ($p = 0.02$), adjusted for covariates including minutes of walking per day. There was no association among men. There also was no association between either fish consumption or minutes of walking with white matter hyperintensities, suggesting that the association was likely not mediated by vascular disease.

In the CHS-Cognition Study, the authors measured fish consumption by FFQ in 1989–1990 and performed MRIs 10 years later (Raji et al., 2014). At the Pittsburgh site, 280 participants were included in a cross-sectional analysis who had an MRI, dietary data and were cognitively normal both in 1992 and 1998. Participants with MCI or AD were excluded from this analysis. Individuals who ate baked or broiled fish at least once per week had larger gray matter volumes (4.3% for baked and 14% for broiled fish) in areas of the brain important to memory and cognition (hippocampus, precuneus, posterior cingulate, and orbital frontal cortex), adjusting for age, sex, race, intracranial volume, education, white matter lesions, diabetes, MRI-identified infarcts, waist-hip ratio, and physical activity (number of city blocks walked in 1 week). In addition, this study showed that brain volumes in the regions of interest were not associated with plasma omega-3 fatty acids, supporting the contention that dietary intake of fish can impact brain volume independently of circulating levels of omega-3s.

The WHIMS-MRI Study investigators calculated an omega-3 index using EPA+DHA in red blood cells and measured total brain and hippocampal volume 8 years later in 1111 postmenopausal women (Pottala et al., 2014). They found that the omega-3 index in the highest quartile compared with the first quartile was associated with greater hippocampal volume. DHA was marginally associated with total brain volume ($p = 0.06$), but ischemic brain lesion volumes were not associated with EPA, DHA or EPA+DHA. These findings were similar to those from the Framingham Offspring Study in which total brain volumes also were associated with RBC omega-3 concentrations (Tan et al., 2012).

CRITIQUE OF THE SINGLE NUTRIENT APPROACH

The single nutrient statistical approach to studying the etiology of disease has been nicely critiqued by Prentice, Sugar, Wang, Neuhouser, and Patterson (2002). These authors point out that the most robust associations between dietary elements and risk of disease come from those for which a biomarker has been identified, e.g., plasma lipids and CHD or calcium concentrations and risk of bone fracture. In many large-scale studies, such blood measures are unaffordable or are conducted only once despite the fact that long-term dietary habits are relevant. It is unlikely that a single nutrient will provide a "magic bullet" for a chronic disease such as AD, CHD, or cancer, yet the failure of trials to "prove" associations does not imply that diet is unimportant (Willett, 2013) when we consider problems related to the age of the sample, sample size, compliance, attrition, dose, and length of the trial. Prentice et al. also raise many issues related to precision of dietary measurement, confounding of nutrients (and likely interactions with other nutrients, and other variables, including genetic ones), "healthy person" bias, and issues of "competing exposures" within an individual (e.g., if I always have skim milk, I am unlikely to ever have whole milk). RCTs of single nutrients have generally not shown the same results as those from observational cohort studies. Part of the explanation for this may be that the two study designs ask different questions and study different exposures. Although the usual criticism of observational studies is that they can only show associations and not necessarily "causal" associations, RCTs cannot study effects of the long-term diet, the true exposure for which we wish to establish temporal sequence and causality.

Because of these and other issues, nutritional epidemiologists advise that all methods should be combined to study diet, including single nutrients, foods, and dietary patterns (Willett, 2013). If different study approaches yield consistent results, we can be more confident that we are observing something real. Therefore, the examination of dietary patterns is one other method to pursue, and this approach has the benefit of being able to recommend (or not) a way of practicing a more healthy lifestyle.

CALORIC RESTRICTION (CR)

A number of experimental studies have found that reducing the number of calories in the diet of transgenic animals significantly reduces accumulation of Aβ plaques [by 40–55% in one study (Patel et al., 2005)] and that the antiamyloidogenic role of caloric restriction (CR) is specifically associated with an increase in α-secretase activity (vs β-secretase) (Wang et al., 2005). In addition to increasing insulin sensitivity, reducing levels of proinflammatory cytokines and reactive oxygen species, CR has also been touted to be an example of hormesis, in which excessive amounts of a condition result in a detrimental response but small insults or exposures over a long time period that are still above normal evoke a mild stress that is beneficial (Murphy et al., 2014). For example, one study in rats showed that the combination of CR and exercise increased hippocampal BDNF and improved performance on the Morris Water Maze task in which the rat must find a platform it can stand on in the middle of a pool (Kishi & Sunagawa, 2012).

Human studies of caloric intake have led to mixed findings. In WHICAP, participants in the highest quartile of calorie intake had an increased risk for AD (HR = 1.5, 95% CI 1.0–2.2), which was more pronounced among ε4 carriers (HR = 2.3, 95% CI 1.1–4.7). In the Three-City Study, no association was present between dementia risk and total energy intake (Barberger-Gateau et al., 2007).

In a clinical trial of 50 cognitively normal overweight subjects aged 60.5 on average, groups were stratified (not randomized) to three groups: a 30% caloric reduction group (n = 20), a 20% increased unsaturated fatty acids group (n = 20) and a no-intervention group (n = 10) (Witte, Fobker, Gellner, Knecht, & Floel, 2009). Only the CR group showed an effect, an increase by 20% in verbal memory scores ($p<0.001$), which was accompanied by decreases in fasting plasma insulin levels and C-reactive protein, a marker of inflammation. However, this study should only be considered preliminary, because there was no randomization of participants to intervention groups.

DIETARY PATTERNS (DP)

Due to the complexity of how dietary components interact with one another and are statistically correlated, the last decade has seen the emergence of analyses that look at DP instead of single nutrients. The first study to examine DP with respect to the risk for AD was the WHICAP study. Scarmeas and his colleagues noted that the Mediterranean diet (MeDi) had already shown beneficial effects for other outcomes, such as cardiovascular disease, certain cancer types, and overall mortality (Scarmeas, Stern, Tang, Mayeux, & Luchsinger, 2006). They therefore became interested in testing this diet as a protective factor for AD.

The MeDi is more of a cultural DP from countries bordering the Mediterranean Sea than a specific "diet" in the way we think of diets in the United States. It is characterized by a high intake of fruit, vegetables, legumes, complex carbohydrates, and a moderate intake of fish. Olive oil is the primary source of fats and red wine is typically drunk during the meal (Sofi, Macchi, Abbate, Gensini, & Casini, 2010). The MeDi diet contains a healthy mix of antioxidant vitamins, polyphenols, B vitamins, MUFAs, PUFAs, and a moderate intake of alcohol.

In WHICAP, Scarmeas et al. followed 2,258 nondemented participants with a mean age of 77 for 4 years, 262 of whom converted to AD. Diet was measured using the Harvard FFQ comprising 61 items consumed over the past year. When a food was considered beneficial, a point was given for seven food groups, including dairy, meat, fruits, vegetables, legumes, cereals, and fish. A point also was given if consumption was below the median for foods that were considered adverse (Trichopoulou, Costacou, Bamia, & Trichopoulos, 2003). Fat intake and alcohol intake were similarly scored. Adjusting for cohort, age, sex, ethnicity, education, APOE-ε4, caloric intake, smoking, comorbidity, and BMI, the HRs were statistically significant whether the MeDi diet was treated as a continuous (linear) variable or was analyzed in tertiles (HR for the middle compared with the lowest tertile = 0.85, 95% CI = 0.63–1.16; HR for the highest compared with the lowest tertile = 0.60, 95% CI = 0.42–0.87, $p_{\text{for trend}} = 0.007$). When analyzed separately, none of the nine food types was associated with incident AD. Therefore, the authors concluded that the additive or synergistic effects of foods in the MeDi, but *not any specific food component or nutrient*, accounted for the lowered risk for AD. In addition, this group has shown that the effect of the MeDi diet is not influenced by vascular disease (Scarmeas, Stern, Mayeux, & Luchsinger, 2006), suggesting that the important roles of antioxidant and anti-inflammatory properties of this diet are on the risk for AD. However, we must also consider the limitations of this approach, measuring diet at one point in time, at age 65 or later as well as the possible reduction in healthy eating patterns relatively close to the time of AD diagnosis. This last concern is partially mitigated by another paper by the same group that found similar associations between the MeDi diet and incident MCI (Scarmeas, Stern, et al., 2009). In that analysis, the HRs for MCI were of borderline significance (middle vs lowest tertile HR = 0.83, 95% CI = 0.62–1.12; highest vs lowest tertile HR = 0.72, 95% CI = 0.52–1.0, $p_{\text{for trend}} = 0.05$). MeDi diet significantly predicted the conversion from MCI to AD ($p_{\text{for trend}} = 0.02$). In addition, in yet another paper examining physical activity and MeDi diet together, the same authors reported that both of these protective factors were significant and independent of one another (Scarmeas, Luchsinger, et al., 2009).

In an attempt to replicate these results using the same methods as the studies of Scarmeas et al., the Three-City cohort followed 1,410 individuals with an average age of 76 for 4 years (Feart et al., 2009). Annual decline on the MMSE was greatest among those in the lowest tertile of MeDi diet score ($p = 0.01$), but other cognitive tests were unrelated, and the MeDi score was not predictive of incident dementia ($p = 0.64$). The authors cite a shorter follow-up period in their study compared with WHICAP, which could have obscured associations, as well as different distributions of MeDi diet scores between the studies. For example, they contend that the low fruit and vegetable consumers in France may be equivalent to the high fruit and vegetable consumers in the United States. In addition, factors such as much greater use of dietary supplements in the United States than in France may have contributed to the differences in results.

In 2011, the CHAP compared the MeDi DP with the Healthy Eating Index-2005 (HEI-2005) with respect to cognitive outcomes (Tangney, Kwasny, et al., 2011). They used a slightly different method than the studies of Scarmeas et al. in which a separate score was calculated for wine intake, and the diet score was based on 10 food groups: unrefined cereals, potatoes, fruit, vegetables, legumes, nuts and beans, fish, olive oil, red meat and related products, poultry, and whole fat cheese and other dairy. They also scored the MeDi diet based on intake of the Greek population, rather than using median intakes for the study population. The HEI-2005 summarizes 12-components of quality of the diet with scores based on energy intake: total fruit, whole fruit, total vegetables, dark green and orange vegetables and legumes, total grains, whole grains, milk and related products, meat and beans, oils, saturated fat, sodium, and calories from solid fats, alcoholic drinks, and added sugars. In cross-sectional and longitudinal analyses over a mean of 7.6 years, both the MeDi diet and wine scores were highly statistically significantly protective for better performance on a *Z*-scored measure of cognitive function including the MMSE, the Symbol Digit Modalities Test, and the East Boston tests of immediate and delayed recall. All four of these tests loaded on a single factor that explained 74% of the variance. The *p*-values for the MeDi Diet score in cross-sectional and longitudinal analyses were 0.001 and 0.0004, respectively; for the Medi Diet wine score they were 0.02 and 0.0009, respectively. For the HEI-2005 score, they were 0.24 and 0.21. The most likely explanation for the difference in findings between the two DP is how the scores are calculated. The HEI-2005 score, for example, gives more weight to full-fat dairy components and red meats than the MeDi diet.

Another analysis comparing two diets, the MeDi and the DASH diet, was performed on data from the Cache County Study in Utah (Wengreen et al., 2013). This study obtained a 142-item self-administered FFQ for 3,580 participants with a mean age of 74. The DASH diet score includes eight components: fruit, vegetables, low-fat dairy products, nuts and legumes, whole grains, low salt intake, sweetened beverages, and red/processed meats. The DASH diet is effective for reducing blood pressure. The two diets were highly correlated ($r = 0.62$, $p \leq 0.001$). For both diets, 3MS scores differed by quintile ($p_{\text{for trend}}$ for DASH =

0.0001, for MeDi, 0.002) and for the comparison of the highest quintile to the lowest (p for DASH = 0.0009, p for MeDi, = 0.001), controlling for age, sex, education, BMI, physical activity, multivitamin and mineral supplement use, alcohol and smoking, and history of diabetes, myocardial infarction and stroke. Individuals in the highest quintile of both diets scored about a point higher on the 3MS in the multivariate models. Although the study supports the protective roles of both diets, it is not known whether adherence to healthy diets reflects lifelong differences in healthy lifestyles, i.e., what we have been referring to as "healthy person bias."

A recent analysis from the Rush MAP comparing the MIND Diet Score to the DASH and MeDi scores found decreasing risks for AD with increasing tertiles for all three diets ($p_{\text{for trend}}$ for adjusted HRs = 0.003 for the MIND Diet Score, $p_{\text{for trend}} = 0.07$ for the DASH Diet score and $p_{\text{for trend}} = 0.01$ for the MeDi score) (Morris et al., 2015). Significant benefits were present among those who adhered only moderately to the MIND diet whereas for the other two diets, only the highest tertile of adherence to the diet was associated with lower risk for AD. The MIND diet, a hybrid of the Mediterranean and Dash diets, does not rate fruits in general as "healthy" (only berries are rated healthy). Emphasis is placed on consumption of green leafy and other vegetables, beans, whole grains, fish, poultry, olive oil, and wine; while red meats, butter and margarine, cheese, pastries, sweets, and fried/fast foods are rated as unhealthy food groups.

Others have not found that the MeDi diet protects against cognitive decline or incidence of AD. In the Nurses' Health Study (Samieri, Okereke, Devore, & Grodstein, 2013), quintiles of adherence to the MeDi diet over more than 13 years were associated with better absolute cognitive scores ($p_{\text{for trend}} < 0.001$ to 0.004) but were not related to the slope of change in cognition (multivariable-adjusted p-value for the TICS = 0.31). Some of the explanations advanced by the authors included a narrower distribution of cognitive function and decline due to the higher education of their sample, the somewhat modest follow-up period, and the low adherence of American populations to the MeDi DP. They also saliently point out that even if the effect of the MeDi diet is modest, it can still have a widespread impact on cognition and other outcomes.

In 2014, Singh et al. published a meta-analysis of the MeDi DP that included six cohorts (Singh et al., 2014). Most of the analyses counted the Scarmeas et al. studies more than once and also collapsed different outcomes (incident AD, incident MCI). Their overall conclusion was that subjects in the highest tertile of the MeDi diet had a 33% lower risk for incident MCI or AD (HR = 0.67, 95% CI = 0.55–0.81) compared with the lowest tertile. They found no significant heterogeneity in their analyses. However, the results were heavily weighted by the Scarmeas et al. studies.

Finally, a novel method that has been applied to other outcomes was used to identify a protective diet for AD (Gu, Nieves, Stern, Luchsinger, & Scarmeas, 2010). With this method, a number of DPs were investigated by reduced rank regression (RRR). The goal was to explain variability in seven sets of nutrients: saturated fatty acids, MUFAs, *n*-3 and *n*-6 PUFAs, vitamin E, vitamin B_{12}, and folate. The analysis included 2,148 participants from WHICAP 1 (recruited in 1992) and WHICAP 2 (recruited in 1999). The authors used 30 preset food groups as predictor variables and seven nutrients as response variables. The RRR identifies linear combinations, or DP scores, of a set of food groups by maximizing the variation explained by the nutrients. The analysis generated seven DP scores for each subject that were uncorrelated, a higher DP score showing that the subject's diet is more strongly representative of that particular diet. The seven DP scores explained almost 77% of total variation in nutrients and about 30% of the variation in food intake. Only one DP score was associated with AD risk in a univariate model (HR = 0.54, 95% CI = 0.39–0.75). This DP was high in *n*-3 and *n*-6 PUFAs, vitamin E, and folate, but low in saturated fats and vitamin B_{12}. It was positively correlated with consumption of salad dressings, fish, tomatoes, poultry, cruciferous vegetables, fruits, and dark and green leafy vegetables and negatively correlated with high-fat dairy products, red meat, organ meat, and butter. The fully adjusted model, controlling for recruitment cohort, age, education, ethnicity, sex, smoking, BMI, caloric intake, comorbidities, and APOE, showed a dose–response trend with increasing adherence to this DP (HR for the middle tertile compared with the lowest tertile = 0.81, 95% CI = 0.59–1.12, HR for the highest tertile compared with the lowest tertile = 0.62, 95% CI = 0.43–0.89, $p_{\text{for trend}} = 0.01$).

DP analysis for AD is an area of intense research at the present time, and is generally considered to be superior to the investigation of individual nutrients. There are still limitations to studying DP in relation to AD and additional research is needed. For AD, there is the problem with reverse causation, where DP are likely to change before dementia is diagnosed. This could be addressed by examining dietary data from early or midlife, but few studies can provide this type of information. Most of the studies to date have used an FFQ administered at one time point, often in populations that are 65 years old and older. Conducting RCTs of DP likely will prove difficult, given the extensive changes that would be required for participants to remain on these diets for a significant length of time. However, the other benefits of diets like the MeDi suggest that conversion to this type of diet is likely to reduce cardiovascular disease and cancer in addition to reducing the risk for AD. Clearly, the earlier this type of diet is adopted, the more likely one is likely to benefit.

Chapter 16

Physical Activity

The Centers for Disease Control in the United States has regularly published guidelines for recommended aerobic and muscle-strengthening activities. The current guidelines recommend 2h and 30min of moderate-intensity aerobic activity, such as brisk walking, or 1h and 15min of vigorous-intensity aerobic activity, such as jogging or running, every week for adults of all ages. In addition, they recommend muscle-strengthening activities on two or more days per week that work all major muscle groups. In 2011, only 21% of Americans met both sets of guidelines (Centers for Disease Control, 2011). This number increased to about 50% for meeting only the aerobic exercise guideline. The strongest predictor of meeting the physical activity guidelines was level of education attained. Sixty-one percent of adults with a college degree met the aerobic exercise guidelines, while only 39% of those with less than high school diploma did. Race and ethnicity also predicted meeting guidelines, with Caucasians more likely to fulfill the guidelines for both forms of exercise than African-Americans or Hispanics. According to the World Health Organization, physical inactivity among adults was highest in the Americas and the Eastern Mediterranean countries and lowest in Southeast Asia (http://www.who.int/dietphysicalactivity/factsheet_inactivity/en/).

METHODS OF ASSESSING PHYSICAL ACTIVITY IN EPIDEMIOLOGIC STUDIES

Epidemiologic studies have ascertained physical activity using a variety of methods including validated questionnaires (Braskie et al., 2014), single or multiple questions (Larson et al., 2006), lists of types of leisure activities engaged in (Verghese et al., 2003), and actigraphy (Buchman et al., 2012). Most attention in the questionnaires has been given to the frequency and duration of activities, usually quantified as times or hours per exercise session or week. Intensity, while occasionally quantified in terms of metabolic equivalents or metabolic equivalent (METs), was usually estimated by the type of activity engaged in or the results of that activity in terms of breathlessness and sweating. Laundry lists of leisure activities have been variable in length, but have generally covered the most common

Alzheimer's Disease. DOI: http://dx.doi.org/10.1016/B978-0-12-804538-1.00016-X

activities engaged in by the populations of interest, who were usually over age 65. Some studies have focused on walking, quantifying the distance walked by the number of city block equivalents (Yaffe, Barnes, Nevitt, Lui, & Covinsky, 2001) or estimated distance walked per day (Abbott et al., 2004).

Because of its multidimensionality, physical activity is difficult to measure accurately. Crude measures can lead to inconsistent findings, and even detailed assessments may not take into account day-to-day and seasonal variability. Given that almost all measures of physical activity are obtained through self-report in epidemiologic studies, limitations of such measures must be considered in interpreting the findings. Two important limitations include social desirability bias, in which over-report of physical exercise can occur, and obtaining information from participants who are close to onset of dementia. With regard to the latter problem, one must be aware of the possibility of reverse causation, where physical exercise is given up as the individual moves toward dementia, as well as problems with recall of physical activities by participants who are beginning to dement that can bias the findings. Because of these measurement problems, it is difficult to compare the strengths of associations across studies. Within studies, if the method is valid, the rank order of exercise participation is likely to reflect the relative level of physical exercise. However, if the physical exercise measure is dependent upon performing one or more activities in a list, the omission of an exercise activity in which the subject participated will lead to an underestimate of that person's exercise activities. Finally, most questionnaires have been developed to assess leisure exercise activities. Other forms of physical exercise, such as those involved in getting to work or in carrying out occupational activities, are usually not considered.

PHYSICAL ACTIVITY AND COGNITIVE PERFORMANCE

The association between physical activity and cognitive performance has been extensively studied in humans in cross-sectional and cohort studies as well as in randomized clinical trials (Blondell, Hammersley-Mather, & Veerman, 2014). The general picture that has emerged is that greater physical activity is associated with less cognitive decline and a reduced risk for dementia (Carvalho, Rea, Parimon, & Cusack, 2014). The magnitude of this effect is evident from cohort studies of dementia. In a meta-analysis of eight large cohort studies assessing physical activity in relation to incident AD, greater physical activity was found to be associated with lower risk for AD [pooled RR = 0.58 (95% CI = 0.49–0.70) with little heterogeneity in findings among studies ($Q = 3.2$, $p = 0.867$)] (Figure 16.1) (Beydoun et al., 2014). Given the pooled relative risk and frequency of high and low physical activity in these studies, the PAF or proportion of dementia cases attributable to lower physical activity was 31.9% (95% CI = 22.7%–41.2%), larger than that for low education (24%) and lower fish consumption (21.9%). These findings suggest that physical exercise, a low-cost intervention with multiple health benefits, could offer a simple and healthful preventive strategy for AD.

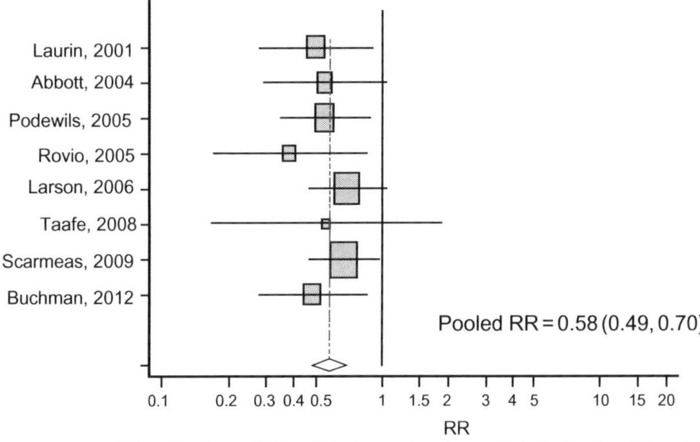

FIGURE 16.1 Pooled meta-analysis of physical activity and incident AD from eight cohort studies. *Reprinted from Beydoun et al. (2014).*

Although the general finding across studies has been that physical exercise is associated with improved cognition and lower risk for dementia, it is important to note that a few epidemiologic studies did not find an association between history of physical exercise and risk of dementia (Morgan et al., 2012; Verghese et al., 2003). It also is possible that because AD pathology is present for years or decades before clinical expression, reverse causation (incipient AD leading to reduction in physical activity) could explain the association in some cohort studies (Abbott et al., 2004; Buchman et al., 2012; Larson et al., 2006; Laurin, Verreault, Lindsay, MacPherson, & Rockwood, 2001; Podewils et al., 2005; Ravaglia et al., 2008; Scarmeas, Luchsinger, et al., 2009; Taaffe et al., 2008) where the mean follow-up period from assessment of physical activity to dementia was less than 10 years.

Because of the possibility of reverse causation, it is of interest to examine the effects of physical exercise in midlife and earlier on the risk of dementia in old age. Using data from a longitudinal study that spanned midlife and old age, Rovio et al. (2005) reported that midlife physical activity had a strong protective effect on dementia over two decades later. Andel et al. (2008) examined the association between level of exercise during midlife in Swedish twins and presence of AD an average of 31 years later. Using a case-control design, they found that twins who regularly exercised in midlife compared to those who did not exercise were significantly less likely to have AD in late life (OR = 0.34, 95% CI = 0.14–0.86). Another study that relied on retrospective reporting of earlier physical activity found a *stronger* association of physical exercise in the teenage years than later in adult life with cognitive impairment in old age (Middleton, Barnes, Lui, & Yaffe, 2010), suggesting that early physical activity may build up a reserve that protects one against cognitive impairment and dementia in later life. In Chapter 23, we return to this intriguing question and consider the possibility of "banking" brain tissue early in life for use as a buffer against dementia in late life.

ANIMAL STUDIES OF PHYSICAL ACTIVITY AND COGNITION

Studies in rodents have demonstrated strong beneficial effects of physical exercise on cognitive tasks dependent on hippocampal function (Berchtold, Castello, & Cotman, 2010). Findings related to physical exercise included enhanced long-term potentiation in the dentate gyrus of the hippocampus (Farmer et al., 2004) and increases in brain-derived neurotrophic factor (BDNF) in this region of the brain (Berchtold, Kesslak, & Cotman, 2002; Farmer et al., 2004; Garza, Ha, Garcia, Chen, & Russo-Neustadt, 2004; Neeper, Gomez-Pinilla, Choi, & Cotman, 1995), which can result in increased neurogenesis (Kim et al., 2004; van Praag, Christie, Sejnowski, & Gage, 1999; van Praag, Shubert, Zhao, & Gage, 2005). In addition, increased levels of dopamine (Poulton & Muir, 2005), acetylcholine (Fordyce & Farrar, 1991), and serotonin (Blomstrand, Perrett, Parry-Billings, & Newsholme, 1989), as well as circulating levels and brain uptake of insulin-like growth factor (Carro, Trejo, Busiguina, & Torres-Aleman, 2001; Trejo, Carro, & Torres-Aleman, 2001), fibroblast growth factor (Gomez-Pinilla, So, & Kesslak, 1998), and vascular endothelial growth factor (Vital et al., 2014) have been observed. Structurally, exercise has been shown to promote both synaptogenesis and angiogenesis (Black, Isaacs, Anderson, Alcantara, & Greenough, 1990).

Human studies have also demonstrated beneficial effects of physical exercise on cognition. For example, a meta-analysis of 29 short-term randomized clinical trial (RCTs) of adults without dementia demonstrated significant benefits of physical exercise interventions on a variety of cognitive outcomes, including memory, attention, and executive function (P. J. Smith et al., 2010).

PHYSICAL FITNESS

Although *physical or aerobic fitness* is a potential measure of the benefits of physical exercise in individuals, its association with cognitive performance is unclear. A meta-analysis of aerobic fitness and cognition failed to show an association between the magnitude of increases in aerobic fitness and size of improvements in cognitive performance in training studies with a pre-post design (Etnier, Nowell, Landers, & Sibley, 2006). In fact, this meta-analysis reported that individuals who had *smaller* gains in fitness showed *greater* improvements in cognitive measures, opposite to what one might expect given the greater improvements in cardiovascular function resulting from more intensive exercise programs. On the other hand, there is abundant evidence that on average more aerobically fit people have better cognitive skills compared with less fit people (Colcombe et al., 2004; Etnier et al., 2006). One of the reasons for the possible discrepancy in these findings relates to an inverse association between exercise intensity and serum levels of BDNF discussed below.

PHYSICAL ACTIVITY AND BRAIN VOLUME

A number of cross-sectional studies have shown that more physically fit older adults with and without AD have larger cortical gray matter volumes (Burns et al., 2008; Colcombe et al., 2003; Honea et al., 2009) as well as greater hippocampal volumes (Erickson et al., 2009). Similar findings have been obtained in middle-aged adults (Boots et al., 2014), where a continuous measure of cardiorespiratory fitness was found to be associated with larger gray matter volumes in the hippocampus, amygdala, precuneus, supramarginal gyrus, and rostral middle frontal gyrus. In addition, this study showed a strong association of greater cardiorespiratory fitness with reductions in white matter lesion burden, consistent with the associations of cardiorespiratory fitness with several indicators of vascular risk, including hypertension, C-reactive protein, and total cholesterol.

Associations between physical exercise and brain volumes are consistent in showing that those who exercise more have larger brain volumes (Erickson, Leckie, & Weinstein, 2014). These findings in cross-sectional studies have been replicated in cohort and case-control studies, establishing temporal relationships between physical exercise and brain volume. For example, Erickson, Raji, et al. (2010) found that increased walking distances per week in older adults were associated with greater gray matter volumes of the frontal, occipital, entorhinal, and hippocampal regions 9 years after this exposure measurement was obtained, after adjusting for age, sex, total intracranial volume, white matter hyperintensity (WMH) grade, MCI, race, and education. In a study of 45 women with a mean age of 75.7, we found that greater minutes of walking per day at age 50 was significantly associated with larger whole brain volumes 25 years later, adjusted for age and fish consumption at age 50 (Mortimer et al., 2013). However, no association was evident between walking at age 50 and WMH volume in the same women. Because brain volume adjusted for intracranial volume indicates how much atrophy has taken place, these findings suggest that atrophy, an important correlate of dementia, can be reduced through physical exercise across the life course. These findings are consistent with effects of lifetime physical exercise on reducing dementia risk.

Finally, randomized clinical trials in older individuals have shown that aerobic exercise training leads to significant increases in brain volumes (Colcombe et al., 2006; Erickson et al., 2011; Ruscheweyh et al., 2011). Increases in hippocampal volume have been shown to be related to increased aerobic fitness as well as higher serum levels of BDNF (Erickson et al., 2011).

MECHANISMS

Physical exercise may be beneficial to cognitive outcomes in two different ways: (1) by reducing the rate of accumulation of Alzheimer and vascular pathology and (2) by increasing the level of neurotrophins in the brain leading to growth of brain tissue and formation of synapses in regions that atrophy in AD.

Effects of Exercise on Reduction of Alzheimer and Vascular Pathology

Alzheimer Pathology

Moderate exercise has long been known to reduce inflammation. While major focus has been placed on the role of chronic moderate level exercise in reducing C-reactive protein, lowering of IL-6 and IL-1β has also been observed (Latta, Brothers, & Wilcock, 2014). The latter effects may be important for Alzheimer's disease, because levels of both IL-6 and IL-1β have been shown to be higher in Alzheimer patients than age-matched controls (Swardfager et al., 2010). For many decades, we have understood that inflammation accompanies Alzheimer pathology, possibly contributing to the acceleration of brain atrophy. In fact, "activated" microglia, the brain's immune cells, were first described by Alois Alzheimer in his original report on Auguste D. as surrounding plaques and tangles (Chapter 1). Neuroinflammation may play a beneficial role early in the disease process through targeting of β-amyloid from the brain and a harmful role later as neurofibrillary tangles develop and atrophy accelerates (Latta et al., 2014). It is unclear at present whether Alzheimer pathology leads to inflammation, inflammation causes increases in Alzheimer pathology, or the association between these processes is bidirectional. If inflammation increases the amount of Alzheimer pathology, then moderate exercise might be expected to reduce the severity of Alzheimer lesions. If inflammation leads to the accelerated removal of β-amyloid from the brain, the opposite association might be present.

Findings from animal studies have shown variable effects of physical exercise on Alzheimer lesions. Voluntary exercise has been shown to significantly decrease β-amyloid load in transgenic mouse models of AD (Adlard, Perreau, Pop, & Cotman, 2005; Lazarov et al., 2005), consistent with accelerated removal and degradation of this protein in exercising animals. Transgenic mice exposed to 5 months of voluntary physical exercise beginning at age 1 month or less showed decreases in amyloid plaque counts in the hippocampus and cortex (Adlard et al., 2005). In the second study, 1-month old mice were randomized to enriched versus standard environments for 5 months. Those in the enriched group showed reduced brain amyloid. Other studies failed to find any effect of aerobic exercise in amyloid precursor protein (APP) transgenic mice on levels of β-amyloid in the brain (Xu et al., 2013) or tau pathology (Marlatt, Potter, Bayer, van Praag, & Lucassen, 2013). An important difference between positive and null studies was that in positive studies the exercise intervention was begun at a much earlier age, suggesting that timing of physical exercise could be an important predictor of reduction in Alzheimer neuropathology in the transgenic mice. In a particularly interesting study, exercise in pregnant mothers of transgenic mice was found to be associated with reduced amyloid deposition in their nonexercised offspring (Herring et al., 2012), consistent with exercise effects on Alzheimer pathology occurring even before birth. These findings are consistent with human studies that suggest that exercise earlier in life may be more effective in preventing Alzheimer's disease than exercise later in life.

One study (Liang et al., 2010) assessed the level of cerebrospinal fluid (CSF) and positron emission tomography (PET) biomarkers for AD in relation to exercise during the previous 10 years in cognitively normal people. Nonsignificant trends for lower Alzheimer biomarkers with higher exercise levels were seen, but the causal direction (preclinical AD leads to lower exercise vs more exercise leads to lower biomarker levels) could not be determined. A subsequent study by the same investigators (Head et al., 2012) showed that exercise significantly reduced levels of AD neuropathologic markers, but only in individuals carrying one or more Apolipoprotein E (APOE)-ε4 alleles.

Vascular Brain Pathology

As we noted in Chapter 14, the prevalence of dementia among individuals with AD pathology is strongly influenced by cerebrovascular lesions. Lifelong physical exercise, particularly vigorous exercise in early adulthood, is an important preventive risk factor for stroke (Paganini-Hill & Perez Barreto, 2001; Shinton & Sagar, 1993). In nondemented elderly, WMHs are associated with a variety of risk factors for vascular disease, including hypertension as well as high levels of glycated hemoglobin and cholesterol. Middle-aged adults with greater cardiovascular fitness have been found to have fewer WMH (Boots et al., 2014), indicative of less vascular damage at this stage of life. Although the precise mechanisms by which physical exercise reduce the risk for AD through modulation of cerebrovascular function are unknown, likely possibilities include reduction of WMHs, lacunar infarctions, and cerebral microhemorrhages, all known risk factors for dementia (Viswanathan, Rocca, & Tzourio, 2009).

EFFECTS OF EXERCISE ON NEUROTROPHINS

Brain-Derived Neurotrophic Factor

Among neurotrophins, BDNF has been most well-studied in relation to exercise. Numerous animal studies have shown an increase in brain BDNF release and expression with physical exercise (Ahlskog, Geda, Graff-Radford, & Petersen, 2011). Because BDNF is rapidly transported across the blood brain barrier in both directions (Pan, Banks, Fasold, Bluth, & Kastin, 1998), serum levels can be used to judge brain concentrations. The absence of a consistent association between fitness, *chronic* aerobic exercise and BDNF concentrations in humans

(Baker et al., 2010; Currie, Ramsbottom, Ludlow, Nevill, & Gilder, 2009; Goekint et al., 2010; Nofuji et al., 2008; Rasmussen et al., 2009; Schiffer, Schulte, Hollmann, Bloch, & Struder, 2009) suggests that *long-term* aerobic exercise interventions may not be effective in increasing BDNF. An alternative explanation is that some of the positive associations observed may be the result of concomitant mental stimulation independent of physical exercise. A recent RCT in which seniors were randomly assigned to a pure physical exercise (cycling) and a combined mental and physical exercise (cycling combined with decision-making using a virtual reality display) showed that the increase in BDNF levels over the course of the intervention was almost five times greater in the group with combined mental and physical exercise than it was in the group with physical exercise alone ($p<0.05$) (Anderson-Hanley et al., 2012). Both groups expended the same amount of energy, providing a control for the effect of aerobic exercise on BDNF. Although the mechanism behind this finding is unknown, it suggests that mental stimulation can have important modulatory effects on growth factors related to aerobic physical exercise.

BDNF is highly concentrated in the hippocampus (Murer, Yan, & Raisman-Vozari, 2001), where it is thought to contribute to neurogenesis in the dentate gyrus (Benraiss, Chmielnicki, Lerner, Roh, & Goldman, 2001). Studies of aging humans show that lower serum concentrations of BDNF mediate age-related decline in hippocampal volume (Erickson, Prakash, et al., 2010) consistent with findings from adult primates where increased production of BDNF reverses neuronal atrophy in this region (Nagahara et al., 2009).

BDNF Polymorphism

Because of the role of BDNF in growing brain tissue in the hippocampus, there has been considerable interest in BDNF genetic polymorphisms as risk factors for AD and as effect-modifiers of the association between physical activity and brain growth. The most well-studied of these polymorphisms is the single nucleotide polymorphism at nucleotide 196, commonly referred to as Val66Met (rs6265), which results in an amino acid substitution of valine (VAL) to methionine (MET). The human genotype for BDNF can be homozygous for VAL at this locus (VAL,VAL); homozygous for MET (MET, MET) or heterozygous (VAL, MET). In US populations, around 80% of the population are VAL homozygotes, while in Asia, this percentage is much lower (approximately 33%) (Shimizu, Hashimoto, & Iyo, 2004). Because there are considerable data suggesting that older MET carriers have smaller hippocampi (Hajek, Kopecek, & Hoschl, 2012), there could be important ethnic differences in brain growth potential, which might influence the risk for AD. It is important to note that while the pooled difference in mean hippocampal volumes was highly significant between MET carriers and VAL homozygotes in a meta-analysis of seven studies including 399 subjects, 36% of whom were MET carriers (Hajek et al., 2012), the size of the effect was relatively modest, with only a 0.4 standard deviation difference in mean volumes between MET carriers and VAL homozygotes. An effect of this size corresponds to a reduction of hippocampal volume seen with an increase in a single Braak stage at death, for example, III-IV or IV-V (Gosche, Mortimer, Smith, Markesbery, & Snowdon, 2001). As such, it has the potential to contribute to increased memory impairment and risk for AD.

The role of this polymorphism in the causation of Alzheimer's disease and cognitive impairment has been the subject of extensive debate. Most studies have not shown an increased risk for dementia with possession of one or more MET alleles. However, in nondemented older subjects at risk for AD by virtue of carrying an APOE-ε4 allele (Lim, Villemagne, Laws, Pietrzak, et al., 2014; Ward et al., 2014) or having an elevated level of β-amyloid on PET scans (Lim, Villemagne, Laws, Ames, et al., 2014), possession of one or more MET alleles was associated with reduced hippocampal volume (Lim, Villemagne, Laws, Ames, et al., 2014) and a more rapid decline in episodic memory (Lim, Villemagne, Laws, Ames, et al., 2014; Lim, Villemagne, Laws, Pietrzak, et al., 2014; Ward et al., 2014). The BDNF Val66Met polymorphism has been shown not to be related to the severity of AD pathology on PET scans (Lim et al., 2013) and therefore is unlikely to influence the rate of accumulation of aggregated β-amyloid. This polymorphism appears to have a major effect on synaptic growth in the hippocampus in response to activation (Egan et al., 2003). While the VAL form of BDNF colocalizes with synaptic proteins, the MET form aggregates mainly in the cell body instead of the dendrites, where it would have little effect on the long-term potentiation and the laying down of new memories during the life course.

Two studies have considered the role of the Val66Met polymorphism in modifying the effects of exercise on cognitive function and brain volumes. Kim et al. (2011) studied the incidence of dementia with respect to intensity of physical activity at baseline and the Val66Met polymorphism. Although lower baseline physical activity was associated with greater incidence of dementia, the Val66Met was not significantly associated with this outcome. However, the strength of association between lower physical activity and incident dementia increased with the number of MET alleles. Closer inspection of the findings demonstrated no difference in incidence risk between MET carriers and VAL-VAL homozygotes among individuals with high to moderate physical activity at baseline, but a marked increase in risk in MET carriers who did not exercise (nonexerciser incidence for MET-MET = 40% vs MET-VAL = 18% vs VAL-VAL = 0%). A similar finding was obtained for working memory performance among 1,032 participants in the University of Pittsburgh Adult Health and Behavior Project (Erickson et al., 2013), who were an average of 44.6 years old at the time of testing. Again, differences between MET carriers and VAL-VAL homozygotes were most apparent in those who exercised least, with little difference among those who exercised vigorously and regularly. Greater amounts of physical activity mitigated poorer working memory performance in MET carriers, but had minimal effects on working memory function in VAL homozygotes.

Given the strong interaction of the APOE and BDNF polymorphisms in cognitive decline, these findings would suggest that individuals who carry an APOE-ε4 allele and are MET carriers for BDNF would benefit from regular physical exercise across the lifespan. Because moderate exercise is beneficial for the cardiovascular system, VAL-VAL homozygotes who carry an ε4 allele might show some benefit as well.

INTENSITY AND DURATION VERSUS VARIETY OF EXERCISE

Strenuous running in rodents, which is associated with substantial improvements in aerobic fitness, has been found to be associated with *decreases* rather than increases in BDNF (Soya et al., 2007). Similarly, comparison of young men who participated in vigorous training in single sports with nonexercisers the same age showed *lower* mean levels of serum BDNF in the chronic exercisers (Nofuji et al., 2008). Moreover, an inverse correlation ($r = 0.51$, $p < 0.05$) was observed between the intensity of the exercise and the level of serum BDNF in this study. These findings suggest that growth in brain volume may not be simply related to the intensity of physical exercise and level of aerobic fitness attained. Although short episodes of high-intensity aerobic exercise lead to transient increases in serum BDNF, resting levels of this neurotrophic factor are *inversely* related to the level of aerobic fitness and higher levels of habitual physical activity, those with higher aerobic fitness having *lower* resting levels of BDNF (Currie et al., 2009). This finding may be related to the modification of the association of physical exercise at baseline with incident dementia seen in the ACT Study (Larson et al., 2006). A greater risk reduction of dementia by physical exercise was seen in participants who were less fit at baseline. By contrast, in individuals who had high levels of physical performance at baseline, greater exercise had little effect on their later dementia risk.

An alternative explanation for the growth of brain with exercise is that it is not the intensity, but rather the *variety* of exercise that is responsible. Such a finding was obtained in the CHS, in which the number of different physical exercise activities was associated with lower future risk of dementia (HR = 0.51, 95% CI = 0.33–0.79 for participation in four or more activities vs one or fewer, $p_{\text{for trend}} = 0.004$), but the intensity of physical exercise was not (HR = 0.85, 95% CI = 0.61–1.19 for the highest quartile of physical energy expenditure vs the lowest quartile, $p_{\text{for trend}} = 0.11$) (Podewils et al., 2005). Many brain exercise programs stress novelty and challenge, for example, using the left hand to perform a normally right-handed task. Such tasks as well as novel physical exercise programs that provide continuing cognitive as well as physical challenges may be more effective in stimulating the release of BDNF and other neurotrophins. In the RCT that we conducted in Shanghai, China comparing T'ai Chi with fast walking, significant increases in brain volume were seen with T'ai Chi (+0.47%, $p < 0.05$), but not with walking (–0.15%, not significance (NS))

(Mortimer et al., 2012). The walking activity consisted of three times per week walking around a fixed course and offered little challenge to participants, who complained that the activity was boring. By contrast, participants in the T'ai Chi intervention continually learned and practiced new sequences of movement and posture.

Because the release of growth factors is a dynamic process related to apparent need, a certain amount of stress is likely to be beneficial. This concept, which we have already discussed, is referred to as hormesis, a condition in which responses to low exposures to toxins and other stressors result in more favorable outcomes through activation of enzymatic pathways to deal with these types of exposures. For example, in aging, stressors such as food restriction and exposure to certain spices such as curcumin at moderate levels have been shown to prevent disease and extend life. These findings suggest that *frequent changes in physical exercise programs, such as cross-training, may be more beneficial in growing brain than developing a high level of aerobic fitness through a single form of exercise*. Although this may be true from the viewpoint of induction of brain growth factors, the other benefits of aerobic fitness on the vascular system and Type 2 diabetes cannot be overlooked. It is likely that an optimal exercise program from brain health will include both variety and aerobic fitness.

THE ROLE OF EXERCISE IN THE PREVENTION OF AD—AN UPDATE

A National Institutes of Health State-of-the-Science Statement published in 2010 concluded that the quality of evidence for an association of physical activity with a reduced risk of AD was low (Williams et al., 2010). In a review of the literature cited in the accompanying document, the authors used nine cohort studies to examine the association between baseline physical exercise measures and risk for incident AD. Hazard ratios from some of the individual studies used in this analysis, particularly those showing a higher risk of AD with more exercise, were not based on adequate measures of physical activity at baseline. One example of this problem is the study of Ravaglia et al. (2008), where the estimate selected was kilocalories expended per week walking (HR = 1.42, 95% CI = 0.68–2.97) versus total kilocalories expended in all activities per week (HR = 0.70, 95% CI = 0.33–1.49). Use of the less robust exposure estimate from this study biased the pooled HR toward 1.0 and substantially increased measures of heterogeneity. A second study did not assess intensity of physical exercise at all, but simply added the time spent per day on three activities with some, but likely very limited physical effort [doing odds jobs, taking a walk (length not specified) and gardening] (Akbaraly et al., 2009). The HR for AD associated with this exposure was 1.29. If this study, based on questionable exposure measurement were eliminated from the analysis, the pooled estimate for physical exercise would have been more protective and heterogeneity decreased further.

The meta-analysis shown in Figure 16.1 contained many of the same studies as those in the meta-analysis conducted in preparation for the NIH statement, but did not include studies in which the exposure was measured inappropriately.

The authors of the NIH statement based their conclusion that the quality of evidence for an association of physical activity with a reduced risk of AD was low primarily on the basis of the type of study. Observational studies were assigned a low rating, randomized controlled trials a high rating. As discussed in this chapter, the effects of physical exercise on AD likely spans many decades. Randomized trials of this duration are impractical, making reliance on observational studies necessary. It is important to note that randomized trials in nondemented adults have demonstrated effects of physical exercise on both memory as well as whole brain and hippocampal volumes in individuals at risk for dementia, consistent with the reduction in AD risk with greater physical activity seen in observational studies. Furthermore, plausible mechanisms, such as increased secretion of BDNF and other growth factors and in some instances reduction in Aβ accumulation, have been shown to occur in both humans and animals following physical exercise, providing support for exercise per se rather than other elements of a healthy lifestyle as the likely cause of reduction in risk of AD and dementia. Given the low risk of physical exercise, presently available data support its use in maintaining critical brain tissue and reducing the risk of dementia.

Chapter 17

Cognitive Activity

Epidemiologic studies of the association of mental exercise and intellectual ability with risk for Alzheimer's disease (AD) have either used proxies of measurements, such as attained education, IQ, or occupational complexity, or have employed questionnaires asking to what extent people participated in several different activities with varying amounts of cognitive demand. Unlike physical activity where the degree of aerobic or strength demands can be quantified using standardized scales, mental exercise is more difficult to quantify. To what extent does 2h of reading equate to a defined amount of mental activity? It probably depends on what is being read and the degree to which the reader is actively intellectually engaged in the activity. Given that mental exercise is often quantified by adding together durations of several different types of activities, each of which provides unknown levels of intellectual involvement, the indices obtained are unlikely to be as valid as a measure of the number of blocks walked per week is for physical exercise, for example. Although large differences in intellectual activity estimated from participation in a list of activities likely are important for separating those with active intellectual lives from those with little intellectual stimulation, small differences are likely to have less validity.

The use of randomized controlled trials (RCTs) in which individuals are trained to perform specific cognitive tasks is clearly more valid than recall of participation in intellectually stimulating activities, but provides only a limited snapshot of the potential changes in cognitive function that could occur over a lifetime and does not address the association of cognitive training or exercise with the incidence of dementia or minor cognitive impairment (MCI).

In this chapter, we will consider cohort and case–control designs first, followed by a review of randomized trials of mental exercise. We will then review the mechanisms through which cognitive stimulation can produce beneficial effects. As with physical exercise, RCTs have utilized measures of change in both the physical structure of and connections within the brain as outcomes.

Alzheimer's Disease. DOI: http://dx.doi.org/10.1016/B978-0-12-804538-1.00017-1

COHORT AND CASE–CONTROL STUDIES

Education

In Chapter 11, we reviewed the role of education and IQ in predicting the risk of incident AD and dementia. Higher education and IQ had strong inverse associations with incident dementia in a large number of studies. Given that higher education is frequently associated with more cognitively challenging occupations and that higher educated individuals are more likely to have lifestyles in which intellectual activity plays a more important role, education is likely to be a reasonable surrogate, albeit indirect, for an adult lifetime of mental exercise. Whereas physical fitness is related to both cognitive outcomes and regional or total brain volumes, IQ and global measures of cognitive ability may play a similar role with mental exercise.

Occupation

Up to this point, we have not reviewed the association of cognitively stimulating or challenging occupations with risk for AD. The earliest study to examine occupation was that of Stern et al. (1994). Stratifying occupations into high (manager, professional, or technical) and low (unskilled/semiskilled, skilled, or clerical) attainment, they reported a higher risk for incident AD among those with low occupational attainment adjusting for age (RR = 2.25, 95% CI = 1.32–3.84). Later studies showed trends in the same direction, but often the risk estimates were not significant (Helmer, Joly, Letenneur, Commenges, & Dartigues, 2001; Scarmeas, Levy, Tang, Manly, & Stern, 2001). Although occupational attainment is likely to reflect the amount of intellectual involvement, better measures of the latter have been developed. Smyth et al. (2004), using a factor analysis of measures developed by the US Department of Labor identified one factor related to mental occupational demand. In a case–control study, they found that occupations held by future AD cases had significantly lower levels of mental demands in comparison with those of controls, adjusting for race, sex, year of birth, and education. Andel et al. (2005) using the population-based study of Swedish Twins examined complexity of occupation with regard to people, data, or things. They reported that greater complexity of work with people (OR = 0.80, 95% CI = 0.68–0.93), but not with data (OR = 0.94, 95% CI = 0.85–1.05) or things (OR = 1.06, 95% CI 0.98–1.15), was associated with decreased risk for AD. A subsequent study using incidence data from the CSHA (Kroger et al., 2008) found that increased complexity of work with people (HR = 0.66, 95% CI = 0.44–0.98) and things (HR = 0.72, 95% CI = 0.52–0.99), but not with data (HR = 1.14, 95% CI = 0.79–1.64) was associated with decreased incidence for dementia. The findings were particularly strong for occupations held for long periods of time. Finally, using incident dementia as the outcome, Karp et al. (2009) reported that the risk for dementia among participants in the Kungsholmen Study was lower in those who had occupations with higher complexity of work with people

(HR = 0.88, 95% CI = 0.80–0.97) and data (HR = 0.85, 95% CI = 0.77–0.95). Although not entirely consistent, these studies suggest that more complex work, especially that involving people, is associated with lower risk for dementia. The interpretations of these findings are facilitated by examining outcomes related to decline in cognitive abilities with aging. Jonaitis et al. (2013) reported that greater complexity of work with data was associated with reduced loss of speed and flexibility, but not with change in memory-related functions, in a middle-aged sample of nondemented adults at risk for AD.

Cognitive Activities

A number of cohort studies have utilized questionnaires to obtain measures of leisure-related cognitive activities, particularly those that were thought to be intellectually stimulating or cognitively demanding. These studies have shown that nondemented older adults who became demented within 5 years participated less in cognitively stimulating activities at baseline than those who did not become demented within this time span (Akbaraly et al., 2009; Pillai et al., 2011; Verghese et al., 2003; Wilson, Bennett, et al., 2002; Wilson, Mendes De Leon, et al., 2002). Because intellectually demanding activities are very likely to be given up during the preclinical period of AD, significant associations of cognitive activities in the 10-year period before diagnosis may well reflect reverse associations, where impending dementia leads to reduction of intellectual activity. For example, Hall et al. (2009) followed 488 cognitively intact individuals in the Bronx Aging Study for up to 15 years, 101 of whom became demented. Among the latter, the median time from baseline to dementia was 4.4 years. Change point analysis revealed that among those reporting more cognitive activities at baseline, memory performance began to decline more quickly around 5 years *prior* to dementia diagnosis compared to 2 years among those reporting less cognitive ability at baseline. Given the proximity of the cognitive activity assessment to the onset of dementia, the simplest explanation that can be given to these findings is that individuals begin to give up cognitive activities at about the same time they begin to decline, consistent with an inverse association in which impending dementia leads to reduced cognitive activities.

A better assessment of the possible role of cognitive activity in preventing or delaying onset of dementia is provided by studies in which information about cognitive activities in childhood, young adulthood and middle age was obtained among cohort participants followed for development of dementia. The first study to obtain data on intellectual activity in early adulthood (20s and 30s) and middle age (40s and 50s) in relation to risk for AD in late life employed a case–control design in which information was obtained from surrogates for cases and from controls themselves (Friedland et al., 2001). Controls were friends or neighbors of the cases or participants in organizations to which the cases belonged. The researchers reported that controls participated in intellectual activities a significantly higher total hours per month than cases in both early adulthood and midlife, with ORs ranging from 2.65 to 5.58 and *p*-values <0.001. One limitation of this study is that proxy respondents for cases only had to have known the case for 10 years to qualify. It is not clear how many of these respondents would have had difficulty in reporting on case intellectual activities up to 60 years prior to the time of the interview. Lack of familiarity with the case's behavior earlier in life could have led to underreporting of case intellectual activity. This explanation is supported by a substudy that was carried out in which intellectual intensity measures were administered to 49 controls and 49 people they indicated were "well-acquainted with their past and present activities." Only 59% of the proxy respondents specifically selected because they were well acquainted with the past and present activities of the controls were able to complete the questionnaire regarding intellectual activities in early-life and 78% for intellectual activities in midlife.

In the Rush MAP (Wilson, Scherr, Schneider, Tang, & Bennett, 2007), investigators queried 775 well-educated nondemented participants with a mean age of 80.4 years at baseline about their cognitive activity at five different ages during their lifetimes (age 6, 12, 18, 40, and current) using a structured questionnaire that rated activity frequency or presence of the activity at specific ages. Adjusting for baseline age, sex, and education, a lower risk for incident AD during 5 years of follow-up was associated with higher values on a cognitive activity measure reflecting recalled cognitive activities at 40 years of age or less (RR = 0.56, 95% CI = 0.36–0.88). It is important to recognize that detailed information about past cognitive activities (including those at age 6) were obtained from participants who would become demented within 5 years as well as for those who would remain nondemented. Given the fact that individuals who would become demented are likely to recall details about their past lives less well, it is entirely possible that they would underreport the frequency of presence of cognitive activities in early-life in comparison with those who would remain nondemented. This would produce an apparent protective effect of such activities in those who did not become demented.

To control for possible recall bias, studies in which cognitive activities were documented much earlier in life and individuals followed for dementia incidence decades later would be preferred. Very few studies have collected data on cognitive activities prospectively two or more decades before the onset of dementia. Crowe, Andel, Pedersen, Johansson, and Gatz (2003) examined participation in "intellectual-cultural" leisure activities among Swedish twins in relation to their risk for AD. Exposure data were acquired from a questionnaire administered in 1967 and dementia outcomes were determined between 1987 and 1991. One hundred and seven same-sex twin pairs were identified where one twin had AD and the other did not. Adjusting for education, twins with AD were less likely to have reported participation in intellectual activities 20 years earlier (OR = 0.55, 95% CI = 0.28–1.08), with a significant difference apparent in female twin pairs (OR = 0.42, 95% CI = 0.18–1.00). Al-Najjar et al. (2015) reported that greater participation in total cognitive activity during midlife was associated with a reduced risk of AD (HR = 0.42, 95% CI = 0.25–0.73) an average of 38 years later when the female study participants were 70–84 years old.

COGNITIVE TRAINING AND COGNITIVE STIMULATION IN HEALTHY OLDER ADULTS

A number of studies have examined the effect of cognitive training or stimulation on memory as well as other cognitive domains in older adults with normal cognition. These studies have generally reported improvement in the *trained domain*, but for the most part have failed to demonstrate generalization to other cognitive domains or to everyday functioning. Because of cost, most of these studies are small and of relatively short duration, limiting their power to show differences. In addition, because of their relatively brief duration, none of the intervention studies was able to assess differences in clinical outcomes, such as MCI and dementia. However, improvements in cognitive performance could contribute to cognitive reserve, possibly delaying the onset of dementia. Systematic reviews and meta-analyses of intervention studies (Martin, Clare, Altgassen, Cameron, & Zehnder, 2011; Papp, Walsh, & Snyder, 2009; Reijnders, van Heugten, & van Boxtel, 2013; Tardif & Simard, 2011) showed modest improvements in memory, executive function, processing speed, and attention. The quality of studies varied widely with few employing an active control group, raising the possibility that some of the improvements seen could be attributed to nonspecific improvements related to increased attention.

The largest intervention study to date is the ACTIVE trial (Ball et al., 2002), in which 2,832 volunteers aged 65–94 years with normal cognition were randomized to four groups: a memory training group, a reasoning training group, a speed of processing training group, and a no-contact control group. Training consisted of 10 sessions over 6 weeks. Sixty percent of the participants received booster training 11 months after the first 6-week training period. Immediately after training and after 1- and 2-year follow-ups, significant improvements were found in the trained domain. However, the untrained domains did not show any change. No effect was found on everyday problem-solving or instrumental activities of daily functioning (IADL). A 5-year follow-up of the participants (Willis et al., 2006) continued to show improvements in performance only in the trained domains. *Self-reported* improved performance on IADLs was seen in one of the three training groups, but no alteration was apparent on *performance-based* IADL measures. Finally, a 10-year follow-up (Rebok et al., 2014) demonstrated persistence of relative improvements in the specific areas trained. Again, *self-reported* performance on instrumental activities was seen in all three training groups in comparison to the no-contact control group. However, no differences were seen when performance-based IADL measures were evaluated.

Participants in a novel brain plasticity-based computerized cognitive training program (Brain Fitness Program, Posit Science) included 487 cognitively normal seniors randomized to receive a computerized cognitive training program or a novelty- and intensity-matched general cognitive stimulation program for 1 h per day, 5 days a week, for 8 weeks (Smith et al., 2009). At the end of the trial, those in the brain fitness program showed significantly greater improvement on auditory memory and attention in comparison with the active control group. Although the authors suggest that performance improvements generalized to untrained standardized measures of memory and attention, the training program involved auditory memory and attention, and the tests that showed improvement were administered orally requiring similar skills to those that were trained.

Generalization to multiple areas of cognition and function from training in a single domain has been characterized as near transfer (improvements in cognitive tests closely related to the training task) and far transfer (improvements in tests not closely related to the training task). Ideally, cognitive training should lead to far transfer. However, with few exceptions, only near transfer has been demonstrated. In those studies claiming far transfer (Jaeggi, Buschkuehl, Jonides, & Perrig, 2008; Smith et al., 2009), the training tasks usually share much with the tests that are used to assess improvement. Data from 5- and 10-year follow-ups of the ACTIVE cohort are consistent with the authors' conclusions that "a main lesson of the ACTIVE study and other cognitive intervention trials is that *the benefits of cognitive training are specific to the cognitive ability trained*" (Rebok et al., 2014).

It is of interest to compare cognitive training with aerobic physical exercise. In contrast to cognitive training, aerobic exercise appears to have a more global impact on cognitive performance. As we shall see below, this is reflected in imaging studies where physical exercise has a more global influence on brain growth than cognitive training, which appears to impact only the growth of brain regions closely related to the tasks being trained.

Whether longer durations or more intense cognitive training would result in larger or more persistent gains of function that have been documented in the ACTIVE study is unclear. In one of the few studies in which this has been examined, longer training appeared to increase performance (Jaeggi, Buschkuehl, Jonides, & Perrig, 2008), but it is unclear whether longer or more intense training leads to greater *persistence* of improved function.

COGNITIVE ACTIVITY AND CHANGES IN BRAIN VOLUME

While cognitive training has been shown to lead to improved performance on specific cognitive activities, imaging studies have provided important information regarding the mechanisms through which this occur. Structural MRI scans provide clear evidence of brain plasticity in relation to learning new skills. Because they are not affected by day-to-day fluctuations in attention and motivation, they offer much more sensitive, objective, and reliable measures of change in brain function than cognitive outcomes.

In the seminal study in this area, Maguire et al. (2000) reported that London taxi drivers had significantly larger posterior hippocampal gray matter volumes in comparison to a group of sex- and age-matched males who did not drive taxis. In addition, the length of time driving a taxi was positively correlated with the volume of the right posterior hippocampus. Importantly, no other region of the brain showed increases in volume, consistent with functional neuroimaging studies demonstrating the importance of the posterior human hippocampus to spatial memory and navigation (Maguire, Burgess, & O'Keefe, 1999). This association was later confirmed by a longitudinal study of 79 individuals training over 3 years to become licensed London taxi drivers (Woollett & Maguire, 2011). At baseline, no differences in posterior hippocampal volume were evident between trainees and a group of men of similar age and education. After 3 years of training, significant and highly selective increases in gray matter in the posterior hippocampus were seen in trainees who qualified as London taxi drivers, but not in those who failed to qualify or in the group of controls. Because posterior hippocampal size among those who qualified did not differ from those who failed to qualify at the time of enrollment in the study, the findings could not be explained by differences in the volume of this part of the brain at baseline.

Studies by the same research group also have documented *decreases* in anterior hippocampal brain volume paralleling the increases in posterior brain volume in taxi drivers (Woollett & Maguire, 2011). In addition, tests that rely on anterior hippocampal brain volume, such as learning new associations concerning the spatial location of objects, were performed less well by taxi drivers after training. The growth of one part of the hippocampus *at the expense of another* suggests that specific cognitive training may produce both benefits and deficits in neuropsychological performance. This potential trade-off must be taken into account in cognitive interventions to prevent or delay Alzheimer symptoms.

Several other studies have focused on both gray and white matter increases through training of specific skills. Draganski et al. (2004) showed that learning juggling was associated with increases in gray matter volume in areas that govern visual motion processing, while Bezzola, Merillat, Gaser, and Jancke (2011) reported that 40h of golf practice in novices resulted in gray matter volume increases in task-relevant regions of the brain. Other studies have shown modifications of white matter integrity with training, consistent with increased myelination (Engvig et al., 2012). Another study by Draganski et al. (2006) of 38 medical students showed an increase in gray matter volume in the posterior and lateral parietal cortex as well as an increase in the volume of the posterior hippocampus, particularly on the right side, for 3 months while they were studying for an examination. Of interest, the volume increases were maintained in the cortex, but continued to increase in the posterior hippocampus for 3 months following the exam. It is tempting to suggest that the longer duration increase in posterior hippocampal volume in comparison with the parietal cortex was associated with neurogenesis in the hippocampus (Eriksson et al., 1998) versus synaptogenesis in the parietal cortex, consistent with the growth of new neurons in the hippocampus that can take several months in comparison to a rapid increase in synaptogenesis that is evident almost immediately (Zhao, Teng, Summers, Ming, & Gage, 2006).

Studies of older adults have largely confirmed those in younger people, demonstrating that brain plasticity is maintained with aging during skill acquisition (Valkanova, Eguia Rodriguez, & Ebmeier, 2014). Similar to younger adults, increases in hippocampal volume were maintained for 4 months after the end of training in one study (Lovden et al., 2012), while those involving growth in cortical regions were lost over a 3-month period following termination of training in another (Boyke, Driemeyer, Gaser, Buchel, & May, 2008).

MECHANISMS

Human studies are limited in the degree to which they can establish mechanisms for brain growth and improved cognition after cognitive training. Much of the information we have comes from studies of transgenic mice with increased expression of brain amyloid and tau.

Reduction in β-Amyloid and Tau

Combined amyloid and tau transgenic mice improved their performance in learning after water-maze spatial training and also showed reductions in both amyloid beta and tau neuropathology (Billings, Green, McGaugh, & LaFerla, 2007). While the effects were transient, reductions in amyloid-β oligomers and plaque formation were evident. In another experiment, transgenic mice in enriched versus standard environments showed a reduction of amyloid deposition, but this reduction appeared to be related to time spent running, a physical activity (Lazarov et al., 2005). Cracchiolo et al. (2007) studied transgenic Alzheimer mice raised in four environments (impoverished, social, social + physical, complete enrichment) and found reduced β-amyloid deposition only among those raised in the complete enrichment environment. They argued that the addition of novel cognitive stimulation was necessary to produce increased synaptogenesis and reductions in β-amyloid deposition in the hippocampus and entorhinal cortex. Because environmental enrichment does not influence brain amyloid precursor protein levels in the brain (Lazarov et al., 2005), it is likely that increased stimulation led to either increased sequestration of amyloid-β or its accelerated removal from the brain (Cracchiolo et al., 2007). Finally, a recent study (Mainardi et al., 2014) showed that environmental enrichment may act by reducing Aβ oligomers and increased synthesis of the Aβ-degrading enzyme neprilysin. The difficulty in separating cognitive from physical activity in environmental enrichment leaves open the question of whether it is increased physical activity, increased mental activity or a combination of the two that is responsible for reducing Aβ oligomers and Aβ deposition in rodent models. Other recent animal studies (Bo et al., 2014; Liu, Zhao, Zhang, & Shi, 2013; Yu, Xu, Song, Ji, & Zhang, 2013) suggest that treadmill exercise without additional cognitive or social stimulation may be sufficient to lower β-amyloid expression when it is prolonged and repeated over several weeks, suggesting that physical exercise when it is more intense may be sufficient to reduce Aβ.

In a human study, Landau et al. (2012) studied the association between retrospectively-determined cognitive engagement using a 25-item questionnaire and β-amyloid deposition in 65 healthy older adults with a mean age of 76. They found that individuals who reported greater early- and middle-life cognitive activity had lower amyloid uptake on PiB, suggesting that cognitive activities earlier in life may be associated with slower deposition of β-amyloid. In another study of 118 normal individuals with a mean age of 76, Wirth, Villeneuve, La Joie, Marks, and Jagust (2014) reported that higher lifetime cognitive activity was associated with a significant reduction in PiB PET β-amyloid deposition in APOE-ε4 carriers. The animal studies cited above are consistent with the effect of cognitive/environmental stimulation in the reduction of β-amyloid load as well as soluble β-amyloid oligomers that are the precursors of aggregated beta seen on PET scans. It is likely that this effect occurs through accelerated removal of β-amyloid, since it has been shown in animal studies that increased synaptic and neuronal activity results in increased production of β-amyloid, not its reduction (Jagust & Mormino, 2011).

Increased Brain-Derived Neurotrophic Factor

The association of increased secretion of brain-derived neurotrophic factor (BDNF) with cognitive stimulation is probably best illustrated by the RCT we discussed earlier in which individuals who cycled with virtual reality tours (cyber-cyling) experienced greater cognitive benefits and significantly higher increase in plasma BDNF compared to those without virtual reality who had similar amounts of physical activity (Anderson-Hanley et al., 2012). One explanation for this finding was the additional mental exercise required in the cybercyling group as compared to the regular cycling group. It is important to note that in this study, only executive function was improved by the cybercyling intervention. No changes were seen in verbal and visuospatial memory, figure copying, verbal fluency, or psychomotor speed. The addition of the requirement of navigating a 3D landscape, anticipating turns and making decisions to the physical activity of cycling depends on executive function. The findings of this study are consistent with the benefits of training being specific to the cognitive ability trained.

ARE PHYSICAL AND MENTAL EXERCISE SYNERGISTIC?

Physical as well as mental exercise have been shown to result in brain growth in MRI structural imaging studies. The difference between these two types of exercise appears to be in the specificity of the brain region affected by the activity. Aerobic exercise has been found to lead to increases in the volumes of numerous regions of the brain, including the hippocampus (Erickson et al.,

2011; Pajonk et al., 2010), cingulate gyrus, middle frontal gyrus, superior temporal lobe, and anterior white matter tracts (Colcombe et al., 2006; Floel et al., 2010) as well as in total brain volume (Braskie et al., 2014). These brain regions do not represent activity-related associations with the demands of the exercise. For example, there is little memory demand in most aerobic exercise programs; however, the hippocampus grows substantially in volume. Conversely, mental exercise has repeatedly been shown to lead to growth of brain tissue very specific to the activity being trained.

The specificity of growth in mental exercise is likely to be related to activation of specific pathways and neurons in the brain associated with the exercise being performed. Secretion of BDNF from both pre- and postsynaptic sites occurs in response to neuronal activity, which is likely to contribute to *local* growth of brain tissue (Balaratnasingam & Janca, 2012). On the other hand, aerobic exercise results in induction of a myokine, FNDC5, that when secreted into the circulation results in upregulation of BDNF expression in the hippocampus (Wrann et al., 2013), but not other parts of the brain. Other investigators using a more intense exercise program demonstrated aerobic exercise upregulation of expression of PGC-1a, which regulates the expression of FNDC5 in brain tissue and is related to BDNF secretion, throughout the brain. Additional metabolic regulatory proteins released during aerobic exercise (Ding, Vaynman, Akhavan, Ying, & Gomez-Pinilla, 2006) might also result in increased BDNF secretion in the brain. In all of these cases, the effect of exercise on the secretion of BDNF in the brain is expected to be nonspecific, so that potentially aerobic exercise could lead to growth throughout the brain.

It is easy to imagine how mental and physical exercise might lead to synergistic effects mediated by BDNF, with local secretion in response to neuronal activity and more global secretion resulting from aerobic exercise combining to increase the volume of brain tissue in areas of higher neuronal activity. The much larger increase in BDNF seen when a mental demand was added to stationary cycling illustrates this type of synergy. If there is synergy between mental and physical exercise, then an optimum program for delaying AD might include memory training combined with regular aerobic exercise.

Chapter 18

Social Engagement

That the benefits of activity, be they physical, cognitive, or social, on cognition are related more to being in a fulfilling and dynamic environment than engaging in the activity without personal meaning and intention is becoming evident from the social engagement literature. Early in the study of social engagement, Berkman remarked, "…the power of engagement and the deep sense of affiliation and worthiness it provides may be the critical pathway through which social networks influence the onset of dementias or cognitive decline. Being alone is what is risky, not living alone" (Berkman, 2000). Berkman's commentary was based on a publication from the Kungsholmen Project in Sweden that reported higher adjusted RRs for dementia associated with living alone (RR = 1.5, 95% CI = 1.0–2.1), living without close social ties (RR = 1.5, 95% CI = 1.0–2.4) and living alone as single people (RR = 1.9, 95% CI = 1.2–3.1) compared with married people living with someone else (Fratiglioni, Wang, Ericsson, Maytan, & Winblad, 2000). The notion that "being" alone was more important than living alone was illustrated by the finding in this study that when people had frequent contact with children that was *not* satisfying (compared with frequent contact that was satisfying), the RR for dementia was 2.0 (95% CI = 1.2–3.4). A dose-response gradient (from extensive to moderate to limited to poor social network) also emerged from this study.

METHODOLOGICAL PROBLEMS IN STUDYING SOCIAL ENGAGEMENT AS A RISK FACTOR FOR AD

The principal methodological problem of many cohort studies investigating the role of social engagement on risk for Alzheimer's disease (AD) is inadequate follow-up time. In case-control studies, it is clear that recall bias on the part of proxy informants (either exaggerating or underreporting the patients' social activities in earlier life) can move the OR away or toward the null value. In cohort studies, it is likely that prodromal AD symptoms may cause a person to become more reclusive and withdraw from social activities. For example, a study of 236 mild-moderate AD patients found that 52% reported subjective word-finding difficulties and that such difficulties were selectively associated

Alzheimer's Disease. DOI: http://dx.doi.org/10.1016/B978-0-12-804538-1.00018-3

with social but not nonsocial activities (Farrell et al., 2014). Reverse causality is therefore an important problem in the interpretation of cohort studies' findings regarding social engagement and cognition.

SOCIAL ENGAGEMENT AS A CONTRIBUTOR TO RESERVE

One finding that reinforces the biologic plausibility of social engagement being important in the expression of cognitive symptoms and AD is that social network size has been found to be an effect-modifier of the association between pathology and cognitive function. This was seen in the Rush Memory and Aging Project in which 89 older participants without dementia who had annual clinical evaluations came to autopsy. Social networks were measured by the number of children, family, and friends that the participant had and how many times per month they saw them. Participants with larger networks performed better on tests of cognitive function, specifically in the areas of episodic, semantic, and working memory, given similar levels of pathology, compared with participants with smaller networks. The finding was especially strong for neurofibrillary tangles. The authors suggest that enhanced social networks may give rise to increased reserve, which may buffer cognitive impairment despite AD pathology (Bennett, Schneider, Tang, Arnold, & Wilson, 2006).

FINDINGS IN SELECTED COHORT STUDIES

An early cohort study of 2812 community-dwelling participants age 65 and older at the New Haven, Connecticut site of the Established Populations for Epidemiology Studies of the Elderly (EPESE) with a long follow-up period (up to 12 years) (Bassuk, Glass, & Berkman, 1999) found that people with no social connections were 2.37 times more likely (95% CI = 1.07–4.88) to develop incident cognitive decline compared with those with 5–6 social connections. The ORs for decline were similar at 3 year follow-up (OR = 2.24, 95% CI = 1.40–3.58) and at 6 year follow-up (OR = 1.91, 95% CI = 1.14–3.18). Although the follow-up in this study was longer than in many later studies, no adjustments were made for other activities, such as physical and cognitive activities that could confound the association (Bassuk et al., 1999).

A 15-year follow-up from the PAQUID study (Amieva et al., 2010) examined six social network variables (marital status, network size, ratio of friends to family, satisfaction with relationships, feeling or being understood by most or all versus some of the people in the network, and a subjective assessment of reciprocity in social exchanges (I received more from others than I gave; I gave more to others than I received; I received from others as much as I gave to them). Only two variables were significantly associated with dementia or AD in Cox models adjusted for age, sex, education, Mini-Mental State Examination (MMSE) score, Center for Epidemiologic Studies Depression Scale (CES-D) score, instrumental activities of daily livings (IADLs), and presence of other chronic diseases. Those who were satisfied with their interactions with other people were significantly less likely to experience incident dementia (RR = 0.77, 95% CI = 0.6–0.9) and the perception of having received more than was given was associated with a reduced risk for dementia and AD (RR = 0.47, 95% CI = 0.2–1.0). These findings point to the *quality* of social interactions as being more important than the quantity. In addition, the follow-up period was 15 years, which helps to address the reverse causality issue. Amieva et al. interpreted their findings in terms of "socioemotional selectivity theory" proposed by Carstensen (Carstensen, Isaacowitz, & Charles, 1999). This theory holds that older people seek satisfying relationships, and with increasing age limit their interactions to satisfying ones. When an older person reports not having satisfying relationships, this implies that their social network is not providing the type of support that is needed.

MARRIAGE, WIDOWHOOD, AND LIVING ALONE

Although marriage can have both satisfying and nonsatisfying components, it is interesting to examine the literature on marital status, which obviously is only one component of social engagement, albeit an important one. Living as a couple and the quality of the relationship are positively associated with other health outcomes and with longevity (Kiecolt-Glaser & Newton, 2001). In 1992, this question was addressed with regard to AD in a matched case-control study in Olmsted County, MN using the Rochester Epidemiology Project data (Beard, Kokmen, Offord, & Kurland, 1992). This study was unable to confirm that marital status was a risk factor for AD. Another study that failed to find an association between marital status and risk for AD is the Hisayama Study (Yoshitake et al., 1995). However, this study had only 42 incident cases of AD and was likely underpowered to observe this association.

Men are known to suffer more emotionally when they become widowed and are at increased risk for depression (Lee, DeMaris, Bavin, & Sullivan, 2001). The FINE Study, a longitudinal investigation of 1,042 men from the Seven Countries Study was used to address the question of transition in marital status and cognition (van Gelder et al., 2006). Three groups were studied: those who were married in 1985–1990 and became unmarried during the following 10 years, those who were married in 1985–1990 and remained married during the following 10 years and those who were unmarried in both time periods. Decline in the score on the MMSE was used as the outcome variable in mixed random effects models. Men who lost a partner or who were unmarried in both time periods had about double the risk for global cognitive decline over the ensuing decade. When viewed from the perspective of living alone, men who began living alone during the study period had a twofold risk for decline, and those who lived alone in both periods declined 3.5 times as fast as those who lived with others in both periods. This analysis did not distinguish between those who were unmarried for different reasons (i.e., always single, divorced, or widowed).

In the AGES-Reykjavik Study in Iceland, widowed people were compared with married people from 1978 to 2002–2006 in relation to the prevalence rates of dementia and mild cognitive impairment (MCI) in late-life (Vidarsdottir et al., 2014). No association was found for any widowed group (men or women, APOE-ε4+ or APOE-ε4–) with regard to MCI ($n = 404$) or dementia ($n = 281$). This study had a large sample size, and the exposure was ascertained from national records, along with documented changes in marital status during the follow-up. The sample was significantly older, though, with a mean age of 76.8, and issues related to marital status and mortality may have already affected the cohort.

In PAQUID, never-married people (single) had an adjusted RR for AD of 2.71 (95% CI = 1.51–4.86) compared with people from married couples or couples living together (Helmer et al., 1999). In the CAIDE study, marital status was assessed at age 50 and MCI and AD were diagnosed 21 years later (Hakansson et al., 2009). Because widowhood before age 50 is an unexpected and traumatizing event, different from being single or divorced, the authors compared widowhood ($n = 174$), being single ($n = 166$), and separated/divorced ($n = 97$) to a reference group (married, $n = 1{,}270$). Being single or divorced was associated with elevated ORs (between 1.50 and 1.78), but these were not statistically significant. Being widowed was associated with a significantly elevated risk for MCI (OR = 3.3, 95% CI = 1.6–6.9). People living without a partner at midlife were at about a twofold risk for developing MCI or AD, after adjusting for age, education, sex, APOE, BMI, systolic blood pressure, cholesterol, occupation, physical activity at work, region of residence, smoking, and depression. Because widowhood was present almost exclusively among women (95.7% of widows were female compared with 56.4% of married people) and widows were substantially older than those in other marital subgroups, the authors examined the OR for either MCI and AD among midlife noncohabitants compared with cohabitants. The OR among women noncohabitants was 1.87 (95% CI = 1.1–3.3) and among men noncohabitants, 2.59 (95% CI = 1.0–6.7). For transitioners from cohabitation in midlife to noncohabitation in late-life, the OR was nonsignificant among women (1.28), but significant for men (2.38, 95% CI = 1.0–5.7). The highest risks for MCI and AD were associated with those who did not have a partner either in midlife or in late-life (OR = 3.17, 95% CI = 1.7–6 for MCI, OR = 2.83, 95% CI = 1.1–7.4 for AD). In addition, there appeared to be strong effect-modification between being widowed or divorced both in mid- and late-life and carrying an APOE-ε4 allele (OR = 25 for ε4+/widowed or divorced in mid- and late-life; OR = 4 for ε4+ and cohabiting with a partner both in mid- and late-life; OR = 3 for ε4– and widowed or divorced both in mid- and late-life, compared with the reference group (OR = 1 for ε4– and cohabiting with a partner both in mid- and late life). The authors suggested that widowhood could be a "triggering" event, resulting in stress and declines in immunological functioning. They also pointed out that if living alone is the true risk factor, their study would have found that single individuals had the highest risk. Instead, they found that being widowed carried the highest risk, implying that some risk factor is related to becoming widowed or that lifestyle changes following the loss of a spouse, such as poor nutrition, stress, obesity, vascular diseases, physical inactivity, smoking, alcohol consumption, and depression, may play a role. We do not yet know at what point in time changes in marital status make a difference for cognitive impairment in older age. This study only looked at widowhood at age 50, which may be different from widowhood at age 80, for example.

Other important difficulties in positing that being married is causally related to lowering the risk for AD include the possibility that factors related to becoming married versus remaining single may be risk factors for this illness. The ability of observational studies to control for known and unknown confounders related to marital status is limited.

SOCIAL ENGAGEMENT AND DEMENTIA: IS THE ASSOCIATION DUE TO REVERSE CAUSATION?

Data from the Honolulu-Asia Aging Study (HAAS) (Saczynski et al., 2006) were used to address this important question. In this study, an index of midlife social engagement (gathered in 1968–1970), based on information collected an average of almost 28 years before dementia diagnoses were ascertained was found to have no association with dementia ($p_{\text{for trend}}$ was not significant), but the same index based on data collected in late-life (1991–1993) showed a highly statistically significant increasing risk with decreasing number of social ties ($p<0.001$). The midlife social engagement index was a composite of five variables (marital status, living arrangement, participation in group activities, and participation in social events or outings with coworkers weekly or more frequently, and whether the participant had a confidant relationship). Each of the five variables was coded 1 or 0 and then summed. Scores were stratified as low, medium-low, medium-high, and high. In late-life, the variables were similar, except that the item about social events and outings with coworkers was replaced by an item about the number of in-person or telephone contacts with close friends each month (≥5 was coded as 1, fewer as 0). When the authors analyzed changes in social engagement from mid- to late-life as risk factors for dementia (not AD), compared to those with consistently high social engagement in mid- and late-life, those whose levels had decreased (high to low) had an HR for dementia of 1.87 (95% CI = 1.12–3.13), and those with persistently low levels had a HR of 1.65 (95% CI = 0.94–2.90). The authors concluded that low social engagement in late-life may be a prodromal symptom of dementia, and that findings of an inverse association between social engagement and risk for dementia or AD were likely due to reverse causality. The authors of the CAIDE study (Hakansson et al., 2009) dispute this, because their findings showed effects on MCI and dementia from marital status assessed 21 years earlier, reducing the probability of reverse causality. While the issue is not yet settled, several other studies also support the finding that social *dis*engagement is associated with increased risk for AD.

LONELINESS

In 2007, the Rush Memory and Aging Program published findings on loneliness and dementia risk from a cohort of 823 nondemented individuals recruited from senior housing in and around Chicago, IL (Wilson, Krueger, et al., 2007). They used the de Jong-Gierveld Loneliness Scale (de Jong-Gierveld, 1987) but modified it in several ways, excluding items used to assess social loneliness, since they were trying to measure emotional loneliness. Scores ranged from 1 to 5, with higher values indicating more loneliness. Annual exams were conducted to ascertain cognition (using 20 tests that were *Z*-scored to represent global cognitive decline) and incident AD by standard NINCDS-ADRDA criteria. In addition, neuropathologic results were available for 90 participants who died and had a brain autopsy. When adjusting for only demographic factors (age, sex, and education), the association between loneliness and risk for incident AD was 1.5 (95% CI = 1.06–2.14) for each point on the de Jong-Gierveld Loneliness Scale. This would translate into a risk of about 2 for someone in the 90th percentile (score 3.2) of loneliness compared with the 10th percentile (score 1.4). One of this study's strengths was that the authors measured physical, cognitive, and social activity, and so were able to examine the independent effect of loneliness on incident AD controlling for these variables. Controlling hierarchically for social network and social activity changed the RR for incident dementia little (1.45, 95% CI = 1.01–2.09). Controlling for cognitive activity also led to only a modest change in the association with loneliness (RR = 1.41, 95% CI = 0.99–2.01). Adjustment for physical activity did not change the estimate either (RR = 1.54, 95% CI = 1.08–2.19). One of the problems in the epidemiology of physical, cognitive, and social activities is that many questionnaires include queries that involve two or all three of these domains (e.g., visiting friends or relatives, going for walks, going to movies, restaurants, and sports events, doing unpaid community volunteer work, playing cards, attending religious services) (Scarmeas, Levy, Tang, Manly, & Stern, 2001). These kinds of questionnaires do not allow us to easily disentangle the three types of activities.

In the Wilson et al. study, loneliness was inversely associated with not only baseline function on all cognitive tests, but also with more rapid decline in global cognitive performance, semantic memory performance, perceptual speed, and visuospatial ability. Since feeling lonely is related to depression, the authors also controlled for the CES-D score, which led to a slight attenuation of the loneliness finding (RR = 1.41, 95% CI = 0.97–2.06). The single item on the CES-D that asks about feeling lonely predicted an increase in the probability of incident AD (RR = 1.86, 95% CI = 1.1–3.1), and the authors proposed that loneliness may be an important aspect of how depression is associated with AD.

Measures of AD pathology were not related to loneliness, showing that loneliness is likely an "enabling" factor, contributing to reduced reserve, rather than a direct risk factor for AD pathology. Although mechanisms are difficult to tease out in humans, rats subjected to social isolation shortly after birth had fewer synapses in the prefrontal cortex and hippocampus, therefore possibly reducing connectivity of the brain, one aspect of brain reserve (Silva-Gomez, Rojas, Juarez, & Flores, 2003). In the study of Wilson et al., frequent participation in social activities decreased the risk for AD, but the size of the social network did not. They concluded that both the *quantity and the quality* of social patterns are important in the etiology of dementia and cognitive decline (Wilson, Krueger, et al., 2007).

Another cohort study conducted in Amsterdam, the Netherlands (The Amsterdam Study of the Elderly, AMSTEL) followed 5,666 older persons randomly selected from 30 general practice registers in the city (Holwerda et al., 2014). Social isolation was defined as living alone, or never or no longer being married, or not having social support. Feelings of loneliness were measured by asking the question, "Do you feel lonely or do you feel very lonely?" Clinical dementia was measured using the Geriatric Mental State (GMS) Automated Geriatric Examination for Computer Assisted Taxonomy (AGECAT), which has a kappa of 0.88 for "organic illness" or dementia. Feelings of loneliness were reported by almost 20% of the sample. Based on 2,173 participants free of dementia at baseline, the OR for incident dementia was 1.64 (95% CI = 1.05–2.56) after adjustment for living alone, never/no longer married, no social support, age, sex, education, depression, comorbid conditions, head injury, cognitive impairment-no dementia, MMSE, and ADL/IADLs. When similar models were run for never/no longer being married, the adjusted OR was 1.23 (95% CI = 0.61–2.50), for living alone, 0.96 (95% CI = 0.48–1.93), and for no social support, 1.06 (95% CI = 0.70–1.60). Therefore, the significant finding was *limited to subjective feelings of loneliness.* The authors correctly note that their finding could be due to reverse causality, particularly with the short follow-up time. An alternative explanation advanced by the authors is that feelings of loneliness may be related to a maladaptive personality, such as low conscientiousness, extraversion and openness, and high neuroticism. Controlling for social isolation, the Odds Ratio associated with loneliness was only slightly attenuated. In this study, even among married people receiving social support, feelings of loneliness increased the risk for dementia. Like the study of Wilson et al., when the investigators controlled for depression, the OR was only slightly affected.

SOCIAL ENGAGEMENT AND ATROPHY

To examine whether high social engagement is associated with less brain atrophy, 305 former lead manufacturing workers and 43 population-based individuals age 48–82 were imaged with a T1-weighted structural MRI (James et al.,

2012). Higher social engagement was defined using a 20-item scale measuring enacted functional performance in daily life. Confirmatory factor analysis led to eight items that loaded into one factor representing social engagement. Scores on the social engagement scale were significantly associated with total brain volume ($p = 0.01$), total gray matter volume ($p = 0.007$), temporal and occipital gray matter volume ($p = 0.009$ and 0.048, respectively), and corpus callosum ($p = 0.004$) volume, adjusting for age, education, intracranial volume, race/ethnicity, hypertension, diabetes, handedness, and control status (lead worker or not). The authors proposed that social engagement may result in larger brain volumes by reducing neuronal death or atrophy, increasing neurogenesis in certain parts of the brain, increasing dendritic spine growth or by axonal rearrangement (James et al., 2012). In this study, the authors also examined change in brain volumes over the 5 year period prior to measurement of social engagement and noted that changes in brain volumes were not related to the level of social engagement. Two explanations can be given for the latter finding. First, socially engaged people in middle and old age were likely socially engaged throughout their lives. Therefore, social engagement can influence brain growth over many decades affecting brain volumes observed in old age. If this effect is not very strong, it may take several decades to see the differences in brain volumes that were observed. By contrast, changes in brain volumes over 5 years could be relatively modest, making it difficult to see an association over this relatively short duration of time. Second, as people grow older, it is likely that at least some of them may become less socially engaged. The decline in social engagement with age may lead to smaller effects on changes in brain volume later in life.

SCHEMA FOR SOCIAL ENGAGEMENT

A summary schema of the types of variables that have been studied in relation to social engagement is shown in Figure 18.1. All of these have been shown to be useful in delaying cognitive symptoms in older age, but not all

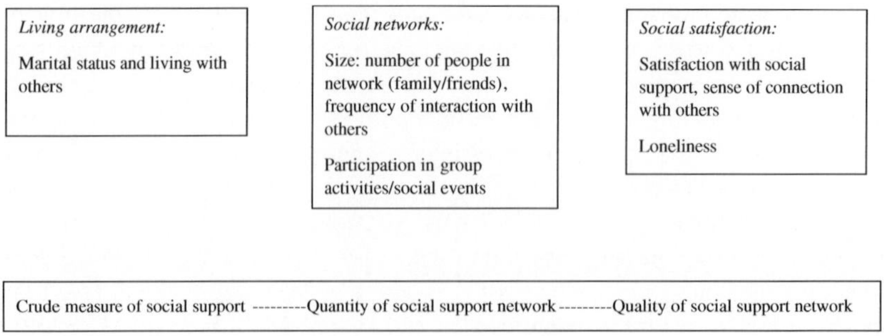

Living arrangement:	*Social networks:*	*Social satisfaction:*
Marital status and living with others	Size: number of people in network (family/friends), frequency of interaction with others Participation in group activities/social events	Satisfaction with social support, sense of connection with others Loneliness

Crude measure of social support ---------Quantity of social support network---------Quality of social support network

FIGURE 18.1 Schema of social engagement variables from crude measures to quantity and quality of relationships.

studies yielded positive findings. To our knowledge, no meta-analysis has been conducted of the association between social engagement variables and risk for cognitive decline, dementia, or dementia subtypes. The fact that social variables are defined differently across studies would make such an analysis challenging. It also is important to note that social engagement variables are "soft" variables. Their reports are usually subjective and based on subjects' recall and willingness to divulge relatively sensitive information. Nevertheless, the findings are sufficiently intriguing that investigators are pursuing social engagement as one part of a multifaceted prevention effort.

A MULTIMODAL PREVENTION STUDY

Social intervention is part of the multidomain Finnish Geriatric Intervention Study to Prevent Cognitive Impairment and Disability (FINGER). The population for FINGER is based on the FINRISK and CAIDE studies, which have collected data on participants since 1972. The main purpose of FINGER was to examine, among older people at increased risk for cognitive decline, how well a multidomain intervention could reduce cognitive impairment over a 2-year intervention period. The domains being tested were nutritional guidance, exercise, cognitive training, social stimulation, and intensive monitoring and management of metabolic and vascular risk factors (Kivipelto et al., 2013). The sample consisted of 1,200 individuals age 60–77 living in six cities in Finland. Persons were eligible if they screened positive on the CAIDE Dementia Risk Score (Kivipelto et al., 2006) (see Chapter 22), which includes age, sex, education, BMI, blood pressure, total cholesterol, and physical activity (Kivipelto et al., 2013). To enter FINGER, a potential participant had to score at least 6 out of 15 on the Dementia Risk Score. To increase the chances that participants are at risk for dementia, they were further required to score at the mean or slightly below the mean in performance on a number of neuropsychological tests, but without showing substantial cognitive decline. Potential participants were excluded if they had conditions that would preclude them from participating in intervention components, prevalent cognitive impairment, or loss of hearing, vision, or ability to speak. Two randomized groups of equal size were followed for 2 years. The intervention group received all four components of the intervention and the placebo group received health advice on a regular basis. Social activities were increased by using group meetings to deliver intervention components and participants were given information about the value of an active lifestyle and social connections. The primary outcomes for FINGER were performance on the modified Neuropsychological Test Battery (mNTB) composite Z-score, the Stroop test, and Trailmaking Tests (A and B). Secondary outcomes included the incidence of dementia and AD according to DSM-IV and NINCDS-ADRDA criteria, but at least 7 years of follow-up will be necessary to have sufficient power to evaluate this outcome. There are a number of other secondary and exploratory outcomes, one of which is MRI on about 100 participants. Enrollment began in September 2009, and of 5,500 invitees, 48% participated. Enrollment was achieved and subjects were randomized to intervention versus nonintervention groups in 2011. Initial findings from this study (Ngandu et al., 2015) showed that those randomized to the intervention performed significantly better on a global measure of cognition ($p = 0.03$) and did better on specific tests of executive function ($p = 0.04$) and speed of cognitive processing ($p = 0.03$) (Ngandu et al., 2015). Unfortunately, because the social engagement component was part of a large set of interventions, it is impossible to know how important social engagement was to the cognitive improvement that occurred.

REMAINING QUESTIONS

The difficulty in disentangling the role of social engagement from cognitive stimulation remains a major problem with studying the role of social engagement in preserving cognition in old age. How much of the social engagement is a result of the cognitive stimulation that comes from social interaction? A second question relevant to cohort studies is how many of the observed associations are due to reverse causation with withdrawal from social interaction in those at high risk for dementia? Finally, the question is raised whether objective measures of social engagement or subjective perceptions are more important for risk of dementia or AD. The data generally show that subjective perceptions on the quality of social interaction are likely to be more important for dementia risk than objective measures such a social network size. This view is reinforced by the findings on loneliness, which differs from living alone. As Berkman (2000) proposed, the perception of being alone is likely more important that the fact of living alone.

Chapter 19

Nonsteroidal Anti-Inflammatory Drugs, Hormone Replacement Therapy, and Anticholinergic Medications

NONSTEROIDAL ANTI-INFLAMMATORY DRUGS

Historically, the brain has been considered an immunologically privileged area because of the existence of the blood–brain barrier. This view has been changing since the 1980s, when microglia were discovered to play critical roles in the innate immune/inflammatory response in Alzheimer's disease (AD) and other neurologic disorders. During development of the brain, microglia help to remodel the brain by eliminating redundant, dying neurons. Aβ deposition elicits a strong microglial response, with accumulations of microglia occurring around plaques, cytokines being elicited as an acute reaction and stimulation of the complement cascade (in t' Veld et al., 2001). Today, microglial activation is seen on a continuum, with cytokines such as Th2, IL-4, IL-10, IL-13, and TGF-β acutely released as inflammatory responses to pathogens and injury and with lower levels being secreted on a long-term basis if the insults persist over time. Inflammation can be a double-edged sword—beneficial in some situations and harmful in others. Early in the AD process, microglia may be beneficial in removing Aβ deposits. However, continued presence of Aβ can lead to chronic stimulation of inflammatory pathways leading to increased formation of neurofibrillary tangles and neuronal death.

Mitigation of inflammatory pathways may be achieved by inhibiting the enzyme cyclooxygenase (COX), which has a direct role in the production of prostaglandins (Wyss-Coray & Rogers, 2012). It has been proposed that nonsteroidal anti-inflammatory drugs (NSAIDs), some of which have direct COX-2 inhibitory effects, could diminish the inflammatory milieu in AD, reduce apoptosis due to glutamate-mediated excitotoxicity, and reduce neuritic plaque formation by downregulating the amount of circulating β-amyloid that comes from platelets (Szekely et al., 2004).

Alzheimer's Disease. DOI: http://dx.doi.org/10.1016/B978-0-12-804538-1.00019-5

In the United States, every day, over 30 million people take over-the-counter and prescription NSAIDs for pain, headaches, and osteo- and rheumatoid arthritis. Early case-control studies, including our own (Graves et al., 1990b), examined arthritis and rheumatoid arthritis as potential risk factors for AD. While our study and one other (Breitner et al., 1994) were null, perhaps owing to low statistical power, others did find statistically significant inverse associations (McGeer, Schulzer, & McGeer, 1996). Meta-analyses (using a fixed model) of case-control studies of AD for arthritis and rheumatoid arthritis in addition to NSAIDs showed strong inverse associations with AD (OR = 0.56, 95% CI = 0.44–0.70) for arthritis without significant heterogeneity and OR = 0.19 (95% CI = 0.09–0.41) for rheumatoid arthritis with heterogeneity (only two studies) (McGeer et al., 1996). For studies of NSAIDs, or NSAIDs plus steroids (seven studies), the meta-analyzed ORs were around 0.50 and were highly statistically significant as well. McGeer et al. attribute the stronger OR for rheumatoid arthritis to the fact that these patients have likely used these drugs for a longer period than patients without arthritis. The duration effect became a point of interest in the prospective cohort studies and the randomized clinical trials (RCTs) that would follow.

The first population-based analysis of NSAIDs and AD was from the baseline data of the Rotterdam Study (Andersen et al., 1995). NSAID use was measured (by interviewer visualization of all medications) within a week before the interview. The sample consisted of 6,258 participants and 228 prevalent dementia patients (155 with AD by standard clinical criteria). Two comparisons were made: the first of all NSAID users to nonusers, and the second of NSAID users to nonusers who were also users of topical medications for eye, ear, or dermatologic indications. This second group was selected in order to examine the effect of "indication bias," in which people with a condition such as AD might have a different prescribing pattern than those without AD. This is likely in our situation, because AD patients may be less likely to communicate pain to their doctor, or the doctor may not be looking for it as intensively as s/he would in a person with another condition. Such indication bias could produce an inverse association. The OR for AD in the first analysis was 0.38 (95% CI= 0.15–0.93) adjusting for age, sex, education, and benzodiazepine use (which was more common among NSAID users). For the second analysis, the point estimate was similar (0.54) but the 95% CI was not significant (0.16–1.78). However, for this analysis, the sample size was reduced from 5,893 to 365, which might account for the lack of statistical significance. The use of prevalent cases in this analysis also brings up the problem of reverse causality—that cases may decrease their NSAID use due to their disease. An early meta-analysis of case-control and cross-sectional data demonstrated an OR from seven studies of 0.51 (95% CI= 0.40–0.66) with no statistical heterogeneity (Szekely et al., 2004).

Because the case-control studies were fairly uniform in their findings, NSAIDs became an early target of investigation in prospective cohort studies and RCTs. An early RCT of indomethacin for 6 months in 44 probable AD patients with an Mini-Mental State Examination (MMSE) score greater than 16 found better cognitive performance at the end of the trial in the treated group compared with the placebo group (Rogers et al., 1993).

Prospective Cohort Studies

NSAID findings from a flurry of prospective studies were published in the 1990s. In 1997, the Baltimore Longitudinal Study of Aging (BLSA), a study of 1,686 mostly white and highly educated volunteers followed for dementia outcomes between 1980 and 1995, reported that more than 2 years of NSAID use (RR = 0.40, 95% CI = 0.19–0.84), but not aspirin (RR = 0.74, 95% CI = 0.46–1.18) or acetaminophen (RR = 1.35, 95% CI = 0.79–2.30), was associated with lower risk for AD (Stewart, Kawas, Corrada, & Metter, 1997). For those with less than 2 years of NSAID use, the RR = 0.65 (95% CI = 0.33–1.29). These authors relied on self-report of all medications, so their finding of no association with acetaminophen (a medication with very few anti-inflammatory properties) boosted the authors' confidence that the inverse association with NSAIDs was not spurious. The follow-up was over 15 years, and exposures were defined as time-dependent covariates. The authors proposed that aspirin was not significant in this analysis because many older people were taking it prophylactically in very small doses to prevent heart disease.

The most important study in this area was published in the *New England Journal of Medicine* in 2001 by investigators from the Rotterdam Study (in t' Veld et al., 2001). This analysis was remarkable for its sample size (N = 6,989 nondemented at baseline with 394 incident dementia cases and 293 AD cases), ability to measure NSAID use from pharmacy records, use of time-dependent exposures in more than dichotomous form, adjustment for multiple covariates, and relatively long follow-up (mean of 6.8 years). The annual rate of NSAID use was stable over time, at about 37–40 days of use per 1,000 person-days. Although the comparison of use of "any" NSAID to nonuse did not yield a statistically significant result (HR for incident AD = 0.86, 95% CI = 0.66–1.09), the dose-response associations showed a decreasing HR with increasing NSAID use duration compared with no NSAID use (≤1 month: HR = 0.95, 95% CI = 0.70–1.29; 1–23 months: HR = 0.83, 95% CI = 0.62–1.11; ≥24 months: HR = 0.20, 95% CI = 0.05–0.83) ($p_{\text{for trend}} = 0.05$). Covariates that were adjusted included age, sex, education, smoking, apolipoprotein E (APOE) genotype, use of histamine H2 receptor antagonists, hypoglycemic and antihypertensive medications, and aspirin. No trend was evident for the outcome of vascular dementia or for either AD or vascular dementia with the use of aspirin. Neither age nor APOE status modified the association between NSAID use and AD. By virtue of examining pharmacy records to document exposure, this analysis is free from biases that might occur as a result of under- or overreporting among individuals destined to become demented in the ensuing years.

Nonaspirin NSAIDs and aspirin also were studied in the Canadian Study of Health and Aging (CSHA), where a similar trend was found, except here, any use of NSAIDs was statistically significantly associated with incident AD in a nested case-base design of 156 incident AD cases and 3,299 controls (OR = 0.65, 95% CI = 0.44–0.95) (Lindsay et al., 2002). Aspirin products again were not associated with AD (OR = 0.85, 95% CI = 0.55–1.31). There were two important limitations in this study. First, medication use was gathered from participants by self-report at baseline, and second, 5 years elapsed between the baseline and the follow-up wave. If individuals who used NSAIDs and in addition had underlying AD were less likely to survive the 5-year follow-up in comparison to those without AD using NSAIDs, NSAID use could be underrepresented in the surviving incident AD cases, resulting in the finding. In fact, the 18% of the cohort that died between the two visits had lower education, were generally older and had more chronic diseases than those who completed the 5-year follow-up. This potential bias in the study's results was acknowledged by the authors.

One of the tactics used by many researchers to examine reverse causality is to exclude cases that occurred at the beginning of the follow-up period—to provide a "lag" time to avoid those cases with incipient dementia. Although such a sensitivity analysis may be useful on one level, it reduces the number of incident cases, decreasing statistical power. It also probably does not affect the findings much, not because reverse causality is not a problem, but rather because the disease has such a long prodromal period that even 2 years lag time is unlikely to cover the entire period during which incipient dementia is having an effect on NSAID usage. Other strategies include excluding new cases that had poor cognitive scores at baseline, but this also will result in a loss of sample size. In the CSHA, when decedents between baseline and follow-up were included in the analyses by coding any death that was due to dementia as AD and any death that was not due to dementia as a control, the ORs were close to 1.0 for both NSAIDs and were no longer statistically significant, implying that the finding could have been due to survival bias.

In the Cache County Study in Utah (Zandi et al., 2002), participants were asked at baseline about their prescription and over-the-counter medications and requested to produce the pill bottles for documentation. In this study, 185 incident dementia cases (104 with definite, probable or possible AD by NINCDS-ADRDA criteria) were identified after about 3 years of follow-up of over 3000 who participated at baseline. Six classes of drugs were investigated for their relationship to dementia and AD [nonaspirin NSAIDs, histamine type 2 receptor antagonists (H_2RA) such as Tagamet and Zantac, aspirin products, non-NSAID pain relievers (acetaminophen (Tylenol), allopurinol, propoxyphene, and other opioids), simple antacids/antiflatulents, and other non-H_2RA stomach remedies such as omeprazole]. Only the first three were of interest—the latter three were included as "dummy" exposures to conceal the exposures of interest. This is done quite often in epidemiologic studies to control for recall bias in sensitivity analyses. Covariates included age, the squared deviation of age from the sample's median value, sex, education, presence of at least one APOE-ε4 alleles and an interaction term between age and APOE. The adjusted HR for AD associated with ever use of nonaspirin NSAIDs was 0.67 (95% CI = 0.40–1.06);

there was no association for any of the other types of medications. There was no interaction with APOE-ε4, but an interaction for NSAIDs with age showed that with increasing age, the protective effect of NSAIDs diminished. Like the previous studies, the point estimates for people who used NSAIDs for more than 2 years were reduced compared with those who used them less, but these were not statistically significant likely because of low statistical power. Individuals who used NSAIDs at baseline (regardless of length of exposure) ($n = 557$) did not have a reduced risk for AD (HR = 0.85, 95% CI = 0.47–1.44), whereas former-users ($n = 389$) did (HR = 0.42, 95% CI = 0.16–0.90). The authors note the potential misclassification of exposure ascertainment in their study, as well as the relatively brief follow-up.

Many of these publications concluded with a statement about how only randomized controlled trials can definitively answer the question of whether an exposure can delay or prevent the onset of AD. Although this is obviously true, the idea that RCTs can provide the answers to all epidemiologic questions is flawed. When RCTs fail to show effects, observational studies showing significant associations are criticized because it is assumed that their results can be explained by potential biases. As we have discussed in earlier chapters, RCTs have their own methodological challenges, such as biased samples, inadequate sample size, as well as inadequate duration to detect significant effects. If prolonged exposure long before the onset age of AD is critical, choosing a sample of older participants including some with mild cognitive impairment (MCI) or early AD is unlikely to show an effect. For such an exposure, cohort studies that begin in midlife or earlier offer the best assessment.

It is important to note that some cohort studies with relatively long follow-up periods did not find that NSAID use affects the risk for AD or found an effect unrelated to dose. The Religious Orders Study (Arvanitakis et al., 2008) examined over 1,000 participants' medication bottles annually and found no association with incident AD (NSAIDs vs no NSAIDs: HR = 1.19, 95% CI = 0.87–1.62), change in cognition (all $p > 0.14$) or global AD pathology in 12 years of follow-up (Arvanitakis et al., 2008). In the Cardiovascular Health Study (Szekely, Breitner, et al., 2008), with a larger sample size and over about 10 years of follow-up, the use of NSAIDs was found to be inversely associated with incident AD (HR = 0.63, 95% CI = 0.45–0.88). However, no dose-response effect was evident in this study. NSAIDs were examined by viewing medication bottles at baseline and divided into those that selectively lowered $A\beta_{42}$ production in animal studies (diclofenac, fenoprofen, flurbiprofen, ibuprofen, indomethacin, meclofenamate, piroxicam, and sulindac) and non-$A\beta_{42}$-lowering NSAIDs (celecoxib, naproxen, ketoprofen, ketorolac, mefanimic acid, nabumetone, naproxen, and phenylbutazone). Aspirin and acetaminophen use were examined as separate groups and neither one was associated with incident AD in adjusted models. A strong interaction was present with APOE-ε4, with the reduction in AD risk being present only among those carrying an ε4 allele (HR = 0.34, 95% CI = 0.18–0.65) and no association being evident in those without this allele (HR = 0.99, 95% CI = 0.79–1.24). In addition to interaction with APOE-ε4, these investigators found an interaction with age, such that the inverse association between NSAID use and AD was present only among individuals who were taking NSAIDs before age 75. No difference in the magnitude of risk was found for the two different types of NSAIDs, indicating no advantage of the $A\beta_{42}$-lowering NSAIDs in the prevention of AD.

To our knowledge only one large prospective cohort study has found that NSAIDs *increase* the risk for AD. This analysis was done within the ACT cohort, and included 3,392 nondemented participants from Group Health Cooperative, an HMO in King County, WA (Breitner et al., 2009). The investigators examined time-dependent measures of NSAID exposure based on the pharmacy records and another combining the pharmacy records with self-reported use. Adjusting for age, sex, APOE status, education, hypertension, diabetes, BMI, osteoarthritis, and regular exercise, HRs for AD increased with increasing use of NSAIDs [1.0 for non- or low-users, 1.26 (95% CI = 0.97–1.65) for moderate users and 1.57 (95% CI = 1.10–2.23) for heavy users]. The major difference between this and other studies is that the ACT cohort cases were old (median age of 83.5 at dementia onset) compared with participants in studies that showed protective effects in younger cohorts (where the median age at onset was almost 10 years younger). The authors propose an interesting hypothesis to account for their findings: that if NSAID exposure delays the onset of AD to later ages, those cases that manifest this illness in late-old age will be enriched for NSAID use. Therefore, this study may not contradict the inverse associations seen in some other studies.

Meta-Analyses

There have been a number of systematic reviews and meta-analyses on this topic (Etminan, Gill, & Samii, 2003; Szekely et al., 2004; Szekely, Green, et al., 2008). The latest one, published in 2014 (Wang, Tan, et al., 2014) used a random effects model and covered the last 20 years of studies. The authors showed the forest plot for effect measures of NSAIDs and AD (Figure 19.1). The pooled effect sizes agreed quite well for the cohort and case-control studies. For cohort studies, RR = 0.69 (95% CI = 0.56–0.86) and for case-control studies, OR = 0.75 (95% CI = 0.68–0.84). Among long-term users, the RR was more pronounced (RR = 0.36, 95% CI = 0.17–0.74). Interestingly, the effect of aspirin use was also significant (RR = 0.77, 95% CI = 0.63–0.95) in this meta-analysis. No publication bias was found, but substantial heterogeneity of studies was reported. The authors posit that this heterogeneity might be partly explained by the differing quality of studies, their age distributions, dosages of drugs, as well as differing covariates used in their analyses.

Randomized Clinical Trials

RCTs of NSAIDs in people who already have AD have been equivocal. For 10 such RCTs, a Cochrane review and meta-analysis (Jaturapatporn, Isaac,

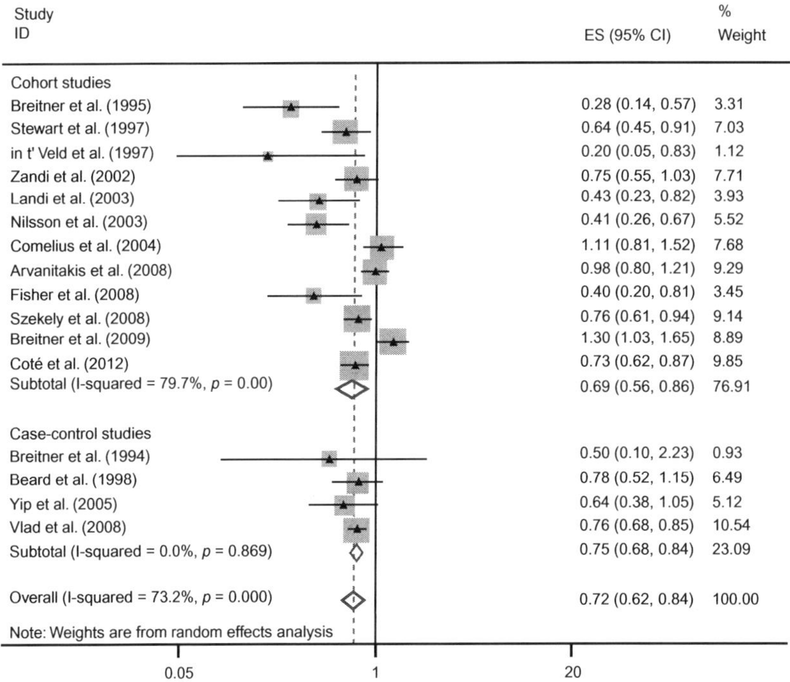

FIGURE 19.1 Forest plot of risk for AD with NSAID use. *Adapted from Wang et al. (2014).*

McCleery, & Tabet, 2012) found that, despite a trend toward protection, no statistically significant differences existed between the NSAID group and the placebo group on ADAS-cog scores (mean difference = −1.41, 95% CI = −3.13 to 0.32).

Only one RCT has been conducted among older (≥70) *cognitively unimpaired* individuals. The Alzheimer's Disease Anti-inflammatory Prevention Trial (ADAPT) (Adapt Research Group, 2006) began in 2001 and was designed to examine incidence of AD in a randomized, double-blind RCT with three arms: a conventional NSAID (naproxen, 220 mg twice daily), a COX-2 inhibitor (celecoxib, 200 mg twice daily), and placebo. The study was conducted at six sites and enrolled over 2,500 participants with a family history of AD. Planned follow-up was 7 years. However, in February 2005, Celebrex (celecoxib) was withdrawn from the market because another study investigating celecoxib's effect on colon polyp prevention showed elevated risks for cardiovascular events (Nissen, 2006). The National Institutes of Health (NIH) decided to stop the ADAPT trial, and in November 2006 the ADAPT investigators published adverse event data by treatment group. Although the HRs were elevated for cardiovascular deaths (n = 10, HR for celecoxib vs placebo = 1.96 and 1.48 for naproxen vs placebo) and cancer deaths (n = 13, HR for celecoxib vs placebo = 1.49 and 1.86 for naproxen vs placebo), none of these HRs was statistically significant. The ADAPT investigators observationally monitored the participants until 2007 (Alzheimer's Disease Anti-inflammatory Prevention Trial Research Group, 2013) and showed that among 161 incident AD cases (48 on celecoxib, 43 on naproxen, and 70 on placebo), those randomized to celecoxib versus placebo had no reduction in risk for AD (HR = 1.03, 95% CI = 0.72–1.50), nor did those randomized to naproxen versus placebo (HR = 0.92, 95% CI = 0.62–1.35). Risk of death also was not elevated for the two treatment groups compared with placebo. This RCT has been critiqued on the basis of its highly selected population (very low participation rate) and poor adherence to study medications for the period in which participants were actively followed (Williams, Plassman, Burke, Holsinger, & Benjamin, 2010).

Conclusions Regarding NSAIDs

Where do these results leave us? There is consensus in the literature that NSAIDs likely do not provide protection when given over a short time period or in people who already have clinical AD. On the other hand, with more long-term usage, particularly earlier in life, NSAIDs may reduce the risk for AD. The very strong effect modification by APOE-ε4 in the CHS study suggests that NSAIDS are likely to be most beneficial in those prone to greater AD pathology at earlier ages. Methodological issues affecting observational studies of NSAIDs are well recognized. These include recall bias, confounding bias (in particular confounding by indication), and insufficient follow-up time. RCTs are affected by insufficient follow-up time and enrollment of individuals with signs of the disease or at advanced ages. It is likely that NSAIDs are effective among those who take them at younger age and who carry an APOE-ε4 allele (Szekely & Zandi, 2010). NSAIDs may not be useful in *treating* AD, but may *prevent* it in those treated sufficiently early.

HORMONE REPLACEMENT THERAPY

Cross-sectional data from the National Health and Nutrition Examination Survey (NHANES) between 1999 and 2010 show that the prevalence of oral postmenopausal hormone replacement therapy (HRT) declined precipitously from 22.4% in 1999–2002 to 4.7% in 2009–2010 among women over the ages of 40 (Sprague, Trentham-Dietz, & Cronin, 2012). This decline began in non-Hispanic whites in 2003–2004, and in other racial/ethnic groups about 2 years later. In 2010, more non-Hispanic whites took HRT (5.4%) compared with non-Hispanic blacks (1.6%) and Hispanics (2.2%). Factors associated with HRT use include a history of hysterectomy, non-Hispanic white race/ethnicity and higher income (Sprague et al., 2012). In the last decade, most of the decline in HRT use likely can be attributed to the published results of the Women's Health Initiative (WHI) studies (Women's Health Initiative Study Group, 1998), which showed increased risks for a number of outcomes, including dementia, with HRT use.

HRT has been shown to be effective for a number of indications among postmenopausal women (Panay et al., 2013). Short-term effects that have been found to be beneficial include vasomotor symptoms associated with hot flashes, mood, sexual function, vaginal atrophy, and urinary frequency. In addition, HRT has a protective effect on connective tissue metabolism in the bone matrix, skin, and invertebral disks. Long-term beneficial effects include higher bone density and prevention of osteoporosis and osteoporosis-related fractures. HRT's effect on cardiovascular disease has a mixed history, as it does for AD. In the Danish Osteoporosis Study, 500 women age 45–58 were randomized to HRT and 500 to placebo (Schierbeck et al., 2012). After about 10 years of treatment, participants were encouraged to discontinue use following the publications of the WHI trial results. They were followed for an additional 5.7 years. In this study, HRT was protective for mortality due to heart failure or myocardial infarction (HR = 0.48, 95% CI = 0.26–0.87). Among women who were under age 50 at time of HRT initiation, the protective HR was a bit more pronounced (HR = 0.35, 95% CI = 0.13–0.89). Beneficial effects were restricted to women who had a hysterectomy (not those with an intact uterus). When mortality was considered alone, there was no effect of HRT. These trends remained at the 16-year follow-up, except the point estimate for women under 50 increased to 0.55 (95% CI = 0.29–1.05). A similar inverse trend was seen for incidence of breast cancer when HRT was initiated before age 50 (HR = 0.50, 95% CI = 0.22–1.14), albeit this was not significant; whereas no association was present after this age.

In contrast to these largely positive findings, the WHI found no association between the use of HRT and the risk for CHD among women who began HRT immediately after menopause. There was a tendency for increased risk for stroke in the same women (Prentice et al., 2009), while women with an intact uterus who began HRT immediately after menopause had a lower risk for hip fracture. Women exposed to HRT also had an increased risk for invasive breast cancer in this study. Similar to the Danish study, no effect from hormone replacement was found for mortality (Rossouw et al., 2002).

Current recommendations are not to take HRT to prevent chronic conditions (Nelson, Walker, Zakher, & Mitchell, 2012). However, the nine studies on which this report is based come mostly from the WHI. Despite the fact that the WHI was a "once-in-a-lifetime" landmark study, it has received a good deal of criticism, owing to the selected nature of the sample, the age at which women were enrolled into the study, the drugs selected for study (which some hypothesized may have negated the protective effect of estrogen on CHD and cerebral vascular disease) (Klaiber, Vogel, & Rako, 2005), and the appropriateness of the analyses (e.g., the use of the relative and not the attributable risk, the latter which was very small), among other concerns (Clark, 2006; Stevenson & Whitehead, 2002).

The WHI was a huge undertaking, and it is recognized that another trial of this size and scope will not happen again. A few more details about its design are useful before we discuss the results for the cognition outcome studies. Initially begun in 1992, the WHI enrolled postmenopausal women age 50–79 at

40 clinical centers in the United States into an RCT ($N = 64{,}500$) or an observational study ($N = 100{,}000$) (1998). The RCT had a dietary modification arm and a HRT arm ($N = 27{,}500$). Women who were ineligible or unwilling to participate in the RCT were invited to enroll in the observational study. A third arm was to test calcium and vitamin D in another component of the study.

Originally both designs would follow the women for about 9 years. The primary outcome of interest was coronary heart disease incidence with hip and other bone fractures as secondary outcomes. Other outcomes, including breast cancer and mortality, also were studied. The study was double-blinded for 0.625 mg/day of conjugated equine estrogen (CEE) versus placebo for women who had a hysterectomy and 0.625 mg/day of CEE plus 2.5 mg/day of medroxyprogesterone versus placebo for women with an intact uterus. Ten percent of the sample was to be between the ages of 50 and 54, when most women are perimenopausal. Higher proportions of older women were enrolled to maximize the statistical power of the study. Women who were already taking HRT went through a 3-month washout period before being randomized. One interesting observation is that the participants in the two HRT trials were different from one another at baseline. Those in the estrogen-alone trial had more risk factors for cardiovascular disease, including high BMI, history of previous myocardial infarction, stroke, higher blood pressure, and more treatment for hypertension and diabetes. They also had risk factors that reduced the risk for breast cancer, including more with prior hysterectomies and bilateral oophorectomies, fewer nulliparous women and fewer first pregnancies at age 30 and over. Therefore, we cannot compare the trials to one another on a "head-to-head" basis for estrogen-only versus estrogen plus progestin (E+P) (Nelson, 2012).

Cognition in the WHI

The cognition papers were published in four publications in the *Journal of the American Medical Association (JAMA)* for a substudy called the Women's Health Initiative Memory Study (WHIMS). Analyses included one for each treatment: estrogen-only (Shumaker et al., 2004) and estrogen plus progestin (E+P) (Shumaker et al., 2003) with regard to risk for probable dementia and MCI. A second set of analyses focused on global cognitive function [estrogen-only (Espeland et al., 2004) and E+P (Rapp et al., 2003)]. The primary outcome for the first set of analyses was all-cause dementia; MCI and global cognition were secondary outcomes. WHIMS included only women who were age 65 and older (Shumaker et al., 2003). The trial was designed to last 8.5 years, but was discontinued after 5.6 years because women in the E+P arm experienced a higher rate of heart disease, stroke, pulmonary embolism and breast cancer compared with the placebo group. Of 4,894 invited participants in WHI, 4,532 enrolled in WHIMS and 2,229 were randomized to E+P with 1,464 randomized to estrogen only. Intent-to-treat analyses were conducted, but adherence in the two groups was significantly different, with adherence being much better in the placebo group. Over a mean follow-up of about 4 years, the HR for probable dementia (DSM-IV criteria) in the E+P analysis was 2.05 (95% CI = 1.21–3.48), and for MCI, it was 1.07 (95% CI = 0.74–1.55). For the estrogen-only study, the HR for probable dementia over about 5 years of follow-up was 1.49 (95% CI = 0.83–2.66) (n = 47 incident cases) and for MCI it was 1.34 (95% CI = 0.95–1.89) (n = 76 incident cases). Although neither of the point estimates for MCI was statistically significant, the authors pooled the two outcomes and derived a statistically significant HR for either probable dementia or MCI in the estrogen-only trial (HR = 1.38, 95% CI = 1.01–1.89, p = 0.04) and a strong trend of 1.37 (95% CI = 0.99–1.89) in the E+P trial. The numbers of events in the trials were quite small. For E+P, there were between 4 and 11 events each year and for placebo between 2 and 9 events. For MCI, the numbers of incident cases were almost all above 5 but smaller than 18. Thus, all HRs lacked power, except that for E+P and incident probable dementia. No analyses were conducted stratifying on the age at which HRT commenced. When the two treatment arms were compared head-to-head, there was no significant difference in the risk for all-cause dementia, and subsequently, the WHIMS investigators considered both treatments similarly despite their differences (Maki, 2013).

The Modified Mini-Mental State Test (3MSE) (out of 100 points) was used to measure global cognitive function in the WHIMS. The first publication on the combined E+P treatment (Rapp et al., 2003) reported slightly increasing mean 3MSE scores with increasing number of years since randomization in treatment and placebo groups. Using a random effects model, the increase in mean 3MSE total score was attenuated in the treatment group (0.149, SD = 0.021) compared with the placebo group (0.213, SD = 0.02) (p = 0.03). The differences were small and considered clinically insignificant. Timing from the last menstrual period did not affect these results. A clinically important decline on the 3MSE ($\geq$2 SD) was seen in 6.7% of the E+P group and 4.8% of the placebo group (p = 0.008). Despite these small differences, the combined treatment did not *improve* cognition compared with placebo, as originally hypothesized.

In the estrogen-alone trial, similar results were seen. Women in the estrogen-alone group were 1.47 times (95% CI = 1.04–2.07) more likely to experience a 10-point decline in 3MSE scores (>2 SD) than those on placebo. In both trials, women with lower baseline 3MSE scores were especially affected by treatment. No differential treatment effect was seen in women with baseline scores higher than 95/100, but the mean decrement increased with progressively lower baseline 3MSE scores. The largest decrements were seen in women who were below study 3MSE screening cut-points. The authors speculated that these women, though not having probable dementia by study exclusion criteria, may have had an underlying neurodegenerative process that was accelerated by hormone treatment (Espeland et al., 2004). The acceleration of neurodegenerative processes by HRT could be through the proinflammatory effects of CEEs (Straub, 2007). Such a process is more likely to be occurring in older, postmenopausal women.

A subsequent MRI study 3 years after the termination of the E + P trial and 1.4 years after the termination of the estrogen-alone trial showed that women in the treatment arm had smaller brain volumes in the frontal lobe and hippocampus compared with women in the placebo arm. The reduction in brain volume was strongest in women with low cognitive performance on the screening test before randomization (Resnick et al., 2009). One of the explanations advanced by WHIMS investigators was that treatment with E+P increased the vascular burden in the brain in people who already had substantial neurodegeneration (Shumaker et al., 2004).

Beneficial Effects of Estrogen

The results of the WHIMS were surprising to the scientific community. For years, the benefits of estrogen from animal studies had been touted in the literature (see Pike, Carroll, Rosario, & Barron, 2009). For example, animal studies showed that estrogen protects against neuronal loss induced by Aβ through regulation of apoptosis, excitotoxicity, inflammation, and oxidative stress. Its antioxidative effects are regulated through estrogen-receptor pathways, where estrogen acts as a free radical scavenger due to its phenolic structure. Estrogen also may repress reactive glial cell function and increase arborization and synaptogenesis of astrocytes. Of interest, anti-inflammatory benefits of estrogen may be limited to early AD pathology, because estrogen is unable to rescue cells after inflammatory reactions have taken place. However, when estrogen is given prior to inflammatory insults, it can reduce microglial activation. With regard to tau, both estrogen and progesterone can alter kinase and phosphatase activities, which regulate tau phosphorylation activity through glycogen synthase kinase-3β pathways. Most of the effects of estrogen occur through the activation of estrogen receptors, which are distributed throughout the brain, including areas important to AD (hippocampus, frontal cortex, amygdala). Other evidence exists to show that estrogen may attenuate accumulation of amyloid precursor protein (APP) as well as Aβ by promoting the nonamyloidogenic cleavage of APP, and by enhancing clearance of Aβ. Experimental research also shows that although there is some degree of neuroprotection afforded by estrogen in aging animals, its effect is attenuated with increasing age.

Observational epidemiologic studies suggest that estrogen is neuroprotective for the brain. As reviewed in Chapter 7, some incidence studies have shown a higher incidence of AD among women, raising the possibility that hormonal influences, particularly loss of estrogen, may be responsible. Early case-control studies and later cohort studies generally found significantly reduced risk for AD among HRT-exposed women (Henderson, 2010), although studies in which exposures were documented from pharmacy or medical records generally did not find statistically significant inverse associations. Two early meta-analyses (Hogervorst, Williams, Budge, Riedel, & Jolles, 2000; Yaffe, Sawaya, Lieberburg, & Grady, 1998) demonstrated about a 30–40% decreased risk. By 2000, the suggestion that

HRT effects may depend on age (and type of menopause) was advanced. It also was noted that, before the WHIMS results came out, observational studies showed a stronger protective effect compared with the RCTs. The suggestion was made that this might be due to confounding by the healthy-person bias. It is known that women who begin HRT after menopause are healthier (in terms of vascular risk factors, plasma lipids, alcohol consumption, and physical activity), more highly educated, and younger than women who do not go on HRT (Hogervorst et al., 2000). It also is known that healthier women tend to seek out and comply with hormone treatment (Hulley & Grady, 2004). Therefore, healthy-person bias may be at least partially responsible for the inverse association between hormone therapy and dementia and AD seen in observational studies.

The most important weakness in the WHIMS design was the restriction of the study to women aged 65 and over. This restriction was made for logistical reasons. Studying a cohort of younger, perimenopausal women would have required years of follow-up to gain sufficient statistical power for late-life outcomes such as dementia. Because WHIMS was limited to women taking HRT who were many years postmenopausal, the application of its findings regarding dementia risk to women taking HRT at around the time of menopause has been questioned. The Danish Osteoporosis Study randomized women who were 48–55 at baseline and found opposite effects on cardiovascular risk than WHIMS. Although cognition was not assessed in this study, the findings raise the possibility that the effects of HRT may depend on the age at which it is given.

The Critical Window Hypothesis

Proponents of the estrogen hypothesis propose that after menopause, neurons may not be sensitive to sex steroid hormones, and that they must be administered during a "critical window" to achieve benefit (Pike et al., 2009; Whitmer, Quesenberry, Zhou, & Yaffe, 2011). In a review of the critical window hypothesis, Maki (2013) discussed 18 observational studies examining "ever" use of HRT and AD. Most of these were case-control in design and are subject to issues in recall of HRT use. Four were prospective cohort studies, and these showed a significant reduction in AD incidence with ever-use of HRT in the range of 29–44% in meta-analysis. None of these studies showed an *increase* in risk for AD. In the Cache County Study, the inverse association with ever-use of HRT with AD was 0.59 (95% CI = 0.36–0.96). The association was limited to former-users (HR = 0.33, 95% CI = 0.15–0.65). Current HRT use was not associated with AD (HR = 1.08, 95% CI = 0.59–1.91). Women with more than 10 years of HRT use had a similar hazard for AD to men, which attenuated the increased risk associated with being female (Zandi et al., 2002). In this study, the use of multivitamins and calcium supplements were not associated with a reduced risk, which suggests that the inverse association with HRT is likely not explained by healthy-person bias. An editorial on this publication proposed that given rapid depletion of estrogen during the early postmenopausal years, the protective effect found in this study with "ever" use is consistent with a critical period in which HRT is most beneficial (Resnick & Henderson, 2002).

Three studies have specifically examined the critical window hypothesis for HRT and AD. The first was a case-control study from the Multi-Institutional Research in Alzheimer Genetic Epidemiology (MIRAGE) investigators. The study enrolled 532 female probable or definite AD cases and 819 female controls who were first-degree relatives or spouses of cases matched on the year of disease onset in the case (to prevent collection of data after the disease began). Exposure was ascertained by self-report. The OR adjusting for age, education, and ethnicity was statistically significant for the entire sample (OR = 0.70, 95% CI = 0.51–0.95) and for women who took HRT between the ages of 50 and 63 (OR = 0.35, 95% CI = 0.19–0.66). ORs in higher age group tertiles (64–71 and 72–99) were below 1 but were not statistically significant (Henderson et al., 2005). However, several biases, including using proxy informants for cases but not controls and using self-reported or proxy-reported HRT in the analyses may have led to apparent protective effects.

The second study (Whitmer et al., 2011) used a survey conducted in 1964 at a mean age of 49 and pharmacy records at a mean age of 76 to test the midlife versus late-life effect of HRT on dementia. Diagnoses were made by ICD-9 codes (AD and vascular dementia (VaD)) from inpatient and outpatient visits to the Department of Neurology and Neuropsychology and Internal Medicine at Kaiser Permanente medical centers and clinics in Northern California (Whitmer et al., 2011). Of 7,758 women, 1,524 were diagnosed with dementia from 1999 to 2008. Cox proportional hazards models adjusted for age, education, race, BMI, number of children, and co-morbidities found that women taking HRT at midlife (but not in late-life) had a HR of 0.74 (95% CI = 0.58–0.94), while those taking HRT in late-life (but not in midlife) had an increased risk (HR = 1.48, 95% CI = 1.10–1.98). Women who took HRT at both periods in life had a similar risk as nonusers in both periods (HR = 1.02, 95% CI = 0.78–1.34). These results are consistent with the WHIMS trial, which found an increased risk for women who initiated HRT in older age.

The last study was a reanalysis of data from the Cache County Study (Shao et al., 2012). This cohort is characterized by very high use of HRT (62.5% of 1,768 women), with an average age of 73.4 (SD = 5.6) in exposed and 76.7 (SD = 6.9) in unexposed women. While "any" HRT use had an adjusted HR of 0.80, missing statistical significance, HRT (of any type) initiated within 5 years of menopause yielded a HR of 0.70 (95% CI = 0.49–0.99). Unopposed HRT was associated with an HR of 0.70 (95% CI = 0.49–1.01), although statistical power was an issue in the stratified analysis. When unopposed use within 5 years of menopause was analyzed separately, the HR declined to 0.65 (95% CI = 0.43–0.98). In agreement with the WHIMS findings, an increased risk for AD (HR = 1.93, 95% CI = 0.94–3.96) was associated with use within 3 years before the baseline of the study when the women were older than 70 on average. Although healthy-person bias and other confounding could still be a problem in this cohort study, the authors stated that adjustments for confounders affected the point estimates negligibly.

Estrogen, BDNF, and the Cholinergic System

Animal studies have shown that hormones can strongly influence the expression of brain-derived neurotrophic factor (BDNF) (Sohrabji & Lewis, 2006). When estrogen replacement was administered to young adult female rats that had their ovaries removed, the expression of BDNF was increased in the olfactory bulb, hippocampus, cortex, amygdala, and other brain areas. In old female rats without ovaries as well as in gonadectomized male mice, estrogen increased BDNF and other growth factors (nerve growth factor and neurotrophin-3) in the hippocampus. When estrogen was administered acutely or long-term, BDNF mRNA levels increased in select regions of the cortex. However, high endogenous levels of estrogen during the estrus cycle were associated with reduced BDNF mRNA in the hippocampus and prefrontal cortex (Cavus & Duman, 2003; Gibbs, 1998; Sohrabji & Lewis, 2006). Relevant to AD, which is primarily a disease affecting the cholinergic neurotransmitter system, both estrogen and neurotrophins have shared functions in the forebrain. For example, they both regulate choline acetyltransferase and high affinity choline uptake in the forebrain. A critical period has also been suggested in animal experiments. For example, in the forebrain, estrogen replacement increases BDNF and trkB protein expression in young adult rats but not in old female rats (Sohrabji & Lewis, 2006).

Testosterone in Men

In men, androgens (testosterone) have similar actions to estrogen (Pike et al., 2009). A number of case-control studies have found that dementia cases have lower testosterone levels than controls, particularly among older men age 80 and above (Hogervorst, Williams, Budge, Barnetson, Combrinck, & Smith, 2001; Hogervorst, Bandelow, Combrinck, & Smith, 2004; Holland, Bandelow, & Hogervorst, 2011). Several studies found associations between levels of free testosterone (FT) and verbal, visual, and working memory, but others found no association after controlling for age. A curvilinear dose-response effect has been seen between total testosterone (TT) or FT levels and verbal and working memory, attention, and global cognition (Holland et al., 2011). Of six prospective cohort studies reviewed in Holland et al., only two showed positive results between FT and cognitive performance and only change in performance on a visual memory test was associated with incident dementia among men with low FT over time (Moffat et al., 2002). In the MRC Healthy Aging Study

(Hogervorst, Matthews, & Brayne, 2010), optimal TT concentrations at baseline predicted higher MMSE scores after a 2-year follow-up. There is also a suggestion that APOE-ε4 may modify the relationship between testosterone levels and global cognition (Burkhardt et al., 2006). Cognitively healthy older people with one or more ε4 alleles have been shown to have lower TT than those without this allele (Hogervorst, Combrinck, & Smith, 2003).

The "Take Home" Message

What is the "take home" message regarding HRT? The consensus of studies is that HRT when given initially many years after menopause is likely associated with an increased risk for AD and dementia. Conversely, there is strong evidence that HRT given close to the time of menopause is likely to have beneficial effects in reducing dementia risk. However, this effect appears to be time-limited, suggesting that it is probably not useful to continue giving HRT begun around menopause for many years. CEEs may increase neuroinflammation in women with an established Alzheimer pathologic process, a condition that is more likely to be present in later life after menopause. This inflammation could accelerate the formation of neurofibrillary tangles and increase the risk for dementia.

ANTICHOLINERGIC DRUGS AND THE RISK FOR INCIDENT DEMENTIA

Medications with anticholinergic effects are commonly used by older persons. These include antidepressants, antihistaminics, and cardiovascular medications, among others. Short-term administration of anticholinergic drugs is well known to trigger delirium (Moore & O'Keeffe, 1999), but associations with dementia have been less studied. An RCT showed a greater effect on reduced memory performance after acute anticholinergic administration in carriers of the APOE-ε4 allele compared to noncarriers (Pomara, Willoughby, Wesnes, & Sidtis, 2004). In the Three-City Study described in Chapter 15, anticholinergic use was examined as a risk factor for dementia in a 4 year follow-up of 6,912 participants over age 65 (Carriere et al., 2009). Adjusting for age, sex, education, BMI, alcohol and tobacco use, caffeine intake, hypercholesterolemia, APOE-ε4, diabetes, depression, Parkinson's disease, ischemic vascular disease, and hypertension, continuous use of anticholinergic drugs throughout the follow-up period was associated with an increased risk for dementia (HR = 1.65, 95% CI = 1.00–2.73). However, patients who discontinued use of these medications during this period did not show a significant association with dementia (HR = 1.28, 95% CI = 0.59–2.76). These data suggest that anticholinergic use may have compromised cognition sufficiently to disclose underlying disease. Because the duration of usage was unknown in this study, the data do not provide information on the association between long-term usage and dementia or AD risk.

Section IV

Epidemiologic and Biologic Markers

Chapter 20

Prodromal Markers of Disease or Causal Risk Factors? Depression, Olfaction, and Subjective Memory Complaints

We can define two major types of "risk factors," markers of disease (tracking underlying pathology) and causal risk factors (contributing to increased incidence of disease). Causal risk factors and markers manifest in the same way, as a significant Odds Ratio or Relative Risk. How then do we distinguish a marker from a causal risk factor? One way to distinguish causal risk factors from markers would be to reduce the level of the factor and determine whether this reduction affects the frequency of the outcome. Reducing the level of a marker would not be expected to lead to reduced frequency of the outcome, whereas reduction in a causal risk factor should. Unfortunately, this test is difficult to apply to most markers, an exception being depression, one of the three potential markers considered in this chapter.

Markers of pathology by definition should track the underlying pathology of the disease of interest over the life course. However, because the severity of AD pathology cannot be easily tracked, this criterion is often difficult to evaluate. Although amyloid imaging with PiB and CSF Aβ and tau offers the possibility of this type of validation (see Chapter 21), repeat studies within individuals are costly and difficult to perform. One alternative would be to cross-sectionally examine the association between a potential marker and the results of amyloid imaging or CSF markers in groups of participants at different ages, but this strategy offers limited information due to the loss of information about individual trajectories.

Because AD pathology is cumulative, it also might be expected that associations between markers and incident disease would become stronger the closer one gets to a disease. However, this criterion is also satisfied by the causal genetic risk factor, APOE-ε4, which is more strongly associated with dementia than MCI. Clearly, causal risk factors that are not associated with the severity of pathology as

Alzheimer's Disease. DOI: http://dx.doi.org/10.1016/B978-0-12-804538-1.00020-1

indexed by amyloid positron emissions tomography (PET) or autopsy findings are not markers for the disease. For example, as discussed earlier in this book, head circumference is not associated with the severity of AD pathology. Therefore, it is not a biomarker for the underlying disease. However, idea density is associated with the severity of pathology at autopsy and therefore can be considered a marker for the disease. Finally, the issue of biological plausibility, which is a criterion in determining whether a risk factor is likely causal, can be used to help distinguish causal risk factors from markers. It is difficult to imagine how having low idea density would be causally associated with AD pathology, for example, whereas hippocampal volume shrinkage associated with depression could be a risk factor for atrophy, one of the main features of AD pathology.

It is important to note that a variable can be both a marker *and* a causal risk factor at the same time. Depression is a good example. It has generally been shown that midlife depression is associated with about a two-fold increase in risk for AD (Byers, Covinsky, Barnes, & Yaffe, 2012), although the timing of depression associated with increased risk is still being debated in the literature (Barnes et al., 2012). Depression causes stress and cortisol to be released, which can result in hippocampal atrophy (Sapolsky, 2000). Together with neurodegenerative damage, hippocampal atrophy caused by depression can lead to earlier attainment of the clinical threshold for dementia. In addition, depression is associated with vascular risks, possibly contributing to earlier attainment of the dementia threshold. Therefore, depression is likely a causal risk factor for AD, because of its contributions to earlier manifestation (and increased incidence) of disease. Depression may also be a marker, because as patients begin to lose cognitive capabilities, they may have insight into their cognitive failures, resulting in depression. This type of depression generally disappears later in the disease course when such insight is lost.

Another example of a variable that may be a causal risk factor as well as a marker is education. Since education reduces reserve across the life course, it is a causal risk factor. However, it can also be viewed as a marker. As we saw in Chapter 11, children at age 12 who carry an ε4 allele voluntarily leave school earlier than children who do not carry this allele. Since ε4 is the primary genetic risk factor for late-onset AD, the neurodegenerative process in this case may be driving the exposure of lower achieved education.

The other examples that we will discuss in this chapter – olfaction and subjective memory complaints – are likely to be markers rather than causal risk factors. Examples of variables that are causal risk factors and not markers include genes, infarcts, and head/brain size.

DEPRESSION

Using NHANES data 2007–2010, the Centers for Disease Control noted that among people 60 years and over, 5% of men and 7% of women reported current depression. Rates were higher in every other age group, and highest in those age 40–59 (Centers for Disease Control and Prevention, 2012). Estimated prevalence of a *history* of depression in contrast to current depression is higher. In a paper in that estimated the population attributable fractions for seven risk factors (Norton et al., 2014), the prevalence of depression derived from population-based studies (Barnes, 2011) was defined as lifetime occurrence of major depressive disorder using Diagnostic and Statistical Manual (DSM) or International Classification of Diseases (ICD) criteria. According to these criteria, the prevalence of a history of depression was 19.2% in the U.S. and 13.2% globally.

One of the problems in the study of depression as a risk factor for AD is the variability of definitions used in different studies. Depression has been defined as a history of meeting clinical criteria at some point in the past, having been hospitalized for depression, self-reported depression, taking anti-depressants, or meeting a certain cut-point or score on a scale measuring depressive symptomatology. For example, in epidemiologic studies, the score on the Center for Epidemiologic Studies Depression Scale (CES-D) is frequently used. There are different versions of this scale, and epidemiologic studies will generally use a version that is appropriate for the length of the in-person examination in that study so as not to unduly burden subjects. Therefore, the psychometric properties of the same scale may vary from study to study. Due to heterogeneity of the definition of depression, meta-analyses can yield mixed findings. A second problem is the gap between onset of depression and onset of cognitive symptoms, dementia or AD. Does long-standing depression have a direct impact on AD risk or neuropathology, or is depression a prodromal marker?

In 1991, we published a meta-analysis of original data from select case-control studies in collaboration with the EURODEM group in which we reported an OR of 2.44 (95% CI = 1.36–4.36) for depression, which was present only for "late-onset" AD (Jorm et al., 1991). Since that time, there has been an evolving consensus that late-life depression is a risk factor for dementia and its subtypes (AD and vascular dementia (VaD)). In one meta-analysis using scores from depression scales such as the CES-D, the HR for AD was 1.65 (95% CI = 1.42–1.92) (Diniz, Butters, Albert, Dew, & Reynolds, 2013), and in another, it was 1.66 (95% CI = 1.29–2.14) (Gao et al., 2013). In both meta-analyses, RRs were also statistically elevated for VaD, any dementia and MCI, with RRs ranging from 1.55 to 2.52. The median follow-up time in the meta-analyzed studies was only five years. Others have shown only a modest increase in depressive symptoms prior to AD onset. Three years after diagnosis of MCI or AD, depressive symptoms had changed very little (Wilson et al., 2010).

A meta-analysis in 2006 (Ownby, Crocco, Acevedo, John, & Loewenstein, 2006) reported very similar ORs and HRs for case-control (pooled OR = 2.03, 95% CI = 1.73–2.38) and cohort studies (pooled HR = 1.90, 95% CI = 1.55–2.33), despite methodological problems in case-control studies associated with recall and informant report of depressive symptoms and histories. In this article, the authors examined the timing of depression by examining the gap between the diagnosis of depression and diagnosis of dementia. They hypothesized that if the length of the gap were inversely associated with AD risk, i.e., shorter gaps showed stronger associations, this would favor an interpretation of depression being a prodromal marker of AD. Conversely, if the length of the gap were positively associated with AD risk, it would favor the interpretation that depression is a causal risk factor. The data supported a positive association, consistent with depression being a causal risk factor.

In a paper from the Framingham Study published after this meta-analysis, Saczynski and colleagues reported that over a 17-year follow-up period, those who scored 16 or higher on the 20-item CES-D (13% of the sample), consistent with a higher likelihood of depression, were at a 1.76-fold increased risk (95% CI = 1.03–3.01) for incident AD compared with those who scored lower (Saczynski et al., 2010). The statistical significance of the effect depended on the definition of depression. When CES-D ≥16 or the use of antidepressant medication (from medical records) was used, the HR remained elevated but lost statistical significance (HR = 1.57, 95% CI = 0.94–2.62). To examine reverse causality, the investigators excluded participants with possible MCI, and in the smaller sample, the HR for AD was statistically significant regardless of the definition of depression. The results changed little when vascular risk factors, smoking, alcohol consumption and APOE-ε4 were adjusted in addition to age, sex and education. However, these investigators did not adjust for other potential confounders, such as diet, physical activity, social engagement and sleep patterns. Duration of depression or adherence to anti-depressant medications also were not assessed.

In the CHS Cognition Study, depressive symptoms were assessed for incident MCI using the 10-item CES-D, and classified as no depressive symptoms (0–2 points), low (3–7 points) and moderate or high (≥8 points). Four U.S. communities, including 2,220 subjects participated and incident MCI was ascertained over a six-year follow-up. MCI was diagnosed if subjects had a baseline Modified Mini-Mental State Test (3MS) score of at least 90 (of 100) in 1992–3 and at follow-up in 1998 did not show dementia but demonstrated "poor cognitive function that reflected a decline from a prior level" (Barnes, Alexopoulos, Lopez, Williamson, & Yaffe, 2006). After adjustment for demographic variables and vascular disease seen on MRI, there remained a strong dose-response association between the category of depressive symptoms and the risk for MCI, with the full model showing an OR of about 2.0 for the highest category of depressive symptoms compared to the lowest category, and the middle category an OR of about 1.4 (both were statistically significant).

At the Mayo Clinic in Rochester, MN over a shorter follow-up period of 3.5 years, 840 clinic-based patients from the Alzheimer's Disease Patient Registry were assessed for depression on the short Geriatric Depression Scale, and those who scored six points or higher were compared to the non-depressed cohort (Geda et al., 2006) for risk of MCI. A similar strength of association with MCI was noted (HR = 2.2, 95% CI = 1.2–4.1), adjusting for age, sex and education, and treating dementia as a competing risk. Interestingly, these investigators found a multiplicative interaction between APOE genotype (ε3ε3 versus ε3ε4) and depression (HR = 5.1, 95% CI = 1.9–13.6) for MCI risk. However, an earlier study of late-onset depression in 142 veteran twins did not find any interaction with APOE-ε4 (Steffens et al., 1997). That study also found decreasing RRs with increasing intervals between the onset of depression and AD, indicating that the association was more likely prodromal.

That similar magnitudes of risk exist for the conversion from MCI to dementia has likewise been found in smaller and more selected samples of depressed and non-depressed participants (Modrego & Ferrandez, 2004) (Gabryelewicz et al., 2007) as well as in population-based samples (e.g., in the Kungsholmen Study) (Palmer et al., 2007).

Depression and Hippocampal Volume

A meta-analysis (Koolschijn, van Haren, Lensvelt-Mulders, Hulshoff Pol, & Kahn, 2009) reported large reductions in volume in frontal regions of the brain, particularly in the anterior cingulate and orbitofrontal cortex, associated with depression. Moderate reductions were observed in the hippocampus, putamen and caudate nucleus. The ages of the individuals in the studies that were meta-analyzed were not discussed, except that participants were over age 18. If these studies contained many older people, the possibility cannot be excluded that many of them would have dementia, which would be an important confounder of the depression-hippocampal volume association and not adjusting for this would overestimate the association. Another publication (Vythilingam et al., 2002) pointed out that severe stress in early life has been associated with smaller hippocampal volumes, and in their study, left (but not right) hippocampal volume was significantly reduced by 18% only among women with current major depression who also were severely abused as children for a protracted amount of time. Women who were depressed but not abused had similar mean left hippocampal volumes as healthy non-depressed women.

It is known that stressful life events elevate the risk for depression (Kendler, Karkowski, & Prescott, 1999) and it is believed that mechanisms such as overproduction of glucocorticoids due to stress underlie changes in structure in the hippocampus due to depression (Sapolsky, 2000). Such stress induces dendritic retraction and neuronal death, in addition to suppression of neurogenesis. Use of anti-depressants, or recovery from depression, conversely, can reverse this atrophy, presumably through growth of existing neurons and increased neurogenesis. In the laboratory, mid- to old-age animals, who already have lower levels of neurogenesis, are particularly susceptible to the effects of stress. Therefore, it is possible that a chains-of-risk or accumulation model of stress throughout the life course applies to a common pathway of brain atrophy, in which age also plays a role. Although the exact mechanisms responsible for the reduced hippocampal size in depressed patients are unknown, it is unlikely that it is due to massive neuronal loss or reduced adult neurogenesis, since this would have to be extreme to result in a 10–15% loss of hippocampal size that is typically seen in depression (Czeh & Lucassen, 2007). Other mechanisms, such as loss of connectivity and shrinkage of the neuropil are likely responsible. Czeh and Lucassen conclude that "depression is a disorder of neuroplasticity and cellular resistance, and not a neurodegenerative disease" (Czeh & Lucassen, 2007). This is important for our discussion, because this would imply that depression acts as a risk factor for the clinical expression of AD but does not affect AD neuropathology. This view is supported by findings from the Religious Orders Study that neither the amount of depressive symptomatology nor changes in depressive symptoms over an eight-year follow-up period were associated with any AD neuropathologic measure (Wilson et al., 2014). There may be a modest increase in depressive symptomatology prior to disease onset, but this is transient, and does not appear to persist as the disease progresses into its middle stages (Wilson et al., 2010).

Using the RR from the meta-analysis by Gao et al. (2013), which was considered more comprehensive than that by Diniz et al. (2013), Population Attributable Fraction (PAFs) were calculated for depression, adjusting for midlife hypertension and obesity, physical inactivity, diabetes and smoking (Norton et al., 2014). In the U.S., the PAF for AD associated with depression (at any time point) was estimated to be 11.1% (95% CI = 7.5–15%), in comparison with 10.7% in Europe (95% CI = 7.2–14.5%) and 7.9% (95% CI = 5.3–10.8%) globally. While few studies are able to specifically distinguish between early- and late-onset depression, studies with relatively few years of follow-up, as well as those with longer follow-up, support the role of depression in the etiology of AD. Whereas in earlier life depression may act as a risk factor for clinical expression of disease, in later life it may accompany the emergence of AD symptoms and be a prodromal marker as well.

OLFACTION

Loss of the sense of smell is common with increasing age, with an estimated prevalence of about 14% in people over age 65 and a higher prevalence in men (Schubert et al., 2012). As early as the early 1980s, it was recognized that AD plaques and neurofibrillary tangles as well as cell loss are numerous in the anterior olfactory nuclei in autopsied patients with AD (Averback, 1983) (Esiri & Wilcock, 1984). The CA1 and CA3 regions of the hippocampus are early targets of AD and are actively engaged in odor recognition memory processing. Olfactory receptors are ciliated nerve cells that project to the olfactory bulb. Preliminary olfactory processing occurs in the olfactory bulb on the inferior surface of the frontal lobe. The next stage of processing occurs in the primary olfactory cortex, located in the medial temporal lobe and the amygdala, which projects to the entorhinal cortex and CA1 and CA3 areas of the hippocampus.

The first case-control comparison of olfaction using a standardized test, the 40-item University of Pennsylvania Smell Identification Test (UPSIT, higher scores are better), showed that among 17 early-stage AD cases from a Veterans Administration Medical Center, the mean score was 20.5 (±7.4) versus 30.2 (±6.9) among 17 age- and sex-matched controls ($p < 0.001$) (Warner, Peabody, Flattery, & Tinklenberg, 1986). In 1987, Doty and colleagues reported from a small matched case-control study of prevalent AD that cases not only had lower UPSIT scores compared with controls, but that their odor threshold also was much higher ($p < 0.001$) (Doty, Reyes, & Gregor, 1987), i.e., they were unable to detect the odor until the concentration of the odor was higher.

The most common type of olfactory identification tests are scratch-and-sniff tests in which the subject or an interviewer scratches off an embedded microencapsulated scent and the subject states what the scent smelled like using a multiple choice response format, e.g., four different scents, such as fruit, cinnamon, wood, or coconut. The most widely used scratch-and-sniff test is the 40-item UPSIT developed by Doty (Doty, Shaman, Kimmelman, & Dann, 1984), for which reference scores based on over 4,000 normal individuals are available by age and sex. The normal UPSIT score for people in their 60s is about 37, declining to 34 in the 70s and 26 in the 80s (Doty, Shaman, Applebaum, et al., 1984). Another way to test olfaction is by testing the lowest level at which a stimulus can be detected. This method is rarely used in epidemiologic studies of AD, mainly because the UPSIT and its modifications are more convenient for research use. However, correct administration of the UPSIT is necessary so that the test remains one of olfaction and not of memory, i.e., it is important that the subject has a way to continuously view all possible choices so they do not have to recall the interviewer's stated choices. In our research, we always use a show card listing all possibilities for the subject to refer to before having to make their final choice.

That olfactory threshold tests are associated with the stage of AD has also been shown. Olfactory dysfunction appears to track with disease severity (Murphy, Gilmore, Seery, Salmon, & Lasker, 1990) (Serby, Larson, & Kalkstein, 1991) and reduction in detection acuity occurs after reduction in identification acuity (Graves et al., 1999). However, the presence of olfactory deficits is not unique to AD. It has been found in many other neurodegenerative disorders, including idiopathic Parkinson's disease, Huntington's chorea, Korsakoff's syndrome, frontal-temporal dementia, the parkinsonian-dementia complex of Guam, multiple sclerosis and amyotrophic lateral sclerosis (Mesholam, Moberg, Mahr, & Doty, 1998) (Doty, Li, Mannon, & Yousem, 1997). However, worsening of olfaction with severity of the clinical illness does not appear to occur with most other diseases, such as Parkinson's (Mesholam et al., 1998).

Despite the lack of specificity of olfactory deficits in AD, several other findings indicate that it may be a good marker for its underlying pathology. In one study, 28 first-degree relatives of AD patients over age 65 were compared with 28 controls recruited from senior citizen centers or from spouses of the AD patients of the same age. Controls were individually matched to a first-degree relative by age, sex and Mini-Mental State Examination (MMSE) score (Serby et al., 1996). The mean UPSIT score in the first-degree relatives was 31.93 (±5.94) and in the controls, 35.43 (±4.04). The authors also noted that 28% of the first-degree relatives scored below 30 (of 40), the optimum cut-score, and that 25–30% of these first-degree relatives would develop AD in their 80s if they lived that long, indicating that olfactory dysfunction may be a very early sign of disease expression (Mohs, Breitner, Silverman, & Davis, 1987). In the Beaver Dam Offspring Study, a study of sensory disorders and aging in which participants were 2,837 adult children of people enrolled in the population-based Epidemiology of Hearing Loss Study, the San Diego Odor Identification test (SDOIT) was used. This test has eight odorants (Schubert et al., 2013). Among middle-aged participants aged 35–64 ($n = 2,403$, mean age 49), olfactory deficits were associated with poorer performance on three cognitive tests: Trail Making-A, Trail Making-B, and the Grooved Pegboard test, all tests of processing speed. Although the differences were not clinically large (a mean of 4–12 seconds), they were statistically significant and suggest that worse performance on odor identification in midlife may already be associated with differences in cognitive ability.

The association between performance on a short version of the UPSIT called the B-SIT was compared with the severity of AD pathology in 77 deceased participants of the Rush Memory and Aging Program (Wilson, Arnold, Schneider, Tang, & Bennett, 2007). After adjusting for age, sex and education, it was found that over 12% of the variation in odor identification could be attributed to a composite measure of AD neuropathology. Tau tangle density decreased with increasing numbers of correct points on the B-SIT and the association was particularly strong for the entorhinal cortex and the CA1 region and subiculum of the hippocampus. However, performance on the B-SIT was not associated with tangle density in other regions of the cerebral cortex. These results suggest that poor olfactory performance is due in part to the accumulation of tangle pathology in areas central to olfactory processing in the brain, which are among the first to be affected in AD.

The first study to longitudinally examine the association between olfaction and cognitive decline was the *Kame* Project (Graves et al., 1999). At baseline, we administered a 12-item test modified and harmonized to the Japanese culture by Dr. Doty (the Cross-Cultural Smell Identification Test (CC-SIT)) (Figure 20.1). This test has good test-retest reliability ($r = 0.71$) (Doty, Marcus, & Lee, 1996). Cognitive decline was defined as a decline on the CASI of greater than 5.15/100 points in two years. Of 1,836 non-demented participants at baseline, 1,604 were re-screened with the CASI at two-year follow-up. Compared with normosmics (individuals with no olfaction abnormality), the OR for cognitive decline, adjusted for age, sex, education, smoking, baseline CASI score and length of follow-up, was 1.25 (95% CI = 0.83–1.89) for microsmics (some impaired olfaction) and 1.92 (95% CI = 1.06–3.47) for anosmics (those with

OLFACTION TEST					
Now I will be testing your sense of smell. I will scratch the surface of the scent strip and hand it to you. Smell the area and select the scent you think it is. Make your best guess.					
(A)	1: fruit	2: cinnamon	3: woody	4: coconut	9: Don't know
(B)	1: turpentine	2: soap	3: dog	4: black pepper	9: Don't know
(C)	1: motor oil	2: garlic	3: rose	4: lemon	9: Don't know
(D)	1: apple	2: grass	3: smoke	4: grape	9: Don't know
(E)	1: lemon	2: chocolate	3: strawberry	4: black pepper	9: Don't know
(F)	1: mint	2: rose	3: lime	4: fruit	9: Don't know
(G)	1: watermelon	2: peanut	3: rose	4: paint thinner	9: Don't know
(H)	1: banana	2: garlic	3: cherry	4: motor oil	9: Don't know
(I)	1: smoke	2: whiskey	3: pineapple	4: onion	9: Don't know
(J)	1: rose	2: lemon	3: apple	4: gasoline	9: Don't know
(K)	1: soap	2: black pepper	3: chocolate	4: peanut	9: Don't know
(L)	1: chocolate	2: banana	3: onion	4: fruit	9: Don't know

FIGURE 20.1 Choices on the 12-item Cross-Cultural Smell Identification Test (CC-SIT), *Kame* Project forms (Doty, Marcus & Lee, 1996).

complete loss of smell). In our analysis, there was a strong interaction with APOE-ε4, with carriers of this allele showing much greater decline, implying that loss of olfaction among genetically at-risk individuals is more important for cognitive decline than those who are not at genetic risk. Others (Murphy, Bacon, Bondi, & Salmon, 1998) have found that ε4 carriers perform worse on olfactory tests than non-carriers, although one study of old twins and singletons did not find this (Doty, Petersen, Mensah, & Christensen, 2011).

Subsequent work from the parent study of older adults in Beaver Dam, Wisconsin (the Epidemiology of Hearing Loss Study, EHLS) examined five-year incident cognitive impairment, defined as a score of less than 24 of 30 on the MMSE or a self- or proxy-report of AD or dementia when an MMSE score was unavailable, in relation to olfactory scores on the SDOIT test among 1,920 participants (Schubert et al., 2008). Those with olfactory impairments were 3.33 fold (95% CI = 2.04–5.42) more likely to show five-year incident cognitive impairment. Given that the SDOIT has only eight odorants and the definition of the outcome was less rigorous than desired, the results from this study suggest a strong association with future cognitive impairment.

Few studies have examined olfactory performance in relation to clinical dementia outcomes. The Rush Memory and Aging Program reported that over a 5.5 year follow-up (mean = 2.7, SD = 1.4), 155 of 471 participants developed MCI, and each higher point of 12 points on the baseline B-SIT score predicted an HR for MCI of 0.87 (95% CI 0.81–0.94) (Wilson et al., 2009). This effect measure was adjusted for APOE-ε4 and performance on an episodic memory task. In a mixed-effects model predicting a composite episodic memory measure, adjusting for age, sex, education, ε4 and initial level of episodic memory, lower olfactory scores predicted a faster decline than higher scores ($p < 0.001$). They also predicted a higher level of AD pathology in a subsample of 34 people who died without cognitive impairment, suggesting that impaired olfaction is an early marker for underlying AD pathology in people who do not yet have the clinical disease.

In the *Kame* Project, among 116 incident probable or possible AD cases, baseline CC-SIT scores were 7.3 (SD = 2.9) out of 12, and 9.3 (SD = 2.4) for 1,717 unaffected individuals. Adjusting for age, sex and education, APOE-ε4 and baseline CASI score, individuals who were microsmic at baseline had a 1.92 (95% CI = 1.00–3.67) increased risk for AD, and those who were anosmic at baseline had a 2.55 (95% CI = 1.08–6.04) increased risk (Graves & Wu, 2002). Deficits in olfaction also predict the transition from normal cognition to MCI (Wilson et al., 2009) and from MCI to AD (Devanand et al., 2000).

The association between regional brain volumes and olfactory deficits has been explored in one study in which hippocampal volume, but not entorhinal cortex volume, correlated with 40-item UPSIT scores ($p < 0.0001$ and 0.45, respectively) (Devanand et al., 2010). Another study that investigated associations between amyloid PET scan findings and olfactory dysfunction found no differences with regard to olfactory performance between aMCI patients who were Aβ-positive and Aβ-negative on such scans (Bahar-Fuchs et al., 2010). This may have been due to small sample size or could have reflected that fact that neurofibrillary tangles play a more important role than amyloid plaques in olfaction. The Harvard Brain Aging Study cross-sectionally examined correlations between hippocampal volumes and entorhinal cortex (EC) thickness from MRI, amyloid burden using PiB PET, and UPSIT-40 scores among 215 cognitively normal older individuals residing in the community (Growdon et al., 2015). In crude models, amyloid burden was marginally associated with UPSIT-40 scores ($p = 0.06$), hippocampal volume ($p < 0.0001$) and EC thickness ($p = 0.003$). In multivariate analyses, those who were amyloid positive showed a strong association between thinner EC and poorer olfactory performance ($p = 0.004$), with no association found between EC thickness and olfaction among amyloid negative individuals. Therefore, in this study, performance in olfactory identification was associated with biologic markers of neurodegeneration.

An interesting question is to what extent does olfaction predict incident AD alone and in combination with other epidemiologic markers? To examine this, we can use the area under the curve (AUC) calculated from receiver-operator characteristic (ROC) curves to look at the performance of olfaction (a continuous variable by virtue of its score) and other variables in discriminating between incident AD cases and individuals who did not develop AD. If the marker does no better than chance in discriminating the case from the control group, the AUC from an ROC analysis will be 0.50. In a logistic regression model in which we included age, sex, education, APOE-ε4, baseline CASI score and olfaction, the AUC for seven-year incident AD for APOE-ε4 alone was 0.61 (95% CI = 0.54–0.68). For olfaction alone, it was 0.68 (95% CI = 0.60–0.76). With all six variables included, the composite AUC was 0.83 (95% CI = 0.76–0.89) (Borenstein, 2002, unpublished data). The high degree of accuracy in predicting future dementia suggests that easily obtained markers in epidemiologic studies, including olfaction, can be used to distinguish individuals who will develop AD from those who will not (Chapter 22). Although biomarkers, derived from CSF analyses and from PET and MRI analyses are likely to be slightly more predictive, they require more invasive procedures and are more expensive to obtain.

SUBJECTIVE MEMORY COMPLAINTS

Meta-memory is the ability of a person to have insight into or be aware of the status of their own memory. Other terms for meta-memory include anosgnosia, disordered awareness, subjective memory complaints (SMC), subjective cognitive complaints and subjective cognitive impairment. In this chapter, we will use SMC to refer to the awareness of individuals that there is something wrong with their memory. In Chapter 1, we noted Dr Alzheimer's description of August D. that she was "unable to understand her situation." Loss of episodic memory is the early hallmark neuropsychological signature of AD related to neuropathologic lesions in the hippocampus (Hyman, Van Hoesen, Damasio, & Barnes, 1984). However, there appears to be a large variability between people in meta-memory, which is as yet not completely understood. Some of this variability may be explained by concomitant depression, premorbid personality characteristics, and coping styles, as well as the extent of interactions with other people (Consentino, Metcalfe, Butterfield, & Stern, 2007). Although most people who develop dementia will recognize that their memory and cognitive function is declining in the early stages, the positive predictive value (PPV) of SMC may not be high, since many people complain about their memory and do not go on to develop the disease, or they do not complain until after they express clinical symptoms. On the other hand, the negative predictive value (NPV) may not be that high either, since there will likely be many people who will develop dementia but deny their symptoms (Table 20.1). Denial of symptoms may also be culturally dependent. A meta-analysis of the PPV and NPV from studies conducted up to 2008 found that for SMC and a clinical diagnosis of MCI, the pooled PPV was 31.4% and the NPV was 86.9%, based on a prevalence of MCI of 16.8% (Mitchell, 2008).

There has been much variability in how SMC is measured. Some studies have used single questions, others have used validated questionnaires that include several questions, and still others were based on physician questioning of the patient and informant. Complaints have been elicited through many different questionnaires, including meta-memory, instrumental activities of daily living (IADL) function, as well as validated and non-validated complaints questionnaires (Roberts, Clare, & Woods, 2009). To the extent that studies have consistently found effects when both exposure (SMC) and outcome (MCI or other cognitive tests/decline/impairment) are non-uniformly defined bodes well for the validity of the existence of this association. On the other hand, lack of standardization of definitions of SMC and outcomes means that the results of meta-analyses may be difficult to interpret.

TABLE 20.1 Positive and Negative Predictive Values for Subjective Memory Complaints and Incident Dementia

	Incident Dementia	No Incident Dementia
Subjective memory complaints	a	b
No subjective memory complaints	c	d

Positive predictive value = a/a+ b.Negative predictive value = d/c+ d.

In addition to understanding the predictive value of SMCs for incipient MCI or AD, other interesting questions about SMC include whether individuals can detect meta-memory problems *before* objective cognitive testing demonstrates impairment, and whether SMCs are related to underlying AD neuropathology.

In Chapter 2, we described the clinical criteria for MCI. The first criterion is that the patient and the informant have a "memory complaint." This is appropriate for potential MCI cases that come into a clinic in a passive case-identification approach. However, in epidemiologic studies of communities, the investigators are actively screening populations to detect all the cases in that sample. Thus, for example, in the Three City Study in France only 18% of individuals had a memory concern (Auriacombe et al., 2010), compared with 100% in clinic-based studies where SMC is required to meet MCI criteria (Petersen, 2010). Petersen has argued convincingly that patients coming to medical attention voluntarily will generally be in a more advanced clinical stage than individuals who are recruited directly from the community (Petersen, 2009). Therefore, it may make sense in population-based epidemiologic studies to drop this criterion from the definition of MCI. Others contend that SMC requirements for MCI can lead to misclassification of MCI subjects. For example, in the Alzheimer's Disease Neuroimaging Initiative (ADNI), there was no association between SMC and objective cognitive performance, but SMC was associated with depression (Edmonds et al., 2014). The ADNI sample is a highly educated, primarily white group of volunteers, so these results may not be applicable in population-based studies that include other ethnic groups. In the Nurses' Health Study, strong dose-response associations were found between worsening cognitive performance and increasing numbers of a total of seven memory complaints, adjusting for age and depressive symptoms ($p < 0.001$) (Amariglio, Townsend, Grodstein, Sperling, & Rentz, 2011). The fact that SMC and level of education, depression and other comorbid conditions are closely linked requires that confounding be tightly controlled in studies of SMC and dementia. This can be difficult if the variables are highly intercorrelated.

The validity of SMC in predicting incipient AD has been questioned. Some studies find that SMCs precede cognitive decline or dementia, while others find that they are associated more with depression, anxiety and neuroticism (Jorm,

Christensen, Korten, Jacomb, & Henderson, 2001). Many of these studies were limited by their methodology. For example, they may have been cross-sectional in design, excluded individuals with objective cognitive impairment or lacked a comparison group (Schofield, Marder, et al., 1997). In a registry study of patients from Northern Manhattan, individuals reporting new SMCs over a one-year follow-up were 4.5 times more likely (95% CI = 1.3–15.4) to have questionable dementia or dementia and to decline on the Visual Recognition Test ($p = 0.01$) and the Delayed Recall Test ($p = 0.05$) (Schofield, Jacobs, Marder, Sano, & Stern, 1997). However, it does not appear that these results were adjusted for depressive symptoms.

In Amsterdam, the AMSTEL Study followed over 4,000 participants in 1990–1991 and asked a single question about memory complaints, "Do you have complaints with your memory?" Answers were coded as no, sometimes but is no problem, yes and is a problem, and yes and is a serious problem (Geerlings, Jonker, Bouter, Ader, & Schmand, 1999). Three years later, a two-phase design identified dementia cases using DSM-IV criteria. Because time-to-the-event was short, the authors used multivariate logistic regression for incident dementia. Even though only one question was used to ascertain SMC, complaints were present in a relatively small proportion of the cohort (10.8%). SMCs were more common in older versus younger cohort members, but the crude OR was not significantly elevated for depression (present versus absent, OR = 1.41, 95% CI = 0.73–2.71). People with lower education were more than twice as likely to report SMC (OR = 2.14, 95% CI = 1.32–3.46). In analyses adjusted for age, sex, education and depression, SMCs were associated with incident AD (OR = 1.95, 95% CI = 1.07–3.53) and in models stratified for initial cognition, the association was present only among those with normal cognition at baseline. This strength of association (about a doubling of the risk with impaired SMC) is consistent with other population-based cohort studies of dementia (Borenstein, 2005) (Palmer, Backman, Winblad, & Fratiglioni, 2003). The authors concluded that their results suggest that SMCs may precede the discovery of impairment from objective cognitive testing. This would imply that it is one of the first and most subtle symptoms of the disease and might be useful for early detection. In earlier studies of SMC and incident dementia or AD, the inclusion of subjects with MCI did not permit determination of whether memory complaints preceded this earlier manifestation of impending dementia. The utility of SMC as a marker for AD would be increased if it could be shown that memory complaints precede the earliest signs of AD, i.e., that they can be detected before onset of MCI.

Several studies have examined SMC as a risk factor for incident MCI. In the Massachusetts Alzheimer's Disease Research Center, 559 individuals were recruited from the community and from specialty clinics into a longitudinal study begun in 2005 (Donovan et al., 2014). SMC was defined as cognitively normal individuals with self- or informant-reported cognitive complaints who did not meet criteria for MCI because of normal performance on neuropsychological testing. The study compared 338 normal controls without SMC to 65 participants with SMC. Those with an SMC diagnosis at baseline had a four-fold risk for progressing to MCI compared with normal controls without this complaint (HR = 4.1, 95% CI = 2.1–7.7).

Investigators from PAQUID used a nested case-control study of 350 incident cases and 350 unaffected controls matched by age (±5 years), sex and education to examine the trajectory of cognitive, functional, and depressive instruments over a 14-year follow-up before AD diagnosis (Amieva et al., 2008). SMCs were measured by a questionnaire that asked participants to rate their level of cognitive difficulty with forgetfulness in daily tasks, learning new information and finding words. Seven to eight years prior to the onset of dementia, SMCs of those who developed dementia diverged significantly from those who did not develop dementia. Changes in scores on neuropsychological tests (objective impairments) were evident somewhat earlier or about the same time as SMC.

In the Biologically Resilient Adults in Neurological Studies (BRAiNS) at the University of Kentucky's Alzheimer's Disease Center, the authors measured risk factors for incident SMC, MCI, dementia or death without dementia in 531 volunteers, half of whom came to autopsy (Kryscio et al., 2014). All participants were cognitively intact at study baseline, and transitions using a semi-Markov model described the movement of participants through SMC, MCI, dementia and to death. SMC was measured by asking only one question at each examination: "Have you noticed any change in memory since your last visit?" The date at which the participant endorsed this question with "Yes" was the date of SMC diagnosis. Over a mean of 10 annual follow-ups, 80% of the participants entered the SMC state. Of these, subsequent annual queries confirmed 70%. Clinically, "incident" SMC increased the odds for developing MCI or dementia (compared with the transition to death, which was used because of competing risks) with an OR = 2.8 (95% CI = 1.9–4.2). From entry into the cohort, it took a mean of 8.3 years for subjects to endorse a change in their memory since the last visit; the transition from SMC to MCI took a mean of 9.2 years; an additional 2.9 years occurred before the transition from MCI to dementia. This study supports the notion that SMC is a precursor of MCI and identifies a "pre-MCI" stage of disease.

If SMCs indeed represent the beginning of a pre-MCI stage, the identification of individuals with SMCs could be used to enrich samples for outcomes in clinical trials. Because there will always be a substantial misclassification of SMCs (false-positives as well as false-negatives), observations of associations between biomarkers and SMC would bolster the argument that SMCs are in fact predictive of the evolution of dementia.

Subjective Memory Complaints and Pathology

In the Rush Memory and Aging Project (Barnes, Schneider, Boyle, Bienias, & Bennett, 2006), SMCs were assessed by two questions, each rated on a 5-point

Likert scale: 1) How often do you have trouble remembering things? (very often to never) and 2) How is your memory compared to 10 years ago (much worse to much better)? The answers to these questions were summed to create a composite score. Mean age at death was 89.9 among AD cases ($n = 23$), and 86.1 among non-AD cases ($n = 67$); about half were women. Linear regression predicting SMC scores showed statistically significant associations for a composite measure of AD pathology ($p = 0.002$), which remained significant after adjustment for depressive symptoms and chronic health problems ($p = 0.003$ and 0.006, respectively). Furthermore, significant associations were seen for both amyloid ($p = 0.01$) and tangles ($p < 0.001$). When the analysis was restricted to non-demented persons, the association between SMC and pathology remained ($p = 0.05$). When demented persons were analyzed separately, there was *no* association with the composite measure of pathology ($p = 0.44$) or with amyloid ($p = 0.12$), but there was with tangles ($p = 0.02$). These results suggest that older persons without dementia can have insight into an underlying pathological process.

A similar finding was reported from the Honolulu-Asia Aging Study (Jorm et al., 2004), based on four questions about memory (ability to remember the names of people you have just met; faces of people you have just met, names of close friends and relatives, and appointments correctly) scored on a Likert scale (definitely, slightly improved; no change; slightly or definitely deteriorated). Of 3,734 Japanese American men aged 71–93 in 1991–1993, 237 who had died and come to autopsy were included in this analysis. SMCs were averaged across the four items and scores ≥4 were categorized as having complaints. Prediction of neuropathologic diagnoses for AD by CERAD criteria or by NIA-Reagan Institute (RI) criteria yielded similar adjusted ORs (about 3.0 for CERAD and about 5.0 for NIA-RI, adjusted for age, education, depression and CASI score).

In the BRAiNs study that we discussed above (Kryscio et al., 2014), 243 of 531 participants came to autopsy. The investigators created four groups of SMC individuals among those who had died: 1) those without SMC and cognitive impairment ($n = 56$), 2) those with SMC but no cognitive impairment ($n = 120$), 3) those without SMC but cognitively impaired ($n = 17$) and 4) those with both SMC and cognitive impairment ($n = 50$). Among cognitively normal participants, those with SMCs had higher mean neuritic plaques (NP) in the medial temporal lobe and neocortex ($p < 0.03$ for both regions). Among those with SMCs, mean NP and NFT counts were lower in those who were cognitively unimpaired compared with those who were impaired ($p < 0.001$ in the same regions). The proportion of autopsies rated at CERAD NP levels 3 and 4 increased from 23.2% in those with neither SMC nor cognitive impairment, to 36.7% in those with SMC but without cognitive impairment, to 58.8% in those without SMC who were cognitively impaired, and to 76% in those with both SMC and cognitive impairment. This "dose-response" effect is consistent with an evolution from normality to awareness of cognitive impairment to objective cognitive impairment.

Does SMC add to the predictive power of APOE-ε4 in identifying individuals who will cognitively decline over time? Dik et al. in the population-based Longitudinal Aging Study in Amsterdam reported that the combined effect of SMC and APOE-ε4 was additive in predicting the slope of cognitive change over six years compared with people who had neither risk factor (Dik et al., 2001).

Studies have also looked at how biomarkers differ among SMC positive and SMC negative individuals. A study from New York University (Mosconi et al., 2008) examined cerebral metabolic rates for glucose with FDG-PET in 13 cognitively normal ε4 carriers and 15 cognitively normal non-carriers in their 50s and 60s. About half in each group reported significant SMCs. Even with the small sample size, significantly lower metabolic rates in the parietotemporal and parahippocampal gyrus were seen in those who reported SMC in comparison with those who did not.

In a case-control comparison of 20 SMC subjects and 28 controls, those with SMCs had smaller left hippocampal volumes compared with controls ($p < 0.01$) (van der Flier et al., 2004). One potential explanation for this difference is the presence of depression, which was not adjusted due to small sample size. Similar findings in 14 controls, 12 SMC cases, 15 MCI and 13 AD cases were observed for the entorhinal cortex (EC), with EC volumes being smaller in SMC cases compared with controls (Jessen et al., 2006). Volume reduction was greatest in AD, followed by MCI and then SMC cases. This study also reported smaller volumes in the left hippocampus in the SMC group, but this was not quite statistically significant ($p = 0.07$). Entorhinal cortical volumes were 18% smaller and hippocampal volumes 6% smaller in SMC cases.

Other studies have shown effect-modification of the association between SMC and dementia with stronger associations evident in those with higher education (van Oijen, de Jong, Hofman, Koudstaal, & Breteler, 2007) (Borenstein, 2005), higher intelligence (Merema, Speelman, Kaczmarek, & Foster, 2012), female sex (Peres et al., 2011) and higher baseline cognitive scores (Borenstein, 2005), as well as in those of younger age (Wang et al., 2004). These subgroups may be more sensitive to detecting changes in their memory and cognitive function.

In summary, SMC is likely to be a useful marker for early identification of risk of impending MCI and AD. It appears to identify risk at about the same time or earlier than changes in objective neuropsychological performance. It is important to note that at baseline, data on change in cognitive performance are not available for individuals, and one must rely on whether individual scores on a neuropsychological test fall within the normal range or outside of that range. SMC may offer very useful information on AD risk in individuals who are scoring low but are not yet cognitively impaired. Because of high rates of false positives, SMC is most likely to be of benefit when combined with other risk factors and markers, such as APOE-ε4 status, olfactory function and objective cognitive assessment.

Chapter 21

Fluid, Imaging, and Cognitive Biomarkers

Biomarkers are measurable indicators of the presence or severity of disease pathology that can be observed during life or at autopsy. In Chapter 4 we considered biomarkers observed at autopsy, those which define Alzheimer's disease (AD) neuropathologically. Other biomarkers for Alzheimer pathology include genes (Chapter 10), linguistic indicators (idea density, Chapter 11), early signs of the disease, including depression, olfactory dysfunction, and subjective memory complaints (Chapter 20), and unexplained weight loss (Chapter 14).

In this chapter, we will consider fluid, imaging, and cognitive biomarkers that can be observed during life. Such biomarkers serve two purposes. First, they can improve differential diagnosis in symptomatic individuals, and second they can provide preclinical indicators of the presence of underlying disease pathology in asymptomatic people. In this chapter, we will focus on the latter. Early detection of AD by biomarkers is very important, because by the time this illness is clinically diagnosed a great deal of brain damage has already occurred and the probability of successful treatment is likely to be markedly reduced.

An ideal biomarker used for detection of preclinical disease will have both high sensitivity and high specificity, preferably long before the first symptoms appear. Presently, the closest approximations to such markers are cerebrospinal fluid (CSF) assays of $A\beta_{1-42}$ and tau, positron emission tomography (PET) scans for detecting aggregated Aβ in the brain, and atrophy of key regions affected early in Alzheimer's such as the hippocampus. These biomarkers appear to be able to identify carriers of Alzheimer pathology 15–25 years prior to the Alzheimer diagnosis (Bateman et al., 2012). Combinations of biomarkers may permit even earlier detection of the Alzheimer pathology, particularly combinations of apolipoprotein E (APOE)-ε4 genotypes with other biomarkers thought to reflect changes in the brain occurring in AD. We consider such combinations later in this chapter. Because the emergence of neuritic plaques (aggregated β-amyloid) follows the oligomerization of β-amyloid (Walsh & Selkoe, 2007), detection of β-amyloid oligomers could offer an earlier indication of the AD disease process. Currently, work is underway to develop specific ligands for

Alzheimer's Disease. DOI: http://dx.doi.org/10.1016/B978-0-12-804538-1.00021-3

β-amyloid oligomers that can be used in human imaging studies (Viola et al., 2015). Detection of neurofibrillary tangles in the limbic system, an earlier event than plaque formation, is further advanced and may offer the first opportunity for detection of incipient disease three or more decades before its clinical expression (Ariza, Kolb, Moechars, Rombouts, & Andres, 2015).

PRESENT STATUS OF BIOMARKERS

Fluid biomarkers include those obtained from the CSF, blood, or urine. For AD, the most important biomarkers of this type are proteins assayed in the CSF. Given the difficulty of routinely obtaining CSF specimens, especially in large epidemiologic studies, blood markers would be preferable. However, the validity and reliability of such markers remains questionable. Imaging biomarkers offer the possibility of imaging the Alzheimer lesions directly or the brain atrophy that accompanies the Alzheimer pathologic process. In addition, functional imaging can provide insight into the consequences of Alzheimer lesions for brain and cognitive functioning. Finally, performance on cognitive tests can provide sensitive measures of underlying pathology more than two decades before onset of dementia. However, despite the fact that groups of subjects who become demented and do not become demented in the future can be discriminated on the basis of mean performance on specific cognitive tests, the overlap of cognitive performance between these groups is large. Therefore, the utility of these measures for predicting risk within any single individual is likely to be low.

Jack (Jack et al., 2010) has proposed a temporal model for the cascade of events leading to dementia (Figure 4.9). It is important to understand that this model reflects the ability of biomarkers to be detected reliably, which may or may not reflect the relative timing of actual events preceding dementia. As we shall see, the earliest cognitive event in AD may not be the impairment of delayed memory commonly used to define the earliest cognitive change in this illness. Changes in performance on other cognitive tests may predate delayed memory impairment by decades, but despite their greater sensitivity, they are not useful in the diagnosis of prodromal AD because of their relatively low specificity.

VALIDATION OF ALZHEIMER BIOMARKERS

To be useful, a biomarker should be validated against brain pathology. Because the most reliable measures of Alzheimer pathology are those obtained at autopsy, most biomarkers have relied on associations between biomarkers and autopsy findings. The advent of β-amyloid imaging has provided a marker of disease pathology that is available while the person is alive. Correlates of β-amyloid positivity on PET scans therefore could also serve as markers, although their sensitivity and specificity need to be evaluated with regard to this outcome.

CSF Biomarkers

Because proteins are freely transported between the brain and CSF, levels of core Alzheimer-related proteins, including $A\beta_{1-42}$, *p*-tau, and total tau, can provide measures of Alzheimer brain-related pathology early in the disease course. $A\beta_{1-42}$ is the most abundant form of amyloid beta in plaques. Studies have shown that the level of this protein is reduced in the CSF of individuals with AD in comparison to normal controls (Blennow, Hampel, Weiner, & Zetterberg, 2010). In addition, the level of $A\beta_{1-42}$ in CSF has been shown to correlate inversely with the amyloid plaque load in the brain determined at autopsy (Strozyk, Blennow, White, & Launer, 2003) as well as with amyloid load estimated from PET Aβ imaging (Jagust et al., 2009). The explanation for low levels of CSF $A\beta_{1-42}$ in AD is the sequestration of this protein in brain amyloid plaques, resulting in a reduction in its CSF concentration (Hong et al., 2011). Reduced CSF $A\beta_{1-42}$ is apparent at least 15 years prior to estimated time of onset of symptoms in carriers of genes for familial AD when compared with noncarriers (Bateman et al., 2012).

Tau, a microtubule-associated protein, is assayed in the CSF in two forms, the level of total tau that reflects the severity of neuronal damage, and the level of phosphorylated tau (*p*-tau) that is associated with the density of neurofibrillary tangles in the brain. Both forms of tau are increased in the CSF of patients with AD (Buerger et al., 2006). Levels of *p*-tau have been shown to be associated with AD disease progression (Buerger et al., 2006). Levels of tau have been shown to increase reliably in the CSF about 15 years prior to the estimated symptoms in carriers of familial AD genes (Bateman et al., 2012).

Given the association of decreased CSF $A\beta_{1-42}$ and increased CSF total tau and *p*-tau with AD risk, the ratio of tau to $A\beta_{1-42}$ should be considerably larger in those at higher risk of AD. In a longitudinal study of participants with normal cognition, both the tau to $A\beta_{1-42}$ ratio and the *p*-tau to $A\beta_{1-42}$ ratio predicted conversion of participants with normal cognition from a CDR of 0 to a CDR greater than 0 (Fagan et al., 2007).

Blood Biomarkers

Because of their dependence on blood sampling and storage methods, current measures of Aβ and tau in the plasma are more unreliable in predicting AD than CSF biomarkers (Toledo, Shaw, & Trojanowski, 2013). Although there have been several positive studies, particularly with regard to future onset of AD, the overall picture has been one of mixed findings regarding the utility of such markers (Rosen, Hansson, Blennow, & Zetterberg, 2013). Recently, the association between plasma levels of $A\beta_{1-40}$ and $A\beta_{1-42}$ and incident AD was studied in over 2,000 dementia-free participants in the Framingham Study (Chouraki et al., 2015). The authors reported a highly significant association ($p < 0.0005$) between lower levels of plasma $A\beta_{1-42}$ and higher risk for AD (HR per standard deviation = 0.79, 95% CI = 0.68–0.90 in a model adjusted for age, sex, education, APOE-ε4 status, and vascular risk factors). A meta-analysis in the same publication showed a pooled HR for a low plasma $A\beta_{1-42}/A\beta_{1-40}$ ratio of 1.49 (95% CI = 1.17–1.91). Despite the significance of the findings, plasma levels of Aβ are unlikely to be sufficiently reliable to use them in prediction for AD in individuals. However, as part of a larger marker panel, they could be helpful in predicting future AD in large studies in which CSF and PET-scan studies are not practical.

Imaging Biomarkers

Structural MRI Markers

Brain volumes obtained from Magnetic Resonance (MR) scans that have shown promise in early detection of AD as well as tracking of AD pathologic changes include hippocampal, entorhinal, regional gray and white matter, and whole brain volumes (Dickerson et al., 2001; Johnson, Fox, Sperling, & Klunk, 2012; Reiman & Jagust, 2012). Progressive atrophy is a cardinal feature of the neuropathology of AD, likely reflecting the shrinkage of dendrites and loss of neurons. The volume of the hippocampus, a region of the brain affected early in the disease, has been shown to be strongly related to the severity of neuropathology in the same region. Using postmortem MRI scans from the Nun Study, Gosche (Gosche, Mortimer, Smith, Markesbery, & Snowdon, 2001) found that hippocampal volume was inversely correlated with Braak neurofibrillary stage (Figure 4.7). Surprisingly, this correlation extended to the earliest preclinical Braak neurofibrillary stages with significant differences in volume apparent between those in Stages I and II (Gosche, Mortimer, Smith, Markesbery, & Snowdon, 2002). To examine the association with specific neuropathology in the target region, the mean number of neurofibrillary tangles and senile plaques in the CA-1 region of the hippocampus was calculated and correlations obtained with hippocampal volume. Adjusting for age at death, the partial correlation between hippocampal volume and the mean number of neurofibrillary tangles in CA-1 was 0.67 ($p < 0.001$) and that between hippocampal volume and mean senile plaque count in CA-1 was 0.42 ($p < 0.01$). These findings were later replicated by Jack (Jack et al., 2002), who compared hippocampal volumes from antemortem scans of 23 nondemented and 25 AD patients with Braak neurofibrillary stage at autopsy.

We examined the brains of 32 nuns who were not demented at the time of their deaths (Gosche et al., 2002). Forty-eight percent of these participants fulfilled criteria for neuropathologic AD at autopsy. Using hippocampal volume to predict neuropathologic AD yielded an area under the curve of 0.92, corresponding to a specificity of 0.83 and sensitivity of 1.00. These findings suggest that hippocampal volume, while an indirect measure of the severity of Alzheimer pathology, is a very strong biomarker among nondemented individuals, with sensitivity and specificity comparable to CSF biomarkers compared against autopsy results. Because hippocampal volume appears to track even the earliest pathologic stages of the disease (Braak stages I-II), it may offer a very early indicator of disease pathology. In studies of carriers of genes for autosomal dominantly transmitted AD, reliable differences in hippocampal volume were apparent about 15 years prior to the estimated time of onset of symptoms (Bateman et al., 2012). However, nonsignificant differences in decreases in volume comparing gene carriers to noncarriers were seen as early as 25 years prior to symptom onset (Bateman et al., 2012).

Although the hippocampus has been most well-studied as a volumetric MR marker of AD, the earliest atrophy appears to occur somewhat earlier in the entorhinal cortex (Dickerson et al., 2001; Killiany et al., 2002). Other regions showing early atrophy include the amygdala and parahippocampus (Lehericy et al., 1994). The pattern of atrophy seen on MRI closely follows the spread of neurofibrillary tangles with progression of the disease (Braak & Braak, 1991; Whitwell et al., 2008), with progression to the temporal neocortex and subsequently to all association areas of the neocortex (Chan et al., 2001).

Other structural MRI markers that have been explored include thinning of the neocortex in regions affected early in AD (Dickerson et al., 2011) and reduced fractional anisotropy in the cingulum assessed with diffusion tensor imaging (Zhang et al., 2007). Although neither of these measures is likely to change earlier than hippocampal volume preceding clinical AD, combinations of multiple structural MRI markers may provide higher predictive validity than hippocampal volume alone as well as prevent false-positives such as those due to atrophy from hippocampal sclerosis (Dawe, Bennett, Schneider, & Arfanakis, 2011).

Functional MRI Biomarkers

Functional MRI provides a measure of neuronal activity during rest or during specific tasks activating brain regions. Although differences between normal aging, mild cognitive impairment (MCI), and AD have been demonstrated (Johnson et al., 2012), associations with severity of AD pathology in individuals with normal cognition have not been shown and the time course of changes in normal subjects prior to onset of MCI and dementia remains to be determined.

Fibrillar Amyloid PET

A number of PET ligands are currently available to image fibrillar Aβ in living individuals (McConathy & Sheline, 2014). Because its presence in the brain likely precedes fibrillar Aβ by decades, afibrillar Aβ would be a very valuable target for imaging. Although it is likely that soluble oligomers of Aβ are bound by currently available tracers when they reach a critical size, their low concentration in comparison with plaques makes it difficult for them to be detected (Johnson et al., 2012). The development of specific tracers for Aβ oligomers is an important target, because they are likely to give a much earlier indication of nascent Alzheimer pathology than insoluble fibrillar amyloid. For example, human autopsy studies have shown that soluble amyloid-β trimers are present 30 years or more before the first fibrillar plaques can be seen on Aβ PET scans (Lesne et al., 2013). Aβ trimers are the basic building blocks of the oligomer Aβ*56, which is strongly correlated with pathologic soluble tau (Lesne et al., 2013).

Validation of fibrillar amyloid PET against Alzheimer pathology has included direct comparison with postmortem autopsy distributions of plaques (Driscoll et al., 2012) and amyloid load (Ikonomovic et al., 2008), as well as with decreases in CSF $A\beta_{1-42}$ thought to reflect formation of amyloid plaques in the brain (Johnson et al., 2012). PET scans positive for fibrillar Aβ have been shown to have sensitivities of 82–98% and specificities of 77–95% for detection of Aβ plaques at autopsy (McConathy & Sheline, 2014). Fibrillar amyloid PET has also been evaluated using CSF $A\beta_{1-42}$ as a criterion. These two markers are highly correlated in subjects with normal cognition (Fagan et al., 2006).

PET Imaging of Tau Pathology

Although still under development, tracers for pathological tau could potentially provide signals useful in AD detection (James, Doraiswamy, & Borges-Neto, 2015). In a preliminary study, patients with AD had high retention of the tracer F-18 TKH5105 in the temporal cortex, whereas controls did not (Okamura et al., 2014). This or similar markers potentially could be useful in identifying early Braak neurofibrillary stages, perhaps at the same time or before PET fibrillar β-amyloid tracers show significant β-amyloid accumulation in the brain.

Fluorodeoxyglucose PET

Mild AD has been shown to be associated with reduced glucose utilization in several brain regions, including the precuneous, posterior cingulate, and parietotemporal cortex (Langbaum et al., 2009). Fluorodeoxyglucose (FDG) PET provides an indication of regional brain metabolism, primarily reflecting the amount of synaptic activity (Johnson et al., 2012). FDG uptake also correlates strongly with levels of the synaptic vessel protein, synaptophysin (Rocher, Chapon, Blaizot, Baron, & Chavoix, 2003). Decreased uptake in AD is thought to reflect synaptic dysfunction and loss (Johnson et al., 2012). In studies of carriers of autosomal dominantly transmitted AD compared with noncarriers, reliable differences in FDG-PET are apparent about 10 years prior to the estimated time of onset of symptoms (Bateman et al., 2012).

COGNITIVE BIOMARKERS

There is a general consensus that impairments in delayed recall and memory are the initial cognitive changes that occur in preclinical AD, paralleling the neuropathology, and atrophy of the hippocampus (Mortimer, Gosche, Riley, Markesbery, & Snowdon, 2004). However, prospective studies have identified changes in other cognitive domains as being among the earliest changes seen in people who go on to develop AD. Participants in the Framingham Study were given a screening neuropsychological battery and followed for up to 22 years for incidence of AD (Elias et al., 2000). Lower scores on both memory-related tests as well as tests of abstract reasoning predicted later AD. In the PAQUID longitudinal study, participants were given a brief neuropsychological test battery every 2–3 years for 15 years and followed for onset of AD. Using cognitive data from this study, Amieva et al. (2008) found that the earliest reliable difference in cognitive performance was seen on a test of verbal fluency approximately 12 years prior to diagnosis of incident AD. This was followed at 10 years prior to diagnosis by a reliable difference in the score of the Wechsler Similarities Test. Reliable differences between subjects who went on to become demented and remained nondemented were evident 9 years prior to diagnosis for the Mini-Mental State Examination (MMSE) and 8 years prior to diagnosis for the Benton Visual Retention test. These data would suggest that the earliest reliable changes are not necessarily related to memory, but rather to abstract reasoning. In the PAQUID study, cognitive performance in the group destined to develop AD was well within normal limits at the time when they initially scored worse than the group that remained nondemented, and remained so for the incident AD group until very close to the time of diagnosis. Therefore, *individual* cognitive performance before the onset of dementia is not useful by itself in predicting dementia risk. It is possible that longitudinal differences in individual cognitive performance over 2–3 years may signal the onset of dementia earlier than absolute scores on the tests. However, in neither case does it appear that cognitive biomarkers can be used in isolation to predict dementia prior to the time that CSF and imaging biomarkers change.

COMBINATIONS OF BIOMARKERS

Because all biomarkers are imperfect predictors of underlying AD pathology, combining them could increase their reliability and predictive value. Vemuri et al. (2009) examined the combination of a structural MRI imaging score and the CSF tau to $A\beta_{1-42}$ ratio and showed that addition of the CSF ratio, t-tau/$A\beta_{1-42}$, to structural imaging measures significantly increased the ability to predict conversion of MCI to dementia ($p < 0.01$). In individuals with normal cognition, combinations of imaging, CSF, and cognitive measures could provide more reliable prediction of AD than any of these measures alone. However, systematic studies examining this possibility have yet to be conducted.

Given the association of APOE-ε4 with the severity of AD neuropathology at autopsy (Chapter 4), combinations of this genetic biomarker with other biomarkers might provide indications of risk earlier in life. Using PET-FDG imaging, Reiman et al. (2004) demonstrated that young adult carriers of the APOE-ε4 allele with an average age of 30 showed reduced metabolic rates of glucose utilization in the same brain regions affected early in AD. These findings are consistent with functional MRI studies, which show reduced connectivity among ε4 carriers between 20 and 35 years of age (Filippini et al., 2009). Several other studies point to early effects of APOE-ε4 on preclinical AD. In one study, 11 cognitively normal individuals aged 50–62 who were homozygous for ε4 were matched by age, sex, and education with 22 individuals without this allele but who reported a family history of AD (Reiman et al., 1998). The homozygotes were cognitively normal but had significantly reduced glucose metabolism in the regions that are affected in AD, with the largest effect seen in the posterior cingulate cortex. The authors also reported a trend for the homozygotes to show smaller hippocampal volumes and lower performance on a test of long-term memory. In another study by the same investigators, MRI brain imaging of infants carrying an ε4 allele who were 2–25 months of age showed reduced gray matter volumes and myelination in specific cortical regions affected early in AD in comparison to noncarriers (Dean et al., 2014). A small study (Scarmeas et al., 2005) explored cerebral blood flow in college-age students, four who were ε4 carriers and 16 who were not. No differences were found in cognitive performance, but during a nonverbal memory task, the ε4 carriers showed differential cerebral physiology compared with noncarriers. In another study, reduced cortical thickness in the entorhinal cortex, one of the earliest regions to show Alzheimer pathology (Braak & Braak, 1991), was detected in APOE-ε4 carriers in comparison to noncarriers prior to age 21 (Shaw et al., 2007). However, no difference in hippocampal volume by APOE genotype has been seen at this age (Khan et al., 2014). Taken together, this set of findings suggests that the associations of structural or functional biomarkers may be apparent at a much earlier age among carriers of the ε4 allele who are at higher risk of converting to AD.

THE FUTURE OF BIOMARKER RESEARCH

Established CSF fluid biomarkers, structural and functional imaging biomarkers, and cognitive performance measures provide complementary information about the future risk for AD in cognitively normal adults. Because these markers by themselves are imperfect predictors, combining them may provide better indications of risk than any of them in isolation, particularly when combined with epidemiologic markers (Chapter 20). Among individuals at high risk for AD because of carrying specific AD genes, such as APOE-ε4, fluid and imaging markers may provide earlier and more clear-cut risk estimates.

Section V

Future Steps

Chapter 22

Risk Assessment and Prevention of Alzheimer's Disease

Our target in this book is prevention of clinical Alzheimer's disease (AD). As we have seen, people can satisfy the neuropathologic criteria for AD and remain nondemented. Systematic clinicopathologic studies tell us that approximately one-third of people who die with high likelihood of neuropathologic AD according to Reagan criteria are not demented at the time of their deaths. Therefore, there are likely to be two ways to prevent the disease, by giving interventions to slow the underlying pathologic process and by maintaining or growing reserve in order to "tolerate" the lesions without becoming demented. As we have seen in comparisons of the attributable risks for the severity of AD lesions and the degree of reserve, these factors appear to contribute equally to the risk for dementia. However, atrophy, vascular, and other types of brain lesions occurring during aging can tip the scales in favor of dementia in those carrying a high load of Alzheimer lesions in their brains. In this chapter, we will first consider the possibility of slowing the pathologic process leading to clinical AD. Then, we will revisit the issue of modifiable risk factors and the role that they can play in influencing reserve.

MODIFICATION OF PATHOLOGY

Medications to Slow Alzheimer Pathogenesis

If medications can be shown to be safe and effective in slowing the AD pathological process, they can be given to persons at high risk of AD before initial symptoms appear as a form of primary or secondary prevention. Because such medications can have side effects, it is likely that they will be used initially in people who carry definitive markers or are at clear genetic risk for this illness. The majority of prevention trials focus on the use of monoclonal antibodies targeting Aβ and accelerating its removal from the brain. An earlier clinical trial conducted in Alzheimer patients with active vaccination against Aβ had to be stopped in 2002 because a handful of participants developed brain inflammation (Weiner & Selkoe, 2002). Limited follow-up of participants of that trial suggest

Alzheimer's Disease. DOI: http://dx.doi.org/10.1016/B978-0-12-804538-1.00022-5

that there may have been some benefit (Hock et al., 2003). The use of passive immunization through the administration of antibodies against Aβ addresses two issues. First, the dose of antibodies given are under the control of the investigator. The medication can be terminated in those developing side effects, limiting harm. Second, with an active vaccine the immune system of older people may not make the desired antibodies in the concentrations required. Administration of known quantities of antibodies obviates this problem. Because the amyloid stage of AD occurs before the accumulation of neurofibrillary tangles, Aβ antibodies will likely be most effective if given to persons with normal cognition preferably long before clinical symptoms develop.

Several trials of medications that can modify AD neuropathology among at-risk cognitively normal participants are ongoing. At the time of this writing, there are six studies. The Anti-Amyloid Treatment in Asymptomatic Alzheimer's Study (A4 Study—ClinicalTrials.gov ID NCT02008357) (Sperling et al., 2014) is testing solanezumab, a humanized monoclonal antibody targeting Aβ, for 3 years among 1,150 individuals aged 65–85 with initial MMSE scores of 25–30 and CDR scores of 0 who test positive for aggregated amyloid on PET scan. This trial will assess whether the drug is effective in slowing memory and cognitive decline and reducing the accumulation of amyloid plaques in its participants. The Dominantly Inherited Alzheimer Network Trial (DIAN TU—ClinicalTrials.gov ID NCT01760005) (Mills et al., 2013), is testing solanezumab and gantenerumab, a second monoclonal antibody against Aβ, in 210 individuals aged 18–80 who have autosomal dominant AD mutations (PSEN1, PSEN2, and APP). A third study (ClinicalTrials.gov ID NCT01998841) is testing another monoclonal amyloid antibody called crenezumab among 300 people from a large extended family in two villages of Colombia, South America, who carry a PSEN1 mutation that results in AD onset around age 45 (Reiman et al., 2011). The investigators of this study (Reiman et al., 2011) also direct the Alzheimer's Prevention Initiative and are working in conjunction with DIAN TU to identify patients age 30–60 with the same genetic predisposition in the United States (ClinicalTrials.gov ID NCT01998841). Participants in this trial are cognitively normal or have mild cognitive impairment (MCI) or mild dementia with CDR scores of 0–1. Another trial conducted by the same group will test two antiamyloid treatments, an Aβ vaccine and an oral β-secretase inhibitor, among 1,300 cognitively normal people aged 60–75 who are homozygous for apolipoprotein E (APOE)-ε4 (the Alzheimer's Prevention Initiative APOE4 trial) (Langbaum et al., 2013). The final trial is the TOMMORROW Study (ClinicalTrials.gov ID NCT01931566), in which 5,800 individuals aged 65–83 who carry both APOE and another polymorphism that may interact with ε4, TOMM40 (Roses et al., 2010), will receive for 5 years low doses of pioglitazone, a peroxisome proliferator-activated receptor (PPAR)-gamma agonist commonly prescribed for Type 2 diabetes, to test its effectiveness in slowing transitions from normal cognition to MCI. The earliest results will come from DIAN TU in 2017, and results from the other studies will become available before or in 2020.

In addition to these randomized controlled trials (RCTs) that aim to reduce Alzheimer neuropathology, some observational studies have suggested that insulin may facilitate the removal of Aβ from the brain and that antihypertensive medications may have a beneficial effect on AD neuropathology as well (Chapter 14).

Nonpharmacologic Slowing of AD Pathogenesis

Although animal studies have suggested that increased intake of juices, curcumin, coffee, and DHA lead to reductions of Aβ in transgenic mice (Chapter 15), data from human autopsy studies are lacking, making diet a promising though untested means of modifying AD pathology. Animal studies also have shown that physical exercise, particularly that occurring early in life, may have a favorable effect on aggregation of Aβ in the brains of transgenic animals. Consistent with these findings, a human study utilizing PET amyloid imaging and CSF assays showed lower accumulation of AD biomarkers in people who reported more physical exercise (Chapter 16). Animal studies of cognitive stimulation showed that environmental enrichment was associated with reduction of Aβ oligomers. In humans, using retrospectively collected information on cognitive engagement in early and middle life, lower Aβ on a PET scan in adults with a mean age of 76 was shown to be related to more cognitive engagement in earlier life, suggesting a role for cognitive stimulation in reducing Aβ (Chapter 17).

Although these findings suggest that diet, and mental and physical exercise might influence the risk of AD through modifications of AD pathology, there are considerably more data showing that these interventions affect brain growth contributing to increased reserve. It is entirely possible that both of these effects are occurring simultaneously and that accelerated brain growth is associated with an increased rate of removal of Aβ.

MODIFIABLE RISK FACTORS THAT INFLUENCE RESERVE

A second approach to prevention of AD is to implement interventions based on modifiable risk factors with the aim of building or maintaining reserve. This strategy would delay clinical expression of dementia and AD, thereby reducing the incidence of the disease. Are we ready for this kind of approach?

In an NIH State-of-the-Science statement published in 2010–2011 (Daviglus et al., 2011; Williams, 2010) the authors reviewed observational and human experimental evidence on modifiable risk factors. They concluded that there was "insufficient evidence to support the association of any modifiable risk factor with risk of cognitive decline or AD" (Daviglus et al., 2011). Diabetes mellitus, hyperlipidemia in midlife, and current cigarette smoking were found to increase the risk for AD; while Mediterranean-type diets, folic acid, low or moderate alcohol consumption, and cognitive and physical activities were found to decrease its risk. However, for all these variables, the quality of the data was considered to be low using guidelines from the Grading of Recommendations Assessment, Development, and Evaluation working group (Daviglus et al., 2011). Low-quality evidence under these guidelines indicates that additional research may affect the direction or magnitude of the observed association. However, the authors caution that methodological limitations, including the use of self-reported exposure data, limited knowledge of the natural history of AD (presumably referring to insufficient follow-up periods in many studies, as well as lack of knowledge as to when AD begins and what exposure ascertainment windows should be), and inconsistent use of consensus-based diagnostic criteria for AD could account for their conclusions. The panel recommended that "large-scale, long-term population-based studies and clinical trials are urgently needed to identify risk factors for AD" and "carefully designed future studies may yet establish significant associations between these same factors with prevention of AD. It is hoped that the panel's report will instigate rigorous high-quality research that can provide conclusive evidence" (Daviglus et al., 2011).

Criteria for study inclusion that were used in the Williams, Plassman, Burke, Holsinger, and Benjamin (2010) report included English-language studies from 1984 to 2009 that sampled adults age 50 and older from the general populations of developed countries, sample sizes of at least 300 for cohort studies and 50 for RCTs, use of well-accepted diagnostic criteria, and a lag time of at least 2 years between exposure and diagnosis of dementia. However, as we have seen in this book, many studies' results were likely susceptible to reverse causation stemming from insufficient follow-up periods. If AD develops over the life course, we may need 20 years or more instead of 2 years between exposure ascertainment and clinical onset of dementia commonly found in cohort studies beginning in late-life. In addition, we have shown that many exposures are important for risk of AD only in midlife. Therefore, the findings of the cohort studies conducted in later life that were used in this report may not represent the underlying associations fairly. Many studies used in the Williams et al. report were lacking in their exposure definitions. For example, some studies of physical activity and AD only gathered information on *selected* physical activities. Such misclassification might lead to an underestimation of the RR.

In addition, Williams et al. strictly followed the hierarchy of analytic study designs shown in Figure 9.2. As we have seen, the natural history of AD, including the very slowly evolving pathology, raises important issues regarding this hierarchy. Cohort studies with short follow-ups likely have a serious problem with information bias. In case–control studies of AD, much effort is taken to minimize information bias by matching case proxies to control proxies and not accepting studies where the controls themselves have been interviewed. In a cohort study, such mismatching in sources of information occurs naturally in that individuals who will develop dementia in the ensuing few years are already poor historians at baseline compared to those who will not develop dementia in this time frame. This can lead to underreporting of exposures in the future cases, which for risk factors can bias the RR toward the null value. Case–control studies can sometimes give us answers that cannot be provided from short-term cohort studies, but the report excluded studies with this design. Other issues with this report that we have discussed in this book include differences between studies in variables that were controlled to adjust for confounding. For example, education is only one aspect of socioeconomic status (SES), but in many studies included in the report it was the only measure of SES that was adjusted. Finally, causal inferences are not based on literature reviews, although consistency is one criterion for such conclusions. Inductive inference in epidemiology is based on causal criteria, which was described briefly in the Primer. Even then, none of these criteria is either necessary or sufficient for establishing whether or not an observed association is causal, except the requirement of temporal sequence (Rothman, Greenland, & Lash, 2008).

RCTs were considered the most valid type of study in the Williams et al. report. However, they have problems that do not allow us to draw firm conclusions about causality. For example, the Women's Health Initiative Memory Study (WHIMS) showed that hormone replacement therapy (HRT) in late-life has adverse consequences for dementia, but observational studies showed that when taken around the time of menopause such therapy is likely to reduce dementia risk. From a biological plausibility perspective, it is likely that HRT in the late 40s and early 50s is indeed protective for dementia. Therefore, the observational findings should perhaps carry more weight than the RCT. For other factors like physical activity and smoking, the data supporting their associations with dementia and AD are more robust, and some decry the Williams et al. report as being too negative, when animal, human, and imaging data all support the associations (Flicker, Liu-Ambrose, & Kramer, 2011). In the 5 years since the report was published, there have been many additional studies of the risk and protective factors, and a number of associations have come to light when data were stratified by age, education, or APOE status.

MULTIMODAL PREVENTION

We believe there are important data supporting the associations of almost all of the risk factors covered in this book with either the pathologic process of AD or its clinical expression or both. Those risk and protective factors that affect clinical expression of dementia do so by depleting, maintaining or increasing brain and cognitive reserve. Therefore, an "attack on all fronts" approach is likely necessary, in which multimodal interventions, including improvement of early-life risk factors, diet, physical, cognitive and social activities, and reduction of head trauma, vascular risk, obesity, smoking, and depression are targeted to people at risk for AD. Several studies have taken varied approaches to investigating combined effects of activities on cognition. For example, in one study (Fabre, Chamari, Mucci, Masse-Biron, & Prefaut, 2002), 32 volunteers age 60–76 were randomized to aerobic training, memory training, a combined aerobic and memory training group, and to a no-intervention group (8 in each). After 2 months, the group that did the combined training performed better on a memory test than the other two training groups. Other studies found no effect of a combination of exercise and mental activity (Barnes et al., 2013) or nutrient-dense foods and exercise (de Jong et al., 2001), but these trials were very short in duration (12–17 weeks). Several other studies are in progress (Gates et al., 2011; Legault et al., 2011; O'Dwyer, Burton, Pachana, & Brown, 2007).

One large study that is using a multimodal approach to prevention is the Finnish Geriatric Intervention Study to Prevent Cognitive Impairment and Disability (FINGER). As we noted in Chapter 18, preliminary findings from this study are encouraging in showing that individuals randomized to the comprehensive treatment group showed improvements in several cognitive tests compared to those in the comparison group over the first 2 years of intervention.

Another multidomain intervention study is being conducted in France, the Multidomain Approach for Prevention of Alzheimer's Disease (MAPT) Study (Vellas et al., 2014). In this study, based on 13 memory clinics in four French cities, 1,680 participants age 70 and older (mean age 75.3 and 65% female) were randomized to four groups: (i) omega-3 supplementation; (ii) multidomain intervention; (iii) omega-3+ multidomain intervention; or (iv) placebo. The primary endpoint is change in memory function at 3-year follow-up on the Free and Cued Selective Reminding test. In addition, several secondary outcomes are included that test other cognitive domains. Participants were selected from community-based residents coming to their general practitioner and spontaneously reporting a memory complaint, limitation in one IADL, and slow walking speed (more than 5 s to walk 4 m). Demented subjects as well as those scoring less than 24 on the MMSE were excluded, as were subjects who could not perform the interventions or had been taking omega-3 supplements for the prior 6 months. Participants in the omega-3 intervention take two capsules per day containing a total of 800 mg docosahexaenoic acid (DHA) and 112.5 mg per day of eicosapentenoic acid (EPA) for 3 years. The placebo group receives identical capsules that do not contain DHA and EPA. The multidomain intervention consists of training sessions in nutrition, physical activity, and cognitive training. In addition, subjects receive outpatient visits with the goal of detecting sensory, mood, gait, malnutrition, and vascular disorders. Cognitive training includes reasoning, memory, and mnemonic strategies. Participants were recruited from May 2008 to February 2011 and initial results of this intervention study should be published in the near future.

The Prevention of Dementia by Intensive Vascular Care (PreDIVA) trial also is ongoing (Richard et al., 2009). This study is being conducted by investigators from the Netherlands. Its goal is to determine whether intensive treatment of cardiovascular risk factors prevents dementia or changes in MRI indices of brain disease. This trial, which will last 6 years, randomized about 1,700 healthy participants aged 70–78 to standard care or intensive treatment of hypertension and high cholesterol, smoking cessation, exercise, and adoption of a healthy lifestyle. Preliminary results have found that the intervention results in decreased blood pressure, but results have not yet been published for dementia outcomes or brain atrophy.

European investigators have collaboratively established the European Dementia Prevention Initiative (EDPI) to explore the design and implementation of prevention studies (Richard et al., 2012). This collaboration will enable pooling of data from the three prevention studies we have described as well as the design of studies for future research. These investigators recognize that "the balance between optimal timing of the intervention and incidence of the primary outcome is precarious" (Richard et al., 2012). In addition, they acknowledge that such studies require a long follow-up and a long-term vision on the part of both the investigators and funding agencies. They suggest that such prevention studies should be of a minimum of 4 years duration, but that much longer durations than this might jeopardize the follow-up rate.

In the United States, a prevention registry has been established (http://www.endalznow.org/) that is building a large sample size of healthy people age 18 and older who wish to find out about prevention study opportunities for AD. To date, over 127,000 people have enrolled. However, besides the antiamyloid trials discussed earlier, at the time of this writing only two small multidomain prevention studies are currently in progress in the United States (ClinicalTrials.gov IDs NCT02290912, NCT00979446).

PRECLINICAL DETECTION

In the CAIDE study, 1,449 participants were evaluated at an average age of 50 and followed up 20 years later for dementia (Kivipelto et al., 2006). From this sample, a Mid-Life Dementia Risk Index was developed, that included age, sex, education, BMI, blood pressure, total cholesterol, physical activity, and APOE. Scores were obtained by standardizing β coefficients from the multivariable logistic model and assigning a score of 1 to the lowest β coefficient. Remaining coefficients were multiplied by 1/lowest β coefficient. For example, in this study, the lowest β coefficient was 0.44, so this value was assigned a score of 1. 1/0.44 is approximately 2.5. Therefore, all other β coefficients were multiplied by 2.5. Other risk indices that we will discuss below used a similar approach to weight factors. The scoring is shown in Table 22.1. The Mid-Life Dementia Risk Index had an accuracy of 0.77, judged by the c-statistic or area under the curve in a receiver-operating characteristic curve, where 1.0 is perfect accuracy and 0.50 is no better than chance. When APOE was included in the model, the c-statistic increased to 0.78.

In 2009, Barnes et al. published a Late-Life Dementia Risk Index for prediction of dementia risk strata (low, moderate, or high) in a 6-year follow-up (Barnes et al., 2009). The Cardiovascular Health Cognition Study, nested in the Cardiovascular Health Study (CHS), begun in 1998–1999, included 3608 CHS study participants, all of whom had an MRI scan and Modified Mini-Mental

TABLE 22.1 CAIDE Dementia Risk Score: Probability of Dementia in 20 Years According to Midlife Risk Score Categories

Risk Factor		Points
Age	<47	0
	47–53	3
	>53	4
Education	>10 years	0
	7–9 years	2
	<7 years	3
Gender	Female	0
	Male	1
Blood Pressure	<140 mm Hg	0
	>140 mm Hg	2
Body mass index	<30 kg/m^2	0
	>30 kg/m^2	2
Total cholesterol	<6.5 mmol/L	0
	>6.5 mmol/L	2
Physical activity	Yes	0
	No	1

Total Score	Dementia Risk
0–5	1.0%
6–7	1.9%
8–9	4.2%
10–11	7.4%
12–15	16.4%

Adapted from Kivipelto et al. (2013).

State Examination (3MS) scores in 1991–1994. The population was recruited from randomized Medicare eligibility lists in Forsyth County, NC; Washington County, MD; Sacramento County, CA; and Pittsburgh, PA. The Late-Life Dementia Risk Index targeted to individuals aged 65 and older included the variables shown in Table 22.2. The c-statistic for this index was 0.81

TABLE 22.2 The Late-Life Dementia Risk Index

Risk Factor	Points
Age 75–79	1
Age 80–100	2
Low 3MS score	2
Low DSST (Digit Symbol Substitution Test)	2
BMI <18.5	2
≥1 APOE-ε4 allele	1
MRI white matter disease (grade ≥3)	1
MRI enlarged ventricles (grade ≥4)	1
Internal carotid artery thickness ≥2.2 mm	1
History of coronary bypass surgery	1
Time to put on and button shirt >45 s	1
Lack of alcohol consumption	1

Adapted from Barnes et al. (2009).
Scores range from 0 to 15.

(95% CI = 0.79–0.83), meaning that it classified the outcome correctly in 81% of participants. Among those with low scores in this study, dementia risk within 6 years was 4%, among those with moderate scores, it was 23%, and among those with high scores, it was 56%. Although the Late-Life Dementia Risk Index has somewhat stronger prediction characteristics than the Mid-Life Dementia Risk Index, its purpose was only for a 6-year prediction. In addition, it required information that may not be readily obtained from individuals at the population level, including quantitative MRI analyses. To circumvent this problem, the same investigators pooled data from four cohort studies, the CHS, the Framingham Heart Study (FHS), the Health and Retirement Study (HRS), and the Sacramento Area Latino Study on Aging (SALSA) (Barnes, Beiser, et al., 2014). The index used in this study included age (1 point per year from ages 65–79), less than 12 years of education (9 points), diabetes mellitus (3 points), BMI less than 18.5 (8 points), requires assistance with money or medications (10 points), and depressive symptoms (6 points). Harrell's c-statistic was consistent across studies (CHS, 0.68; FHS, 0.77; HRS, 0.76; SALSA, 0.78). This index was developed for use in primary care to assist clinicians in identifying patients for cognitive screening. Its main advantage is that it can be easily used in older populations.

In a comparison between the Mid-Life and Late-Life Dementia Risk Indices, Barnes and Yaffe (2009) noted that the three variables common to both indices were age, education, and APOE genotype. The remaining variables in the Mid-Life Dementia Risk Index are cardiovascular risk factors, including physical inactivity. Conversely, in the Late-Life Dementia Risk Index, the additional measures were mostly cardiovascular outcomes, and cognitive and functional status.

In 2010, a vascular summary risk score algorithm was published from the Northern Manhattan Study (Reitz et al., 2010b). One thousand and fifty-one nondemented Medicare recipients aged 65 and older living in New York were followed for conversion to dementia. With a median follow-up of 4.2 years, dementia was diagnosed by consensus based on the DSM and NINCDS-ADRDA criteria. Risk scores were evaluated in the same manner as the CAIDE Mid-Life Risk Index (Kivipelto et al., 2006). Quintiles of vascular risk scores were determined using age, sex, education, presence of diabetes, hypertension, current smoking, low HDL-C, and high waist-to-hip ratio. The RR for developing probable AD by NINCDS-ADRDA criteria was 1.0 for individuals scoring 0–14 on the risk index, 3.7 for those scoring 15–18, 3.6 for those scoring 19–22, 12.6 for those scoring 23–28, and 20.5 for those with a score of 28 or higher.

In Australia, Anstey, Cherbuin, and Herath (2013) used a different approach to develop a risk index called the Australian National University Alzheimer's Risk Index (ANU-ADRI) that could be inexpensively applied in populations. This index used the existing literature on dementia and AD risk to select risk factors that could be readily obtained by questionnaire, without clinical assessment, neuropsychological testing, genetic evaluation, or imaging. This approach did not rely on data from only one study, but rather estimated coefficients from existing meta-analyses of risk factors. The use of only self-reported data can be viewed as an advantage in terms of ease of data collection (which was the investigators' main point), but it can also be viewed as a liability in terms of the accuracy of exposure ascertainment. Individual scores were developed using the same technique as Kivipelto et al. (2006), except that the standardized β coefficients were derived from odds ratios of pooled effect sizes from meta-analyses instead of from a single study. Thirty-eight potential risk factors were initially identified, 25 of which were considered to have sufficient evidence to include in the index. These variables included age (for men and women separately), education, BMI, diabetes, depressive symptoms, high cholesterol, head trauma, smoking, alcohol consumption, social engagement, physical activity, cognitive activity, fish intake, and pesticide exposure. External validation of the ANU-ADRI is currently ongoing.

An important external validation of the Mid-Life Dementia Risk Index from CAIDE was conducted in 9,480 patients in the Kaiser Permanente Medical Care Program (KPNC) in Northern California who participated in surveys in 1964 and 1976 (Exalto et al., 2014). In this study, dementia diagnoses were made by searching ICD-9 codes for dementia in the electronic medical records at KPNC, as well as diagnoses confirmed by a medical specialist in a memory clinic or neurology department. In addition to the variables included in the CAIDE risk index, several new variables contained in the KPNC records were added. These were central obesity defined as sagittal abdominal diameter more than 25 cm, depressed mood, diabetes, head trauma, poor lung function defined as the lowest quintile of forced expiratory volumes, and smoking. The original CAIDE midlife dementia risk score performed well in this multiethnic U.S. sample with a follow-up of 40 years. The overall c-statistic was similar to the original CAIDE c-statistic (0.75 versus. 0.78, respectively). In addition, c-statistics varied similarly in racial subgroup analyses (c-statistics for Asians was 0.81, for blacks, 0.75, and for whites, 0.74). None of the new variables improved the predictive power of the risk score. The authors explain this by noting that some of the additional risk factors were highly correlated with the CAIDE predictors (e.g., central obesity and BMI). A second explanation was that some risk factors, such as diabetes and head trauma, are more prevalent in late-life, and the population attributable fraction in midlife may be too low to have a significant influence. The risk for dementia in late-life according to the sum score of the midlife risk score validated in the KNPC population increased from 9% for the lowest score to 29% for the highest score.

Recently, a new risk score algorithm to predict MCI was developed from the Mayo Clinic Study of Aging (Pankratz et al., 2015). The goal of this prediction model was to provide a brief noninvasive and inexpensive tool for risk stratification at the population level, as well as one that would inform the design of intervention trials. Olmsted County, MN residents age 70–89 as of 2004 were identified and randomly sampled, with a participation rate of 62%. All 2,719 participants were clinically and neuropsychologically evaluated, and detailed information was collected on risk factors. There were 1,418 participants who were evaluated every 15 months for a median follow-up time of 4.8 years. Of these, 410 developed incident MCI. Two basic risk models were calculated. The first included basic demographic and medical history characteristics for both sexes, including education, self-reported memory complaints, alcohol problems, history of stroke, diabetes (<age 75 and age 75–84, with more risk points assigned to earlier diabetes), and history of atrial fibrillation. Specific additional factors for women included current smoking, midlife hyperlipidemia, and hypertension. For men, additional variables included maximum adult BMI in excess of 30 kg/m^2 and being never married or widowed. For women, the c-statistic (standard error) was 0.58 (0.03) and for men, 0.62 (0.03). In the augmented clinical model, neuropsychiatric features (presence of agitation, apathy, anxiety) and CDR-Sum of Boxes >0 were added. For women, additional variables included the score on the Short Test of Mental Status, total Unified Parkinson's Disease Rating Scale (UPDRS) score >0, and Functional Activities Questionnaire (FAQ) total score >0. For men, additional variables included slow gait (<0.9 m/s) anxiety, and score on the Short Test of Mental Status. Models were run with and without APOE-ε4 as well. The c-statistics for women and men in the model with APOE-ε4 were 0.69 (standard error = 0.03) and 0.71 (standard error 0.03), respectively. Overall, both women and men with risk scores in the highest sex-specific quartiles of the augmented model incurred a sevenfold risk for MCI, with APOE-ε4 adding to the predictive power (Pankratz et al., 2015).

Other risk models have been developed expressly for diabetics (Exalto et al., 2013) and for transitions from MCI to AD (Lee, Ritchie, Yaffe, Stijacic Cenzer, & Barnes, 2014). Dementia risk indices had c-statistics for available dementia risk algorithms that ranged from 0.49 (chance) to 0.81 (Solomon & Soininen, 2015). A c-statistic between 0.70 and 0.80 is considered adequate for use in public health education programs and awareness campaigns. For example, the Framingham Risk Score (Lloyd-Jones et al., 2004), which has been in use for many years to predict heart disease, meets this standard, with a c-statistic ranging between 0.75 and 0.80. The selection of a particular risk index will depend on the specific purpose for which it will be used. While research to determine which risk algorithm works best in which populations is still in progress, more work needs to done on validating the existing algorithms in diverse populations (Solomon & Soininen, 2015).

In general, risk indices that have been developed to predict dementia work best close in time to its onset, but midlife indices that include cardiovascular risk factors and APOE have good predictive accuracy. Prediction of MCI appears to be more difficult than dementia, likely because the outcome is less rigorous and has considerable variability. For purposes of identifying suitable candidates for interventions with potentially harmful side effects, the existing risk indices are only marginally adequate. Better accuracy would be achieved by evaluating combinations of CSF and imaging markers. The development of more comprehensive indices that incorporate markers and risk factors for Alzheimer and vascular pathology as well as measures of reserve are needed to better define risk in individuals.

Chapter 23

Summary and Recommendations

Although reliable biomarkers for the neuropathology of Alzheimer's disease (AD) can be detected about 20 years before the initial clinical symptoms, there is growing evidence that the disease begins much earlier and that exposures over the entire life course affect the risk of the illness as well as the timing of its initial symptoms. The risk for AD is related to the evolving neuropathologic process as well as its interaction with brain reserve. It is clear that genes play a major role in the lifetime risk for AD and dementia. The primary genetic susceptibility allele, APOE-ε4, has observable effects in infancy through late adulthood. Deprivation in the form of poor nutrition, deficient stimulation, and adverse educational or economic circumstances, as well as the tendency to develop vascular disease and increased exposures to oxidative stress and inflammation aggravate these risks. If Aβ oligomers are responsible for later-developing Aβ plaques, one can argue that the very lengthy neuropathologic process of AD starts with a genetic propensity to lay down this pathology at a certain rate beginning in fetal life, resulting in an individual genetic trajectory that is impacted by the many environmental influences and propensities to develop other chronic conditions that each person encounters in his or her lifetime. Because of this, each person is likely traversing his or her own trajectory, since no two individuals will share all genetic and environmental propensities. This leads to the concept of personalized medicine and personalized prevention, in which it is recognized that such propensities interact with one another, as well as with epigenetic, proteomic, and metabolomic systems, which are the next frontiers in AD science.

TWO APPROACHES TO PREVENTION

There are two ways we can currently tackle the propensity to develop AD. One approach is to slow down the neuropathologic process in people with the disease. RCTs of drug therapies for AD have been disappointing to date (Cummings, Morstorf, & Zhong, 2014; Selkoe, 2013). Pharmacologic treatment trials for MCI have yielded mixed results, but also generally have not been

Alzheimer's Disease. DOI: http://dx.doi.org/10.1016/B978-0-12-804538-1.00023-7

promising (Vega & Newhouse, 2014). We now await the results of the primary and secondary prevention trials discussed in Chapter 22. The second approach is to decrease our vascular risks and increase reserve through nonpharmacologic means. In MCI and in preclinical cognitive impairment, nonpharmacologic treatments have a better track record. Even when disease-modifying drugs become available to prevent AD, we may still want to augment their effects through risk factor modification, such as reducing vascular risks, diet, and exercise. In this regard, prevention of AD will be similar to prevention of diabetes, where combinations of diet, exercise, and medications provide the most effective treatment.

Currently, the single most promising treatment for prevention of AD is physical exercise (Flicker, Liu-Ambrose, & Kramer, 2011; Nagamatsu et al., 2014). Physical exercise has recently been touted as an essential part of healthy aging (Nagamatsu et al., 2014), and it has been estimated that elimination of 25% of physical inactivity worldwide would prevent one million cases of dementia (Barnes and Yaffe, 2011). However, scientists, funding agencies, and the public are slow to accept these recommendations due to the fact that more specific information is needed regarding what type of exercise should be done, for how long, and how to publicize these messages to educate older people about the cognitive benefits of exercise. Many of the cognitively beneficial lifestyle exposures that appear to be protective for AD have few downsides and might be considered by most to be obviously "good for you." Articles discussing these lifestyle changes are slowly making their way into the science press (Deweerdt, 2011).

As noted above, it is likely that both tactics, medications to decrease AD neuropathology and nonpharmacologic approaches to increase reserve, will be used in combination. It is unlikely, though not impossible, that a "silver bullet" will be discovered to treat early AD. Because observational epidemiologic studies can answer different questions from clinical trials, there remains a dire need for observational epidemiology to continue to be funded at a high level in the United States, given the sheer number of aging baby boomers who are predicted to develop AD in the coming decades and the enormous financial and emotional burden that this will bring. As we noted at the beginning of the book, in developing countries, the need to curtail the dementia epidemic is even more pronounced.

In this book, we have shown that approximately one-third of individuals who meet AD based on neuropathologic criteria were not demented during life. Research to determine the underlying brain structure that leads to this compensatory ability has begun (Bartres-Faz & Arenaza-Urquijo, 2011; Perneczky et al., 2006; Sole-Padulles et al., 2009; Stern, 2012), but is still in its infancy. We have reviewed many factors across the life course that are associated with brain and cognitive reserve, such as education, IQ, occupation, physical activity, adherence to certain dietary patterns, cognitive activities, and social engagement, each of which may contribute in a different way to reserve (Foubert-Samier et al., 2012; James et al., 2012). We now have good evidence that pathologies are additive and that the two types of risk factors for AD, those for the pathology and those for its expression, are largely uncorrelated with one another. We also know that brain and cognitive reserve modify the effect of neuropathology on clinical expression of disease, with the net result that the higher an individual's reserve, the longer on average the clinical disease can be delayed. However, once an individual with high reserve presents with clinical symptoms of AD or dementia, they are in a more advanced pathologic state and will decline more rapidly.

Although some risk factors for AD pathology cannot be changed today, such as genes, there are multiple risk factors for clinical expression that we can influence. AD may be similar to cardiovascular disease, in that although we may not be able to prevent it altogether, we may be able to delay its onset, resulting in a large decrease in its incidence over the life course.

THE FUTURE OF OBSERVATIONAL AND EXPERIMENTAL STUDIES OF AD

For future observational and experimental human studies, epidemiologists should recognize that the traditional hierarchy of epidemiologic study design does not apply to all diseases. The natural history of AD forces us to reexamine the questions we are asking and carefully consider the most appropriate design to obtain the most valid answers. Observational cohort studies will remain important to study long-term exposures such as diet, physical, cognitive, and social activities. However, it will be necessary to devise more valid methods for determining exposure than asking individuals who will soon become demented to recall their past exposures. It also will be necessary to consider the issue of reverse causation and to assess its possible contributions to observed associations. Using existing longitudinal exposure data from studies conducted decades before remains an important option if participants in those studies can be traced and their dementia status established, as has been done in the CAIDE Study and the Lothian Birth Cohort Studies. Alternatively, using systematically collected data from medical care providers, such as the Mayo Clinic or the Kaiser Permanente Medical Care Program, provides an option for examining risk factors associated with medical care, such as head trauma or cardiovascular disease.

To capture transitions from normal cognition to dementia, experimental intervention studies would need to include large numbers of participants in the age of risk of AD or be of very long duration. These requirements raise several issues. The cost of trials needed to observe clinical transitions is likely to be very high. As we have discussed in Chapter 22, three large multimodal intervention trials of sufficiently long duration to observe transitions to dementia are being performed in Europe. However, the focus in these trials is on interventions *applied in late life*, a compromise necessary to yield sufficient numbers of transitions to dementia. With this design, interventions that have a critical time window in midlife for maximum beneficial effect, including diabetes treatment, hypertension control, and estrogen replacement therapy, cannot be evaluated validly in short or medium duration RCTs.

An alternative to study the effects of interventions in midlife on the risk of dementia would be to use biomarkers of AD pathology and reserve as outcomes. These might include structural MRI volumes, CSF biomarkers of Aβ and tau, PET markers of Aβ and tau, or glucose utilization. These types of markers are likely to require smaller sample sizes due to their greater precision in comparison with change in scores on cognitive tests, another surrogate for AD that is less valid and much less reliable (Jack et al., 2004). While such studies may not yield reliable data on the prevention of AD *per se*, they may be very useful for exploring the effects of interventions earlier in life on markers that have strong associations with the outcome of interest later in life.

The disappointing results of RCTs to date may in part be due to the utilization of samples of AD patients in which the targeted therapy addressed an earlier pathologic phase of the illness, a "critical window" that is largely over by the time MCI or AD is apparent. The movement toward using agents that target tau rather than Aβ in early AD, for example, illustrates this issue (Medina & Avila, 2014). Finally, the samples used in most intervention trials are not representative of the population in which they are intended to be applied. Utilization of random samples of the general population would increase the external validity of studies. To our knowledge, one of the only studies on AD interventions that recruited a random, community-based sample of participants was our T'ai Chi study described in Chapter 16.

EXPOSURES LIKELY HAVE CRITICAL TIME WINDOWS

In this book, we have portrayed AD as a lifelong illness, beginning at conception with the inheritance of genes that play a dominant role in determining its risk. Upon this genetic background, a lifetime of risk factors influences the development and loss of brain reserve, permitting some carriers of the neuropathology to live out their lives without become demented while others succumb to the disease. Although many of the so-called modifiable risk factors are under the control of the individual who could develop the disease, others reflect at least partially genetic inheritance or are determined by societal influences. For example, parental education and income of the family of origin can influence brain structure in early-life and adolescence, particularly among children in lower income strata, limiting the brain growth and development that determine late-life reserve. Exposures also are likely to have their major effects during critical periods of life. Once past, the associations of such exposures with dementia risk may change and even reverse in effect. Hormone replacement therapy is one example of this phenomenon, but others, e.g., the interaction of physical exercise with estrogen in women, may also be time-limited. Understanding the mechanism through which exposures affect reserve will be critical to deciding how best to prevent AD. For example, in individuals at risk, one may want to combine regular aerobic exercise with specific cognitive training focused on memory to maximize growth in regions of the brain that are most affected early in AD.

As has been shown for hormone replacement therapy, timing of interventions for prevention of AD is likely very important. The issue of when to begin physical exercise, intellectual stimulation, weight control, and a healthy brain diet remains open. Although most would agree that the answer to this question is as early as possible, is it ever too late? The maximum benefit from physical exercise appears to occur in preadulthood. Obesity in midlife and earlier is important to AD risk, but overweight in late life is not. Diabetes in midlife is more consequential for AD than diabetes in late life. Two explanations can be given for the apparently greater effect of healthy brain behaviors when begun early. First, there is some evidence that physical exercise may influence Aβ more when begun at a younger age (Adlard, Perreau, Pop, & Cotman, 2005). If AD results from a progressive pathological process, interference with earlier steps in this process may slow the rate of accumulation of aberrant proteins contributing to neuritic plaques and neurofibrillary tangles. Second, it is possible that growth of brain tissue earlier in life will lead to more functional brain tissue later in life. The concept of a "brain bank" is obvious for brain growth in the first decade of life when the eventual size of the brain and its connectivity is being determined, but may extend to later decades. For example, when physical exercise was evaluated at different times during life, exercise in late adolescence and early adulthood was more strongly related to cognitive decline in old age than exercise later in life (Dik, Deeg, Visser, & Jonker, 2003; Middleton, Barnes, Lui, & Yaffe, 2010). We found that minutes of walking at age 50 in women strongly influenced the amount of brain atrophy over 20 years later (Mortimer et al., 2013). These findings, while preliminary, suggest that behaviors earlier in life may result in brain growth that persists for decades and provides reserve when it is needed much later.

PREVENTION OF AD AT THE POPULATION AND INDIVIDUAL LEVEL

Finally, prevention of AD can be considered at the population or individual level. At the population level, clear and effective communication of the facts regarding risk and protective factors for AD is essential. Different segments of the population defined by age, gender, education, and ethnicity will likely need to receive this information through different types of media, including traditional print and broadcast outlets as well as through the internet, social, and even entertainment media. In many societies, group activities are popular and to the degree possible people should be encouraged to "prevent" together, e.g., to join a walking or discussion group.

The message itself needs to be one that AD is not an inevitable consequence of growing older. The issue of motivation is an important one. In 2006, 93% of Americans over 45 said they had heard of AD (MetLife Mature Market Institute and LifePlans Inc., 2006). In fact, over 60% of older Americans know someone who has it (Roberts, McLaughlin, & Connell, 2014). In a survey of the participants of the Health and Retirement Study, 60% admitted that they would like to know their own chances of getting Alzheimer's in the future (Roberts, McLaughlin, et al., 2014). Remarkably, this group that was representative of the US population at the time of their enrollment in this study, understood that genetics was an important cause of the disease (89%), and that physical (88%) and mental (93%) activity along with a healthy diet (87%) could help to prevent it. Although this is encouraging, the number of older adults who practice what they perceive is beneficial falls far short of these numbers. The ultimate challenge then is to translate this knowledge into action through programs that encourage beginning and sustaining activities and behaviors that can reduce the risk for AD.

It also is very important to publicize the message that AD is a lifelong disease and that early childhood physical and intellectual growth is likely one of the best ways to reduce its incidence in the future. The specific messages regarding physical and mental exercise, diet, control of risk factors for vascular disease must reach adults of all ages, since the earlier healthy brain behaviors are adopted the more likely that people will enter their later years with the brain reserve needed to prevent dementia.

At the individual level, personalized prevention will require assessment of the risk that a person has for developing AD as well as the most likely age at which this would occur. The best way to do this will be to combine epidemiologic markers (such as olfaction and subjective memory complaints) with epidemiologic protective and risk factor profiles, and genetic, neuropsychological, and imaging data when resources permit. New models of risk assessment are needed that will permit a sequential approach to determination of disease risk, beginning with low cost, noninvasive procedures and proceeding to sensitive and specific biomarkers. Much remains to be learned regarding the interaction of genes with exercise and diet, as well as the best ways to reduce inflammation, an important player in the acceleration of Alzheimer's pathology. Finally, individuals who participate in personalized prevention programs need to be monitored for progression of AD to assess efficacy. This will require regular assessments, mostly likely based on imaging, to assess changes in pathology as well as growth and atrophy of the brain.

References

Abbott, R. D., White, L. R., Ross, G. W., Masaki, K. H., Curb, J. D., & Petrovitch, H. (2004). Walking and dementia in physically capable elderly men. *JAMA*, *292*(12), 1447–1453. http://dx.doi.org/10.1001/jama.292.12.1447.

Abbott, R. D., White, L. R., Ross, G. W., Petrovitch, H., Masaki, K. H., & Snowdon, D. A., et al. (1998). Height as a marker of childhood development and late-life cognitive function: The Honolulu-Asia aging study. *Pediatrics*, *102*(3), 602–609. http://dx.doi.org/10.1542/peds.102.3.602.

Abner, E. L., Nelson, P. T., Schmitt, F. A., Browning, S. R., Fardo, D. W., Wan, L., & Kryscio, R. J. (2014). Self-reported head injury and risk of late-life impairment and AD pathology in an AD center cohort. *Dementia and Geriatric Cognitive Disorders*, *37*(5–6), 294–306. http://dx.doi.org/10.1159/000355478.

Adapt Research Group, (2006). Cardiovascular and cerebrovascular events in the randomized, controlled Alzheimer's Disease Anti-Inflammatory Prevention Trial (ADAPT). *PLoS Clinical Trials*, *1*(7), e33. http://dx.doi.org/10.1371/journal.pctr.0010033.

Adlard, P. A., Perreau, V. M., Pop, V., & Cotman, C. W. (2005). Voluntary exercise decreases amyloid load in a transgenic model of Alzheimer's disease. *The Journal of Neuroscience*, *25*(17), 4217–4221. http://dx.doi.org/10.1523/JNEUROSCI.0496-05.2005.

Adlercreutz, H., & Mazur, W. (1997). Phyto-oestrogens and Western diseases. *Annals of Medicine*, *29*(2), 95–120.

Agnew-Blais, J. C., Wassertheil-Smoller, S., Kang, J. H., Hogan, P. E., Coker, L. H., & Snetselaar, L. G., et al. (2014). Folate, vitamin B-6, and vitamin B-12 intake and mild cognitive impairment and probable dementia in the women's health initiative memory study. *Journal of the Academy of Nutrition and Dietetics*. http://dx.doi.org/10.1016/j.jand.2014.07.006.

Ahlskog, J. E., Geda, Y. E., Graff-Radford, N. R., & Petersen, R. C. (2011). Physical exercise as a preventive or disease-modifying treatment of dementia and brain aging. *Mayo Clinic Proceedings*, *86*(9), 876–884. http://dx.doi.org/10.4065/mcp.2011.0252.

Aisen, P. S., Schneider, L. S., Sano, M., Diaz-Arrastia, R., van Dyck, C. H., Weiner, M. F., & Thal, L. J. (2008). High-dose B vitamin supplementation and cognitive decline in Alzheimer disease: A randomized controlled trial. *JAMA*, *300*(15), 1774–1783. http://dx.doi.org/10.1001/jama.300.15.1774.

Akbaraly, T. N., Portet, F., Fustinoni, S., Dartigues, J. F., Artero, S., Rouaud, O., & Berr, C. (2009). Leisure activities and the risk of dementia in the elderly: Results from the Three-City Study. *Neurology*, *73*(11), 854–861. http://dx.doi.org/10.1212/WNL.0b013e3181b7849b.

Albert, M. S., DeKosky, S. T., Dickson, D., Dubois, B., Feldman, H. H., Fox, N. C., & Phelps, C. H. (2011). The diagnosis of mild cognitive impairment due to Alzheimer's disease: Recommendations from the National Institute on Aging-Alzheimer's Association workgroups on diagnostic guidelines for Alzheimer's disease. *Alzheimer's & Dementia: The Journal of the Alzheimer's Association*, *7*(3), 270–279. http://dx.doi.org/10.1016/j.jalz.2011.03.008.

Aliyu, M. H., Jolly, P. E., Ehiri, J. E., & Salihu, H. M. (2005). High parity and adverse birth outcomes: Exploring the maze. *Birth*, *32*(1), 45–59. http://dx.doi.org/10.1111/j.0730-7659.2005.00344.x.

Al-Najjar, J., Skoog, I., Hällström, T., Őstling, S., Gudmundsson, P., & Johansson, L., et al. (2015). Leisure artistic and intellectual engagements and physical activity in midlife are associated with reduced risk of late-life dementia: A 38-year follow-up. *Alzheimer's & Dementia*, *11* (7, Suppl.); P3–254, p. 274.

Altmann, A., Tian, L., Henderson, V. W., Greicius, M. D., & Alzheimer's Disease Neuroimaging Initiative, I. (2014). Sex modifies the APOE-related risk of developing Alzheimer disease. *Annals of Neurology*, *75*(4), 563–573. http://dx.doi.org/10.1002/ana.24135.

Alzheimer, A. (1907). Uber ene eigenartige Erkrankung der Hirnrinde. *Allgemeine Zeitschrift fur Psychiatrie und Psychisch-Gerichtliche Medizin*, *64*, 146–148.

Alzheimer's Association (2012). 2012 Alzheimer's disease facts and figures. *Alzheimers Dement*, *8*(2), 131–168.

Alzheimer's Disease Anti-inflammatory Prevention Trial Research Group (2013). Results of a follow-up study to the randomized Alzheimer's Disease Anti-inflammatory Prevention Trial (ADAPT). *Alzheimer's & Dementia : The Journal of the Alzheimer's Association*, *9*(6), 714–723. http://dx.doi.org/10.1016/j.jalz.2012.11.012.

Amaducci, L. A., Fratiglioni, L., Rocca, W. A., Fieschi, C., Livrea, P., & Pedone, D., et al. (1986). Risk factors for clinically diagnosed Alzheimer's disease: A case-control study of an Italian population. *Neurology*, *36*(7), 922–931.

Amariglio, R. E., Townsend, M. K., Grodstein, F., Sperling, R. A., & Rentz, D. M. (2011). Specific subjective memory complaints in older persons may indicate poor cognitive function. *Journal of the American Geriatrics Society*, *59*(9), 1612–1617. http://dx.doi.org/10.1111/j.1532-5415.2011.03543.x.

American Psychiatric Association (2000). *Diagnostic and statistical manual of mental disorders*. Washington, D.C.: American Psychiatric Association. (4th ed., text rev.)

American Psychiatric Association (2013). *Diagnostic and statistical manual of mental disorders* (5th ed.). Arlington, VA: American Psychiatric Publishing.

Amieva, H., Le Goff, M., Millet, X., Orgogozo, J. M., Peres, K., Barberger-Gateau, P., & Dartigues, J. F. (2008). Prodromal Alzheimer's disease: Successive emergence of the clinical symptoms. *Annals of Neurology*, *64*(5), 492–498. http://dx.doi.org/10.1002/ana.21509.

Amieva, H., Stoykova, R., Matharan, F., Helmer, C., Antonucci, T. C., & Dartigues, J. F. (2010). What aspects of social network are protective for dementia? Not the quantity but the quality of social interactions is protective up to 15 years later. *Psychosomatic Medicine*, *72*(9), 905–911. http://dx.doi.org/10.1097/PSY.0b013e3181f5e121.

Andel, R., Crowe, M., Pedersen, N. L., Fratiglioni, L., Johansson, B., & Gatz, M. (2008). Physical exercise at midlife and risk of dementia three decades later: A population-based study of Swedish twins. *The Journals of Gerontology Series A, Biological Sciences and Medical Sciences*, *63*(1), 62–66.

Andel, R., Crowe, M., Pedersen, N. L., Mortimer, J., Crimmins, E., & Johansson, B., et al. (2005). Complexity of work and risk of Alzheimer's disease: A population-based study of Swedish twins. *The Journals of Gerontology Series B, Psychological Sciences and Social Sciences*, *60*(5), P251–258.

Andersen, K., Launer, L. J., Ott, A., Hoes, A. W., Breteler, M. M., & Hofman, A. (1995). Do non-steroidal anti-inflammatory drugs decrease the risk for Alzheimer's disease? The Rotterdam Study. *Neurology*, *45*(8), 1441–1445.

Anderson-Hanley, C., Arciero, P. J., Brickman, A. M., Nimon, J. P., Okuma, N., Westen, S. C., & Zimmerman, E. A. (2012). Exergaming and older adult cognition: A cluster randomized clinical trial. *American Journal of Preventive Medicine*, *42*(2), 109–119. http://dx.doi.org/10.1016/j.amepre.2011.10.016.

Annweiler, C., & Beauchet, O. (2011). Vitamin D-mentia: Randomized clinical trials should be the next step. *Neuroepidemiology*, *37*(3–4), 249–258. http://dx.doi.org/10.1159/000334177.

Annweiler, C., Dursun, E., Feron, F., Gezen-Ak, D., Kalueff, A. V., Littlejohns, T., & Beauchet, O. (2014). 'Vitamin D and cognition in older adults': Updated international recommendations. *Journal of Internal Medicine*. http://dx.doi.org/10.1111/joim.12279.

Annweiler, C., Llewellyn, D. J., & Beauchet, O. (2012). Low serum vitamin D concentrations in Alzheimer's disease: A systematic review and meta-analysis. *Journal of Alzheimer's Disease*, *33*, 659–674.

Anstey, K. J., Cherbuin, N., Budge, M., & Young, J. (2011). Body mass index in midlife and late-life as a risk factor for dementia: A meta-analysis of prospective studies. *Obesity Reviews: An Official Journal of the International Association for the Study of Obesity*, *12*(5), e426–437. http://dx.doi.org/10.1111/j.1467-789X.2010.00825.x.

Anstey, K. J., Cherbuin, N., & Herath, P. M. (2013). Development of a new method for assessing global risk of Alzheimer's disease for use in population health approaches to prevention. *Prevention Science: The Official Journal of the Society for Prevention Research*, *14*(4), 411–421. http://dx.doi.org/10.1007/s11121-012-0313-2.

Anstey, K. J., Jorm, A. F., Reglade-Meslin, C., Maller, J., Kumar, R., von Sanden, C., & Sachdev, P. (2006). Weekly alcohol consumption, brain atrophy, and white matter hyperintensities in a community-based sample aged 60 to 64 years. *Psychosomatic Medicine*, *68*(5), 778–785. http://dx.doi.org/10.1097/01.psy.0000237779.56500.af.

Anstey, K. J., von Sanden, C., Salim, A., & O'Kearney, R. (2007). Smoking as a risk factor for dementia and cognitive decline: A meta-analysis of prospective studies. *American Journal of Epidemiology*, *166*(4), 367–378. http://dx.doi.org/10.1093/aje/kwm116.

Anttila, T., Helkala, E. L., Viitanen, M., Kareholt, I., Fratiglioni, L., Winblad, B., & Kivipelto, M. (2004). Alcohol drinking in middle age and subsequent risk of mild cognitive impairment and dementia in old age: A prospective population based study. *BMJ*, *329*(7465), 539. http://dx.doi.org/10.1136/bmj.38181.418958.BE.

Arab, L., Biggs, M. L., O'Meara, E. S., Longstreth, W. T., Crane, P. K., & Fitzpatrick, A. L. (2011). Gender differences in tea, coffee, and cognitive decline in the elderly: The cardiovascular health study. *Journal of Alzheimer's Disease*, *27*(3), 553–566. http://dx.doi.org/10.3233/JAD-2011-110431.

Arendash, G. W., & Cao, C. (2010). Caffeine and coffee as therapeutics against Alzheimer's disease. *Journal of Alzheimer's Disease*, *20*(Suppl. 1), S117–126. http://dx.doi.org/10.3233/JAD-2010-091249.

Ariza, M., Kolb, H. C., Moechars, D., Rombouts, F., & Andres, J. I. (2015). Tau Positron Emission Tomography (PET) imaging: Past, present, and future. *Journal of Medicinal Chemistry*. http://dx.doi.org/10.1021/jm5017544.

Ariza, M., Serra-Grabulosa, J. M., Junque, C., Ramirez, B., Mataro, M., Poca, A., & Sahuquillo, J. (2006). Hippocampal head atrophy after traumatic brain injury. *Neuropsychologia*, *44*(10), 1956–1961. http://dx.doi.org/10.1016/j.neuropsychologia.2005.11.007.

Arvanitakis, Z., Grodstein, F., Bienias, J. L., Schneider, J. A., Wilson, R. S., Kelly, J. F., & Bennett, D. A. (2008). Relation of NSAIDs to incident AD, change in cognitive function, and AD pathology. *Neurology*, *70*(23), 2219–2225. http://dx.doi.org/10.1212/01.wnl.0000313813.48505.86.

Arvanitakis, Z., Leurgans, S. E., Barnes, L. L., Bennett, D. A., & Schneider, J. A. (2011). Microinfarct pathology, dementia, and cognitive systems. *Stroke*, *42*(3), 722–727. http://dx.doi.org/10.1161/STROKEAHA.110.595082.

Auriacombe, S., Helmer, C., Amieva, H., Berr, C., Dubois, B., & Dartigues, J. F. (2010). Validity of the free and cued selective reminding test in predicting dementia: The 3C study. *Neurology, 74*(22), 1760–1767. http://dx.doi.org/10.1212/WNL.0b013e3181df0959.

Averback, P. (1983). Two new lesions in Alzheimer's disease. *Lancet, 2*(8360), 1203.

Axelsen, P. H., Komatsu, H., & Murray, I. V. (2011). Oxidative stress and cell membranes in the pathogenesis of Alzheimer's disease. *Physiology (Bethesda), 26*(1), 54–69. http://dx.doi.org/10.1152/physiol.00024.2010.

Bachman, D. L., Wolf, P. A., Linn, R., Knoefel, J. E., Cobb, J., Belanger, A., & White, L. R. (1992). Prevalence of dementia and probable senile dementia of the Alzheimer type in the Framingham Study. *Neurology, 42*(1), 115–119.

Bahar-Fuchs, A., Chetelat, G., Villemagne, V. L., Moss, S., Pike, K., Masters, C. L., & Savage, G. (2010). Olfactory deficits and amyloid-beta burden in Alzheimer's disease, mild cognitive impairment, and healthy aging: A PiB PET study. *Journal of Alzheimer's disease, 22*(4), 1081–1087. http://dx.doi.org/10.3233/JAD-2010-100696.

Baker, L. D., Frank, L. L., Foster-Schubert, K., Green, P. S., Wilkinson, C. W., McTiernan, A., & Craft, S. (2010). Effects of aerobic exercise on mild cognitive impairment: A controlled trial. *Archives of Neurology, 67*(1), 71–79. http://dx.doi.org/10.1001/archneurol.2009.307.

Balaratnasingam, S., & Janca, A. (2012). Brain derived neurotrophic factor: A novel neurotrophin involved in psychiatric and neurological disorders. *Pharmacology & Therapeutics, 134*(1), 116–124. http://dx.doi.org/10.1016/j.pharmthera.2012.01.006.

Ball, K., Berch, D. B., Helmers, K. F., Jobe, J. B., Leveck, M. D., Marsiske, M., & Vital Elderly Study Group, (2002). Effects of cognitive training interventions with older adults: A randomized controlled trial. *JAMA, 288*(18), 2271–2281.

Bannerman, E., Reilly, J. J., MacLennan, W. J., Kirk, T., & Pender, F. (1997). Evaluation of validity of British anthropometric reference data for assessing nutritional state of elderly people in Edinburgh: Cross sectional study. *BMJ, 315*(7104), 338–341.

Barberger-Gateau, P., Jutand, M. A., Letenneur, L., Larrieu, S., Tavernier, B., & Berr, C., et al. (2005). Correlates of regular fish consumption in French elderly community dwellers: Data from the Three-City study. *European Journal of Clinical Nutrition, 59*(7), 817–825. http://dx.doi.org/10.1038/sj.ejcn.1602145.

Barberger-Gateau, P., Letenneur, L., Deschamps, V., Peres, K., Dartigues, J. F., & Renaud, S. (2002). Fish, meat, and risk of dementia: Cohort study. *BMJ, 325*(7370), 932–933.

Barberger-Gateau, P., Raffaitin, C., Letenneur, L., Berr, C., Tzourio, C., & Dartigues, J. F., et al. (2007). Dietary patterns and risk of dementia: The Three-City cohort study. *Neurology, 69*(20), 1921–1930. http://dx.doi.org/10.1212/01.wnl.0000278116.37320.52.

Barker, D. J. (1998). In utero programming of chronic disease. *Clinical Science (London, England: 1979), 95*(2), 115–128.

Barker, D. J., Larsen, G., Osmond, C., Thornburg, K. L., Kajantie, E., & Eriksson, J. G. (2012). The placental origins of sudden cardiac death. *International Journal of Epidemiology, 41*(5), 1394–1399. http://dx.doi.org/10.1093/ije/dys116.

Barker, D. J., & Thornburg, K. L. (2013). Placental programming of chronic diseases, cancer and lifespan: A review. *Placenta, 34*(10), 841–845. http://dx.doi.org/10.1016/j.placenta.2013.07.063.

Barker, D. J., Winter, P. D., Osmond, C., Margetts, B., & Simmonds, S. J. (1989). Weight in infancy and death from ischaemic heart disease. *Lancet, 2*(8663), 577–580.

Barker, D. J. P. (2004). The developmental origins of well-being. *Philosophical Transactions of the Royal Society of London B, 359*, 1359–1366.

Barnes, D. E., Alexopoulos, G. S., Lopez, O. L., Williamson, J. D., & Yaffe, K. (2006). Depressive symptoms, vascular disease, and mild cognitive impairment: Findings from the Cardiovascular

Health Study. *Archives of General Psychiatry*, *63*(3), 273–279. http://dx.doi.org/10.1001/archpsyc.63.3.273.

Barnes, D. E., Beiser, A. S., Lee, A., Langa, K. M., Koyama, A., Preis, S. R., & Weir, D. R. (2014). Development and validation of a brief dementia screening indicator for primary care. *Alzheimer's & Dementia: The Journal of the Alzheimer's Association*, *10*(6), 656–665.e1. http://dx.doi.org/10.1016/j.jalz.2013.11.006.

Barnes, D. E., Covinsky, K. E., Whitmer, R. A., Kuller, L. H., Lopez, O. L., & Yaffe, K. (2009). Predicting risk of dementia in older adults: The late-life dementia risk index. *Neurology*, *73*(3), 173–179. http://dx.doi.org/10.1212/WNL.0b013e3181a81636.

Barnes, D. E., Kaup, A., Kirby, K. A., Byers, A. L., Diaz-Arrastia, R., & Yaffe, K. (2014). Traumatic brain injury and risk of dementia in older veterans. *Neurology*, *83*(4), 312–319. http://dx.doi.org/10.1212/WNL.0000000000000616.

Barnes, D. E., Santos-Modesitt, W., Poelke, G., Kramer, A. F., Castro, C., & Middleton, L. E., et al. (2013). The Mental Activity and eXercise (MAX) trial: A randomized controlled trial to enhance cognitive function in older adults. *JAMA Internal Medicine*, *173*(9), 797–804. http://dx.doi.org/10.1001/jamainternmed.2013.189.

Barnes, D. E., & Yaffe, K. (2009). Predicting dementia: Role of dementia risk indices. *Future Neurology*, *4*(5), 555–560. http://dx.doi.org/10.2217/fnl.09.43.

Barnes, D. E., & Yaffe, K. (2011). The projected impact of risk factor reduction on Alzheimer's disease prevalence. *Lancet Neurology*, *10*(9), 819–828.

Barnes, D. E., Yaffe, K., Byers, A. L., McCormick, M., Schaefer, C., & Whitmer, R. A. (2012). Midlife vs late-life depressive symptoms and risk of dementia: Differential effects for Alzheimer disease and vascular dementia. *Archives of General Psychiatry*, *69*(5), 493–498. http://dx.doi.org/10.1001/archgenpsychiatry.2011.1481.

Barnes, L. L., Schneider, J. A., Boyle, P. A., Bienias, J. L., & Bennett, D. A. (2006). Memory complaints are related to Alzheimer disease pathology in older persons. *Neurology*, *67*(9), 1581–1585. http://dx.doi.org/10.1212/01.wnl.0000242734.16663.09.

Bartres-Faz, D., & Arenaza-Urquijo, E. M. (2011). Structural and functional imaging correlates of cognitive and brain reserve hypotheses in healthy and pathological aging. *Brain Topography*, *24*(3–4), 340–357. http://dx.doi.org/10.1007/s10548-011-0195-9.

Bassuk, S. S., Glass, T. A., & Berkman, L. F. (1999). Social disengagement and incident cognitive decline in community-dwelling elderly persons. *Annals of Internal Medicine*, *131*(3), 165–173.

Bateman, R. J., Xiong, C., Benzinger, T. L., Fagan, A. M., Goate, A., Fox, N. C., & Dominantly Inherited Alzheimer Network, (2012). Clinical and biomarker changes in dominantly inherited Alzheimer's disease. *The New England Journal of Medicine*, *367*(9), 795–804. http://dx.doi.org/10.1056/NEJMoa1202753.

Baty, J., & Morris, J. C. (2011). *Calculation of global clinical dementia rating score (Form B4: CDRGLOB). The NIA Alzheimer's Disease Centers Program.* <https://www.alz.washington.edu/cdmacc.html> Accessed 03.07.13.

Beard, C. M., Kokmen, E., Offord, K. P., & Kurland, L. T. (1992). Lack of association between Alzheimer's disease and education, occupation, marital status, or living arrangement. *Neurology*, *42*(11), 2063–2068.

Beeri, M. S., Davidson, M., Silverman, J. M., Noy, S., Schmeidler, J., & Goldbourt, U. (2005). Relationship between body height and dementia. *The American Journal of Geriatric Psychiatry: Official Journal of the American Association for Geriatric Psychiatry*, *13*(2), 116–123. http://dx.doi.org/10.1176/appi.ajgp.13.2.116.

Benedictus, M. R., van Harten, A. C., Scheltens, P., Barkhof, F., Prins, N., & van der Flier, W. M. (2014). White matter hyperintensities predict mild cognitive impairment and dementia in patients with subjective cognitive complaints. *Alzheimer's & Dementia (Abstract)*, *10*(4), 42–43.

Bennett, D. A., Schneider, J. A., Arvanitakis, Z., Kelly, J. F., Aggarwal, N. T., & Shah, R. C., et al. (2006). Neuropathology of older persons without cognitive impairment from two community-based studies. *Neurology*, *66*(12), 1837–1844. http://dx.doi.org/10.1212/01.wnl.0000219668.47116.e6.

Bennett, D. A., Schneider, J. A., Arvanitakis, Z., & Wilson, R. S. (2012). Overview and findings from the religious orders study. *Current Alzheimer Research*, *9*(6), 628–645.

Bennett, D. A., Schneider, J. A., Buchman, A. S., Barnes, L. L., Boyle, P. A., & Wilson, R. S. (2012). Overview and findings from the rush memory and aging project. *Current Alzheimer Research*, *9*(6), 646–663.

Bennett, D. A., Schneider, J. A., Tang, Y., Arnold, S. E., & Wilson, R. S. (2006). The effect of social networks on the relation between Alzheimer's disease pathology and level of cognitive function in old people: A longitudinal cohort study. *Lancet Neurology*, *5*(5), 406–412. http://dx.doi.org/10.1016/S1474-4422(06)70417-3.

Bennett, D. A., Schneider, J. A., Wilson, R. S., Bienias, J. L., & Arnold, S. E. (2004). Neurofibrillary tangles mediate the association of amyloid load with clinical Alzheimer disease and level of cognitive function. *Archives of Neurology*, *61*(3), 378–384. http://dx.doi.org/10.1001/archneur.61.3.378.

Bennett, D. A., Wilson, R. S., Schneider, J. A., Evans, D. A., Mendes de Leon, C. F., Arnold, S. E., & Bienias, J. L. (2003). Education modifies the relation of AD pathology to level of cognitive function in older persons. *Neurology*, *60*(12), 1909–1915. http://dx.doi.org/10.1212/01.wnl.0000069923.64550.9f.

Bennett, D. A., Yu, L., Yang, J., Srivastava, G. P., Aubin, C., & De Jager, P. L. (2015). Epigenomics of Alzheimer's disease. *Translational Research: The Journal of Laboratory and Clinical Medicine*, *165*(1), 200–220. http://dx.doi.org/10.1016/j.trsl.2014.05.006.

Benraiss, A., Chmielnicki, E., Lerner, K., Roh, D., & Goldman, S. A. (2001). Adenoviral brain-derived neurotrophic factor induces both neostriatal and olfactory neuronal recruitment from endogenous progenitor cells in the adult forebrain. *The Journal of Neuroscience*, *21*(17), 6718–6731.

Berchtold, N. C., Castello, N., & Cotman, C. W. (2010). Exercise and time-dependent benefits to learning and memory. *Neuroscience*, *167*(3), 588–597. http://dx.doi.org/10.1016/j.neuroscience.2010.02.050.

Berchtold, N. C., Kesslak, J. P., & Cotman, C. W. (2002). Hippocampal brain-derived neurotrophic factor gene regulation by exercise and the medial septum. *Journal of Neuroscience Research*, *68*(5), 511–521. http://dx.doi.org/10.1002/jnr.10256.

Berkman, L. F. (2000). Which influences cognitive function: Living alone or being alone? *Lancet*, *355*(9212), 1291–1292. http://dx.doi.org/10.1016/S0140-6736(00)02107-3.

Bertram, L., McQueen, M. B., Mullin, K., Blacker, D., & Tanzi, R. E. (2007). Systematic meta-analyses of Alzheimer disease genetic association studies: The AlzGene database. *Nature Genetics*, *39*(1), 17–23. http://dx.doi.org/10.1038/ng1934.

Beydoun, M. A., Beydoun, H. A., Gamaldo, A. A., Teel, A., Zonderman, A. B., & Wang, Y. (2014). Epidemiologic studies of modifiable factors associated with cognition and dementia: Systematic review and meta-analysis. *BMC Public Health*, *14*(1), 643. http://dx.doi.org/10.1186/1471-2458-14-643.

Beydoun, M. A., Beydoun, H. A., & Wang, Y. (2008). Obesity and central obesity as risk factors for incident dementia and its subtypes: A systematic review and meta-analysis. *Obesity Reviews: An Official Journal of the International Association for the Study of Obesity*, *9*(3), 204–218. http://dx.doi.org/10.1111/j.1467-789X.2008.00473.x.

Bezzola, L., Merillat, S., Gaser, C., & Jancke, L. (2011). Training-induced neural plasticity in golf novices. *The Journal of Neuroscience*, *31*(35), 12444–12448. http://dx.doi.org/10.1523/JNEUROSCI.1996-11.2011.

Bierer, L. M., Hof, P. R., Purohit, D. P., Carlin, L., Schmeidler, J., & Davis, K. L., et al. (1995). Neocortical neurofibrillary tangles correlate with dementia severity in Alzheimer's disease. *Archives of Neurology*, *52*(1), 81–88.

Bieswal, F., Ahn, M. T., Reusens, B., Holvoet, P., Raes, M., & Rees, W. D., et al. (2006). The importance of catch-up growth after early malnutrition for the programming of obesity in male rat. *Obesity (Silver Spring)*, *14*(8), 1330–1343. http://dx.doi.org/10.1038/oby.2006.151.

Billings, L. M., Green, K. N., McGaugh, J. L., & LaFerla, F. M. (2007). Learning decreases A beta*56 and tau pathology and ameliorates behavioral decline in 3xTg-AD mice. *The Journal of Neuroscience*, *27*(4), 751–761. http://dx.doi.org/10.1523/JNEUROSCI.4800-06.2007.

Bird, T. D., Lampe, T. H., Nemens, E. J., Sumi, S. M., Nochlin, D., & Schellenberg, G. D., et al. (1989). Characteristics of familial Alzheimer's disease in nine kindreds of Volga German ancestry. *Progress in Clinical and Biological Research*, *317*, 229–234.

Black, J. E., Isaacs, K. R., Anderson, B. J., Alcantara, A. A., & Greenough, W. T. (1990). Learning causes synaptogenesis, whereas motor activity causes angiogenesis, in cerebellar cortex of adult rats. *Proceedings of the National Academy of Sciences of the United States of America*, *87*(14), 5568–5572.

Blennow, K., Hampel, H., Weiner, M., & Zetterberg, H. (2010). Cerebrospinal fluid and plasma biomarkers in Alzheimer disease. *Nature Reviews Neurology*, *6*(3), 131–144. http://dx.doi.org/10.1038/nrneurol.2010.4.

Blennow, K., Hardy, J., & Zetterberg, H. (2012). The neuropathology and neurobiology of traumatic brain injury. *Neuron*, *76*(5), 886–899. http://dx.doi.org/10.1016/j.neuron.2012.11.021.

Blomstrand, E., Perrett, D., Parry-Billings, M., & Newsholme, E. A. (1989). Effect of sustained exercise on plasma amino acid concentrations and on 5-hydroxytryptamine metabolism in six different brain regions in the rat. *Acta Physiologica Scandinavica*, *136*(3), 473–481. http://dx.doi.org/10.1111/j.1748-1716.1989.tb08689.x.

Blondell, S. J., Hammersley-Mather, R., & Veerman, J. L. (2014). Does physical activity prevent cognitive decline and dementia?: A systematic review and meta-analysis of longitudinal studies. *BMC Public Health*, *14*, 510. http://dx.doi.org/10.1186/1471-2458-14-510.

Bo, H., Kang, W., Jiang, N., Wang, X., Zhang, Y., & Ji, L. L. (2014). Exercise-induced neuroprotection of hippocampus in APP/PS1 transgenic mice via upregulation of mitochondrial 8-oxoguanine DNA glycosylase. *Oxidative Medicine and Cellular Longevity*, *2014*, 834502. http://dx.doi.org/10.1155/2014/834502.

Bonaiuto, S., Rocca, W. A., Lippi, A., Giannandrea, E., Mele, M., & Cavarzeran, F., et al. (1995). Education and occupation as risk factors for dementia: A population-based case-control study. *Neuroepidemiology*, *14*(3), 101–109.

Boothby, L. A., & Doering, P. L. (2005). Vitamin C and vitamin E for Alzheimer's disease. *The Annals of Pharmacotherapy*, *39*(12), 2073–2080. http://dx.doi.org/10.1345/aph.1E495.

Boots, E. A., Schultz, S. A., Oh, J. M., Larson, J., Edwards, D., Cook, D., & Okonkwo, O. C. (2014). Cardiorespiratory fitness is associated with brain structure, cognition, and mood in a middle-aged cohort at risk for Alzheimer's disease. *Brain Imaging and Behavior*. http://dx.doi.org/10.1007/s11682-014-9325-9.

Borenstein, A. R., Dahlquist, E., Wu, Y., Larson, E. B., & Teng, E. L. (2007). Education, reaction time and the National Adult Reading Test as predictors of incident dementia: The Kame Project. *Alzheimer's & Dementia*, *3*(Suppl. 2), S181–182.

Borenstein, A. R., Mortimer, J. A., Ding, D., Schellenberg, G. D., DeCarli, C., Qianhua, Z., & Zhen, H. (2010). Effects of apolipoprotein E-epsilon4 and -epsilon2 in amnestic mild cognitive impairment and dementia in Shanghai: SCOBHI-P. *American Journal of Alzheimer's Disease and Other Dementias*, *25*(3), 233–238. http://dx.doi.org/10.1177/1533317509357736.

Borenstein, A. R., Mortimer, J. A., & Larson, E. B. (2014). Population attributable fraction for incident dementia related to brain reserve, Alzheimer's disease, and vascular disease: Brain reserve is most important. *Alzheimer's & Dementia*, *10*(4 Suppl.), P230–231.

Borenstein, A. R., Mortimer, J. A., & Larson, E. B. (2014). Factor scores for brain reserve, Alzheimer and vascular pathology are independent risk factors for dementia in a population-based cohort study. *Neurology*. http://www.abstracts2view.com/aan/view.php?nu=AAN14L_1_S58.006.

Borenstein, A. R., Mortimer, J. A., Wu, Y., Jureidini-Webb, F. M., Fallin, M. D., Small, B. J., & Crawford, F. C. (2006). Apolipoprotein E and cognition in community-based samples of African Americans and Caucasians. *Ethnicity & Disease*, *16*(1), 9–15.

Borenstein, A. R., Wu, Y., Bowen, J. D., McCormick, W. C., Uomoto, J., McCurry, S. M., & Larson, E. B. (2014). Incidence rates of dementia, Alzheimer disease, and vascular dementia in the Japanese American Population in Seattle, WA: The Kame Project. *Alzheimer Disease and Associated Disorders*, *28*(1), 23–29. http://dx.doi.org/10.1097/WAD.0b013e3182a2e32f.

Borenstein, A.R., Wu, Y., Larson, E.B. (2005). *Subjective memory decline predicts dementia in a population-based study: The Kame Project. Neurology* 64 (Suppl 1) March 2005: A318.

Borenstein, A. R., Wu, Y., Mortimer, J. A., Schellenberg, G. D., McCormick, W. C., Bowen, J. D., & Larson, E. B. (2005). Developmental and vascular risk factors for Alzheimer's disease. *Neurobiology of Aging*, *26*(3), 325–334. http://dx.doi.org/10.1016/j.neurobiolaging.2004.04.010.

Borenstein Graves, A. (2004). Alzheimer's disease and vascular dementia. In L. M. Nelson, C. M. Tanner, S. K. Van Den Eeden & V. M. McGuire (Eds.), *Neuroepidemiology: From principles to practice* (pp. 102–130). New York: Oxford University Press.

Borenstein Graves, A., Mortimer, J. A., Bowen, J. D., McCormick, W. C., McCurry, S. M., & Schellenberg, G. D., et al. (2001). Head circumference and incident Alzheimer's disease: Modification by apolipoprotein E. *Neurology*, *57*, 1453–1460.

Bowden, C. L., Kokmen, E., Beard, C. M., Kurland, L. T., Kirkland, L. R., & Jarvik, L. F., et al. (1990). The presence of Alzheimer's disease in a community population. *JAMA*, *263*(18), 2447–2449.

Boyke, J., Driemeyer, J., Gaser, C., Buchel, C., & May, A. (2008). Training-induced brain structure changes in the elderly. *The Journal of Neuroscience*, *28*(28), 7031–7035. http://dx.doi.org/10.1523/JNEUROSCI.0742-08.2008.

Boyle, P. A., Wilson, R. S., Yu, L., Barr, A. M., Honer, W. G., & Schneider, J. A., et al. (2013). Much of late life cognitive decline is not due to common neurodegenerative pathologies. *Annals of Neurology*, *74*(3), 478–489. http://dx.doi.org/10.1002/ana.23964.

Boyle, P. A., Yu, L., Wilson, R. S., Schneider, J. A., & Bennett, D. A. (2013). Relation of neuropathology with cognitive decline among older persons without dementia. *Frontiers Aging Neuroscience*, *5*, 50. http://dx.doi.org/10.3389/fnagi.2013.00050.

Braak, H., & Braak, E. (1991). Neuropathological stageing of Alzheimer-related changes. *Acta Neuropathologica*, *82*(4), 239–259.

Braak, H., & Braak, E. (1997). Frequency of stages of Alzheimer-related lesions in different age categories. *Neurobiology of Aging*, *18*(4), 351–357.

Braak, H., Braak, E., Yilmazer, D., de Vos, R. A., Jansen, E. N., & Bohl, J. (1997). Neurofibrillary tangles and neuropil threads as a cause of dementia in Parkinson's disease. *Journal of Neural Transmission Supplementum*, *51*, 49–55.

Braskie, M. N., Boyle, C. P., Rajagopalan, P., Gutman, B. A., Toga, A. W., Raji, C. A., & Thompson, P. M. (2014). Physical activity, inflammation, and volume of the aging brain. *Neuroscience*, *273*, 199–209. http://dx.doi.org/10.1016/j.neuroscience.2014.05.005.

Brayne, C., Richardson, K., Matthews, F. E., Fleming, J., Hunter, S., Xuereb, J. H., & Cambridge City Over-75s Cohort Cc75c Study Neuropathology Collaboration. (2009). Neuropathological correlates of dementia in over-80-year-old brain donors from the population-based Cambridge city over-75s cohort (CC75C) study. *Journal of Alzheimer's Disease*, *18*(3), 645–658. http://dx.doi.org/10.3233/JAD-2009-1182.

Breitner, J. C., Gau, B. A., Welsh, K. A., Plassman, B. L., McDonald, W. M., & Helms, M. J., et al. (1994). Inverse association of anti-inflammatory treatments and Alzheimer's disease: Initial results of a co-twin control study. *Neurology*, *44*(2), 227–232.

Breitner, J. C., Haneuse, S. J., Walker, R., Dublin, S., Crane, P. K., & Gray, S. L., et al. (2009). Risk of dementia and AD with prior exposure to NSAIDs in an elderly community-based cohort. *Neurology*, *72*(22), 1899–1905. http://dx.doi.org/10.1212/WNL.0b013e3181a18691.

Breitner, J. C., Wyse, B. W., Anthony, J. C., Welsh-Bohmer, K. A., Steffens, D. C., Norton, M. C., & Khachaturian, A. (1999). APOE-epsilon4 count predicts age when prevalence of AD increases, then declines: The cache county study. *Neurology*, *53*(2), 321–331.

Breteler, M. M. (2000). Vascular risk factors for Alzheimer's disease: An epidemiologic perspective. *Neurobiology of Aging*, *21*(2), 153–160.

Bretsky, P. M., Buckwalter, J. G., Seeman, T. E., Miller, C. A., Poirier, J., Schellenberg, G. D., & Henderson, V. W. (1999). Evidence for an interaction between apolipoprotein E genotype, gender, and Alzheimer disease. *Alzheimer Disease and Associated Disorders*, *13*(4), 216–221.

Brickman, A. M., Zahodne, L. B., Guzman, V. A., Narkhede, A., Meier, I. B., Griffith, E. Y., & Mayeux, R. (2014). Reconsidering harbingers of dementia: Progression of parietal lobe white matter hyperintensities predicts Alzheimer's disease incidence. *Neurobiology of Aging*. http://dx.doi.org/10.1016/j.neurobiolaging.2014.07.019.

Brodaty, H., Seeher, K., & Gibson, L. (2012). Dementia time to death: A systematic literature review on survival time and years of life lost in people with dementia. *International Psychogeriatrics/IPA*, *24*(7), 1034–1045. http://dx.doi.org/10.1017/S1041610211002924.

Brody, J. A., & Schneider, E. L. (1986). Diseases and disorders of aging: An hypothesis. *Journal of Chronic Diseases*, *39*(11), 871–876.

Brondino, N., Re, S., Boldrini, A., Cuccomarino, A., Lanati, N., & Barale, F., et al. (2014). Curcumin as a therapeutic agent in dementia: A mini systematic review of human studies. *Scientific World Journal*, *2014*, 174282. http://dx.doi.org/10.1155/2014/174282.

Brookmeyer, R., Evans, D. A., Hebert, L., Langa, K. M., Heeringa, S. G., & Plassman, B. L., et al. (2011). National estimates of the prevalence of Alzheimer's disease in the United States. *Alzheimer's & Dementia: The Journal of the Alzheimer's Association*, *7*(1), 61–73. http://dx.doi.org/10.1016/j.jalz.2010.11.007.

Brookmeyer, R., Gray, S., & Kawas, C. (1998). Projections of Alzheimer's disease in the United States and the public health impact of delaying disease onset. *American Journal of Public Health*, *88*(9), 1337–1342.

Brookmeyer, R., Johnson, E., Ziegler-Graham, K., & Arrighi, H. M. (2007). Forecasting the global burden of Alzheimer's disease. *Alzheimer's & Dementia: The Journal of the Alzheimer's Association*, *3*(3), 186–191. http://dx.doi.org/10.1016/j.jalz.2007.04.381.

Brust, J. C. (2010). Ethanol and Cognition: Indirect effects, neurotoxicity and neuroprotection: A review. *International Journal of Environmental Research and Public Health*, *7*(4), 1540–1557. http://dx.doi.org/10.3390/ijerph7041540.

Buchman, A. S., Boyle, P. A., Yu, L., Shah, R. C., Wilson, R. S., & Bennett, D. A. (2012). Total daily physical activity and the risk of AD and cognitive decline in older adults. *Neurology*, *78*(17), 1323–1329. http://dx.doi.org/10.1212/WNL.0b013e3182535d35.

Buerger, K., Ewers, M., Pirttila, T., Zinkowski, R., Alafuzoff, I., Teipel, S. J., & Hampel, H. (2006). CSF phosphorylated tau protein correlates with neocortical neurofibrillary pathology in Alzheimer's disease. *Brain, 129*(Pt 11), 3035–3041. http://dx.doi.org/10.1093/brain/awl269.

Burkhardt, M. S., Foster, J. K., Clarnette, R. M., Chubb, S. A., Bruce, D. G., Drummond, P. D., & Yeap, B. B. (2006). Interaction between testosterone and apolipoprotein E epsilon4 status on cognition in healthy older men. *The Journal of Clinical Endocrinology and Metabolism, 91*(3), 1168–1172. http://dx.doi.org/10.1210/jc.2005-1072.

Burns, J. M., Cronk, B. B., Anderson, H. S., Donnelly, J. E., Thomas, G. P., Harsha, A., & Swerdlow, R. H. (2008). Cardiorespiratory fitness and brain atrophy in early Alzheimer disease. *Neurology, 71*(3), 210–216. http://dx.doi.org/10.1212/01.wnl.0000317094.86209.cb.

Byers, A. L., Covinsky, K. E., Barnes, D. E., & Yaffe, K. (2012). Dysthymia and depression increase risk of dementia and mortality among older veterans. *The American Journal of Geriatric Psychiatry: Official Journal of the American Association for Geriatric Psychiatry, 20*(8), 664–672. http://dx.doi.org/10.1097/JGP.0b013e31822001c1.

Caamano-Isorna, F., Corral, M., Montes-Martinez, A., & Takkouche, B. (2006). Education and dementia: A meta-analytic study. *Neuroepidemiology, 26*(4), 226–232. http://dx.doi.org/10.1159/000093378.

Cai, Y., Xiong, K., Zhang, X. M., Cai, H., Luo, X. G., Feng, J. C., & Yan, X. X. (2010). Beta-Secretase-1 elevation in aged monkey and Alzheimer's disease human cerebral cortex occurs around the vasculature in partnership with multisystem axon terminal pathogenesis and beta-amyloid accumulation. *The European Journal of Neuroscience, 32*(7), 1223–1238. http://dx.doi.org/10.1111/j.1460-9568.2010.07376.x.

Calleja-Agius, J., Muscat-Baron, Y., & Brincat, M. P. (2007). Skin ageing. *Menopause International, 13*(2), 60–64.

Canadian Study of Health and Aging Investigators, (1994). The Canadian study of health and aging: Risk factors for Alzheimer's disease in Canada. *Neurology, 44*(11), 2073–2080.

Cao, Y., Lu, L., Liang, J., Liu, M., Li, X., Sun, R., & Zhang, P. (2014). Omega-3 fatty acids and primary and secondary prevention of cardiovascular disease. *Cell Biochemistry and Biophysics*. http://dx.doi.org/10.1007/s12013-014-0407-5.

Carmelli, D., Cardon, L. R., & Fabsitz, R. (1994). Clustering of hypertension, diabetes and obesity in adult male twins: Same genes or same environments? *American Journal of Human Genetics, 55*(3), 566–573.

Carriere, I., Fourrier-Reglat, A., Dartigues, J. F., Rouaud, O., Pasquier, F., & Ritchie, K., et al. (2009). Drugs with anticholinergic properties, cognitive decline, and dementia in an elderly general population: The 3-city study. *Archives of Internal Medicine, 169*(14), 1317–1324. http://dx.doi.org/10.1001/archinternmed.2009.229.

Carro, E., Trejo, J. L., Busiguina, S., & Torres-Aleman, I. (2001). Circulating insulin-like growth factor I mediates the protective effects of physical exercise against brain insults of different etiology and anatomy. *The Journal of Neuroscience, 21*(15), 5678–5684.

Carstensen, L. L., Isaacowitz, D. M., & Charles, S. T. (1999). Taking time seriously. A theory of socioemotional selectivity. *The American Psychologist, 54*(3), 165–181.

Carvalho, A., Rea, I. M., Parimon, T., & Cusack, B. J. (2014). Physical activity and cognitive function in individuals over 60 years of age: A systematic review. *Clinical Interventions in Aging, 9*, 661–682. http://dx.doi.org/10.2147/CIA.S55520.

Cavus, I., & Duman, R. S. (2003). Influence of estradiol, stress, and 5-HT2A agonist treatment on brain-derived neurotrophic factor expression in female rats. *Biological Psychiatry, 54*(1), 59–69.

Centers for Disease Control (2013). Adult participation in aerobic and muscle-strengthening physical activities - United States, 2011. In Centers for Disease Control (Ed.), *United States morbidity and mortality weekly report* 62(17):326–330.

Centers for Disease Control and Prevention (2012). Prevalence of current depression among persons aged > =12 years, by age group and sex—United States, National Health and Nutrition Examination Survey, 2007–2010. *Morbidity and Mortality Weekly Report (MMWR)* <http://www.cdc.gov/mmwr/preview/mmwrhtml/mm6051a7.htm?s_cid=mm6051a7_w#x2013;%20United%20States,%20National%20Health%20and%20Nutrition%20Examination%20Survey,%202007-2010%3C/a%3E> Accessed 13.01.15.

Chan, D., Fox, N. C., Scahill, R. I., Crum, W. R., Whitwell, J. L., Leschziner, G., & Rossor, M. N. (2001). Patterns of temporal lobe atrophy in semantic dementia and Alzheimer's disease. *Annals of Neurology*, *49*(4), 433–442.

Chandra, V., Bharucha, N. E., & Schoenberg, B. S. (1986). Patterns of mortality from types of dementia in the United States, 1971 and 1973–1978. *Neurology*, *36*(2), 204–208.

Chandra, V., Ganguli, M., Pandav, R., Johnston, J., Belle, S., & DeKosky, S. T. (1998). Prevalence of Alzheimer's disease and other dementias in rural India: The Indo-US Study. *Neurology*, *51*, 1000–1008.

Chandra, V., Ganguli, M., Ratcliff, G., Pandav, R., Sharma, S., Belle, S., & Nath, L. (1998). Practical issues in cognitive screening of elderly illiterate populations in developing countries. The Indo-US Cross-National Dementia Epidemiology Study. *Aging (Milano)*, *10*(5), 349–357.

Chandra, V., Pandav, R., Dodge, H. H., Johnston, J. M., Belle, S. H., & DeKosky, S. T., et al. (2001). Incidence of Alzheimer's disease in a rural community in India: The Indo-US study. *Neurology*, *57*(6), 985–989.

Chandra, V., Philipose, V., Bell, P. A., Lazaroff, A., & Schoenberg, B. S. (1987). Case-control study of late onset "probable Alzheimer's disease". *Neurology*, *37*(8), 1295–1300.

Chase, H. P. (1973). The effects of intrauterine and postnatal undernutrition on normal brain development. *Annals of the New York Academy of Sciences*, *205*, 231–244.

Chernausek, S. D. (2012). Update: Consequences of abnormal fetal growth. *The Journal of Clinical Endocrinology and Metabolism*, *97*(3), 689–695. http://dx.doi.org/10.1210/jc.2011-2741.

Cherubini, A., Martin, A., Andres-Lacueva, C., Di Iorio, A., Lamponi, M., Mecocci, P., & Ferrucci, L. (2005). Vitamin E levels, cognitive impairment and dementia in older persons: The InCHIANTI study. *Neurobiology of Aging*, *26*(7), 987–994. http://dx.doi.org/10.1016/j.neurobiolaging.2004.09.002.

Chetelat, G., La Joie, R., Villain, N., Perrotin, A., de La Sayette, V., & Eustache, F., et al. (2013). Amyloid imaging in cognitively normal individuals, at-risk populations and preclinical Alzheimer's disease. *Neuroimage Clinical*, *2*, 356–365. http://dx.doi.org/10.1016/j.nicl.2013.02.006.

Chiu, C. C., Su, K. P., Cheng, T. C., Liu, H. C., Chang, C. J., Dewey, M. E., & Huang, S. Y. (2008). The effects of omega-3 fatty acids monotherapy in Alzheimer's disease and mild cognitive impairment: A preliminary randomized double-blind placebo-controlled study. *Progress in Neuro-Psychopharmacology & Biological Psychiatry*, *32*(6), 1538–1544. http://dx.doi.org/10.1016/j.pnpbp.2008.05.015.

Cholerton, B., Baker, L. D., & Craft, S. (2013). Insulin, cognition, and dementia. *European Journal of Pharmacology*, *719*(1–3), 170–179. http://dx.doi.org/10.1016/j.ejphar.2013.08.008.

Chouraki, V., Beiser, A., Younkin, L., Preis, S. R., Weinstein, G., Hansson, O., & Seshadri, S. (2015). Plasma amyloid-beta and risk of Alzheimer's disease in the Framingham Heart Study. *Alzheimer's & Dementia: The Journal of the Alzheimer's Association*, *11*(3), 249–257.e241. http://dx.doi.org/10.1016/j.jalz.2014.07.001.

Chui, H. C., Zheng, L., Reed, B. R., Vinters, H. V., & Mack, W. J. (2012). Vascular risk factors and Alzheimer's disease: Are these risk factors for plaques and tangles or for concomitant vascular pathology that increases the likelihood of dementia? An evidence-based review. *Alzheimers Research & Therapy*, *4*(1), 1. http://dx.doi.org/10.1186/alzrt98.

Cimini, A., Gentile, R., D'Angelo, B., Benedetti, E., Cristiano, L., Avantaggiati, M. L., & Desideri, G. (2013). Cocoa powder triggers neuroprotective and preventive effects in a human Alzheimer's disease model by modulating BDNF signaling pathway. *Journal of Cellular Biochemistry, 114*(10), 2209–2220. http://dx.doi.org/10.1002/jcb.24548.

Clare, P., Bradford, D., Courtney, R. J., Martire, K., & Mattick, R. P. (2013). The relationship between socioeconomic status and 'hardcore' smoking over time-greater accumulation of hardened smokers in low-SES than high-SES smokers. *Tobacco Control*. http://dx.doi.org/10.1136/tobaccocontrol-2013-051436.

Clark, G. M., Zamenhof, S., Van Mathens, E., Grauel, L., & Kruger, L. (1973). The effect of prenatal malnutrition on dimensions of cerebral cortex. *Brain Research, 54*, 397–402.

Clark, J. H. (2006). A critique of Women's Health Initiative Studies (2002–2006). *Nuclear Receptor Signaling, 4*, e023. http://dx.doi.org/10.1621/nrs.04023.

Clarke, R., Bennett, D., Parish, S., Lewington, S., Skeaff, M., Eussen, S. J., & Grodstein, F. (2014). Effects of homocysteine lowering with B vitamins on cognitive aging: Meta-analysis of 11 trials with cognitive data on 22,000 individuals. *The American Journal of Clinical Nutrition, 100*(2), 657–666. http://dx.doi.org/10.3945/ajcn.113.076349.

Clayton, D. (1991). The EURODEM collaborative re-analysis of case-control studies of Alzheimer's disease: Some methodological considerations. *International Journal of Epidemiology, 20*(Suppl 2), S62–64.

Codemo, A., Corti, M. C., & Mazzetto, G., et al. (2000). Education, APOE status and cognitive impairment in elderly: An epidemiological study in a rural setting. *Neurobiology of Aging, 2*, S246.

Colcombe, S. J., Erickson, K. I., Raz, N., Webb, A. G., Cohen, N. J., & McAuley, E., et al. (2003). Aerobic fitness reduces brain tissue loss in aging humans. *The Journals of Gerontology Series A, Biological Sciences and Medical Sciences, 58*(2), 176–180.

Colcombe, S. J., Erickson, K. I., Scalf, P. E., Kim, J. S., Prakash, R., McAuley, E., & Kramer, A. F. (2006). Aerobic exercise training increases brain volume in aging humans. *The Journals of Gerontology Series A, Biological Sciences and Medical Sciences, 61*(11), 1166–1170.

Colcombe, S. J., Kramer, A. F., Erickson, K. I., Scalf, P., McAuley, E., Cohen, N. J., & Elavsky, S. (2004). Cardiovascular fitness, cortical plasticity, and aging. *Proceedings of the National Academy of Sciences of the United States of America, 101*(9), 3316–3321. http://dx.doi.org/10.1073/pnas.0400266101.

Cole, G. M., Ma, Q. L., & Frautschy, S. A. (2009). Omega-3 fatty acids and dementia. *Prostaglandins, Leukotrienes, and Essential Fatty Acids, 81*(2–3), 213–221. http://dx.doi.org/10.1016/j.plefa.2009.05.015.

Cole, G. M., Teter, B., & Frautschy, S. A. (2007). Neuroprotective effects of curcumin. *Advances in Experimental Medicine and Biology, 595*, 197–212. http://dx.doi.org/10.1007/978-0-387-46401-5_8.

Colsher, P. L., & Wallace, R. B. (1991). Longitudinal application of cognitive function measures in a defined population of community-dwelling elders. *Annals of Epidemiology, 1*, 215–230.

Commenges, D., Scotet, V., Renaud, S., Jacqmin-Gadda, H., Barberger-Gateau, P., & Dartigues, J. F. (2000). Intake of flavonoids and risk of dementia. *European Journal of Epidemiology, 16*(4), 357–363.

Consentino, S., Metcalfe, J., Butterfield, B., & Stern, Y. (2007). Objective metamemory testing captures awareness of deficit in Alzheimer's disease. *Cortex, 43*, 1004–1019.

Corder, E. H., Ghebremedhin, E., Taylor, M. G., Thal, D. R., Ohm, T. G., & Braak, H. (2004). The biphasic relationship between regional brain senile plaque and neurofibrillary tangle distributions: Modification by age, sex, and APOE polymorphism. *Annals of the New York Academy of Sciences*, *1019*, 24–28. http://dx.doi.org/10.1196/annals.1297.005.

Corder, E. H., Saunders, A. M., Strittmatter, W. J., Schmechel, D. E., Gaskell, P. C., Small, G. W., & Pericak-Vance, M. A. (1993). Gene dose of apolipoprotein E type 4 allele and the risk of Alzheimer's disease in late onset families. *Science*, *261*(5123), 921–923.

Corey-Bloom, J., Thal, L. J., & Galasko, D., et al. (1995). Diagnosis and evaluation of dementia. *Neurology*, *45*, 211–218.

Corrada, M. M., Brookmeyer, R., Berlau, D., Paganini-Hill, A., & Kawas, C. H. (2008). Prevalence of dementia after age 90: Results from the 90+ study. *Neurology*, *71*(5), 337–343. http://dx.doi.org/10.1212/01.wnl.0000310773.65918.cd.

Corrada, M. M., Brookmeyer, R., Paganini-Hill, A., Berlau, D., & Kawas, C. H. (2010). Dementia incidence continues to increase with age in the oldest old: The 90+ study. *Annals of Neurology*, *67*(1), 114–121. http://dx.doi.org/10.1002/ana.21915.

Correia, S. C., Santos, R. X., Carvalho, C., Cardoso, S., Candeias, E., Santos, M. S., & Moreira, P. I. (2012). Insulin signaling, glucose metabolism and mitochondria: Major players in Alzheimer's disease and diabetes interrelation. *Brain Research*, *1441*, 64–78. http://dx.doi.org/10.1016/j.brainres.2011.12.063.

Corsellis, J. A. N. (1975). Posttraumatic dementia. In R. Katzman, R. D. Terry, & K. L. Bick (Eds.). *Alzheimer's disease: Senile dementia and related disorders* (Vol. 7, pp. 125–133). New York: Raven Press.

Corsellis, J. A. N., & Brierley, J. B. (1959). Observations on the pathology of insidious dementia following head injury. *The Journal of Mental Science*, *105*, 714–720.

Cowie, C. C., Rust, K. F., Byrd-Holt, D. D., Eberhardt, M. S., Flegal, K. M., Engelgau, M. M., & Gregg, E. W. (2006). Prevalence of diabetes and impaired fasting glucose in adults in the U.S. population: National health and nutrition examination survey 1999–2002. *Diabetes Care*, *29*(6), 1263–1268. http://dx.doi.org/10.2337/dc06-0062.

Cracchiolo, J. R., Mori, T., Nazian, S. J., Tan, J., Potter, H., & Arendash, G. W. (2007). Enhanced cognitive activity—over and above social or physical activity—is required to protect Alzheimer's mice against cognitive impairment, reduce Abeta deposition, and increase synaptic immunoreactivity. *Neurobiology of Learning and Memory*, *88*(3), 277–294. http://dx.doi.org/10.1016/j.nlm.2007.07.007.

Craft, S. (2009). The role of metabolic disorders in Alzheimer disease and vascular dementia: Two roads converged. *Archives of Neurology*, *66*(3), 300–305. http://dx.doi.org/10.1001/archneurol.2009.27.

Craft, S., Baker, L. D., Montine, T. J., Minoshima, S., Watson, G. S., Claxton, A., & Gerton, B. (2012). Intranasal insulin therapy for Alzheimer disease and amnestic mild cognitive impairment: A pilot clinical trial. *Archives of Neurology*, *69*(1), 29–38. http://dx.doi.org/10.1001/archneurol.2011.233.

Crane, P. K., Walker, R., Hubbard, R. A., Li, G., Nathan, D. M., Zheng, H., & Larson, E. B. (2013). Glucose levels and risk of dementia. *The New England Journal of Medicine*, *369*(6), 540–548. http://dx.doi.org/10.1056/NEJMoa1215740.

Crews, W. D., Jr., Harrison, D. W., & Wright, J. W. (2008). A double-blind, placebo-controlled, randomized trial of the effects of dark chocolate and cocoa on variables associated with neuropsychological functioning and cardiovascular health: Clinical findings from a sample of healthy, cognitively intact older adults. *The American Journal of Clinical Nutrition*, *87*(4), 872–880.

Critchley, M. (1957). Medical aspects of boxing, particularly from a neurological standpoint. *British Medical Journal*, *1*(5015), 357–362.

Crowe, M., Andel, R., Pedersen, N. L., Johansson, B., & Gatz, M. (2003). Does participation in leisure activities lead to reduced risk of Alzheimer's disease? A prospective study of Swedish twins. *The Journals of Gerontology Series B, Psychological Sciences and Social Sciences*, *58*(5), P249–255.

Cummings, J. L., Dubois, B., Molinuevo, J. L., & Scheltens, P. (2013). International work group criteria for the diagnosis of Alzheimer disease. *The Medical Clinics of North America*, *97*, 363–368.

Cummings, J. L., Morstorf, T., & Zhong, K. (2014). Alzheimer's disease drug-development pipeline: Few candidates, frequent failures. *Alzheimers Research & Therapy*, *6*(4), 37. http://dx.doi.org/10.1186/alzrt269.

Currie, J., Ramsbottom, R., Ludlow, H., Nevill, A., & Gilder, M. (2009). Cardio-respiratory fitness, habitual physical activity and serum brain derived neurotrophic factor (BDNF) in men and women. *Neuroscience Letters*, *451*(2), 152–155. http://dx.doi.org/10.1016/j.neulet.2008.12.043.

Czeh, B., & Lucassen, P. J. (2007). What causes the hippocampal volume decrease in depression? Are neurogenesis, glial changes and apoptosis implicated? *European Archives of Psychiatry and Clinical Neuroscience*, *257*(5), 250–260. http://dx.doi.org/10.1007/s00406-007-0728-0.

Dahl, A. K., Fauth, E. B., Ernsth-Bravell, M., Hassing, L. B., Ram, N., & Gerstof, D. (2013). Body mass index, change in body mass index, and survival in old and very old persons. *Journal of the American Geriatrics Society*, *61*(4), 512–518. http://dx.doi.org/10.1111/jgs.12158.

Dai, Q., Borenstein, A. R., Wu, Y., Jackson, J. C., & Larson, E. B. (2006). Fruit and vegetable juices and Alzheimer's disease: The Kame Project. *The American Journal of Medicine*, *119*(9), 751–759. http://dx.doi.org/10.1016/j.amjmed.2006.03.045.

Dams-O'Connor, K., Gibbons, L. E., Bowen, J. D., McCurry, S. M., Larson, E. B., & Crane, P. K. (2013). Risk for late-life re-injury, dementia and death among individuals with traumatic brain injury: A population-based study. *Journal of Neurology, Neurosurgery, and Psychiatry*, *84*(2), 177–182. http://dx.doi.org/10.1136/jnnp-2012-303938.

Dartigues, J. F., Gagnon, M., & Michel, P., et al. (1991). Le programme de recherche PAQUID sur l'epidemiologie de la demence: Methodes et resultats initiaux. *Revue Neurologique (Paris)*, *147*, 225–230.

Daviglus, M. L., Plassman, B. L., Pirzada, A., Bell, C. C., Bowen, P. E., Burke, J. R., & Williams, J. W., Jr. (2011). Risk factors and preventive interventions for Alzheimer disease: State of the science. *Archives of Neurology*, *68*(9), 1185–1190. http://dx.doi.org/10.1001/archneurol.2011.100.

Dawe, R. J., Bennett, D. A., Schneider, J. A., & Arfanakis, K. (2011). Neuropathologic correlates of hippocampal atrophy in the elderly: A clinical, pathologic, postmortem MRI study. *PLoS One*, *6*(10), e26286. http://dx.doi.org/10.1371/journal.pone.0026286.

Dawodu, S. T. (2015). Traumatic Brain Injury (TBI)—Definition, epidemiology, pathophysiology. *Drugs & Diseases* <http://emedicine.medscape.com/article/326510-overview>.

Dean, D. C., III, Jerskey, B. A., Chen, K., Protas, H., Thiyyagura, P., Roontiva, A., & Reiman, E. M. (2014). Brain differences in infants at differential genetic risk for late-onset Alzheimer disease: A cross-sectional imaging study. *JAMA Neurology*, *71*(1), 11–22. http://dx.doi.org/10.1001/jamaneurol.2013.4544.

Deary, I. J., & Caryl, P. G. (1997). Neuroscience and human intelligence differences. *Trends in Neurosciences*, *20*(8), 365–371.

Deary, I. J., Gow, A. J., Taylor, M. D., Corley, J., Brett, C., Wilson, V., & Starr, J. M. (2007). The Lothian Birth Cohort 1936: A study to examine influences on cognitive ageing from age 11 to age 70 and beyond. *BMC Geriatrics*, *7*, 28. http://dx.doi.org/10.1186/1471-2318-7-28.

Deaton, A. (2007). Height, health, and development. *Proceedings of the National Academy of Sciences*, *104*(33), 13232–13237.

Debette, S., & Markus, H. S. (2010). The clinical importance of white matter hyperintensities on brain magnetic resonance imaging: Systematic review and meta-analysis. *BMJ*, *341*, c3666. http://dx.doi.org/10.1136/bmj.c3666.

De Braekeleer, M., Froda, S., Gautrin, D., Tetreault, H., & Gauvreau, D. (1988). Parental age and birth order in Alzheimer's disease: A case-control study in the Saguenay-Lac-St-Jean area (Quebec, Canada). *The Canadian Journal of Neurological Sciences Le Journal Canadien des Sciences Neurologiques*, *15*(2), 139–141.

de Bruin, E. A., Hulshoff Pol, H. E., Schnack, H. G., Janssen, J., Bijl, S., Evans, A. C., & Verbaten, M. N. (2005). Focal brain matter differences associated with lifetime alcohol intake and visual attention in male but not in female non-alcohol-dependent drinkers. *Neuroimage*, *26*(2), 536–545. http://dx.doi.org/10.1016/j.neuroimage.2005.01.036.

DeCarli, C. (2013). Clinically asymptomatic vascular brain injury: A potent cause of cognitive impairment among older individuals. *Journal of Alzheimer's Disease*, *33*(Suppl. 1), S417–426. http://dx.doi.org/10.3233/JAD-2012-129004.

De Felice, F. G., Lourenco, M. V., & Ferreira, S. T. (2014). How does brain insulin resistance develop in Alzheimer's disease? *Alzheimer's & Dementia*, *10*, S26–32.

de Groot, R. H., Stein, A. D., Jolles, J., van Boxtel, M. P., Blauw, G. J., & van de Bor, M., et al. (2011). Prenatal famine exposure and cognition at age 59 years. *International Journal of Epidemiology*, *40*(2), 327–337. http://dx.doi.org/10.1093/ije/dyq261.

de Jager, C. A. (2014). Critical levels of brain atrophy associated with homocysteine and cognitive decline. *Neurobiology of Aging*, *35*(Suppl. 2), S35–39. http://dx.doi.org/10.1016/j.neurobiolaging.2014.03.040.

de Jager, C. A., Oulhaj, A., Jacoby, R., Refsum, H., & Smith, A. D. (2012). Cognitive and clinical outcomes of homocysteine-lowering B-vitamin treatment in mild cognitive impairment: A randomized controlled trial. *International Journal of Geriatric Psychiatry*, *27*(6), 592–600. http://dx.doi.org/10.1002/gps.2758.

de Jong-Gierveld, J. (1987). Developing and testing a model of loneliness. *Journal of Personality and Social Psychology*, *53*(1), 119–128.

de Jong, N., Chin, A., Paw, M. J., de Groot, L. C., Rutten, R. A., & Swinkels, D. W., et al. (2001). Nutrient-dense foods and exercise in frail elderly: Effects on B vitamins, homocystein, methylmalonic acid, and neuropsychological functioning. *American Journal of Clinical Nutrition*, *73*(2), 338–346.

DeKosky, S. T., Abrahamson, E. E., Ciallella, J. R., Paljug, W. R., Wisniewski, S. R., & Clark, R. S., et al. (2007). Association of increased cortical soluble abeta42 levels with diffuse plaques after severe brain injury in humans. *Archives of Neurology*, *64*(4), 541–544. http://dx.doi.org/10.1001/archneur.64.4.541.

de la Torre, J. C. (2013). Vascular risk factors: A ticking time bomb to Alzheimer's disease. *American Journal of Alzheimer's Disease and Other Dementias*, *28*. http://dx.doi.org/10.1177/1533317513494457.

Delisle, H. (2002). Programming of chronic disease by impaired fetal nutrition: Evidence and implications for policy and intervention strategies. WHO/NHD/02.3. WHO/NPH/02.1. World Health Organization, Department of Nutrition for Health and Development and Department of Noncommunicable Disease Prevention and Health Promotion, Geneva, Switzerland.

de Rooij, S. R., Wouters, H., Yonker, J. E., Painter, R. C., & Roseboom, T. J. (2010). Prenatal undernutrition and cognitive function in late adulthood. *Proceedings of the National Academy of Sciences of the United States of America*, *107*(39), 16881–16886. http://dx.doi.org/10.1073/pnas.1009459107.

Deschaintre, Y., Richard, F., Leys, D., & Pasquier, F. (2009). Treatment of vascular risk factors is associated with slower decline in Alzheimer disease. *Neurology*, *73*(9), 674–680. http://dx.doi.org/10.1212/WNL.0b013e3181b59bf3.

Devanand, D. P., Michaels-Marston, K. S., Liu, X., Pelton, G. H., Padilla, M., Marder, K., & Mayeux, R. (2000). Olfactory deficits in patients with mild cognitive impairment predict Alzheimer's disease at follow-up. *The American Journal of Psychiatry*, *157*(9), 1399–1405.

Devanand, D. P., Tabert, M. H., Cuasay, K., Manly, J. J., Schupf, N., Brickman, A. M., & Mayeux, R. (2010). Olfactory identification deficits and MCI in a multi-ethnic elderly community sample. *Neurobiology of Aging*, *31*(9), 1593–1600. http://dx.doi.org/10.1016/j.neurobiolaging.2008.09.008.

Deweerdt, S. (2011). Prevention: Activity is the best medicine. *Nature*, *475*(7355), S16–17. http://dx.doi.org/10.1038/475S16a.

Diamond, B. J., Shiflett, S. C., Feiwel, N., Matheis, R. J., Noskin, O., & Richards, J. A., et al. (2000). Ginkgo biloba extract: Mechanisms and clinical indications. *Archives of Physical Medicine and Rehabilitation*, *81*(5), 668–678.

Dickerson, B. C., Goncharova, I., Sullivan, M. P., Forchetti, C., Wilson, R. S., Bennett, D. A., & deToledo-Morrell, L. (2001). MRI-derived entorhinal and hippocampal atrophy in incipient and very mild Alzheimer's disease. *Neurobiology of Aging*, *22*(5), 747–754.

Dickerson, B. C., Stoub, T. R., Shah, R. C., Sperling, R. A., Killiany, R. J., Albert, M. S., & Detoledo-Morrell, L. (2011). Alzheimer-signature MRI biomarker predicts AD dementia in cognitively normal adults. *Neurology*, *76*(16), 1395–1402. http://dx.doi.org/10.1212/WNL.0b013e3182166e96.

Dickstein, D. L., Walsh, J., Brautigam, H., Stockton, S. D., Jr., Gandy, S., & Hof, P. R. (2010). Role of vascular risk factors and vascular dysfunction in Alzheimer's disease. *The Mount Sinai Journal of Medicine, New York*, *77*(1), 82–102. http://dx.doi.org/10.1002/msj.20155.

Dietert, R. R., Etzel, R. A., Chen, D., Halonen, M., Holladay, S. D., Jarabek, A. M., & Zoetis, T. (2000). Workshop to identify critical windows of exposure for children's health: Immune and respiratory systems work group summary. *Environmental Health Perspectives*, *108*(Suppl 3), 483–490.

Dik, M., Deeg, D. J., Visser, M., & Jonker, C. (2003). Early life physical activity and cognition at old age. *Journal of Clinical and Experimental Neuropsychology*, *25*(5), 643–653. http://dx.doi.org/10.1076/jcen.25.5.643.14583.

Dik, M. G., Jonker, C., Comijs, H. C., Bouter, L. M., Twisk, J. W., & van Kamp, G. J., et al. (2001). Memory complaints and APOE-epsilon4 accelerate cognitive decline in cognitively normal elderly. *Neurology*, *57*(12), 2217–2222.

Ding, D., Zhao, Q., Guo, Q., Meng, H., Wang, B., Yu, P., & Hong, Z. (2014). The Shanghai aging study: Study design, baseline characteristics, and prevalence of dementia. *Neuroepidemiology*, *43*(2), 114–122. http://dx.doi.org/10.1159/000366163.

Ding, E. L., Hutfless, S. M., Ding, X., & Girotra, S. (2006). Chocolate and prevention of cardiovascular disease: A systematic review. *Nutrition & Metabolism*, *3*, 2. http://dx.doi.org/10.1186/1743-7075-3-2.

Ding, J., Eigenbrodt, M. L., Mosley, T. H., Jr., et al., Hutchinson, R. G., Folsom, A. R., & Harris, T. B., et al. (2004). Alcohol intake and cerebral abnormalities on magnetic resonance imaging in a community-based population of middle-aged adults: The Atherosclerosis Risk in Communities (ARIC) study. *Stroke*, *35*(1), 16–21. http://dx.doi.org/10.1161/01.STR.0000105929.88691.8E.

Ding, Q., Vaynman, S., Akhavan, M., Ying, Z., & Gomez-Pinilla, F. (2006). Insulin-like growth factor I interfaces with brain-derived neurotrophic factor-mediated synaptic plasticity to modulate aspects of exercise-induced cognitive function. *Neuroscience*, *140*(3), 823–833. http://dx.doi.org/10.1016/j.neuroscience.2006.02.084.

Diniz, B. S., Butters, M. A., Albert, S. M., Dew, M. A., & Reynolds, C. F., III (2013). Late-life depression and risk of vascular dementia and Alzheimer's disease: Systematic review and meta-analysis of community-based cohort studies. *The British Journal of Psychiatry: The Journal of Mental Science*, *202*(5), 329–335. http://dx.doi.org/10.1192/bjp.bp.112.118307.

Doets, E. L., Ueland, P. M., Tell, G. S., Vollset, S. E., Nygard, O. K., Van't Veer, P., & Eussen, S. J. (2014). Interactions between plasma concentrations of folate and markers of vitamin B(12) status with cognitive performance in elderly people not exposed to folic acid fortification: The Hordaland Health Study. *The British Journal of Nutrition*, *111*(6), 1085–1095. http://dx.doi.org/10.1017/S000711451300336X.

Donovan, N. J., Amariglio, R. E., Zoller, A. S., Rudel, R. K., Gomez-Isla, T., Blacker, D., & Rentz, D. M. (2014). Subjective cognitive concerns and neuropsychiatric predictors of progression to the early clinical stages of Alzheimer disease. *The American Journal of Geriatric Psychiatry: Official Journal of the American Association for Geriatric Psychiatry*, *22*(12), 1642–1651. http://dx.doi.org/10.1016/j.jagp.2014.02.007.

Doty, R. L., Li, C., Mannon, L. J., & Yousem, D. M. (1997). Olfactory dysfunction in multiple sclerosis. *The New England Journal of Medicine*, *336*(26), 1918–1919. http://dx.doi.org/10.1056/NEJM199706263362617.

Doty, R. L., Marcus, A., & Lee, W. W. (1996). Development of the 12-item Cross-Cultural Smell Identification Test (CC-SIT). *Laryngoscope*, *106*(3 Pt 1), 353–356.

Doty, R. L., Petersen, I., Mensah, N., & Christensen, K. (2011). Genetic and environmental influences on odor identification ability in the very old. *Psychology and Aging*, *26*(4), 864–871. http://dx.doi.org/10.1037/a0023263.

Doty, R. L., Reyes, P. F., & Gregor, T. (1987). Presence of both odor identification and detection deficits in Alzheimer's disease. *Brain Research Bulletin*, *18*(5), 597–600.

Doty, R. L., Shaman, P., Applebaum, S. L., Giberson, R., Siksorski, L., & Rosenberg, L. (1984). Smell identification ability: Changes with age. *Science*, *226*(4681), 1441–1443.

Doty, R. L., Shaman, P., Kimmelman, C. P., & Dann, M. S. (1984). University of Pennsylvania smell identification test: A rapid quantitative olfactory function test for the clinic. *Laryngoscope*, *94*(2 Pt 1), 176–178.

Douaud, G., Refsum, H., de Jager, C. A., Jacoby, R., Nichols, T. E., & Smith, S. M., et al. (2013). Preventing Alzheimer's disease-related gray matter atrophy by B-vitamin treatment. *Proceedings of the National Academy of Sciences of the United States of America*, *110*(23), 9523–9528. http://dx.doi.org/10.1073/pnas.1301816110.

Downey, D. B. (2001). Number of siblings and intellectual development. The resource dilution explanation. *The American Psychologist*, *56*(6–7), 497–504.

Draganski, B., Gaser, C., Busch, V., Schuierer, G., Bogdahn, U., & May, A. (2004). Neuroplasticity: Changes in grey matter induced by training. *Nature*, *427*(6972), 311–312. http://dx.doi.org/10.1038/427311a.

Draganski, B., Gaser, C., Kempermann, G., Kuhn, H. G., Winkler, J., & Buchel, C., et al. (2006). Temporal and spatial dynamics of brain structure changes during extensive learning. *The Journal of Neuroscience*, *26*(23), 6314–6317. http://dx.doi.org/10.1523/JNEUROSCI.4628-05.2006.

Driscoll, I., Troncoso, J. C., Rudow, G., Sojkova, J., Pletnikova, O., Zhou, Y., & Resnick, S. M. (2012). Correspondence between *in vivo* (11)C-PiB-PET amyloid imaging and postmortem, region-matched assessment of plaques. *Acta Neuropathologica*, *124*(6), 823–831. http://dx.doi.org/10.1007/s00401-012-1025-1.

Dubois, B., Feldman, H. H., Jacova, C., Dekosky, S. T., Barberger-Gateau, P., Cummings, J., & Scheltens, P. (2007). Research criteria for the diagnosis of Alzheimer's disease: Revising the NINCDS-ADRDA criteria. *Lancet Neurology*, *6*(8), 734–746. http://dx.doi.org/10.1016/S1474-4422(07)70178-3.

Durazzo, T. C., Mattsson, N., & Weiner, M. W. (2014). Smoking and increased Alzheimer's disease risk: A review of potential mechanisms. *Alzheimer's & Dementia: The Journal of the Alzheimer's Association*, *10*(3 Suppl.), S122–145. http://dx.doi.org/10.1016/j.jalz.2014.04.009.

Durazzo, T. C., Meyerhoff, D. J., & Nixon, S. J. (2010). Chronic cigarette smoking: Implications for neurocognition and brain neurobiology. *International Journal of Environmental Research and Public Health*, *7*(10), 3760–3791. http://dx.doi.org/10.3390/ijerph7103760.

Dysken, M. W., Sano, M., Asthana, S., Vertrees, J. E., Pallaki, M., Llorente, M., & Guarino, P. D. (2014). Effect of vitamin E and memantine on functional decline in Alzheimer disease: The TEAM-AD VA cooperative randomized trial. *JAMA*, *311*(1), 33–44. http://dx.doi.org/10.1001/jama.2013.282834.

Edland, S. D., Rocca, W. A., Petersen, R. C., Cha, R. H., & Kokmen, E. (2002). Dementia and Alzheimer disease incidence rates do not vary by sex in Rochester, Minn. *Archives of Neurology*, *59*(10), 1589–1593.

Edmonds, E. C., Delano-Wood, L., Galasko, D. R., Salmon, D. P., Bondi, M. W., & Alzheimer's Disease Neuroimaging Initiative, (2014). Subjective cognitive complaints contribute to misdiagnosis of mild cognitive impairment. *Journal of the International Neuropsychological Society*, *20*(8), 836–847. http://dx.doi.org/10.1017/S135561771400068X.

Egan, M. F., Kojima, M., Callicott, J. H., Goldberg, T. E., Kolachana, B. S., Bertolino, A., & Weinberger, D. R. (2003). The BDNF val66met polymorphism affects activity-dependent secretion of BDNF and human memory and hippocampal function. *Cell*, *112*(2), 257–269.

Eichner, J. E., Dunn, S. T., Perveen, G., Thompson, D. M., Stewart, K. E., & Stroehla, B. C. (2002). Apolipoprotein E polymorphism and cardiovascular disease: A HuGE review. *American Journal of Epidemiology*, *155*(6), 487–495.

Ekamper, P., van Poppel, F., Stein, A. D., & Lumey, L. H. (2013). Independent and additive association of prenatal famine exposure and intermediary life conditions with adult mortality between age 18–63 years. *Social Science & Medicine*. http://dx.doi.org/10.1016/j.socscimed.2013.10.027.

Elias, M. F., Beiser, A., Wolf, P. A., Au, R., White, R. F., & D'Agostino, R. B. (2000). The preclinical phase of Alzheimer disease: A 22-year prospective study of the Framingham Cohort. *Archives of Neurology*, *57*(6), 808–813.

Elias, M. F., Wolf, P. A., D'Agostino, R. B., Cobb, J., & White, L. R. (1993). Untreated blood pressure level is inversely related to cognitive functioning: The Framingham Study. *American Journal of Epidemiology*, *138*(6), 353–364.

Ellis, W. G., McCulloch, J. R., & Corley, C. L. (1974). Presenile dementia in Down's syndrome. Ultrastructural identity with Alzheimer's disease. *Neurology*, *24*(2), 101–106.

Emmerzaal, T. L., Kiliaan, A. J., & Gustafson, D. R. (2014). 2003–2013: A decade of body mass index, Alzheimer's disease, and dementia. *Journal of Alzheimer's Disease*. http://dx.doi.org/10.3233/JAD-141086.

Engelhart, M. J., Geerlings, M. I., Ruitenberg, A., Van Swieten, J. C., Hofman, A., & Witteman, J. C., et al. (2002). Diet and risk of dementia: Does fat matter?: The Rotterdam study. *Neurology*, *59*(12), 1915–1921.

Engelhart, M. J., Geerlings, M. I., Ruitenberg, A., van Swieten, J. C., Hofman, A., & Witteman, J. C., et al. (2002). Dietary intake of antioxidants and risk of Alzheimer disease. *JAMA*, *287*(24), 3223–3229.

Engelhart, M. J., Ruitenberg, A., Meijer, J., Kiliaan, A., van Swieten, J. C., Hofman, A., & Breteler, M. M. (2005). Plasma levels of antioxidants are not associated with Alzheimer's disease or cognitive decline. *Dementia and Geriatric Cognitive Disorders*, *19*(2–3), 134–139. http://dx.doi.org/10.1159/000082884.

Engelman, M., Agree, E. M., Meoni, L. A., & Klag, M. J. (2010). Propositional density and cognitive function in later life: Findings from the Precursors Study. *The Journals of Gerontology Series B, Psychological Sciences and Social Sciences*, *65*(6), 706–711. http://dx.doi.org/10.1093/geronb/gbq064.

Englund, H., Anneren, G., Gustafsson, J., Wester, U., Wiltfang, J., Lannfelt, L., & Hoglund, K. (2007). Increase in beta-amyloid levels in cerebrospinal fluid of children with Down syndrome. *Dementia and Geriatric Cognitive Disorders*, *24*(5), 369–374. http://dx.doi.org/10.1159/000109215.

Engvig, A., Fjell, A. M., Westlye, L. T., Moberget, T., Sundseth, O., & Larsen, V. A., et al. (2012). Memory training impacts short-term changes in aging white matter: A longitudinal diffusion tensor imaging study. *Human Brain Mapping*, *33*(10), 2390–2406. http://dx.doi.org/10.1002/hbm.21370.

Erickson, K. I., Banducci, S. E., Weinstein, A. M., Macdonald, A. W., III, Ferrell, R. E., Halder, I., & Manuck, S. B. (2013). The brain-derived neurotrophic factor Val66Met polymorphism moderates an effect of physical activity on working memory performance. *Psychological Science*, *24*(9), 1770–1779. http://dx.doi.org/10.1177/0956797613480367.

Erickson, K. I., Leckie, R. L., & Weinstein, A. M. (2014). Physical activity, fitness, and gray matter volume. *Neurobiology of Aging*, *35*(Suppl. 2), S20–28. http://dx.doi.org/10.1016/j.neurobiolaging.2014.03.034.

Erickson, K. I., Prakash, R. S., Voss, M. W., Chaddock, L., Heo, S., McLaren, M., & Kramer, A. F. (2010). Brain-derived neurotrophic factor is associated with age-related decline in hippocampal volume. *The Journal of Neuroscience*, *30*(15), 5368–5375. http://dx.doi.org/10.1523/JNEUROSCI.6251-09.2010.

Erickson, K. I., Prakash, R. S., Voss, M. W., Chaddock, L., Hu, L., Morris, K. S., & Kramer, A. F. (2009). Aerobic fitness is associated with hippocampal volume in elderly humans. *Hippocampus*, *19*(10), 1030–1039. http://dx.doi.org/10.1002/hipo.20547.

Erickson, K. I., Raji, C. A., Lopez, O. L., Becker, J. T., Rosano, C., Newman, A. B., & Kuller, L. H. (2010). Physical activity predicts gray matter volume in late adulthood: The cardiovascular health study. *Neurology*, *75*(16), 1415–1422. http://dx.doi.org/10.1212/WNL.0b013e3181f88359.

Erickson, K. I., Voss, M. W., Prakash, R. S., Basak, C., Szabo, A., Chaddock, L., & Kramer, A. F. (2011). Exercise training increases size of hippocampus and improves memory. *Proceedings of the National Academy of Sciences of the United States of America*, *108*(7), 3017–3022. http://dx.doi.org/10.1073/pnas.1015950108.

Eriksson, P. S., Perfilieva, E., Bjork-Eriksson, T., Alborn, A. M., Nordborg, C., & Peterson, D. A., et al. (1998). Neurogenesis in the adult human hippocampus. *Nature Medicine*, *4*(11), 1313–1317. http://dx.doi.org/10.1038/3305.

Erkinjuntti, T., Ostbye, T., Steenhuis, R., & Hachinski, V. (1997). The effect of different diagnostic criteria on the prevalence of dementia. *The New England Journal of Medicine*, *337*(23), 1667–1674. http://dx.doi.org/10.1056/NEJM199712043372306.

Esiri, M. M., & Wilcock, G. K. (1984). The olfactory bulbs in Alzheimer's disease. *Journal of Neurology, Neurosurgery, and Psychiatry*, *47*(1), 56–60.

Eskelinen, M. H., Ngandu, T., Helkala, E. L., Tuomilehto, J., Nissinen, A., & Soininen, H., et al. (2008). Fat intake at midlife and cognitive impairment later in life: A population-based CAIDE study. *International Journal of Geriatric Psychiatry*, *23*(7), 741–747. http://dx.doi.org/10.1002/gps.1969.

Espeland, M. A., Gu, L., Masaki, K. H., Langer, R. D., Coker, L. H., Stefanick, M. L., & Rapp, S. R. (2005). Association between reported alcohol intake and cognition: Results from the Women's Health Initiative Memory Study. *American Journal of Epidemiology*, *161*(3), 228–238. http://dx.doi.org/10.1093/aje/kwi043.

Espeland, M. A., Rapp, S. R., Shumaker, S. A., Brunner, R., Manson, J. E., Sherwin, B. B., & Women's Health Initiative Memory Study, (2004). Conjugated equine estrogens and global cognitive function in postmenopausal women: Women's Health Initiative Memory Study. *JAMA*, *291*(24), 2959–2968. http://dx.doi.org/10.1001/jama.291.24.2959.

Espinosa, P. S., Kryscio, R. J., Mendiondo, M. S., Schmitt, F. A., Wekstein, D. R., & Markesbery, W. R., et al. (2006). Alzheimer's disease and head circumference. *Journal of Alzheimer's Disease*, *9*(1), 77–80.

Etminan, M., Gill, S., & Samii, A. (2003). Effect of non-steroidal anti-inflammatory drugs on risk of Alzheimer's disease: Systematic review and meta-analysis of observational studies. *BMJ*, *327*(7407), 128. http://dx.doi.org/10.1136/bmj.327.7407.128.

Etnier, J. L., Nowell, P. M., Landers, D. M., & Sibley, B. A. (2006). A meta-regression to examine the relationship between aerobic fitness and cognitive performance. *Brain Research Reviews*, *52*(1), 119–130. http://dx.doi.org/10.1016/j.brainresrev.2006.01.002.

Evans, D. A., Beckett, L. A., Albert, M. S., Hebert, L. E., Scherr, P. A., & Funkenstein, H. H., et al. (1993). Level of education and change in cognitive function in a community population of older persons. *Annals of Epidemiology*, *3*(1), 71–77.

Evans, D. A., Bennett, D. A., Wilson, R. S., Bienias, J. L., Morris, M. C., & Scherr, P. A., et al. (2003). Incidence of Alzheimer disease in a biracial Urban community. *Archives of Neurology*, *60*, 185–189.

Evans, D. A., Funkenstein, H. H., Albert, M. S., Scherr, P. A., Cook, N. R., Chown, M. J., & Taylor, J. O. (1989). Prevalence of Alzheimer's disease in a community population of older persons. Higher than previously reported. *JAMA*, *262*(18), 2551–2556.

Evans, D. A., Smith, L. A., Scherr, P. A., Albert, M. S., Funkenstein, H. H., & Hebert, L. E. (1991). Risk of death from Alzheimer's disease in a community population of older persons. *American Journal of Epidemiology*, *134*(4), 403–412.

Evans, R. M., Emsley, C. L., Gao, S., Sahota, A., Hall, K. S., & Farlow, M. R., et al. (2000). Serum cholesterol, APOE genotype, and the risk of Alzheimer's disease: A population-based study of African Americans. *Neurology*, *54*(1), 240–242.

Exalto, L. G., Biessels, G. J., Karter, A. J., Huang, E. S., Katon, W. J., & Minkoff, J. R., et al. (2013). Risk score for prediction of 10 year dementia risk in individuals with type 2 diabetes: A cohort study. *Lancet Diabetes Endocrinology*, *1*(3), 183–190. http://dx.doi.org/10.1016/S2213-8587(13)70048-2.

Exalto, L. G., Quesenberry, C. P., Barnes, D., Kivipelto, M., Biessels, G. J., & Whitmer, R. A. (2014). Midlife risk score for the prediction of dementia four decades later. *Alzheimer's & Dementia: The Journal of the Alzheimer's Association*, *10*(5), 562–570. http://dx.doi.org/10.1016/j.jalz.2013.05.1772.

Expert Panel on Detection, Evaluation and Treatment of HIgh Blood Cholesterol in Adults, (2001). Executive Summary of the Third Report of the National Cholesterol Education Program (NCEP) Expert Panel on Dection, Evaluation and Treatment of High Blood Cholesterol in Adults (Adult Treatment Panel III). *JAMA*, *285*, 2486–2497.

Faa, G., Marcialis, M. A., Ravarino, A., Piras, M., Pintus, M. C., & Fanos, V. (2014). Fetal programming of the human brain: Is there a link with insurgence of neurodegenerative disorders in adulthood? *Current Medicinal Chemistry*, *21*, 3854–3876.

Fabre, C., Chamari, K., Mucci, P., Masse-Biron, J., & Prefaut, C. (2002). Improvement of cognitive function by mental and/or individualized aerobic training in healthy elderly subjects. *International Journal of Sports Medicine*, *23*(6), 415–421. http://dx.doi.org/10.1055/s-2002-33735.

Faden, A. I., & Loane, D. J. (2014). Chronic neurodegeneration after traumatic brain injury: Alzheimer disease, chronic traumatic encephalopathy, or persistent neuroinflammation? *Neurotherapeutics*. http://dx.doi.org/10.1007/s13311-014-0319-5.

Fagan, A. M., Mintun, M. A., Mach, R. H., Lee, S. Y., Dence, C. S., Shah, A. R., & Holtzman, D. M. (2006). Inverse relation between *in vivo* amyloid imaging load and cerebrospinal fluid Abeta42 in humans. *Annals of Neurology*, *59*(3), 512–519. http://dx.doi.org/10.1002/ana.20730.

Fagan, A. M., Roe, C. M., Xiong, C., Mintun, M. A., Morris, J. C., & Holtzman, D. M. (2007). Cerebrospinal fluid tau/beta-amyloid(42) ratio as a prediction of cognitive decline in nondemented older adults. *Archives of Neurology*, *64*(3), 343–349. http://dx.doi.org/10.1001/archneur.64.3.noc60123.

Farias, S. T., Chand, V., Bonnici, L., Baynes, K., Harvey, D., Mungas, D., & Reed, B. (2012). Idea density measured in late life predicts subsequent cognitive trajectories: Implications for the measurement of cognitive reserve. *The Journals of Gerontology Series B, Psychological Sciences and Social Sciences*, *67*(6), 677–686. http://dx.doi.org/10.1093/geronb/gbr162.

Farmer, J., Zhao, X., van Praag, H., Wodtke, K., Gage, F. H., & Christie, B. R. (2004). Effects of voluntary exercise on synaptic plasticity and gene expression in the dentate gyrus of adult male Sprague-Dawley rats *in vivo*. *Neuroscience*, *124*(1), 71–79. http://dx.doi.org/10.1016/j.neuroscience.2003.09.029.

Farrell, M. T., Zahodne, L. B., Stern, Y., Dorrejo, J., Yeung, P., & Cosentino, S. (2014). Subjective word-finding difficulty reduces engagement in social leisure activities in Alzheimer's disease. *Journal of the American Geriatrics Society*, *62*(6), 1056–1063. http://dx.doi.org/10.1111/jgs.12850.

Farrer, L. A., Cupples, L. A., Haines, J. L., Hyman, B., Kukull, W. A., Mayeux, R., & van Duijn, C. M. (1997). Effects of age, sex, and ethnicity on the association between apolipoprotein E genotype and Alzheimer disease. A meta-analysis. APOE and Alzheimer disease meta analysis consortium. *JAMA*, *278*(16), 1349–1356.

Feart, C., Samieri, C., Rondeau, V., Amieva, H., Portet, F., Dartigues, J. F., & Barberger-Gateau, P. (2009). Adherence to a Mediterranean diet, cognitive decline, and risk of dementia. *JAMA*, *302*(6), 638–648. http://dx.doi.org/10.1001/jama.2009.1146.

Ferini-Strambi, L., Smirne, S., Garancini, P., Pinto, P., & Franceschi, M. (1990). Clinical and epidemiological aspects of Alzheimer's disease with presenile onset: A case control study. *Neuroepidemiology*, *9*(1), 39–49.

Ferri, C. P., Prince, M., Brayne, C., Brodaty, H., Fratiglioni, L., Ganguli, M., & Scazufca, M. (2005). Global prevalence of dementia: A Delphi consensus study. *Lancet*, *366*(9503), 2112–2117. http://dx.doi.org/10.1016/S0140-6736(05)67889-0.

Filippini, N., MacIntosh, B. J., Hough, M. G., Goodwin, G. M., Frisoni, G. B., Smith, S. M., & Mackay, C. E. (2009). Distinct patterns of brain activity in young carriers of the APOE-epsilon4 allele. *Proceedings of the National Academy of Sciences of the United States of America*, *106*(17), 7209–7214. http://dx.doi.org/10.1073/pnas.0811879106.

Fillenbaum, G. G., Heyman, A., Huber, M. S., Woodbury, M. A., Leiss, J., Schmader, K. E., & Trapp-Moen, B. (1998). The prevalence and 3-year incidence of dementia in older black and white community residents. *Journal of Clinical Epidemiology*, *51*(7), 587–595.

Filley, C. M. (2015). Alzheimer disease prevention: New optimism. *Neurology: Clinical Practice*, *5*, 193–200.

Finkelstein, E. A., Khavjou, O. A., Thompson, H., Trogdon, J. G., Pan, L., & Sherry, B., et al. (2012). Obesity and severe obesity forecasts through 2030. *American Journal of Preventive Medicine*, *42*(6), 563–570. http://dx.doi.org/10.1016/j.amepre.2011.10.026.

Fitzpatrick, A. L., Kuller, L. H., Ives, D. G., Lopez, O. L., Jagust, W., Breitner, J. C., & Dulberg, C. (2004). Incidence and prevalence of dementia in the cardiovascular health study. *Journal of the American Geriatrics Society*, *52*(2), 195–204.

Fitzpatrick, A. L., Kuller, L. H., Lopez, O. L., Diehr, P., O'Meara, E. S., & Longstreth, W. T., et al. (2009). Midlife and late-life obesity and the risk of dementia: Cardiovascular health study. *Archives of Neurology*, *66*(3), 336–342. http://dx.doi.org/10.1001/archneurol.2008.582.

Fleminger, S., Oliver, D. L., Lovestone, S., Rabe-Hesketh, S., & Giora, A. (2003). Head injury as a risk factor for Alzheimer's disease: The evidence 10 years on; a partial replication. *Journal of Neurology, Neurosurgery, and Psychiatry*, *74*(7), 857–862.

Flicker, L., Liu-Ambrose, T., & Kramer, A. F. (2011). Why so negative about preventing cognitive decline and dementia? The jury has already come to the verdict for physical activity and smoking cessation. *British Journal of Sports Medicine*, *45*(6), 465–467. http://dx.doi.org/10.1136/bjsm.2010.077446.

Floel, A., Ruscheweyh, R., Kruger, K., Willemer, C., Winter, B., Volker, K., & Knecht, S. (2010). Physical activity and memory functions: Are neurotrophins and cerebral gray matter volume the missing link? *Neuroimage*, *49*(3), 2756–2763. http://dx.doi.org/10.1016/j.neuroimage.2009.10.043.

Folkow, B., & Svanborg, A. (1993). Physiology of cardiovascular aging. *Physiological Reviews*, *73*(4), 725–764.

Folstein, M. F., Folstein, S. E., & McHugh, P. R. (1975). "Mini-mental state". A practical method for grading the cognitive state of patients for the clinician. *Journal of Psychiatric Research*, *12*(3), 189–198.

Fordyce, D. E., & Farrar, R. P. (1991). Enhancement of spatial learning in F344 rats by physical activity and related learning-associated alterations in hippocampal and cortical cholinergic functioning. *Behavioural Brain Research*, *46*(2), 123–133.

Forette, F., Seux, M. L., Staessen, J. A., Thijs, L., Babarskiene, M. R., Babeanu, S., & Birkenhager, W. H. (2002). The prevention of dementia with antihypertensive treatment: New evidence from the Systolic Hypertension in Europe (Syst-Eur) study. *Archives of Internal Medicine*, *162*(18), 2046–2052.

Foubert-Samier, A., Catheline, G., Amieva, H., Dilharreguy, B., Helmer, C., & Allard, M., et al. (2012). Education, occupation, leisure activities, and brain reserve: A population-based study. *Neurobiology of Aging*, *33*(2) 423.e415-425. http://dx.doi.org/10.1016/j.neurobiolaging.2010.09.023.

Fournier, A., Oprisiu-Fournier, R., Serot, J. M., Godefroy, O., Achard, J. M., Faure, S., & Sato, N. (2009). Prevention of dementia by antihypertensive drugs: How AT1-receptor-blockers and dihydropyridines better prevent dementia in hypertensive patients than thiazides and ACE-inhibitors. *Expert Review of Neurotherapeutics*, *9*(9), 1413–1431. http://dx.doi.org/10.1586/ern.09.89.

Fox, N. C., Kennedy, A. M., Harvey, R. J., Lantos, P. L., Roques, P. K., Collinge, J., & Rossor, M. N. (1997). Clinicopathological features of familial Alzheimer's disease associated with the M139V mutation in the presenilin 1 gene. Pedigree but not mutation specific age at onset provides evidence for a further genetic factor. *Brain*, *120*(Pt 3), 491–501.

Fratiglioni, L., Grut, M., & Forsell, Y., et al. (1991). Prevalence of Alzheimer's disease and other dementias in an elderly urban population: Relationship with age, sex and education. *Neurology*, *41*, 1886–1892.

Fratiglioni, L., Viitanen, M., von Strauss, E., Tontodonati, V., Herlitz, A., & Winblad, B. (1997). Very old women at highest risk of dementia and Alzheimer's disease: Incidence data from the Kungsholmen Project, Stockholm. *Neurology*, *48*, 132–138.

Fratiglioni, L., Wang, H. X., Ericsson, K., Maytan, M., & Winblad, B. (2000). Influence of social network on occurrence of dementia: A community-based longitudinal study. *Lancet*, *355*(9212), 1315–1319. http://dx.doi.org/10.1016/S0140-6736(00)02113-9.

Frecker, M. F., Pryse-Phillips, W. E., & Strong, H. R. (1995). Alzheimer's disease death certificates. *Neurology*, *45*(12), 2298–2299.

Freiherr, J., Hallschmid, M., Frey, W. H., II, et al., Brunner, Y. F., Chapman, C. D., & Holscher, C., et al. (2013). Intranasal insulin as a treatment for Alzheimer's disease: A review of basic research and clinical evidence. *CNS Drugs*, *27*, 505–514.

Friedhoff, L. T., Cullen, E. I., Geoghagen, N. S., & Buxbaum, J. D. (2001). Treatment with controlled-release lovastatin decreases serum concentrations of human beta-amyloid (A beta) peptide. *The International Journal of Neuropsychopharmacology/Official Scientific Journal of the Collegium Internationale Neuropsychopharmacologicum (CINP)*, *4*(2), 127–130. http://dx.doi.org/10.1017/S1461145701002310.

Friedland, R. P., Fritsch, T., Smith, K. A., Koss, E., Lerner, A. J., & Chen, C. H., et al. (2001). Patients with Alzheimer's disease have reduced activities in midlife compared with healthy control-group members. *Proceedings of the National Academy of Sciences of the United States of America*, *98*(6), 3440–3445.

Fritsch, T., Smyth, K. A., McClendon, M. J., Ogrocki, P. K., Santillan, C., & Larsen, J. D., et al. (2005). Associations between dementia/mild cognitive impairment and cognitive performance and activity levels in youth. *Journal of the American Geriatrics Society*, *53*(7), 1191–1196. http://dx.doi.org/10.1111/j.1532-5415.2005.53361.x.

Fujimi, K., Sasaki, K., Noda, K., Wakisaka, Y., Tanizaki, Y., Matsui, Y., & Iwaki, T. (2008). Clinicopathological outline of dementia with Lewy bodies applying the revised criteria: The Hisayama study. *Brain pathology (Zurich, Switzerland)*, *18*(3), 317–325. http://dx.doi.org/10.1111/j.1750-3639.2008.00169.x.

Gabryelewicz, T., Styczynska, M., Luczywek, E., Barczak, A., Pfeffer, A., Androsiuk, W., & Barcikowska, M. (2007). The rate of conversion of mild cognitive impairment to dementia: Predictive role of depression. *International Journal of Geriatric Psychiatry*, *22*(6), 563–567. http://dx.doi.org/10.1002/gps.1716.

Galasko, D., Bennett, D., Sano, M., Ernesto, C., Thomas, R., & Grundman, M., et al. (1997). An inventory to assess activities of daily living for clinical trials in Alzheimer's disease. The Alzheimer's disease cooperative study. *Alzheimer Disease and Associated Disorders*, *11*(Suppl. 2), S33–39.

Gallagher, D., Visser, M., Sepulveda, D., Pierson, R. N., Harris, T., & Heymsfield, S. B. (1996). How useful is body mass index for comparison of body fatness across age, sex, and ethnic groups? *American Journal of Epidemiology*, *143*(3), 228–239.

Ganguli, M., Chandra, V., Kamboh, M. I., Johnston, J. M., Dodge, H. H., Thelma, B. K., & DeKosky, S. T. (2000). Apolipoprotein E polymorphism and Alzheimer disease: The Indo-US cross-national dementia study. *Archives of Neurology*, *57*(6), 824–830.

Ganguli, M., Dodge, H. H., Chen, P., Belle, S., & DeKosky, S. T. (2000). Ten-year incidence of dementia in a rural elderly US community population: The MoVIES project. *Neurology*, *54*(5), 1109–1116.

Gao, S., Hendrie, H. C., Hall, K. S., & Hui, S. (1998). The relationships between age, sex, and the incidence of dementia and Alzheimer disease: A meta-analysis. *Archives of General Psychiatry*, *55*(9), 809–815.

Gao, Y., Huang, C., Zhao, K., Ma, L., Qiu, X., Zhang, L., & Xiao, Q. (2013). Depression as a risk factor for dementia and mild cognitive impairment: A meta-analysis of longitudinal studies. *International Journal of Geriatric Psychiatry*, *28*(5), 441–449. http://dx.doi.org/10.1002/gps.3845.

Gardner, R. C., Valcour, V., & Yaffe, K. (2013). Dementia in the oldest old: A multi-factorial and growing public health issue. *Alzheimers Research & Therapy*, *5*(4), 27. http://dx.doi.org/10.1186/alzrt181.

Garza, A. A., Ha, T. G., Garcia, C., Chen, M. J., & Russo-Neustadt, A. A. (2004). Exercise, antidepressant treatment, and BDNF mRNA expression in the aging brain. *Pharmacology, Biochemistry, and Behavior*, *77*(2), 209–220.

Gates, N. J., Valenzuela, M., Sachdev, P. S., Singh, N. A., Baune, B. T., Brodaty, H., & Fiatarone Singh, M. A. (2011). Study of Mental Activity and Regular Training (SMART) in at risk individuals: A randomised double blind, sham controlled, longitudinal trial. *BMC Geriatrics*, *11*, 19. http://dx.doi.org/10.1186/1471-2318-11-19.

Gatz, M., Pedersen, N. L., Berg, S., Johansson, B., Johansson, K., Mortimer, J. A., & Ahlbom, A. (1997). Heritability for Alzheimer's disease: The study of dementia in Swedish twins. *The Journals of Gerontology Series A, Biological Sciences and Medical Sciences*, *52*(2), M117–125.

Gatz, M., Prescott, C. A., & Pedersen, N. L. (2006). Lifestyle risk and delaying factors. *Alzheimer Disease and Associated Disorders*, *20*(3 Suppl. 2), S84–88.

Gatz, M., Reynolds, C. A., Fratiglioni, L., Johansson, B., Mortimer, J. A., Berg, S., & Pedersen, N. L. (2006). Role of genes and environments for explaining Alzheimer disease. *Archives of General Psychiatry*, *63*(2), 168–174. http://dx.doi.org/10.1001/archpsyc.63.2.168.

Gaugler, J., James, B., Johnson, T., Scholz, K., Weuve, J., & The Alzheimer's Association, (2013). In *2013 Alzheimer's disease facts and figures* (Vol. 9). Chicago, IL: Alzheimer's Association.

Geda, Y. E., Knopman, D. S., Mrazek, D. A., Jicha, G. A., Smith, G. E., Negash, S., & Rocca, W. A. (2006). Depression, apolipoprotein E genotype, and the incidence of mild cognitive impairment: A prospective cohort study. *Archives of Neurology*, *63*(3), 435–440. http://dx.doi.org/10.1001/archneur.63.3.435.

Geddes, J. F., Vowles, G. H., Nicoll, J. A., & Revesz, T. (1999). Neuronal cytoskeletal changes are an early consequence of repetitive head injury. *Acta Neuropathologica*, *98*(2), 171–178.

Geerlings, M. I., Jonker, C., Bouter, L. M., Ader, H. J., & Schmand, B. (1999). Association between memory complaints and incident Alzheimer's disease in elderly people with normal baseline cognition. *The American Journal of Psychiatry*, *156*(4), 531–537.

Gelber, R. P., Launer, L. J., & White, L. R. (2012). The Honolulu-Asia aging study: Epidemiologic and neuropathologic research on cognitive impairment. *Current Alzheimer Research*, *9*(6), 664–672.

Geller, L. N., & Potter, H. (1999). Chromosome missegregation and trisomy 21 mosaicism in Alzheimer's disease. *Neurobiology of Disease*, *6*(3), 167–179. http://dx.doi.org/10.1006/nbdi.1999.0236.

George, S., Duran, N., & Norris, K. (2014). A systematic review of barriers and facilitators to minority research participation among african americans, latinos, asian americans, and pacific islanders. *American Journal of Public Health*, *104*(2), e16–31. http://dx.doi.org/10.2105/AJPH.2013.301706.

Gibbons, W. E., Cedars, M., & Ness, R. B. (2011). Toward understanding obstetrical outcome in advanced assisted reproduction: Varying sperm, oocyte, and uterine source and diagnosis. *Fertility and Sterility*, *95*(5) 1645-1649.e1641. http://dx.doi.org/10.1016/j.fertnstert.2010.11.029.

Gibbs, R. B. (1998). Levels of trkA and BDNF mRNA, but not NGF mRNA, fluctuate across the estrous cycle and increase in response to acute hormone replacement. *Brain Research*, *810* (1–2), 294.

Gilbert, M., Snyder, C., Corcoran, C., Norton, M. C., Lyketsos, C. G., & Tschanz, J. T. (2014). The association of traumatic brain injury with rate of progression of cognitive and functional impairment in a population-based cohort of Alzheimer's disease: The Cache County Dementia

Progression Study. *International Psychogeriatrics/IPA*, *26*(10), 1593–1601. http://dx.doi.org/10.1017/S1041610214000842.

Giunta, B., Obregon, D., Velisetty, R., Sanberg, P. R., Borlongan, C. V., & Tan, J. (2012). The immunology of traumatic brain injury: A prime target for Alzheimer's disease prevention. *Journal of Neuroinflammation*, *9*, 185. http://dx.doi.org/10.1186/1742-2094-9-185.

Glodzik, L., Mosconi, L., Tsui, W., de Santi, S., Zinkowski, R., Pirraglia, E., & de Leon, M. J. (2012). Alzheimer's disease markers, hypertension, and gray matter damage in normal elderly. *Neurobiology of Aging*, *33*(7), 1215–1227. http://dx.doi.org/10.1016/j.neurobiolaging.2011.02.012.

Glushakova, O. Y., Johnson, D., & Hayes, R. L. (2014). Delayed increases in microvascular pathology after experimental traumatic brain injury are associated with prolonged inflammation, blood–brain barrier disruption, and progressive white matter damage. *Journal of Neurotrauma*, *31*(13), 1180–1193. http://dx.doi.org/10.1089/neu.2013.3080.

Goate, A., Chartier-Harlin, M. C., Mullan, M., Brown, J., Crawford, F., & Fidani, L., et al. (1991). Segregation of a missense mutation in the amyloid precursor protein gene with familial Alzheimer's disease. *Nature*, *349*(6311), 704–706. http://dx.doi.org/10.1038/349704a0.

Goekint, M., DePauw, K., Roelands, B., Niemini, R., Bautmans, I., & Mets, T., et al. (2010). Strength training does not influence serum brain-derived neurotrophic factor. *European Journal of Applied Physiology*, *110*(2), 285–293.

Gomez-Pinilla, F., So, V., & Kesslak, J. P. (1998). Spatial learning and physical activity contribute to the induction of fibroblast growth factor: Neural substrates for increased cognition associated with exercise. *Neuroscience*, *85*(1), 53–61.

Gorelick, P. B. (2004). Risk factors for vascular dementia and Alzheimer disease. *Stroke*, *35*(11 Suppl. 1), 2620–2622. http://dx.doi.org/10.1161/01.STR.0000143318.70292.47.

Gorelick, P. B., Scuteri, A., Black, S. E., Decarli, C., Greenberg, S. M., Iadecola, C., & Seshadri, S. (2011). Vascular contributions to cognitive impairment and dementia: A statement for healthcare professionals from the American Heart Association/American Stroke Association. *Stroke*, *42*(9), 2672–2713. http://dx.doi.org/10.1161/STR.0b013e3182299496.

Gosche, K. M., Mortimer, J. A., Smith, C. D., Markesbery, W. R., & Snowdon, D. A. (2001). An automated technique for measuring hippocampal volumes from MR imaging studies. *American Journal of Neuroradiology*, *22*(9), 1686–1689.

Gosche, K. M., Mortimer, J. A., Smith, C. D., Markesbery, W. R., & Snowdon, D. A. (2002). Hippocampal volume as an index of Alzheimer neuropathology: Findings from the Nun Study. *Neurology*, *58*(10), 1476–1482.

Granic, A., Padmanabhan, J., Norden, M., & Potter, H. (2010). Alzheimer Abeta peptide induces chromosome mis-segregation and aneuploidy, including trisomy 21: Requirement for tau and APP. *Molecular Biology of the Cell*, *21*(4), 511–520. http://dx.doi.org/10.1091/mbc.E09-10-0850.

Graves, A. B., Bowen, J. D., Rajaram, L., McCormick, W. C., McCurry, S. M., & Schellenberg, G. D., et al. (1999). Impaired olfaction as a marker for cognitive decline: Interaction with apolipoprotein E epsilon4 status. *Neurology*, *53*(7), 1480–1487.

Graves, A. B., Larson, E. B., Edland, S. D., Bowen, J. D., McCormick, W. C., McCurry, S. M., & Uomoto, J. M. (1996). Prevalence of dementia and its subtypes in the Japanese American population of King County, Washington state. The Kame Project. *American Journal of Epidemiology*, *144*(8), 760–771.

Graves, A. B., Larson, E. B., White, L. R., Teng, E. L., & Homma, A. (1994). Opportunities and challenges in international collaborative epidemiologic research of dementia and its subtypes: Studies between Japan and the U.S. *International Psychogeriatrics/IPA*, *6*(2), 209–223.

Graves, A. B., & Mortimer, J. A. (1994). Does smoking reduce the risks of Parkinson's and Alzheimer's diseases? *Journal of Smoking-Related Disorders, 169*, 79–90.

Graves, A. B., Mortimer, J. A., & Bowen, J. D., et al. (2001). Head circumference and incident Alzheimer's disease: Modification by apolipoprotein E. *Neurology, 57*, 1453–1460.

Graves, A. B., Mortimer, J. A., Larson, E. B., Wenzlow, A., Bowen, J. D., & McCormick, W. C. (1996). Head circumference as a measure of cognitive reserve. Association with severity of impairment in Alzheimer's disease. *The British Journal of Psychiatry, 169*(1), 86–92. http://dx.doi.org/10.1192/bjp.169.1.86.

Graves, A. B., van Duijn, C. M., Chandra, V., Fratiglioni, L., Heyman, A., & Jorm, A. F., et al. (1991). Alcohol and tobacco consumption as risk factors for Alzheimer's disease: A collaborative re-analysis of case-control studies. EURODEM risk factors research group. *International Journal of Epidemiology, 20*(Suppl. 2), S48–57.

Graves, A. B., White, E., Koepsell, T. D., Reifler, B. V., van Belle, G., & Larson, E. B., et al. (1990a). The association between head trauma and Alzheimer's disease. *American Journal of Epidemiology, 131*(3), 491–501.

Graves, A. B., White, E., Koepsell, T. D., Reifler, B. V., van Belle, G., & Larson, E. B., et al. (1990b). A case-control study of Alzheimer's disease. *Annals of Neurology, 28*(6), 766–774. http://dx.doi.org/10.1002/ana.410280607.

Greenberg, S. M., Vernooij, M. W., Cordonnier, C., Viswanathan, A., Al-Shahi Salman, R., Warach, S., & Breteler, M. M. (2009). Cerebral microbleeds: A guide to detection and interpretation. *Lancet Neurology, 8*(2), 165–174. http://dx.doi.org/10.1016/S1474-4422(09)70013-4.

Greendale, G. A., Huang, M. H., Leung, K., Crawford, S. L., Gold, E. B., Wight, R., & Karlamangla, A. S. (2012). Dietary phytoestrogen intakes and cognitive function during the menopausal transition: Results from the study of Women's health across the nation phytoestrogen study. *Menopause, 19*(8), 894–903. http://dx.doi.org/10.1097/gme.0b013e318242a654.

Grimm, M. O., Rothhaar, T. L., Grosgen, S., Burg, V. K., Hundsdorfer, B., Haupenthal, V. J., & Hartmann, T. (2012). Trans fatty acids enhance amyloidogenic processing of the Alzheimer amyloid precursor protein (APP). *The Journal of Nutritional Biochemistry, 23*(10), 1214–1223. http://dx.doi.org/10.1016/j.jnutbio.2011.06.015.

Grodstein, F., Chen, J., & Willett, W. C. (2003). High-dose antioxidant supplements and cognitive function in community-dwelling elderly women. *The American Journal of Clinical Nutrition, 77*(4), 975–984.

Growdon, M. E., Schultz, A. P., Dagley, A. S., Amariglio, R. E., Hedden, T., Rentz, D. M., & Marshall, G. A. (2015). Odor identification and Alzheimer disease biomarkers in clinically normal elderly. *Neurology, 84*(21), 2153–2160. http://dx.doi.org/10.1212/WNL.0000000000001614.

Gu, Y., Nieves, J. W., Stern, Y., Luchsinger, J. A., & Scarmeas, N. (2010). Food combination and Alzheimer disease risk: A protective diet. *Archives of Neurology, 67*(6), 699–706. http://dx.doi.org/10.1001/archneurol.2010.84.

Gu, Y., Scarmeas, N., Short, E. E., Luchsinger, J. A., DeCarli, C., Stern, Y., & Brickman, A. M. (2014). Alcohol intake and brain structure in a multiethnic elderly cohort. *Clinical Nutrition (Edinburgh, Scotland), 33*(4), 662–667. http://dx.doi.org/10.1016/j.clnu.2013.08.004.

Guo, Z., Cupples, L. A., Kurz, A., Auerbach, S. H., Volicer, L., Chui, H., & Farrer, L. A. (2000). Head injury and the risk of AD in the MIRAGE study. *Neurology, 54*(6), 1316–1323.

Guo, Z., Fratiglioni, L., Zhu, L., Fastbom, J., Winblad, B., & Viitanen, M. (1999). Occurrence and progression of dementia in a community population aged 75 years and older: Relationship of antihypertensive medication use. *Archives of Neurology, 56*(8), 991–996.

Guo, Z., Viitanen, M., Fratiglioni, L., & Winblad, B. (1996). Low blood pressure and dementia in elderly people: The Kungsholmen project. *BMJ, 312*(7034), 805–808.

Gupta, S. C., Patchva, S., & Aggarwal, B. B. (2013). Therapeutic roles of curcumin: Lessons learned from clinical trials. *The AAPS Journal*, *15*(1), 195–218. http://dx.doi.org/10.1208/s12248-012-9432-8.

Gureje, O., Ogunniyi, A., Baiyewu, O., Price, B., Unverzagt, F. W., Evans, R. M., & Murrell, J. R. (2006). APOE epsilon4 is not associated with Alzheimer's disease in elderly Nigerians. *Annals of Neurology*, *59*(1), 182–185. http://dx.doi.org/10.1002/ana.20694.

Gurland, B. J. (1981). The borderlands of dementia: The influence of sociocultural characteristics on rates of dementia occurring in the senium. In N. E. Miller & G. D. Cohen (Eds.), *Clinical aspects of Alzheimer's disease and senile dementia* (pp. 61–80). New York: Raven Press.

Gurland, B. J., Wilder, D. E., Lantigua, R., Stern, Y., Chen, J., & Killeffer, E. H., et al. (1999). Rates of dementia in three ethnoracial groups. *International Journal of Geriatric Psychiatry*, *14*(6), 481–493.

Gustafson, D., Rothenberg, E., Blennow, K., Steen, B., & Skoog, I. (2003). An 18-year follow-up of overweight and risk of Alzheimer disease. *Archives of Internal Medicine*, *163*(13), 1524–1528. http://dx.doi.org/10.1001/archinte.163.13.1524.

Haan, M. N., Mungas, D. M., Gonzalez, H. M., Ortiz, T. A., Acharya, A., & Jagust, W. J. (2003). Prevalence of dementia in older latinos: The influence of type 2 diabetes mellitus, stroke and genetic factors. *Journal of the American Geriatrics Society*, *51*(2), 169–177.

Hajek, T., Kopecek, M., & Hoschl, C. (2012). Reduced hippocampal volumes in healthy carriers of brain-derived neurotrophic factor Val66Met polymorphism: Meta-analysis. *The World Journal of Biological Psychiatry: The Official Journal of the World Federation of Societies of Biological Psychiatry*, *13*(3), 178–187. http://dx.doi.org/10.3109/15622975.2011.580005.

Hakansson, K., Rovio, S., Helkala, E. L., Vilska, A. R., Winblad, B., Soininen, H., & Kivipelto, M. (2009). Association between mid-life marital status and cognitive function in later life: Population based cohort study. *BMJ*, *339*, b2462. http://dx.doi.org/10.1136/bmj.b2462.

Hall, C. B., Lipton, R. B., Sliwinski, M., Katz, M. J., Derby, C. A., & Verghese, J. (2009). Cognitive activities delay onset of memory decline in persons who develop dementia. *Neurology*, *73*(5), 356–361. http://dx.doi.org/10.1212/WNL.0b013e3181b04ae3.

Hall, C. B., Verghese, J., Sliwinski, M., Chen, Z., Katz, M., & Derby, C., et al. (2005). Dementia incidence may increase more slowly after age 90: Results from the Bronx Aging Study. *Neurology*, *65*(6), 882–886. http://dx.doi.org/10.1212/01.wnl.0000176053.98907.3f.

Halvorsen, B. L., Holte, K., Myhrstad, M. C., Barikmo, I., Hvattum, E., Remberg, S. F., & Blomhoff, R. (2002). A systematic screening of total antioxidants in dietary plants. *The Journal of Nutrition*, *132*(3), 461–471.

Hamaguchi, T., Ono, K., & Yamada, M. (2010). REVIEW: Curcumin and Alzheimer's disease. *CNS Neuroscience & Therapeutics*, *16*(5), 285–297. http://dx.doi.org/10.1111/j.1755-5949.2010.00147.x.

Hardy, J. (2006). A hundred years of Alzheimer's disease research. *Neuron*, *52*(1), 3–13. http://dx.doi.org/10.1016/j.neuron.2006.09.016.

Hartman, R. E., Shah, A., Fagan, A. M., Schwetye, K. E., Parsadanian, M., Schulman, R. N., & Holtzman, D. M. (2006). Pomegranate juice decreases amyloid load and improves behavior in a mouse model of Alzheimer's disease. *Neurobiology of Disease*, *24*(3), 506–515. http://dx.doi.org/10.1016/j.nbd.2006.08.006.

Harwood, D. G., Barker, W. W., Ownby, R. L., & Duara, R. (2000). Relationship of behavioral and psychological symptoms to cognitive impairment and functional status in Alzheimer's disease. *International Journal of Geriatric Psychiatry*, *15*(5), 393–400.

Havlik, R. J., Izmirlian, G., Petrovitch, H., Ross, G. W., Masaki, K., Curb, J. D., & White, L. (2000). APOE-epsilon4 predicts incident AD in Japanese-American men: The Honolulu-Asia aging study. *Neurology*, *54*(7), 1526–1529.

Head, D., Bugg, J. M., Goate, A. M., Fagan, A. M., Mintun, M. A., Benzinger, T., & Morris, J. C. (2012). Exercise engagement as a moderator of the effects of APOE genotype on amyloid deposition. *Archives of Neurology*, *69*(5), 636–643. http://dx.doi.org/10.1001/archneurol.2011.845.

Hebert, L. E., Scherr, P. A., Beckett, L. A., Albert, M. S., Pilgrim, D. M., Chown, M. J., & Evans, D. A. (1995). Age-specific incidence of Alzheimer's disease in a community population. *JAMA*, *273*(17), 1354–1359.

Hebert, L. E., Scherr, P. A., Bienias, J. L., Bennett, D. A., & Evans, D. A. (2003). Alzheimer disease in the US population: Prevalence estimates using the 2000 census. *Archives of Neurology*, *60*(8), 1119–1122. http://dx.doi.org/10.1001/archneur.60.8.1119.

Hebert, L. E., Scherr, P. A., McCann, J. J., Beckett, L. A., & Evans, D. A. (2001). Is the risk of developing Alzheimer's disease greater for women than for men? *American Journal of Epidemiology*, *153*(2), 132–136.

Hebert, L. E., Weuve, J., Scherr, P. A., & Evans, D. A. (2013). Alzheimer disease in the United States (2010–2050) estimated using the 2010 census. *Neurology*, *80*(19), 1778–1783. http://dx.doi.org/10.1212/WNL.0b013e31828726f5.

Heishman, S. J., Kleykamp, B. A., & Singleton, E. G. (2010). Meta-analysis of the acute effects of nicotine and smoking on human performance. *Psychopharmacology (Berlin)*, *210*(4), 453–469.

Helmer, C., Damon, D., Letenneur, L., Fabrigoule, C., Barberger-Gateau, P., Lafont, S., & Dartigues, J. F. (1999). Marital status and risk of Alzheimer's disease: A French population-based cohort study. *Neurology*, *53*(9), 1953–1958.

Helmer, C., Joly, P., Letenneur, L., Commenges, D., & Dartigues, J. F. (2001). Mortality with dementia: Results from a French prospective community-based cohort. *American Journal of Epidemiology*, *154*(7), 642–648.

Helmer, C., Letenneur, L., Rouch, I., Richard-Harston, S., Barberger-Gateau, P., Fabrigoule, C., & Dartigues, J. F. (2001). Occupation during life and risk of dementia in French elderly community residents. *Journal of Neurology, Neurosurgery, and Psychiatry*, *71*(3), 303–309.

Helmer, C., Stengel, B., Metzger, M., Froissart, M., Massy, Z. A., & Tzourio, C., et al. (2011). Chronic kidney disease, cognitive decline, and incident dementia: The 3C Study. *Neurology*, *77*(23), 2043–2051. http://dx.doi.org/10.1212/WNL.0b013e31823b4765.

Helzner, E. P., Scarmeas, N., Cosentino, S., Tang, M. X., Schupf, N., & Stern, Y. (2008). Survival in Alzheimer disease: A multiethnic, population-based study of incident cases. *Neurology*, *71*(19), 1489–1495. http://dx.doi.org/10.1212/01.wnl.0000334278.11022.42.

Henderson, A. S., Jorm, A. F., Korten, A. E., Creasey, H., McCusker, E., Broe, G. A., & Anthony, J. C. (1992). Environmental risk factors for Alzheimer's disease: Their relationship to age of onset and to familial or sporadic types. *Psychological Medicine*, *22*(2), 429–436.

Henderson, V. W. (2010). Action of estrogens in the aging brain: Dementia and cognitive aging. *Biochimica et Biophysica Acta*, *1800*(10), 1077–1083. http://dx.doi.org/10.1016/j.bbagen.2009.11.005.

Henderson, V. W., Benke, K. S., Green, R. C., Cupples, L. A., Farrer, L. A., & Group, M. S. (2005). Postmenopausal hormone therapy and Alzheimer's disease risk: Interaction with age. *Journal of Neurology, Neurosurgery, and Psychiatry*, *76*(1), 103–105. http://dx.doi.org/10.1136/jnnp.2003.024927.

Henderson, V. W., St John, J. A., Hodis, H. N., Kono, N., McCleary, C. A., Franke, A. A., & Group, W. R. (2012). Long-term soy isoflavone supplementation and cognition in women: A randomized, controlled trial. *Neurology*, *78*(23), 1841–1848. http://dx.doi.org/10.1212/WNL.0b013e318258f822.

Hendrie, H. C., Ogunniyi, A., Hall, K. S., Baiyewu, O., Unverzagt, F. W., Gureje, O., & Hui, S. L. (2001). Incidence of dementia and Alzheimer disease in 2 communities: Yoruba residing in Ibadan, Nigeria, and African Americans residing in Indianapolis, Indiana. *JAMA*, *285*(6), 739–747.

Hendrie, H. C., Osuntokun, B. O., Hall, K. S., Ogunniyi, A. O., Hui, S. L., Unverzagt, F. W., & Musick, B. S. (1995). Prevalence of Alzheimer's disease and dementia in two communities: Nigerian Africans and African Americans. *The American Journal of Psychiatry*, *152*(10), 1485–1492.

Herbst, A. L., Ulfelder, H., & Poskanzer, D. C. (1971). Adenocarcinoma of the vagina. Association of maternal stilbestrol therapy with tumor appearance in young women. *The New England Journal of Medicine*, *284*(15), 878–881. http://dx.doi.org/10.1056/NEJM197104222841604.

Hernan, M. A., Alonso, A., & Logroscino, G. (2008). Cigarette smoking and dementia: Potential selection bias in the elderly. *Epidemiology*, *19*(3), 448–450. http://dx.doi.org/10.1097/EDE.0b013e31816bbe14.

Herring, A., Donath, A., Yarmolenko, M., Uslar, E., Conzen, C., Kanakis, D., & Keyvani, K. (2012). Exercise during pregnancy mitigates Alzheimer-like pathology in mouse offspring. *The FASEB Journal: Official Publication of the Federation of American Societies for Experimental Biology*, *26*(1), 117–128. http://dx.doi.org/10.1096/fj.11-193193.

Heston, L. L. (1985). Clinical genetics of Alzheimer's disease. In J. T. Hutton & A. D. Kenny (Eds.), *Senile dementia of the Alzheimer type* (pp. 197–204). New York: Alan R. Liss.

Heston, L. L., Mastri, A. R., Anderson, V. E., & White, J. (1981). Dementia of the Alzheimer type. Clinical genetics, natural history, and associated conditions. *Archives of General Psychiatry*, *38*(10), 1085–1090.

Heyman, A., Wilkinson, W. E., Stafford, J. A., Helms, M. J., Sigmon, A. H., & Weinberg, T. (1984). Alzheimer's disease: A study of epidemiological aspects. *Annals of Neurology*, *15*(4), 335–341. http://dx.doi.org/10.1002/ana.410150406.

Hill, A. B. (1965). The environment and disease: Association or causation? *Proceedings of the Royal Society of Medicine*, *58*, 295–300.

Hirono, N., Yasuda, M., Tanimukai, S., Kitagaki, H., & Mori, E. (2000). Effect of the apolipoprotein E epsilon4 allele on white matter hyperintensities in dementia. *Stroke*, *31*(6), 1263–1268.

Hock, C., Konietzko, U., Streffer, J. R., Tracy, J., Signorell, A., Muller-Tillmanns, B., & Nitsch, R. M. (2003). Antibodies against beta-amyloid slow cognitive decline in Alzheimer's disease. *Neuron*, *38*(4), 547–554.

Hof, P. R., Bouras, C., Buee, L., Delacourte, A., Perl, D. P., & Morrison, J. H. (1992). Differential distribution of neurofibrillary tangles in the cerebral cortex of dementia pugilistica and Alzheimer's disease cases. *Acta Neuropathologica*, *85*(1), 23–30.

Hoffman, L. B., Schmeidler, J., Lesser, G. T., Beeri, M. S., Purohit, D. P., & Grossman, H. T., et al. (2009). Less Alzheimer disease neuropathology in medicated hypertensive than nonhypertensive persons. *Neurology*, *72*(20), 1720–1726. http://dx.doi.org/10.1212/01.wnl.0000345881.82856.d5.

Hofman, A., Darwish Murad, S., van Duijn, C. M., Franco, O. H., Goedegebure, A., Ikram, M. A., & Vernooij, M. W. (2013). The Rotterdam Study: 2014 objectives and design update. *European Journal of Epidemiology*, *28*(11), 889–926. http://dx.doi.org/10.1007/s10654-013-9866-z.

Hofman, A., Ott, A., Breteler, M. M., Bots, M. L., Slooter, A. J., van Harskamp, F., & Grobbee, D. E. (1997). Atherosclerosis, apolipoprotein E, and prevalence of dementia and Alzheimer's disease in the Rotterdam Study. *Lancet*, *349*(9046), 151–154. http://dx.doi.org/10.1016/S0140-6736(96)09328-2.

Hofman, A., Rocca, W. A., Brayne, C., Breteler, M. M., Clarke, M., & Cooper, B., et al. (1991). The prevalence of dementia in Europe: A collaborative study of 1980–1990 findings. Eurodem Prevalence Research Group. *International Journal of Epidemiology*, *20*(3), 736–748.

Hogervorst, E., Bandelow, S., Combrinck, M., & Smith, A. D. (2004). Low free testosterone is an independent risk factor for Alzheimer's disease. *Experimental Gerontology*, *39*(11–12), 1633–1639. http://dx.doi.org/10.1016/j.exger.2004.06.019.

Hogervorst, E., Combrinck, M., & Smith, A. D. (2003). Testosterone and gonadotropin levels in men with dementia. *Neuro Endocrinology Letters*, *24*(3–4), 203–208.

Hogervorst, E., Matthews, F. E., & Brayne, C. (2010). Are optimal levels of testosterone associated with better cognitive function in healthy older women and men? *Biochimica et Biophysica Acta*, *1800*(10), 1145–1152. http://dx.doi.org/10.1016/j.bbagen.2009.12.009.

Hogervorst, E., Sadjimim, T., Yesufu, A., Kreager, P., & Rahardjo, T. B. (2008). High tofu intake is associated with worse memory in elderly Indonesian men and women. *Dementia and Geriatric Cognitive Disorders*, *26*(1), 50–57. http://dx.doi.org/10.1159/000141484.

Hogervorst, E., Williams, J., Budge, M., Barnetson, L., Combrinck, M., & Smith, A. D. (2001). Serum total testosterone is lower in men with Alzheimer's disease. *Neuroendicronology Letters*, *22*(3), 163–168.

Hogervorst, E., Williams, J., Budge, M., Riedel, W., & Jolles, J. (2000). The nature of the effect of female gonadal hormone replacement therapy on cognitive function in post-menopausal women: A meta-analysis. *Neuroscience*, *101*(3), 485–512.

Holland, J., Bandelow, S., & Hogervorst, E. (2011). Testosterone levels and cognition in elderly men: A review. *Maturitas*, *69*(4), 322–337. http://dx.doi.org/10.1016/j.maturitas.2011.05.012.

Holmgren, S., Molander, B., & Nilsson, L. G. (2006). Intelligence and executive functioning in adult age: Effects of sibship size and birth order. *European Journal of Cognitive Psychology*, *18*(1), 138–158.

Holwerda, T. J., Deeg, D. J., Beekman, A. T., van Tilburg, T. G., Stek, M. L., & Jonker, C., et al. (2014). Feelings of loneliness, but not social isolation, predict dementia onset: Results from the Amsterdam Study of the Elderly (AMSTEL). *Journal of Neurology, Neurosurgery, and Psychiatry*, *85*(2), 135–142. http://dx.doi.org/10.1136/jnnp-2012-302755.

Honea, R. A., Thomas, G. P., Harsha, A., Anderson, H. S., Donnelly, J. E., & Brooks, W. M., et al. (2009). Cardiorespiratory fitness and preserved medial temporal lobe volume in Alzheimer disease. *Alzheimer Disease and Associated Disorders*, *23*(3), 188–197. http://dx.doi.org/10.1097/WAD.0b013e31819cb8a2.

Hong, S., Quintero-Monzon, O., Ostaszewski, B. L., Podlisny, D. R., Cavanaugh, W. T., Yang, T., & Selkoe, D. J. (2011). Dynamic analysis of amyloid beta-protein in behaving mice reveals opposing changes in ISF versus parenchymal Abeta during age-related plaque formation. *The Journal of Neuroscience*, *31*(44), 15861–15869. http://dx.doi.org/10.1523/JNEUROSCI.3272-11.2011.

Horvat, P., Richards, M., Malyutina, S., Pajak, A., Kubinova, R., Tamosiunas, A., & Bobak, M. (2014). Life course socioeconomic position and mid-late life cognitive function in Eastern Europe. *The Journals of Gerontology Series B, Psychological Sciences and Social Sciences*, *69*(3), 470–481. http://dx.doi.org/10.1093/geronb/gbu014.

Hoyert, D. L., & Rosenberg, H. M. (1997). Alzheimer's disease as a cause of death in the United States. *Public Health Reports*, *112*(6), 497–505.

Huang, T. L., Carlson, M. C., Fitzpatrick, A. L., Kuller, L. H., Fried, L. P., & Zandi, P. P. (2008). Knee height and arm span: A reflection of early life environment and risk of dementia. *Neurology*, *70*(19 Pt 2), 1818–1826. http://dx.doi.org/10.1212/01.wnl.0000311444.20490.98.

Huang, T. L., Zandi, P. P., Tucker, K. L., Fitzpatrick, A. L., Kuller, L. H., Fried, L. P., & Carlson, M. C. (2005). Benefits of fatty fish on dementia risk are stronger for those without APOE epsilon4. *Neurology*, *65*(9), 1409–1414. http://dx.doi.org/10.1212/01.wnl.0000183148.34197.2e.

Hughes, C. P., Berg, L., Danziger, W. L., Coben, L. A., & Martin, R. L. (1982). A new clinical scale for the staging of dementia. *The British Journal of Psychiatry*, *140*(6), 566–572. http://dx.doi.org/10.1192/bjp.140.6.566.

Hughes, T. F., Andel, R., Small, B. J., Borenstein, A. R., Mortimer, J. A., Wolk, A., & Gatz, M. (2010). Midlife fruit and vegetable consumption and risk of dementia in later life in Swedish twins. *The American Journal of Geriatric Psychiatry: Official Journal of the American Association for Geriatric Psychiatry*, *18*(5), 413–420. http://dx.doi.org/10.1097/JGP.0b013e3181c65250.

Hughes, T. F., Borenstein, A. R., Schofield, E., Wu, Y., & Larson, E. B. (2009). Association between late-life body mass index and dementia: The Kame Project. *Neurology*, *72*(20), 1741–1746. http://dx.doi.org/10.1212/WNL.0b013e3181a60a58.

Hulley, S. B., & Grady, D. (2004). The WHI estrogen-alone trial—do things look any better? *JAMA*, *291*(14), 1769–1771. http://dx.doi.org/10.1001/jama.291.14.1769.

Hyman, B. T., & Trojanowski, J. Q. (1997). Consensus recommendations for the postmortem diagnosis of Alzheimer disease from the National Institute on Aging and the Reagan Institute Working Group on diagnostic criteria for the neuropathological assessment of Alzheimer disease. *Journal of Neuropathology and Experimental Neurology*, *56*(10), 1095–1097.

Hyman, B. T., Van Hoesen, G. W., Damasio, A. R., & Barnes, C. L. (1984). Alzheimer's disease: Cell-specific pathology isolates the hippocampal formation. *Science*, *225*(4667), 1168–1170.

Hymes, K. B., Greene, J. B., Marcus, A., William, D. C., Cheung, T., & Prose, N. S., et al. (1981). Kaposi's Sarcoma in Homosexual Men—A report of eight cases. *The Lancet*, *318*(8247), 598–600.

Iacono, D., Markesbery, W. R., Gross, M., Pletnikova, O., Rudow, G., & Zandi, P., et al. (2009). The Nun study: Clinically silent AD, neuronal hypertrophy, and linguistic skills in early life. *Neurology*, *73*(9), 665–673. http://dx.doi.org/10.1212/WNL.0b013e3181b01077.

Ikonomovic, M. D., Klunk, W. E., Abrahamson, E. E., Mathis, C. A., Price, J. C., Tsopelas, N. D., & DeKosky, S. T. (2008). Post-mortem correlates of *in vivo* PiB-PET amyloid imaging in a typical case of Alzheimer's disease. *Brain*, *131*(Pt 6), 1630–1645. http://dx.doi.org/10.1093/brain/awn016.

Ikonomovic, M. D., Uryu, K., Abrahamson, E. E., Ciallella, J. R., Trojanowski, J. Q., Lee, V. M., & DeKosky, S. T. (2004). Alzheimer's pathology in human temporal cortex surgically excised after severe brain injury. *Experimental Neurology*, *190*(1), 192–203. http://dx.doi.org/10.1016/j.expneurol.2004.06.011.

Institute of Medicine (IOM). (2009). *Gulf war and health, Volume 7: Long-term consequencies of traumatic brain injury*. Washington, DC: The National Academic Press.

in t' Veld, B. A., Ruitenberg, A., Hofman, A., Launer, L. J., van Duijn, C. M., Stijnen, T., & Stricker, B. H. (2001). Nonsteroidal antiinflammatory drugs and the risk of Alzheimer's disease. *The New England Journal of Medicine*, *345*(21), 1515–1521. http://dx.doi.org/10.1056/NEJMoa010178.

in t' Veld, B. A., Ruitenberg, A., Hofman, A., Stricker, B. H., & Breteler, M. M. (2001). Antihypertensive drugs and incidence of dementia: The Rotterdam study. *Neurobiology of Aging*, *22*(3), 407–412.

Ishige, K., Schubert, D., & Sagara, Y. (2001). Flavonoids protect neuronal cells from oxidative stress by three distinct mechanisms. *Free Radical Biology & Medicine*, *30*(4), 433–446.

Izmirlian, G., Brock, D., & White, L. (2000). Estimating incidence dementia subtypes assessing impact of missed cases. *Statistics in Medicine*, *19*, 1577–1591.

Jack, C. R., Jr., Dickson, D. W., Parisi, J. E., Xu, Y. C., Cha, R. H., O'Brien, P. C., & Petersen, R. C. (2002). Antemortem MRI findings correlate with hippocampal neuropathology in typical aging and dementia. *Neurology*, *58*(5), 750–757.

Jack, C. R., Jr., & Holtzman, D. M. (2013). Biomarker modeling of Alzheimer's disease. *Neuron*, *80*(6), 1347–1358. http://dx.doi.org/10.1016/j.neuron.2013.12.003.

Jack, C. R., Jr., Knopman, D. S., Jagust, W. J., Shaw, L. M., Aisen, P. S., Weiner, M. W., & Trojanowski, J. Q. (2010). Hypothetical model of dynamic biomarkers of the Alzheimer's pathological cascade. *Lancet Neurology*, *9*(1), 119–128. http://dx.doi.org/10.1016/S1474-4422(09)70299-6.

Jack, C. R., Jr., Lowe, V. J., Senjem, M. L., Weigand, S. D., Kemp, B. J., Shiung, M. M., & Petersen, R. C. (2008). 11C PiB and structural MRI provide complementary information in imaging of Alzheimer's disease and amnestic mild cognitive impairment. *Brain, 131*(Pt 3), 665–680. http://dx.doi.org/10.1093/brain/awm336.

Jack, C. R., Jr., Shiung, M. M., Gunter, J. L., O'Brien, P. C., Weigand, S. D., Knopman, D. S., & Petersen, R. C. (2004). Comparison of different MRI brain atrophy rate measures with clinical disease progression in AD. *Neurology, 62*(4), 591–600.

Jack, C. R., Jr., Shiung, M. M., Weigand, S. D., O'Brien, P. C., Gunter, J. L., Boeve, B. F., & Petersen, R. C. (2005). Brain atrophy rates predict subsequent clinical conversion in normal elderly and amnestic MCI. *Neurology, 65*(8), 1227–1231. http://dx.doi.org/10.1212/01.wnl.0000180958.22678.91.

Jack, C. R., Jr., Vemuri, P., Wiste, H. J., Weigand, S. D., Aisen, P. S., Trojanowski, J. Q., & Alzheimer's Disease Neuroimaging Initiative, (2011). Evidence for ordering of Alzheimer disease biomarkers. *Archives of Neurology, 68*(12), 1526–1535. http://dx.doi.org/10.1001/archneurol.2011.183.

Jaeger, M. M. (2009). Sibship size and educational attainment. A joint test of the Confluence Model and the Resource Dilution Hypothesis. *Research in Social Stratification and Mobility, 27*(1), 1–12. http://dx.doi.org/10.1016/j.rssm.2009.01.002.

Jaeggi, S. M., Buschkuehl, M., Jonides, J., & Perrig, W. J. (2008). Improving fluid intelligence with training on working memory. *Proceedings of the National Academy of Sciences of the United States of America, 105*(19), 6829–6833. http://dx.doi.org/10.1073/pnas.0801268105.

Jagust, W. J., Landau, S. M., Shaw, L. M., Trojanowski, J. Q., Koeppe, R. A., Reiman, E. M., & Alzheimer's Disease Neuroimaging Initiative, (2009). Relationships between biomarkers in aging and dementia. *Neurology, 73*(15), 1193–1199. http://dx.doi.org/10.1212/WNL.0b013e3181bc010c.

Jagust, W. J., & Mormino, E. C. (2011). Lifespan brain activity, beta-amyloid, and Alzheimer's disease. *Trends in Cognitive Sciences, 15*(11), 520–526. http://dx.doi.org/10.1016/j.tics.2011.09.004.

James, B. D., Glass, T. A., Caffo, B., Bobb, J. F., Davatzikos, C., & Yousem, D., et al. (2012). Association of social engagement with brain volumes assessed by structural MRI. *Journal of Aging Research, 2012*, 512714. http://dx.doi.org/10.1155/2012/512714.

James, B. D., Leurgans, S. E., Hebert, L. E., Scherr, P. A., Yaffe, K., & Bennett, D. A. (2014). Contribution of Alzheimer disease to mortality in the United States. *Neurology, 82*(12), 1045–1050. http://dx.doi.org/10.1212/WNL.0000000000000240.

James, O. G., Doraiswamy, P. M., & Borges-Neto, S. (2015). PET imaging of Tau pathology in Alzheimer's disease and Tauopathies. *Frontiers in Neurology, 6*, 38. http://dx.doi.org/10.3389/fneur.2015.00038.

Jaturapatporn, D., Isaac, M. G., McCleery, J., & Tabet, N. (2012). Aspirin, steroidal and non-steroidal anti-inflammatory drugs for the treatment of Alzheimer's disease. *Cochrane Database of Systematic Reviews (Online), 2*, CD006378. http://dx.doi.org/10.1002/14651858.CD006378.pub2.

Jeerakathil, T., Wolf, P. A., Beiser, A., Massaro, J., Seshadri, S., & D'Agostino, R. B., et al. (2004). Stroke risk profile predicts white matter hyperintensity volume: The Framingham Study. *Stroke, 35*(8), 1857–1861. http://dx.doi.org/10.1161/01.STR.0000135226.53499.85.

Jenkins, R., Fox, N. C., Rossor, A. M., Harvey, R. J., & Rossor, M. N. (2000). Intracranial volume and Alzheimer disease: Evidence against the cerebral reserve hypothesis. *Archives of Neurology, 57*(2), 220–224.

Jessen, F., Feyen, L., Freymann, K., Tepest, R., Maier, W., Heun, R., & Scheef, L. (2006). Volume reduction of the entorhinal cortex in subjective memory impairment. *Neurobiology of Aging, 27*(12), 1751–1756. http://dx.doi.org/10.1016/j.neurobiolaging.2005.10.010.

Jiang, Q., Lee, C. Y., Mandrekar, S., Wilkinson, B., Cramer, P., Zelcer, N., & Landreth, G. E. (2008). ApoE promotes the proteolytic degradation of Abeta. *Neuron*, *58*(5), 681–693. http://dx.doi.org/10.1016/j.neuron.2008.04.010.

Jicha, G. A., & Markesbery, W. R. (2010). Omega-3 fatty acids: Potential role in the management of early Alzheimer's disease. *Clinical Interventions in Aging*, *5*, 45–61.

Jick, H., Zornberg, G. L., Jick, S. S., Seshadri, S., & Drachman, D. A. (2000). Statins and the risk of dementia. *Lancet*, *356*(9242), 1627–1631.

Johnson, K. A., Fox, N. C., Sperling, R. A., & Klunk, W. E. (2012). Brain imaging in Alzheimer disease. *Cold Spring Harbor Perspectives Medicine*, *2*(4), a006213. http://dx.doi.org/10.1101/cshperspect.a006213.

Johnson, V. E., Stewart, W., & Smith, D. H. (2010). Traumatic brain injury and amyloid-beta pathology: a link to Alzheimer's disease? *Nature Reviews Neuroscience*, *11*(5), 361–370.

Johnson, V. E., Stewart, J. E., Begbie, F. D., Trojanowski, J. Q., Smith, D. H., & Stewart, W. (2013). Inflammation and white matter degeneration persist for years after a single traumatic brain injury. *Brain*, *136*(Pt 1), 28–42. http://dx.doi.org/10.1093/brain/aws322.

Jonaitis, E., La Rue, A., Mueller, K. D., Koscik, R. L., Hermann, B., & Sager, M. A. (2013). Cognitive activities and cognitive performance in middle-aged adults at risk for Alzheimer's disease. *Psychology and Aging*, *28*(4), 1004–1014. http://dx.doi.org/10.1037/a0034838.

Jordan, B. D., Relkin, N. R., Ravdin, L. D., Jacobs, A. R., Bennett, A., & Gandy, S. (1997). Apolipoprotein E epsilon4 associated with chronic traumatic brain injury in boxing. *JAMA*, *278*(2), 136–140.

Jorm, A. F., Christensen, H., Korten, A. E., Jacomb, P. A., & Henderson, A. S. (2001). Memory complaints as a precursor of memory impairment in older people: A longitudinal analysis over 7–8 years. *Psychological Medicine*, *31*(3), 441–449.

Jorm, A. F., & Jacomb, P. A. (1989). The Informant Questionnaire on Cognitive Decline in the Elderly (IQCODE): Socio-demographic correlates, reliability, validity and some norms. *Psychological Medicine*, *19*(4), 1015–1022.

Jorm, A. F., & Jolley, D. (1998). The incidence of dementia: A meta-analysis. *Neurology*, *51*(3), 728–733.

Jorm, A. F., Korten, A. E., & Henderson, A. S. (1987). The prevalence of dementia: A quantitative integration of the literature. *Acta Psychiatrica Scandinavica*, *76*, 465–479.

Jorm, A. F., Masaki, K. H., Davis, D. G., Hardman, J., Nelson, J., Markesbery, W. R., & White, L. R. (2004). Memory complaints in nondemented men predict future pathologic diagnosis of Alzheimer disease. *Neurology*, *63*(10), 1960–1961.

Jorm, A. F., van Duijn, C. M., Chandra, V., Fratiglioni, L., Graves, A. B., & Heyman, A., et al. (1991). Psychiatric history and related exposures as risk factors for Alzheimer's disease: A collaborative re-analysis of case-control studies. EURODEM Risk Factors Research Group. *International Journal of Epidemiology*, *20*(Suppl. 2), S43–47.

Jotheeswaran, A. T., Williams, J. D., Stewart, R., & Prince, M. J. (2011). Could reverse causality or selective mortality explain associations between leg length, skull circumference and dementia? A South Indian cohort study. *International Psychogeriatrics/IPA*, *23*(2), 328–330. http://dx.doi.org/10.1017/S1041610210001171.

Kahn, R. L., Pollack, M., & Goldfarb, A. I. (1961). *Factors related to individual differences in mental status of institutionalized aged*. New York: Grune & Stratton.

Kalaria, R. N., Akinyemi, R., & Ihara, M. (2012). Does vascular pathology contribute to Alzheimer changes? *Journal of the Neurological Sciences*, *322*(1–2), 141–147. http://dx.doi.org/10.1016/j.jns.2012.07.032.

Kalmijn, S., Foley, D., White, L., Burchfiel, C. M., Curb, J. D., Petrovitch, H., & Launer, L. J. (2000). Metabolic cardiovascular syndrome and risk of dementia in Japanese-American elderly men. The Honolulu-Asia aging study. *Arteriosclerosis, Thrombosis, and Vascular Biology, 20*(10), 2255–2260.

Kalmijn, S., Launer, L. J., Ott, A., Witteman, J. C., Hofman, A., & Breteler, M. M. (1997). Dietary fat intake and the risk of incident dementia in the Rotterdam Study. *Annals of Neurology, 42*(5), 776–782. http://dx.doi.org/10.1002/ana.410420514.

Kang, J. H., Ascherio, A., & Grodstein, F. (2005). Fruit and vegetable consumption and cognitive decline in aging women. *Annals of Neurology, 57*(5), 713–720. http://dx.doi.org/10.1002/ana.20476.

Kannel, W. B., & Dawber, T. R. (1972). Atherosclerosis as a pediatric problem. *The Journal of Pediatrics, 80*(4), 544–554.

Kaplan, G. A., Turrell, G., Lynch, J. W., Everson, S. A., Helkala, E. L., & Salonen, J. T. (2001). Childhood socioeconomic position and cognitive function in adulthood. *International Journal of Epidemiology, 30*(2), 256–263.

Karp, A., Andel, R., Parker, M. G., Wang, H. X., Winblad, B., & Fratiglioni, L. (2009). Mentally stimulating activities at work during midlife and dementia risk after age 75: Follow-up study from the Kungsholmen Project. *The American Journal of Geriatric Psychiatry: Official Journal of the American Association for Geriatric Psychiatry, 17*(3), 227–236. http://dx.doi.org/10.1097/JGP.0b013e318190b691.

Kasper, J.D., Freedman, V.A., & Spillman, B.C. (2013). *Classification of persons by dementia status in the National Health and Aging Trends Study: Technical paper #5*. <http://www.nhats.org/scripts/documents/NHATS_Dementia_Technical_Paper_5_Jul2013.pdf> Accessed 05.06.15.

Katz, M. J., Lipton, R. B., Hall, C. B., Zimmerman, M. E., Sanders, A. E., Verghese, J., & Derby, C. A. (2012). Age-specific and sex-specific prevalence and incidence of mild cognitive impairment, dementia, and Alzheimer dementia in blacks and whites: A report from the Einstein Aging Study. *Alzheimer Disease and Associated Disorders, 26*(4), 335–343. http://dx.doi.org/10.1097/WAD.0b013e31823dbcfc.

Katzman, R. (1976). The prevalence and malignancy of Alzheimer disease: A major killer. *Archives of Neurology, 33*, 217–218.

Katzman, R. (1993). Education and the prevalence of dementia and Alzheimer's disease. *Neurology, 43*(1), 13–20.

Katzman, R., Aronson, M., Fuld, P., Kawas, C., Brown, T., Morgenstern, H., & Ooi, W. L. (1989). Development of dementing illnesses in an 80-year-old volunteer cohort. *Annals of Neurology, 25*(4), 317–324. http://dx.doi.org/10.1002/ana.410250402.

Katzman, R., Galasko, D. R., Saitoh, T., Chen, X., Pay, M. M., & Booth, A., et al. (1996). Apolipoprotein-epsilon4 and head trauma: Synergistic or additive risks? *Neurology, 46*(3), 889–891.

Katzman, R., Terry, R., DeTeresa, R., Brown, T., Davies, P., Fuld, P., & Peck, A. (1988). Clinical, pathological, and neurochemical changes in dementia: A subgroup with preserved mental status and numerous neocortical plaques. *Annals of Neurology, 23*(2), 138–144. http://dx.doi.org/10.1002/ana.410230206.

Kawas, C., Segal, J., Stewart, W. F., Corrada, M., & Thal, L. J. (1994). A validation study of the Dementia Questionnaire. *Archives of Neurology, 51*(9), 901–906.

Kehrberg, M. W., Latham, R. H., Haslam, B. T., Hightower, A., Tanner, M., Jacobson, J. A., & Smith, C. B. (1981). Risk factors for staphylococcal toxic-shock syndrome. *American Journal of Epidemiology, 114*(6), 873–879.

Kendler, K. S., Karkowski, L. M., & Prescott, C. A. (1999). Causal relationship between stressful life events and the onset of major depression. *The American Journal of Psychiatry, 156*(6), 837–841.

Khachaturian, A. S., Zandi, P. P., Lyketsos, C. G., Hayden, K. M., Skoog, I., Norton, M. C., & Breitner, J. C. (2006). Antihypertensive medication use and incident Alzheimer disease: The Cache county study. *Archives of Neurology*, *63*(5), 686–692. http://dx.doi.org/10.1001/archneur.63.5.noc60013.

Khachaturian, Z. S. (1985). Diagnosis of Alzheimer's disease. *Archives of Neurology*, *42*(11), 1097–1105.

Khan, W., Giampietro, V., Ginestet, C., Dell'Acqua, F., Bouls, D., Newhouse, S., & Consortium, (2014). No differences in hippocampal volume between carriers and non-carriers of the ApoE epsilon4 and epsilon2 alleles in young healthy adolescents. *Journal of Alzheimer's Disease: JAD*, *40*(1), 37–43. http://dx.doi.org/10.3233/JAD-131841.

Kiecolt-Glaser, J. K., & Newton, T. L. (2001). Marriage and health: His and hers. *Psychological Bulletin*, *127*(4), 472–503.

Killiany, R. J., Hyman, B. T., Gomez-Isla, T., Moss, M. B., Kikinis, R., Jolesz, F., & Albert, M. S. (2002). MRI measures of entorhinal cortex vs hippocampus in preclinical AD. *Neurology*, *58*(8), 1188–1196.

Kim, J., Lee, H. J., & Lee, K. W. (2010). Naturally occurring phytochemicals for the prevention of Alzheimer's disease. *Journal of Neurochemistry*, *112*(6), 1415–1430. http://dx.doi.org/10.1111/j.1471-4159.2009.06562.x.

Kim, J. M., Stewart, R., Bae, K. Y., Kim, S. W., Yang, S. J., Park, K. H., & Yoon, J. S. (2011). Role of BDNF val66met polymorphism on the association between physical activity and incident dementia. *Neurobiology of Aging*, *32*(3) 551.e555-512. http://dx.doi.org/10.1016/j.neurobiolaging.2010.01.018.

Kim, J. M., Stewart, R., Shin, I. S., Kim, S. W., Yang, S. J., & Yoon, J. S. (2008). Associations between head circumference, leg length and dementia in a Korean population. *International Journal of Geriatric Psychiatry*, *23*(1), 41–48. http://dx.doi.org/10.1002/gps.1833.

Kim, J. M., Stewart, R., Shin, I. S., & Yoon, J. S. (2003). Limb length and dementia in an older Korean population. *Journal of Neurology, Neurosurgery, and Psychiatry*, *74*(4), 427–432.

Kim, J. W., Lee, D. Y., Lee, B. C., Jung, M. H., Kim, H., & Choi, Y. S., et al. (2012). Alcohol and cognition in the elderly: A review. *Psychiatry Investigation*, *9*(1), 8–16. http://dx.doi.org/10.4306/pi.2012.9.1.8.

Kim, Y. P., Kim, H., Shin, M. S., Chang, H. K., Jang, M. H., Shin, M. C., & Kim, C. J. (2004). Age-dependence of the effect of treadmill exercise on cell proliferation in the dentate gyrus of rats. *Neuroscience Letters*, *355*(1-2), 152–154.

Kishi, T., & Sunagawa, K. (2012). Exercise training plus calorie restriction causes synergistic protection against cognitive decline via up-regulation of BDNF in hippocampus of stroke-prone hypertensive rats. *Conference Proceedings: Annual International Conference of the IEEE Engineering in Medicine and Biology Society IEEE Engineering in Medicine and Biology Society Conference*, *2012*, 6764–6767. http://dx.doi.org/10.1109/EMBC.2012.6347547.

Kitaguchi, H., Tomimoto, H., Ihara, M., Shibata, M., Uemura, K., Kalaria, R. N., & Takahashi, R. (2009). Chronic cerebral hypoperfusion accelerates amyloid beta deposition in APPSwInd transgenic mice. *Brain Research*, *1294*, 202–210. http://dx.doi.org/10.1016/j.brainres.2009.07.078.

Kittner, S. J., White, L. R., & Farmer, M. E., et al. (1986). Methodological issues in screening for dementia. The problem of education adjustment. *Journal of Chronic Diseases*, *39*, 163–170.

Kivipelto, M., Helkala, E. L., Laakso, M. P., Hanninen, T., Hallikainen, M., Alhainen, K., & Nissinen, A. (2001). Midlife vascular risk factors and Alzheimer's disease in later life: Longitudinal, population based study. *BMJ*, *322*(7300), 1447–1451.

Kivipelto, M., Helkala, E. L., Laakso, M. P., Hanninen, T., Hallikainen, M., Alhainen, K., & Soininen, H. (2002). Apolipoprotein E epsilon4 allele, elevated midlife total cholesterol level, and high midlife systolic blood pressure are independent risk factors for late-life Alzheimer disease. *Annals of Internal Medicine*, *137*(3), 149–155.

Kivipelto, M., Ngandu, T., Fratiglioni, L., Viitanen, M., Kareholt, I., Winblad, B., & Nissinen, A. (2005). Obesity and vascular risk factors at midlife and the risk of dementia and Alzheimer disease. *Archives of Neurology*, *62*(10), 1556–1560. http://dx.doi.org/10.1001/archneur.62.10.1556.

Kivipelto, M., Ngandu, T., Laatikainen, T., Winblad, B., Soininen, H., & Tuomilehto, J. (2006). Risk score for the prediction of dementia risk in 20 years among middle aged people: A longitudinal, population-based study. *Lancet Neurology*, *5*(9), 735–741. http://dx.doi.org/10.1016/S1474-4422(06)70537-3.

Kivipelto, M., Solomon, A., Ahtiluoto, S., Ngandu, T., Lehtisalo, J., Antikainen, R., & Soininen, H. (2013). The Finnish Geriatric Intervention Study to Prevent Cognitive Impairment and Disability (FINGER): Study design and progress. *Alzheimer's & Dementia: The Journal of the Alzheimer's Association*, *9*(6), 657–665. http://dx.doi.org/10.1016/j.jalz.2012.09.012.

Klaiber, E. L., Vogel, W., & Rako, S. (2005). A critique of the Women's Health Initiative hormone therapy study. *Fertility and Sterility*, *84*(6), 1589–1601. http://dx.doi.org/10.1016/j.fertnstert.2005.08.010.

Kloppenborg, R. P., van den Berg, E., Kappelle, L. J., & Biessels, G. J. (2008). Diabetes and other vascular risk factors for dementia: Which factor matters most? A systematic review. *European Journal of Pharmacology*, *585*(1), 97–108. http://dx.doi.org/10.1016/j.ejphar.2008.02.049.

Knickmeyer, R. C., Gouttard, S., Kang, C., Evans, D., Wilber, K., Smith, J. K., & Gilmore, J. H. (2008). A structural MRI study of human brain development from birth to 2 years. *The Journal of Neuroscience*, *28*(47), 12176–12182. http://dx.doi.org/10.1523/JNEUROSCI.3479-08.2008.

Knopman, D. S., Edland, S. D., Cha, R. H., Petersen, R. C., & Rocca, W. A. (2007). Incident dementia in women is preceded by weight loss by at least a decade. *Neurology*, *69*(8), 739–746. http://dx.doi.org/10.1212/01.wnl.0000267661.65586.33.

Knopman, D. S., Jack, C. R., Jr., Wiste, H. J., Weigand, S. D., Vemuri, P., Lowe, V., & Petersen, R. C. (2012). Short-term clinical outcomes for stages of NIA-AA preclinical Alzheimer disease. *Neurology*, *78*(20), 1576–1582. http://dx.doi.org/10.1212/WNL.0b013e3182563bbe.

Knopman, D. S., Petersen, R. C., Cha, R. H., Edland, S. D., & Rocca, W. A. (2006). Incidence and causes of nondegenerative nonvascular dementia: A population-based study. *Archives of Neurology*, *63*(2), 218–221. http://dx.doi.org/10.1001/archneur.63.2.218.

Knopman, D. S., Petersen, R. C., Rocca, W. A., Larson, E. B., & Ganguli, M. (2011). Passive case-finding for Alzheimer's disease and dementia in two U.S. communities. *Alzheimer's & Dementia: The Journal of the Alzheimer's Association*, *7*(1), 53–60. http://dx.doi.org/10.1016/j.jalz.2010.11.001.

Kokmen, E., Beard, C. M., O'Brien, P. C., Offord, K. P., & Kurland, L. T. (1993). Is the incidence of dementing illness changing? A 25-year time trend study in Rochester, Minnesota (1960–1984). *Neurology*, *43*, 1887–1993.

Kolonel, L. N., Henderson, B. E., Hankin, J. H., Nomura, A. M., Wilkens, L. R., Pike, M. C., & Nagamine, F. S. (2000). A multiethnic cohort in Hawaii and Los Angeles: Baseline characteristics. *American Journal of Epidemiology*, *151*(4), 346–357.

Koolschijn, P. C., van Haren, N. E., Lensvelt-Mulders, G. J., Hulshoff Pol, H. E., & Kahn, R. S. (2009). Brain volume abnormalities in major depressive disorder: A meta-analysis of magnetic resonance imaging studies. *Human Brain Mapping*, *30*(11), 3719–3735. http://dx.doi.org/10.1002/hbm.20801.

Kraepelin, E. (1910). Psychiatry: A textbook for Students and Physicians (pp. 593–632). Leipzig: Barth.

Kral, V. A. (1962). Senescent forgetfulness: Benign and malignant. *Canadian Medical Association Journal*, *86*, 257–260.

Kroger, E., Andel, R., Lindsay, J., Benounissa, Z., Verreault, R., & Laurin, D. (2008). Is complexity of work associated wtih risk of dementia? The Canadian Study of Health and Aging. *American Journal of Epidemiology*, *167*(7), 820–830.

Kryscio, R. J., Abner, E. L., Cooper, G. E., Fardo, D. W., Jicha, G. A., Nelson, P. T., & Schmitt, F. A. (2014). Self-reported memory complaints: Implications from a longitudinal cohort with autopsies. *Neurology*, *83*(15), 1359–1365. http://dx.doi.org/10.1212/WNL.0000000000000856.

Kuczmarski, R. J. (1989). Need for body composition information in elderly subjects. *The American Journal of Clinical Nutrition*, *50*(5 Suppl.), 1150–1157. discussion 1231-1155.

Kuh, D., Ben-Shlomo, Y., Lynch, J., Hallqvist, J., & Power, C. (2003). Life course epidemiology. *Journal of Epidemiology and Community Health*, *57*(10), 778–783.

Kukull, W. A., Higdon, R., Bowen, J. D., McCormick, W. C., Teri, L., Schellenberg, G. D., & Larson, E. B. (2002). Dementia and Alzheimer disease incidence: A prospective cohort study. *Archives of Neurology*, *59*(11), 1737–1746.

Lago, R. M., Singh, P. P., & Nesto, R. W. (2007). Diabetes and hypertension. *Nature Clinical Practice Endocrinology & Metabolism*, *3*(10), 667. http://dx.doi.org/10.1038/ncpendmet0638.

Lahiri, D. K., & Maloney, B. (2010). The "LEARn" (Latent Early-life Associated Regulation) model integrates environmental risk factors and the developmental basis of Alzheimer's disease, and proposes remedial steps. *Experimental Gerontology*, *45*(4), 291–296. http://dx.doi.org/10.1016/j.exger.2010.01.001.

Landau, S. M., Marks, S. M., Mormino, E. C., Rabinovici, G. D., Oh, H., O'Neil, J. P., & Jagust, W. J. (2012). Association of lifetime cognitive engagement and low beta-amyloid deposition. *Archives of Neurology*, *69*(5), 623–629. http://dx.doi.org/10.1001/archneurol.2011.2748.

Langa, K. M., Plassman, B. L., Wallace, R. B., Herzog, A. R., Heeringa, S. G., & Ofstedal, M. B., et al. (2005). The aging, demographics and memory study: Study design and methods. *Neuroepidemiology*, *25*, 181–191.

Langbaum, J. B., Chen, K., Lee, W., Reschke, C., Bandy, D., Fleisher, A. S., & Alzheimer's Disease Neuroimaging Initiative, (2009). Categorical and correlational analyses of baseline fluorodeoxyglucose positron emission tomography images from the Alzheimer's Disease Neuroimaging Initiative (ADNI). *Neuroimage*, *45*(4), 1107–1116. http://dx.doi.org/10.1016/j.neuroimage.2008.12.072.

Langbaum, J. B., Fleisher, A. S., Chen, K., Ayutyanont, N., Lopera, F., Quiroz, Y. T., & Reiman, E. M. (2013). Ushering in the study and treatment of preclinical Alzheimer disease. *Nature Reviews Neurology*, *9*(7), 371–381. http://dx.doi.org/10.1038/nrneurol.2013.107.

Larrieu, S., Letenneur, L., Orgogozo, J. M., Fabrigoule, C., Amieva, H., Le Carret, N., & Dartigues, J. F. (2002). Incidence and outcome of mild cognitive impairment in a population-based prospective cohort. *Neurology*, *59*(10), 1594–1599.

Larson, E. B., McCurry, S. M., Graves, A. B., Bowen, J. D., Rice, M. M., McCormick, W. C., & Sasaki, H. (1998). Standardization of the clinical diagnosis of the dementia syndrome and its subtypes in a cross-national study: The Ni-Hon-Sea experience. *The Journals of Gerontology Series A, Biological Sciences and Medical Sciences*, *53*(4), M313–319.

Larson, E. B., Shadlen, M. F., Wang, L., McCormick, W. C., Bowen, J. D., & Teri, L., et al. (2004). Survival after initial diagnosis of Alzheimer disease. *Annals of Internal Medicine*, *140*(7), 501–509.

Larson, E. B., Wang, L., Bowen, J. D., McCormick, W. C., Teri, L., & Crane, P., et al. (2006). Exercise is associated with reduced risk for incident dementia among persons 65 years of age and older. *Annals of Internal Medicine*, *144*(2), 73–81.

Latta, C. H., Brothers, H. M., & Wilcock, D. M. (2014). Neuroinflammation in Alzheimer's disease; a source of heterogeneity and target for personalized therapy. *Neuroscience*. http://dx.doi.org/10.1016/j.neuroscience.2014.09.061.

Launer, L. J. (2002). Demonstrating the case that AD is a vascular disease: Epidemiologic evidence. *Ageing Research Reviews*, *1*(1), 61–77.

Launer, L. J. (2011). Counting dementia: There is no one "best" way. *Alzheimer's & Dementia: The Journal of the Alzheimer's Association*, *7*(1), 10–14. http://dx.doi.org/10.1016/j.jalz.2010.11.003.

Launer, L. J., Andersen, K., Dewey, M. E., Letenneur, L., Ott, A., Amaducci, L. A., & Hofman, A. (1999). Rates and risk factors for dementia and Alzheimer's disease: Results from EURODEM pooled analyses. EURODEM incidence research group and work groups. European studies of dementia. *Neurology*, *52*(1), 78–84.

Launer, L. J., Hughes, T. M., & White, L. R. (2011). Microinfarcts, brain atrophy, and cognitive function: The Honolulu Asia aging study autopsy study. *Annals of Neurology*, *70*(5), 774–780. http://dx.doi.org/10.1002/ana.22520.

Launer, L. J., Masaki, K., Petrovitch, H., Foley, D., & Havlik, R. J. (1995). The association between midlife blood pressure levels and late-life cognitive function. The Honolulu-Asia aging study. *JAMA*, *274*(23), 1846–1851.

Launer, L. J., Miller, M. E., Williamson, J. D., Lazar, R. M., Gerstein, H. C., Murray, A. M., & Bryan, R. N. (2011). Effects of intensive glucose lowering on brain structure and function in people with type 2 diabetes (ACCORD MIND): A randomised open-label substudy. *Lancet Neurology*, *10*(11), 969–977. http://dx.doi.org/10.1016/S1474-4422(11)70188-0.

Launer, L. J., Petrovitch, H., Ross, G. W., Markesbery, W., & White, L. R. (2008). AD brain pathology: Vascular origins? Results from the HAAS autopsy study. *Neurobiology of Aging*, *29*(10), 1587–1590. http://dx.doi.org/10.1016/j.neurobiolaging.2007.03.008.

Launer, L. J., Ross, G. W., Petrovitch, H., Masaki, K., Foley, D., & White, L. R., et al. (2000). Midlife blood pressure and dementia: The Honolulu-Asia aging study. *Neurobiology of Aging*, *21*(1), 49–55.

Laurin, D., Masaki, K. H., Foley, D. J., White, L. R., & Launer, L. J. (2004). Midlife dietary intake of antioxidants and risk of late-life incident dementia: The Honolulu-Asia Aging Study. *American Journal of Epidemiology*, *159*(10), 959–967.

Laurin, D., Verreault, R., Lindsay, J., MacPherson, K., & Rockwood, K. (2001). Physical activity and risk of cognitive impairment and dementia in elderly persons. *Archives of Neurology*, *58*(3), 498–504.

Lazarov, O., Robinson, J., Tang, Y. P., Hairston, I. S., Korade-Mirnics, Z., Lee, V. M., & Sisodia, S. S. (2005). Environmental enrichment reduces Abeta levels and amyloid deposition in transgenic mice. *Cell*, *120*(5), 701–713. http://dx.doi.org/10.1016/j.cell.2005.01.015.

Lee, G. R., DeMaris, A., Bavin, S., & Sullivan, R. (2001). Gender differences in the depressive effect of widowhood in later life. *The Journals of Gerontology Series B, Psychological Sciences and Social Sciences*, *56*(1), S56–61.

Lee, S. J., Ritchie, C. S., Yaffe, K., Stijacic Cenzer, I., & Barnes, D. E. (2014). A clinical index to predict progression from mild cognitive impairment to dementia due to Alzheimer's disease. *PLoS One*, *9*(12), e113535. http://dx.doi.org/10.1371/journal.pone.0113535.

Lee, Y. B., Lee, H. J., & Sohn, H. S. (2005). Soy isoflavones and cognitive function. *The Journal of Nutritional Biochemistry*, *16*(11), 641–649. http://dx.doi.org/10.1016/j.jnutbio.2005.06.010.

Legault, C., Jennings, J. M., Katula, J. A., Dagenbach, D., Gaussoin, S. A., Sink, K. M., & SHARP-P Study Group, (2011). Designing clinical trials for assessing the effects of cognitive training and physical activity interventions on cognitive outcomes: The Seniors Health and Activity

Research Program Pilot (SHARP-P) study, a randomized controlled trial. *BMC Geriatrics*, *11*, 27. http://dx.doi.org/10.1186/1471-2318-11-27.

Lehericy, S., Baulac, M., Chiras, J., Pierot, L., Martin, N., Pillon, B., & Marsault, C. (1994). Amygdalohippocampal MR volume measurements in the early stages of Alzheimer disease. *AJNR American Journal of Neuroradiology*, *15*(5), 929–937.

Lehman, E. J., Hein, M. J., Baron, S. L., & Gersic, C. M. (2012). Neurodegenerative causes of death among retired National Football League players. *Neurology*, *79*(19), 1970–1974. http://dx.doi.org/10.1212/WNL.0b013e31826daf50.

Leibson, C. L., Rocca, W. A., Hanson, V. A., Cha, R., Kokmen, E., & O'Brien, P. C., et al. (1997). The risk of dementia among persons with diabetes mellitus: A population-based cohort study. *Annals of the New York Academy of Sciences*, *826*, 422–427.

Lesne, S. E., Sherman, M. A., Grant, M., Kuskowski, M., Schneider, J. A., & Bennett, D. A., et al. (2013). Brain amyloid-beta oligomers in ageing and Alzheimer's disease. *Brain*, *136*(Pt 5), 1383–1398. http://dx.doi.org/10.1093/brain/awt062.

Letenneur, L. (2004). Risk of dementia and alcohol and wine consumption: A review of recent results. *Biological Research*, *37*(2), 189–193.

Letenneur, L., Proust-Lima, C., Le Gouge, A., Dartigues, J. F., & Barberger-Gateau, P. (2007). Flavonoid intake and cognitive decline over a 10-year period. *American Journal of Epidemiology*, *165*(12), 1364–1371. http://dx.doi.org/10.1093/aje/kwm036.

Li, F. J., Shen, L., & Ji, H. F. (2012). Dietary intakes of vitamin E, vitamin C, and beta-carotene and risk of Alzheimer's disease: A meta-analysis. *Journal of Alzheimer's Disease*, *31*(2), 253–258. http://dx.doi.org/10.3233/JAD-2012-120349.

Li, G., Rhew, I. C., Shofer, J. B., Kukull, W. A., Breitner, J. C., Peskind, E., & Larson, E. B. (2007). Age-varying association between blood pressure and risk of dementia in those aged 65 and older: A community-based prospective cohort study. *Journal of the American Geriatrics Society*, *55*(8), 1161–1167. http://dx.doi.org/10.1111/j.1532-5415.2007.01233.x.

Li, G., Shen, Y. C., & Chen, C. H., et al. (1991). A three-year follow-up study of age-related dementia in an urban area of Beijing. *Acta Psychiatrica Scandinavica*, *83*, 99–104.

Liang, K. Y., Mintun, M. A., Fagan, A. M., Goate, A. M., Bugg, J. M., Holtzman, D. M., & Head, D. (2010). Exercise and Alzheimer's disease biomarkers in cognitively normal older adults. *Annals of Neurology*, *68*(3), 311–318. http://dx.doi.org/10.1002/ana.22096.

Liepelt-Scarfone, I., Graeber, S., Feseker, A., Baysal, G., Godau, J., Gaenslen, A., & Berg, D. (2011). Influence of different cut-off values on the diagnosis of mild cognitive impairment in Parkinson's disease. *Parkinsons Disease*, *2011*, 540843. http://dx.doi.org/10.4061/2011/540843.

Light, L. L. (1991). Memory and aging: Four hypotheses in search of data. *Annual Review of Psychology*, *42*, 333–376. http://dx.doi.org/10.1146/annurev.ps.42.020191.002001.

Lim, G. P., Calon, F., Morihara, T., Yang, F., Teter, B., Ubeda, O., & Cole, G. M. (2005). A diet enriched with the omega-3 fatty acid docosahexaenoic acid reduces amyloid burden in an aged Alzheimer mouse model. *The Journal of Neuroscience*, *25*(12), 3032–3040. http://dx.doi.org/10.1523/JNEUROSCI.4225-04.2005.

Lim, Y. Y., Villemagne, V. L., Laws, S. M., Ames, D., Pietrzak, R. H., Ellis, K. A., & AIBL Research Group, (2013). BDNF Val66Met, Abeta amyloid, and cognitive decline in preclinical Alzheimer's disease. *Neurobiology of Aging*, *34*(11), 2457–2464. http://dx.doi.org/10.1016/j.neurobiolaging.2013.05.006.

Lim, Y. Y., Villemagne, V. L., Laws, S. M., Ames, D., Pietrzak, R. H., Ellis, K. A., & AIBL Research Group, (2014). Effect of BDNF Val66Met on memory decline and hippocampal atrophy in prodromal Alzheimer's disease: A preliminary study. *PLoS One*, *9*(1), e86498. http://dx.doi.org/10.1371/journal.pone.0086498.

Lim, Y. Y., Villemagne, V. L., Laws, S. M., Pietrzak, R. H., Snyder, P. J., Ames, D., & Maruff, P. (2014). APOE and BDNF polymorphisms moderate amyloid beta-related cognitive decline in preclinical Alzheimer's disease. *Molecular Psychiatry*. http://dx.doi.org/10.1038/mp.2014.123.

Lindsay, J., Laurin, D., Verreault, R., Hebert, R., Helliwell, B., & Hill, G. B., et al. (2002). Risk factors for Alzheimer's disease: A prospective analysis from the Canadian Study of Health and Aging. *American Journal of Epidemiology*, *156*(5), 445–453.

Lindsted, K., Tonstad, S., & Kuzma, J. W. (1991). Body mass index and patterns of mortality among Seventh-day Adventist men. *International Journal of Obesity*, *15*(6), 397–406.

Lithgow, S., Jackson, G. A., & Browne, D. (2012). Estimating the prevalence of dementia: Cognitive screening in Glasgow nursing homes. *International Journal of Geriatric Psychiatry*, *27*(8), 785–791. http://dx.doi.org/10.1002/gps.2784.

Littlejohns, T. J., Henley, W. E., Lang, I. A., Annweiler, C., Beauchet, O., Chaves, P. H., & Llewellyn, D. J. (2014). Vitamin D and the risk of dementia and Alzheimer disease. *Neurology*, *83*(10), 920–928. http://dx.doi.org/10.1212/WNL.0000000000000755.

Liu, H. L., Zhao, G., Zhang, H., & Shi, L. D. (2013). Long-term treadmill exercise inhibits the progression of Alzheimer's disease-like neuropathology in the hippocampus of APP/PS1 transgenic mice. *Behavioural Brain Research*, *256*, 261–272. http://dx.doi.org/10.1016/j.bbr.2013.08.008.

Lloyd-Jones, D. M., Wilson, P. W., Larson, M. G., Beiser, A., Leip, E. P., & D'Agostino, R. B., et al. (2004). Framingham risk score and prediction of lifetime risk for coronary heart disease. *The American Journal of Cardiology*, *94*(1), 20–24. http://dx.doi.org/10.1016/j.amjcard.2004.03.023.

Loef, M., & Walach, H. (2012). Fruit, vegetables and prevention of cognitive decline or dementia: A systematic review of cohort studies. *The Journal of Nutrition, Health & Aging*, *16*(7), 626–630.

Lopez, O. L., Becker, J. T., Klunk, W., Saxton, J., Hamilton, R. L., Kaufer, D. I., & DeKosky, S. T. (2000). Research evaluation and diagnosis of possible Alzheimer's disease over the last two decades: II. *Neurology*, *55*(12), 1863–1869.

Lopez, O. L., Kuller, L. H., Fitzpatrick, A., Ives, D., Becker, J. T., & Beauchamp, N. (2003). Evaluation of dementia in the cardiovascular health cognition study. *Neuroepidemiology*, *22*(1), 1–12.

Lovden, M., Schaefer, S., Noack, H., Bodammer, N. C., Kuhn, S., Heinze, H. J., & Lindenberger, U. (2012). Spatial navigation training protects the hippocampus against age-related changes during early and late adulthood. *Neurobiology of Aging*, *33*(3) 620.e629-620.e622. http://dx.doi.org/10.1016/j.neurobiolaging.2011.02.013.

Lowe, V. J., Weigand, S. D., Senjem, M. L., Vemuri, P., Jordan, L., Kantarci, K., & Petersen, R. C. (2014). Association of hypometabolism and amyloid levels in aging, normal subjects. *Neurology*, *82*(22), 1959–1967. http://dx.doi.org/10.1212/WNL.0000000000000467.

Luchsinger, J. A., & Gustafson, D. R. (2009). Adiposity and Alzheimer's disease. *Current Opinion in Clinical Nutrition and Metabolic Care*, *12*(1), 15–21. http://dx.doi.org/10.1097/MCO.0b013e32831c8c71.

Luchsinger, J. A., & Mayeux, R. (2004). Dietary factors and Alzheimer's disease. *Lancet Neurology*, *3*(10), 579–587. http://dx.doi.org/10.1016/S1474-4422(04)00878-6.

Luchsinger, J. A., Tang, M. X., Miller, J., Green, R., & Mayeux, R. (2007). Relation of higher folate intake to lower risk of Alzheimer disease in the elderly. *Archives of Neurology*, *64*(1), 86–92. http://dx.doi.org/10.1001/archneur.64.1.86.

Luchsinger, J. A., Tang, M. X., Shea, S., & Mayeux, R. (2002). Caloric intake and the risk of Alzheimer disease. *Archives of Neurology*, *59*(8), 1258–1263.

Luchsinger, J. A., Tang, M. X., Shea, S., & Mayeux, R. (2003). Antioxidant vitamin intake and risk of Alzheimer disease. *Archives of Neurology*, *60*(2), 203–208.

Luchsinger, J. A., Tang, M. X., Siddiqui, M., Shea, S., & Mayeux, R. (2004). Alcohol intake and risk of dementia. *Journal of the American Geriatrics Society*, *52*(4), 540–546. http://dx.doi.org/10.1111/j.1532-5415.2004.52159.x.

Lunde, A., Melve, K. K., Gjessing, H. K., Skjaerven, R., & Irgens, L. M. (2007). Genetic and environmental influences on birth weight, birth length, head circumference, and gestational age by use of population-based parent-offspring data. *American Journal of Epidemiology*, *165*(7), 734–741.

Luukinen, H., Viramo, P., Herala, M., Kervinen, K., Kesaniemi, Y. A., Savola, O., & Hillbom, M. (2005). Fall-related brain injuries and the risk of dementia in elderly people: A population-based study. *European Journal of Neurology: The Official Journal of the European Federation of Neurological Societies*, *12*(2), 86–92. http://dx.doi.org/10.1111/j.1468-1331.2004.00953.x.

Lye, T. C., & Shores, E. A. (2000). Traumatic brain injury as a risk factor for Alzheimer's disease: A review. *Neuropsychology Review*, *10*(2), 115–129.

Lynch, J., & Smith, G. D. (2005). A life course approach to chronic disease epidemiology. *Annual Review of Public Health*, *26*, 1–35. http://dx.doi.org/10.1146/annurev.publhealth.26.021304.144505.

Magaziner, J., German, P., Zimmerman, S. I., Hebel, J. R., Burton, L., Gruber-Baldini, A. L., & Kittner, S. (2000). The prevalence of dementia in a statewide sample of new nursing home admissions aged 65 and older: Diagnosis by expert panel. Epidemiology of dementia in nursing homes research group. *Gerontologist*, *40*(6), 663–672.

Magnussen, C. G., Smith, K. J., & Juonala, M. (2014). What the long term cohort studies that began in childhood have taught us about the origins of coronary heart disease. *Current Cardiovascular Risk Reports*, *8*, 373–383.

Maguire, E. A., Burgess, N., & O'Keefe, J. (1999). Human spatial navigation: Cognitive maps, sexual dimorphism, and neural substrates. *Current Opinion in Neurobiology*, *9*(2), 171–177.

Maguire, E. A., Gadian, D. G., Johnsrude, I. S., Good, C. D., Ashburner, J., & Frackowiak, R. S., et al. (2000). Navigation-related structural change in the hippocampi of taxi drivers. *Proceedings of the National Academy of Sciences of the United States of America*, *97*(8), 4398–4403. http://dx.doi.org/10.1073/pnas.070039597.

Maillard, P., Seshadri, S., Beiser, A., Himali, J. J., Au, R., Fletcher, E., & DeCarli, C. (2012). Effects of systolic blood pressure on white-matter integrity in young adults in the Framingham Heart Study: A cross-sectional study. *Lancet Neurology*, *11*(12), 1039–1047. http://dx.doi.org/10.1016/S1474-4422(12)70241-7.

Mainardi, M., Di Garbo, A., Caleo, M., Berardi, N., Sale, A., & Maffei, L. (2014). Environmental enrichment strengthens corticocortical interactions and reduces amyloid-beta oligomers in aged mice. *Frontiers in Aging Neuroscience*, *6*, 1. http://dx.doi.org/10.3389/fnagi.2014.00001.

Mak, Z., Kim, J. M., & Stewart, R. (2006). Leg length, cognitive impairment and cognitive decline in an African-Caribbean population. *International Journal of Geriatric Psychiatry*, *21*(3), 266–272. http://dx.doi.org/10.1002/gps.1458.

Maki, P. M. (2013). Critical window hypothesis of hormone therapy and cognition: A scientific update on clinical studies. *Menopause*, *20*(6), 695–709. http://dx.doi.org/10.1097/GME.0b013e3182960cf8.

Malouf, R., & Grimley Evans, J. (2008). Folic acid with or without vitamin B12 for the prevention and treatment of healthy elderly and demented people. *Cochrane Database of Systematic Reviews (Online)*(4), CD004514. http://dx.doi.org/10.1002/14651858.CD004514.pub2.

Manly, J. J., Tang, M. X., Schupf, N., Stern, Y., Vonsattel, J. P., & Mayeux, R. (2008). Frequency and course of mild cognitive impairment in a multiethnic community. *Annals of Neurology*, *63*(4), 494–506. http://dx.doi.org/10.1002/ana.21326.

Manly, J. J., Touradji, P., Tang, M. X., & Stern, Y. (2003). Literacy and memory decline among ethnically diverse elders. *Journal of Clinical and Experimental Neuropsychology*, *25*(5), 680–690. http://dx.doi.org/10.1076/jcen.25.5.680.14579.

Mann, K., Ackermann, K., Croissant, B., Mundle, G., Nakovics, H., & Diehl, A. (2005). Neuroimaging of gender differences in alcohol dependence: Are women more vulnerable? *Alcoholism, Clinical and Experimental Research*, *29*(5), 896–901.

Markesbery, W. R. (1997). Oxidative stress hypothesis in Alzheimer's disease. *Free Radical Biology & Medicine*, *23*(1), 134–147.

Marlatt, M. W., Potter, M. C., Bayer, T. A., van Praag, H., & Lucassen, P. J. (2013). Prolonged running, not fluoxetine treatment, increases neurogenesis, but does not alter neuropathology, in the 3xTg mouse model of Alzheimer's disease. *Current Topics in Behavioral Neurosciences*, *15*, 313–340. http://dx.doi.org/10.1007/7854_2012_237.

Marmot, M. G., Syme, S. L., Kagan, A., Kato, H., Cohen, J. B., & Belsky, J. (1975). Epidemiologic studies of coronary heart disease and stroke in Japanese men living in Japan, Hawaii and California: Prevalence of coronary and hypertensive heart disease and associated risk factors. *American Journal of Epidemiology*, *102*(6), 514–525.

Martin, M., Clare, L., Altgassen, A. M., Cameron, M. H., & Zehnder, F. (2011). Cognition-based interventions for healthy older people and people with mild cognitive impairment. *Cochrane Database of Systematic Reviews (Online)*(1), CD006220. http://dx.doi.org/10.1002/14651858.CD006220.pub2.

Martland, H. (1928). Punch drunk. *Journal of the American Medical Association*, *91*(15), 1103–1107.

Martorell, P., Bataller, E., Llopis, S., Gonzalez, N., Alvarez, B., Monton, F., & Genoves, S. (2013). A cocoa peptide protects Caenorhabditis elegans from oxidative stress and beta-amyloid peptide toxicity. *PLoS One*, *8*(5), e63283. http://dx.doi.org/10.1371/journal.pone.0063283.

Martyn, C. N., Gale, C. R., Sayer, A. A., & Fall, C. (1996). Growth in utero and cognitive function in adult life: Follow up study of people born between 1920 and 1943. *BMJ*, *312*(7043), 1393–1396.

Martyn, C. N., & Pippard, E. C. (1988). Usefulness of mortality data in determining the geography and time trends of dementia. *Journal of Epidemiology and Community Health*, *42*(2), 134–137.

Masaki, K. H., Losonczy, K. G., Izmirlian, G., Foley, D. J., Ross, G. W., Petrovitch, H., & White, L. R. (2000). Association of vitamin E and C supplement use with cognitive function and dementia in elderly men. *Neurology*, *54*(6), 1265–1272.

Matthews, F. E., Arthur, A., Barnes, L. E., Bond, J., Jagger, C., & Robinson, L., et al. (2013). A two-decade comparison of prevalence of dementia in individuals aged 65 years and older from three geographical areas of England: Results of the Cognitive Function and Ageing Study I and II. *Lancet*, *382*(9902), 1405–1412. http://dx.doi.org/10.1016/S0140-6736(13)61570-6.

Maurer, K., Volk, S., & Gerbaldo, H. (1997). Auguste D and Alzheimer's disease. *The Lancet*, *349*, 1546–1549.

Mayeux, R., Ottman, R., Maestre, G., Ngai, C., Tang, M. X., Ginsberg, H., & Shelanski, M. (1995). Synergistic effects of traumatic head injury and apolipoprotein-epsilon 4 in patients with Alzheimer's disease. *Neurology*, *45*(3 Pt 1), 555–557.

Mayeux, R., Ottman, R., Tang, M. X., Noboa-Bauza, L., Marder, K., & Gurland, B., et al. (1993). Genetic susceptibility and head injury as risk factors for Alzheimer's disease among community-dwelling elderly persons and their first-degree relatives. *Annals of Neurology*, *33*(5), 494–501. http://dx.doi.org/10.1002/ana.410330513.

Mayeux, R., Reitz, C., Brickman, A. M., Haan, M. N., Manly, J. J., Glymour, M. M., & Morris, J. C. (2011). Operationalizing diagnostic criteria for Alzheimer's disease and other age-related cognitive impairment-Part 1. *Alzheimer's & Dementia: The Journal of the Alzheimer's Association*, *7*(1), 15–34. http://dx.doi.org/10.1016/j.jalz.2010.11.005.

McConathy, J., & Sheline, Y. I. (2014). Imaging biomarkers associated with cognitive decline: A review. *Biological Psychiatry*. http://dx.doi.org/10.1016/j.biopsych.2014.08.024.

McDowell, I., Xi, G., Lindsay, J., & Tierney, M. (2007). Mapping the connections between education and dementia. *Journal of Clinical and Experimental Neuropsychology*, *29*(2), 127–141. http://dx.doi.org/10.1080/13803390600582420.

McGeer, P. L., Schulzer, M., & McGeer, E. G. (1996). Arthritis and anti-inflammatory agents as possible protective factors for Alzheimer's disease: A review of 17 epidemiologic studies. *Neurology*, *47*(2), 425–432.

McGuinness, B., Todd, S., Passmore, P., & Bullock, R. (2009). Blood pressure lowering in patients without prior cerebrovascular disease for prevention of cognitive impairment and dementia. *Cochrane Database of Systematic Reviews (Online)*(4), CD004034. http://dx.doi.org/10.1002/14651858.CD004034.pub3.

McKee, A. C., Cantu, R. C., Nowinski, C. J., Hedley-Whyte, E. T., Gavett, B. E., Budson, A. E., & Stern, R. A. (2009). Chronic traumatic encephalopathy in athletes: Progressive tauopathy after repetitive head injury. *Journal of Neuropathology and Experimental Neurology*, *68*(7), 709–735. http://dx.doi.org/10.1097/NEN.0b013e3181a9d503.

McKee, A. C., Stern, R. A., Nowinski, C. J., Stein, T. D., Alvarez, V. E., Daneshvar, D. H., & Cantu, R. C. (2013). The spectrum of disease in chronic traumatic encephalopathy. *Brain*, *136*(Pt 1), 43–64. http://dx.doi.org/10.1093/brain/aws307.

McKhann, G., Drachman, D., Folstein, M., Katzman, R., Price, D., & Stadlan, E. M. (1984). Clinical diagnosis of Alzheimer's disease: Report of the NINCDS-ADRDA Work Group under the auspices of Department of Health and Human Services Task Force on Alzheimer's Disease. *Neurology*, *34*(7), 939–944.

McKhann, G. M., Knopman, D. S., Chertkow, H., Hyman, B. T., Jack, C. R., Jr., Kawas, C. H., & Phelps, C. H. (2011). The diagnosis of dementia due to Alzheimer's disease: Recommendations from the National Institute on Aging-Alzheimer's Association workgroups on diagnostic guidelines for Alzheimer's disease. *Alzheimer's & Dementia: The Journal of the Alzheimer's Association*, *7*(3), 263–269. http://dx.doi.org/10.1016/j.jalz.2011.03.005.

Meagher, E. A., Barry, O. P., Lawson, J. A., Rokach, J., & FitzGerald, G. A. (2001). Effects of vitamin E on lipid peroxidation in healthy persons. *JAMA*, *285*(9), 1178–1182.

Medina, L. D., Rodriguez-Agudelo, Y., Geschwind, D. H., Gilbert, P. E., Liang, L. J., & Cummings, J. L., et al. (2011). Propositional density and apolipoprotein E genotype among persons at risk for familial Alzheimer's disease. *Dementia and Geriatric Cognitive Disorders*, *32*(3), 188–192. http://dx.doi.org/10.1159/000333023.

Medina, M., & Avila, J. (2014). New perspectives on the role of tau in Alzheimer's disease. Implications for therapy. *Biochemical Pharmacology*, *88*(4), 540–547. http://dx.doi.org/10.1016/j.bcp.2014.01.013.

Mehta, K. M., Ott, A., Kalmijn, S., Slooter, A. J., van Duijn, C. M., & Hofman, A., et al. (1999). Head trauma and risk of dementia and Alzheimer's disease: The Rotterdam Study. *Neurology*, *53*(9), 1959–1962.

Meng, X., & D'Arcy, C. (2012). Education and dementia in the context of the cognitive reserve hypothesis: A systematic review with meta-analyses and qualitative analyses. *PLoS One*, *7*(6), e38268. http://dx.doi.org/10.1371/journal.pone.0038268.

Meng, X. -F., Yu, J. -T., Wang, H. -F., Tan, M. -S., & Wang, C. (2014). Midlife vascular risk factors and the risk of Alzheimer's disease: A systematic review and meta-analysis. *Journal of Alzheimer's Disease* July 7. Epub ahead of print. http://dx.doi.org/10.3233/JAD-140954.

Merchant, C., Tang, M. X., Albert, S., Manly, J., Stern, Y., & Mayeux, R. (1999). The influence of smoking on the risk of Alzheimer's disease. *Neurology*, *52*(7), 1408–1412.

Merema, M. R., Speelman, C. P., Kaczmarek, E. A., & Foster, J. K. (2012). Age and premorbid intelligence suppress complaint-performance congruency in raw score measures of memory. *International Psychogeriatrics/IPA*, *24*(3), 397–405. http://dx.doi.org/10.1017/S1041610211001918.

Mesholam, R. I., Moberg, P. J., Mahr, R. N., & Doty, R. L. (1998). Olfaction in neurodegenerative disease: A meta-analysis of olfactory functioning in Alzheimer's and Parkinson's diseases. *Archives of Neurology*, *55*(1), 84–90.

MetLife Mature Market Institute and LifePlans, Inc. (2006). *The MetLife study of Alzheimer's disease: The caregiving experience*. <http://www.metlife.com/assets/cao/mmi/publications/studies/mmi-alzheimers-disease-caregiving-experience-study.pdf> Accessed 08.06.15.

Mezzich, J. E. (2002). International surveys on the use of ICD-10 and related diagnostic systems. *Psychopathology*, *35*, 72–75.

Middleton, L. E., Barnes, D. E., Lui, L. Y., & Yaffe, K. (2010). Physical activity over the life course and its association with cognitive performance and impairment in old age. *Journal of the American Geriatrics Society*, *58*(7), 1322–1326. http://dx.doi.org/10.1111/j.1532-5415.2010.02903.x.

Middleton, L. E., Grinberg, L. T., Miller, B., Kawas, C., & Yaffe, K. (2011). Neuropathologic features associated with Alzheimer disease diagnosis: Age matters. *Neurology*, *77*(19), 1737–1744. http://dx.doi.org/10.1212/WNL.0b013e318236f0cf.

Mielke, M. M., Savica, R., Wiste, H. J., Weigand, S. D., Vemuri, P., Knopman, D. S., & Jack, C. R., Jr. (2014). Head trauma and *in vivo* measures of amyloid and neurodegeneration in a population-based study. *Neurology*, *82*(1), 70–76. http://dx.doi.org/10.1212/01.wnl.0000438229.56094.54.

Mielke, M. M., Zandi, P. P., Sjogren, M., Gustafson, D., Ostling, S., & Steen, B., et al. (2005). High total cholesterol levels in late life associated with a reduced risk of dementia. *Neurology*, *64*(10), 1689–1695. http://dx.doi.org/10.1212/01.WNL.0000161870.78572.A5.

Mild Traumatic Brain Injury Committee of the Head Injury Interdisciplinary Special Interest Group of the American Congress of Rehabilitation Medicine, (1993). Definition of mild traumatic brain injury. *The Journal of Head Trauma Rehabilitation*, *8*(3), 86–87.

Miller, R., King, M. A., Heaton, M. B., & Walker, D. W. (2002). The effects of chronic ethanol consumption on neurotrophins and their receptors in the rat hippocampus and basal forebrain. *Brain Research*, *950*(1–2), 137–147.

Mills, S. M., Mallmann, J., Santacruz, A. M., Fuqua, A., Carril, M., Aisen, P. S., & Bateman, R. J. (2013). Preclinical trials in autosomal dominant AD: Implementation of the DIAN-TU trial. *Revue Neurologique*, *169*(10), 737–743. http://dx.doi.org/10.1016/j.neurol.2013.07.017.

Mirra, S. S., Heyman, A., McKeel, D., Sumi, S. M., Crain, B. J., Brownlee, L. M., & Berg, L. (1991). The Consortium to Establish a Registry for Alzheimer's Disease (CERAD). Part II. Standardization of the neuropathologic assessment of Alzheimer's disease. *Neurology*, *41*(4), 479–486.

Mitchell, A. J. (2008). The clinical significance of subjective memory complaints in the diagnosis of mild cognitive impairment and dementia: A meta-analysis. *International Journal of Geriatric Psychiatry*, *23*(11), 1191–1202. http://dx.doi.org/10.1002/gps.2053.

Moceri, V. M., Kukull, W. A., Emanuel, I., van Belle, G., & Larson, E. B. (2000). Early-life risk factors and the development of Alzheimer's disease. *Neurology*, *54*, 415–420.

Moceri, V. M., Kukull, W. A., Emanual, I., van Belle, G., Starr, J. R., Schellenberg, G. D., & Larson, E. B. (2001). Using census data and birth certificates to reconstruct the early-life socioeconomic environment and the relation to the development of Alzheimer's disease. *Epidemiology*, *12*(4), 383–389.

Modrego, P. J., & Ferrandez, J. (2004). Depression in patients with mild cognitive impairment increases the risk of developing dementia of Alzheimer type: A prospective cohort study. *Archives of Neurology*, *61*(8), 1290–1293. http://dx.doi.org/10.1001/archneur.61.8.1290.

Moffat, S. D., Zonderman, A. B., Metter, E. J., Blackman, M. R., Harman, S. M., & Resnick, S. M. (2002). Longitudinal assessment of serum free testosterone concentration predicts memory performance and cognitive status in elderly men. *The Journal of Clinical Endocrinology and Metabolism*, *87*(11), 5001–5007. http://dx.doi.org/10.1210/jc.2002-020419.

Mohs, R. C., Breitner, J. C., Silverman, J. M., & Davis, K. L. (1987). Alzheimer's disease. Morbid risk among first-degree relatives approximates 50% by 90 years of age. *Archives of General Psychiatry*, *44*(5), 405–408.

Mokdad, A. H., Ford, E. S., Bowman, B. A., Dietz, W. H., Vinicor, F., & Bales, V. S., et al. (2003). Prevalence of obesity, diabetes, and obesity-related health risk factors, 2001. *JAMA*, *289*(1), 76–79.

Montagne, A., Barnes, S. R., Sweeney, M. D., Halliday, M. R., Sagare, A. P., Zhao, Z., & Zlokovic, B. V. (2015). Blood–brain barrier breakdown in the aging human hippocampus. *Neuron*, *85*(2), 296–302. http://dx.doi.org/10.1016/j.neuron.2014.12.032.

Montine, T. J., Sonnen, J. A., Montine, K. S., Crane, P. K., & Larson, E. B. (2012). Adult Changes in Thought study: Dementia is an individually varying convergent syndrome with prevalent clinically silent diseases that may be modified by some commonly used therapeutics. *Current Alzheimer Research*, *9*(6), 718–723.

Moore, A. R., & O'Keeffe, S. T. (1999). Drug-induced cognitive impairment in the elderly. *Drugs & Aging*, *15*(1), 15–28.

Moran, C., Phan, T. G., Chen, J., Blizzard, L., Beare, R., Venn, A., & Srikanth, V. (2013). Brain atrophy in type 2 diabetes: Regional distribution and influence on cognition. *Diabetes Care*, *36*(12), 4036–4042. http://dx.doi.org/10.2337/dc13-0143.

Morbelli, S., & Nobili, F. (2014). Cognitive reserve and clinical expression of Alzheimer's disease: Evidence and implications for brain PET imaging. *American Journal of Nuclear Medicine and Molecular Imaging*, *4*(3), 239–247.

Moretti, L., Cristofori, I., Weaver, S. M., Chau, A., Portelli, J. N., & Grafman, J. (2012). Cognitive decline in older adults with a history of traumatic brain injury. *Lancet Neurology*, *11*(12), 1103–1112. http://dx.doi.org/10.1016/S1474-4422(12)70226-0.

Morgan, G. S., Gallacher, J., Bayer, A., Fish, M., Ebrahim, S., & Ben-Shlomo, Y. (2012). Physical activity in middle-age and dementia in later life: Findings from a prospective cohort of men in Caerphilly, South Wales and a meta-analysis. *Journal of Alzheimer's Disease*, *31*(3), 569–580. http://dx.doi.org/10.3233/JAD-2012-112171.

Morris, J. C. (2012). Revised criteria for mild cognitive impairment may compromise the diagnosis of Alzheimer disease dementia. *Archives of Neurology*, *69*(6), 700–708. http://dx.doi.org/10.1001/archneurol.2011.3152.

Morris, M. C. (2009). The role of nutrition in Alzheimer's disease: Epidemiological evidence. *European Journal of Neurology: The Official Journal of the European Federation of Neurological Societies*, *16*(Suppl. 1), 1–7. http://dx.doi.org/10.1111/j.1468-1331.2009.02735.x.

Morris, M. C., Beckett, L. A., Scherr, P. A., Hebert, L. E., Bennett, D. A., & Field, T. S., et al. (1998). Vitamin E and vitamin C supplement use and risk of incident Alzheimer disease. *Alzheimer Disease and Associated Disorders*, *12*(3), 121–126.

Morris, M. C., Evans, D. A., Bienias, J. L., Tangney, C. C., Bennett, D. A., Aggarwal, N., & Scherr, P. A. (2002). Dietary intake of antioxidant nutrients and the risk of incident Alzheimer disease in a biracial community study. *JAMA*, *287*(24), 3230–3237.

Morris, M. C., Evans, D. A., Bienias, J. L., Tangney, C. C., Bennett, D. A., Wilson, R. S., & Schneider, J. (2003). Consumption of fish and n-3 fatty acids and risk of incident Alzheimer disease. *Archives of Neurology*, *60*(7), 940–946. http://dx.doi.org/10.1001/archneur.60.7.940.

Morris, M. C., Evans, D. A., Tangney, C. C., Bienias, J. L., & Wilson, R. S. (2006). Associations of vegetable and fruit consumption with age-related cognitive change. *Neurology*, *67*(8), 1370–1376. http://dx.doi.org/10.1212/01.wnl.0000240224.38978.d8.

Morris, M. C., & Tangney, C. C. (2014). Dietary fat composition and dementia risk. *Neurobiology of Aging*, *35*(Suppl. 2), S59–64. http://dx.doi.org/10.1016/j.neurobiolaging.2014.03.038.

Morris, M. C., Tangney, C. C., Wang, Y., Sacks, F. M., Bennett, D. A., & Aggarwal, N. T. (2015). MIND diet associated with reduced incidence of Alzheimer's disease. *Alzheimer's & Dementia: The Journal of the Alzheimer's Association*. http://dx.doi.org/10.1016/j.jalz.2014.11.009.

Mortimer, J. A. (1988). *Do psychosocial risk factors contribute to Alzheimer's disease?* Chichester: John Wiley and Sons.

Mortimer, J. A. (1995). The continuum hypothesis of Alzheimer's disease and normal aging: The role of brain reserve. *Alzheimer Research*, *1995*(1), 67–70.

Mortimer, J. A. (2009). Important role of brain reserve in lowering the risk of Alzheimer's disease. *Future Neurology*, *4*, 1–4.

Mortimer, J. A. (2012). The Nun Study: Risk factors for pathology and clinical-pathologic correlations. *Current Alzheimer Research*, *9*(6), 621–627.

Mortimer, J. A., & Borenstein, A. R. (2014). Brain reserve is as important as Alzheimer's and vascular pathology in determining dementia status: The Nun Study. *Alzheimer's & Dementia*, *10*(4, Suppl.), P230–231.

Mortimer, J. A., Borenstein, A. R., Ding, D., Decarli, C., Zhao, Q., Copenhaver, C., & Hong, Z. (2010). High normal fasting blood glucose is associated with dementia in Chinese elderly. *Alzheimer's & Dementia: The Journal of the Alzheimer's Association*, *6*(6), 440–447. http://dx.doi.org/10.1016/j.jalz.2010.03.017.

Mortimer, J. A., Borenstein, A. R., Ding, D., Zhao, Q., Chus, S., & Gao, S., et al. (2013). Fish consumption and exercise in midlife are associated with decreased brain atrophy in women. *Alzheimer's and Dementia*, *9*, P632–633.

Mortimer, J. A., Borenstein, A. R., Gosche, K. M., & Snowdon, D. A. (2005). Very early detection of Alzheimer neuropathology and the role of brain reserve in modifying its clinical expression. *Journal of Geriatric Psychiatry and Neurology*, *18*(4), 218–223. http://dx.doi.org/10.1177/0891988705281869.

Mortimer, J. A., Ding, D., Borenstein, A. R., DeCarli, C., Guo, Q., Wu, Y., & Chu, S. (2012). Changes in brain volume and cognition in a randomized trial of exercise and social interaction in a community-based sample of non-demented Chinese elders. *Journal of Alzheimer's Disease*, *30*(4), 757–766. http://dx.doi.org/10.3233/JAD-2012-120079.

Mortimer, J. A., Fortier, I., Rajaram, L., & Gauvreau, D. (1998). Higher education and socio economic status in childhood protect individuals at genetic risk of AD from expressing symptoms in late life: The Saguenay-Lac-Saint-Jean Health and Aging Study. *Neurobiology of Aging*, *19*, S215.

Mortimer, J. A., French, L. R., Hutton, J. T., & Schuman, L. M. (1985). Head injury as a risk factor for Alzheimer's disease. *Neurology*, *35*(2), 264–267.

Mortimer, J. A., French, L. R., Hutton, J. T., & Schuman, L. M. (1983). Reported head trauma in an epidemiologic study of Alzheimer's disease. Abstract. *Neurology*, *33*(Suppl. 2), 85.

Mortimer, J. A., Gosche, K. M., Riley, K. P., Markesbery, W. R., & Snowdon, D. A. (2004). Delayed recall, hippocampal volume and Alzheimer neuropathology: Findings from the Nun Study. *Neurology*, *62*(3), 428–432.

Mortimer, J. A., & Graves, A. B. (1993). Education and other socioeconomic determinants of dementia and Alzheimer's disease. *Neurology*, *43*(Suppl. 4), S39–S44.

Mortimer, J. A., Schuman, L. M., & French, L. R. (1981). Epidemiology of dementing illness. In J. A. Mortimer & L. M. Schuman (Eds.), *The epidemiology of dementia* (pp. 3–23). New York: Oxford University Press.

Mortimer, J. A., Snowdon, D. A., & Markesbery, W. R. (2003). Head circumference, education and risk of dementia: Findings from the Nun Study. *Journal of Clinical and Experimental Neuropsychology*, *25*(5), 671–679. http://dx.doi.org/10.1076/jcen.25.5.671.14584.

Mortimer, J. A., Snowdon, D. A., & Markesbery, W. R. (2008). Small head circumference is associated with less education in persons at risk for Alzheimer disease in later life. *Alzheimer Disease and Associated Disorders*, *22*(3), 249–254. http://dx.doi.org/10.1097/WAD.0b013e318170d455.

Mortimer, J. A., Snowdon, D. A., & Markesbery, W. R. (2009). The effect of APOE-epsilon4 on dementia is mediated by Alzheimer neuropathology. *Alzheimer Disease and Associated Disorders*, *23*(2), 152–157.

Mortimer, J. A., van Duijn, C. M., Chandra, V., Fratiglioni, L., Graves, A. B., & Heyman, A., et al. (1991). Head trauma as a risk factor for Alzheimer's disease: A collaborative re-analysis of case-control studies. EURODEM Risk Factors Research Group. *International Journal of Epidemiology*, *20*(Suppl. 2), S28–35.

Mosconi, L., De Santi, S., Brys, M., Tsui, W. H., Pirraglia, E., Glodzik-Sobanska, L., & de Leon, M. J. (2008). Hypometabolism and altered cerebrospinal fluid markers in normal apolipoprotein E E4 carriers with subjective memory complaints. *Biological Psychiatry*, *63*(6), 609–618. http://dx.doi.org/10.1016/j.biopsych.2007.05.030.

Mucke, L., & Selkoe, D. J. (2012). Neurotoxicity of amyloid beta-protein: Synaptic and network dysfunction. *Cold Spring Harbor Perspectives Medicine*, *2*(7), a006338. http://dx.doi.org/10.1101/cshperspect.a006338.

Mukamal, K. J., Kuller, L. H., Fitzpatrick, A. L., Longstreth, W. T., Jr., Mittleman, M. A., & Siscovick, D. S. (2003). Prospective study of alcohol consumption and risk of dementia in older adults. *JAMA*, *289*(11), 1405–1413.

Mukamal, K. J., & Rimm, E. B. (2001). Alcohol's effects on the risk for coronary heart disease. *Alcohol Research & Health: The Journal of the National Institute on Alcohol Abuse and Alcoholism*, *25*(4), 255–261.

Muller, M., Sigurdsson, S., Kjartansson, O., Gunnarsdottir, I., Thorsdottir, I., & van Buchem, M., et al. (2014). Birth weight, mid-life hypertension, and late-life brain tissue loss: A life-course approach. *Alzheimer's & Dementia*, *10*(Suppl. 4), p294. <http://alzheimersanddementiajournal.net/article/S1552-5260%2814%2900616-5/abstract>.

Muller, M., Sigurdsson, S., Kjartansson, O., Jonsson, P. V., Garcia, M., von Bonsdorff, M. B., & Launer, L. J. (2014). Birth size and brain function 75 years later. *Pediatrics*, *134*(4), 761–770. http://dx.doi.org/10.1542/peds.2014-1108.

Munoz, D. G., Ganapathy, G. R., Eliasziw, M., & Hachinski, V. (2000). Educational attainment and socioeconomic status of patients with autopsy-confirmed Alzheimer disease. *Archives of Neurology*, *57*(1), 85–89.

Murer, M. G., Yan, Q., & Raisman-Vozari, R. (2001). Brain-derived neurotrophic factor in the control human brain, and in Alzheimer's disease and Parkinson's disease. *Progress in Neurobiology*, *63*(1), 71–124.

Murphy, C., Bacon, A. W., Bondi, M. W., & Salmon, D. P. (1998). Apolipoprotein E status is associated with odor identification deficits in nondemented older persons. *Annals of the New York Academy of Sciences*, *855*, 744–750.

Murphy, C., Gilmore, M. M., Seery, C. S., Salmon, D. P., & Lasker, B. R. (1990). Olfactory thresholds are associated with degree of dementia in Alzheimer's disease. *Neurobiology of Aging*, *11*(4), 465–469.

Murphy, S. L., Xu, J., & Kochanek, K. D. (2013). In *Deaths: Final data for 2010. National Vital Statistics Reports* (Vol. 61). Hyattsville, MD: National Center for Health Statistics.

Murphy, T., Dias, G. P., & Thuret, S. (2014). Effects of diet on brain plasticity in animal and human studies: Mind the gap. *Neural Plasticity*, *2014*, 563160. http://dx.doi.org/10.1155/2014/563160.

Murray, A. D., McNeil, C. J., Salarirad, S., Whalley, L. J., & Staff, R. T. (2014). Early life socio-economic circumstance and late life brain hyperintensities—A population based cohort study. *PLoS One*, *9*(2), e88969. http://dx.doi.org/10.1371/journal.pone.0088969.

Murray, M. D., Lane, K. A., Gao, S., Evans, R. M., Unverzagt, F. W., & Hall, K. S., et al. (2002). Preservation of cognitive function with antihypertensive medications: A longitudinal analysis of a community-based sample of African Americans. *Archives of Internal Medicine*, *162*(18), 2090–2096.

Murrell, J. R., Price, B., Lane, K. A., Baiyewu, O., Gureje, O., Ogunniyi, A., & Hall, K. S. (2006). Association of apolipoprotein E genotype and Alzheimer disease in African Americans. *Archives of Neurology*, *63*(3), 431–434. http://dx.doi.org/10.1001/archneur.63.3.431.

Nagahara, A. H., Merrill, D. A., Coppola, G., Tsukada, S., Schroeder, B. E., Shaked, G. M., & Tuszynski, M. H. (2009). Neuroprotective effects of brain-derived neurotrophic factor in rodent and primate models of Alzheimer's disease. *Nature Medicine*, *15*(3), 331–337. http://dx.doi.org/10.1038/nm.1912.

Nagai, M., Hoshide, S., & Kario, K. (2010). Hypertension and dementia. *American Journal of Hypertension: Journal of the American Society of Hypertension*, *23*(2), 116–124. http://dx.doi.org/10.1038/ajh.2009.212.

Nagamatsu, L. S., Flicker, L., Kramer, A. F., Voss, M. W., Erickson, K. I., & Hsu, C. L., et al. (2014). Exercise is medicine, for the body and the brain. *British Journal of Sports Medicine*, *48*(12), 943–944. http://dx.doi.org/10.1136/bjsports-2013-093224.

Naik, M., & Nygaard, H. A. (2008). Diagnosing dementia—ICD-10 not so bad after all: A comparison between dementia criteria according to DSM-IV and ICD-10. *International Journal of Geriatric Psychiatry*, *23*(3), 279–282.

Naj, A. C., Jun, G., Beecham, G. W., Wang, L. S., Vardarajan, B. N., Buros, J., & Schellenberg, G. D. (2011). Common variants at MS4A4/MS4A6E, CD2AP, CD33 and EPHA1 are associated with late-onset alzheimer's disease. *Nature Genetics*, *43*(5), 436–441. http://dx.doi.org/10.1038/ng.801.

Neeper, S. A., Gomez-Pinilla, F., Choi, J., & Cotman, C. (1995). Exercise and brain neurotrophins. *Nature*, *373*(6510), 109. http://dx.doi.org/10.1038/373109a0.

Nehlig, A., Daval, J. L., & Debry, G. (1992). Caffeine and the central nervous system: Mechanisms of action, biochemical, metabolic and psychostimulant effects. *Brain Research Brain Research Reviews*, *17*(2), 139–170.

Nelson, C. A., III, Zeanah, C. H., Fox, N. A., Marshall, P. J., Smyke, A. T., & Guthrie, D. (2007). Cognitive recovery in socially deprived young children: The Bucharest Early Intervention Project. *Science*, *318*(5858), 1937–1940. http://dx.doi.org/10.1126/science.1143921.

Nelson, H. D., Walker, M., Zakher, B., & Mitchell, J. (2012). Menopausal hormone therapy for the primary prevention of chronic conditions: Systematic review to udate the 2002 and 2005 U.S. preventive services task force recommendations. In *Evidence synthesis, No. 93*. Rockville, MD: Agency fo Healthcare Research and Quality. Report No. A. P. N. 12-05168-EF-1.

Nelson, L. M., Longstreth, W. T., Jr, Koepsell, T. D., & van Belle, G. (1990). Proxy respondents in epidemiologic research. *Epidemiologic Reviews*, *12*, 71–86.

Nelson, P. T., Smith, C. D., Abner, E. A., Schmitt, F. A., Scheff, S. W., Davis, G. J., & Markesbery, W. R. (2009). Human cerebral neuropathology of Type 2 diabetes mellitus. *Biochimica et Biophysica Acta*, *1792*(5), 454–469. http://dx.doi.org/10.1016/j.bbadis.2008.08.005.

Nemetz, P. N., Leibson, C., Naessens, J. M., Beard, M., Kokmen, E., & Annegers, J. F., et al. (1999). Traumatic brain injury and time to onset of Alzheimer's disease: A population-based study. *American Journal of Epidemiology*, *149*(1), 32–40.

Neuropathology Group of the Medical Research Council Cognitive Function and Aging Study (MRC-CFAS), (2001). Pathologic correlates of late onset dementia in a multicentre, community based population in England and Wales. *Lancet*, *357*, 169–175.

Ng, T. P., Chiam, P. C., Lee, T., Chua, H. C., Lim, L., & Kua, E. H. (2006). Curry consumption and cognitive function in the elderly. *American Journal of Epidemiology*, *164*(9), 898–906. http://dx.doi.org/10.1093/aje/kwj267.

Ngandu, T., Lehtisalo, J., Solomon, A., Levalahti, E., Ahtiluoto, S., Antikainen, R., & Kivipelto, M. (2015). A 2 year multidomain intervention of diet, exercise, cognitive training, and vascular risk monitoring versus control to prevent cognitive decline in at-risk elderly people (FINGER): A randomised controlled trial. *Lancet*. http://dx.doi.org/10.1016/S0140-6736(15)60461-5.

Nicoll, J. A., Roberts, G. W., & Graham, D. I. (1995). Apolipoprotein E epsilon 4 allele is associated with deposition of amyloid beta-protein following head injury. *Nature Medicine*, *1*(2), 135–137.

Nissen, S. E. (2006). ADAPT: The wrong way to stop a clinical trial. *PLoS Clinical Trials*, *1*(7), e35. http://dx.doi.org/10.1371/journal.pctr.0010035.

Noble, K. G., Houston, S. M., Brito, N. H., Bartsch, H., Kan, E., Kuperman, J. M., & Sowell, E. R. (2015). Family income, parental education and brain structure in children and adolescents. *Nature Neuroscience*. http://dx.doi.org/10.1038/nn.3983.

Nofuji, Y., Suwa, M., Moriyama, Y., Nakano, H., Ichimiya, A., Nishichi, R., & Kumagai, S. (2008). Decreased serum brain-derived neurotrophic factor in trained men. *Neuroscience Letters*, *437*(1), 29–32. http://dx.doi.org/10.1016/j.neulet.2008.03.057.

Nordstrom, P., Michaelsson, K., Gustafson, Y., & Nordstrom, A. (2014). Traumatic brain injury and young onset dementia: A nationwide cohort study. *Annals of Neurology*, *75*(3), 374–381.

Norton, S., Matthews, F. E., Barnes, D. E., Yaffe, K., & Brayne, C. (2014). Potential for primary prevention of Alzheimer's disease: An analysis of population-based data. *Lancet Neurology*, *13*(8), 788–794. http://dx.doi.org/10.1016/S1474-4422(14)70136-X.

Notkola, I. L., Sulkava, R., Pekkanen, J., Erkinjuntti, T., Ehnholm, C., Kivinen, P., & Nissinen, A. (1998). Serum total cholesterol, apolipoprotein E epsilon 4 allele, and Alzheimer's disease. *Neuroepidemiology*, *17*(1), 14–20.

Nurk, E., Refsum, H., Drevon, C. A., Tell, G. S., Nygaard, H. A., & Engedal, K., et al. (2009). Intake of flavonoid-rich wine, tea, and chocolate by elderly men and women is associated with better cognitive test performance. *The Journal of Nutrition*, *139*(1), 120–127. http://dx.doi.org/10.3945/jn.108.095182.

Nurminen, M. L., Niittynen, L., Korpela, R., & Vapaatalo, H. (1999). Coffee, caffeine and blood pressure: A critical review. *European Journal of Clinical Nutrition*, *53*(11), 831–839.

O'Brien, J. T., Erkinjuntti, T., Reisberg, B., Roman, G., Sawada, T., Pantoni, L., & DeKosky, S. T. (2003). Vascular cognitive impairment. *Lancet Neurology*, *2*(2), 89–98.

O'Brien, R. J., Resnick, S. M., Zonderman, A. B., Ferrucci, L., Crain, B. J., Pletnikova, O., & Troncoso, J. C. (2009). Neuropathologic studies of the Baltimore Longitudinal Study of Aging (BLSA). *Journal of Alzheimer's Disease*, *18*(3), 665–675. http://dx.doi.org/10.3233/JAD-2009-1179.

O'Dwyer, S. T., Burton, N. W., Pachana, N. A., & Brown, W. J. (2007). Protocol for fit bodies, fine minds: A randomized controlled trial on the affect of exercise and cognitive training on cognitive functioning in older adults. *BMC Geriatrics*, *7*, 23. http://dx.doi.org/10.1186/1471-2318-7-23.

Office of Communications. (2003). *Agriculture fact book 2001–2002*. Washington, DC: United States Department of Agriculture.

Ogden, C. L., Carroll, M. D., Curtin, L. R., McDowell, M. A., Tabak, C. J., & Flegal, K. M. (2006). Prevalence of overweight and obesity in the United States, 1999–2004. *JAMA*, *295*(13), 1549–1555. http://dx.doi.org/10.1001/jama.295.13.1549.

Oinas, M., Polvikoski, T., Sulkava, R., Myllykangas, L., Juva, K., & Notkola, I. L., et al. (2009). Neuropathologic findings of dementia with lewy bodies (DLB) in a population-based Vantaa 85+ study. *Journal of Alzheimers Disease*, *18*(3), 677–689.

Okamura, N., Furumoto, S., Fodero-Tavoletti, M. T., Mulligan, R. S., Harada, R., Yates, P., & Villemagne, V. L. (2014). Non-invasive assessment of Alzheimer's disease neurofibrillary pathology using 18F-THK5105 PET. *Brain*, *137*(Pt 6), 1762–1771. http://dx.doi.org/10.1093/brain/awu064.

Oksman, M., Iivonen, H., Hogyes, E., Amtul, Z., Penke, B., Leenders, I., & Tanila, H. (2006). Impact of different saturated fatty acid, polyunsaturated fatty acid and cholesterol containing diets on beta-amyloid accumulation in APP/PS1 transgenic mice. *Neurobiology of Disease*, *23*(3), 563–572. http://dx.doi.org/10.1016/j.nbd.2006.04.013.

Oleckno, W. A. (2008). *Epidemiology: Concepts and methods*. Long Grove, IL: Waveland Press, Inc.

Omalu, B. (2014). Chronic traumatic encephalopathy. *Progress in Neurological Surgery*, *28*, 38–49. http://dx.doi.org/10.1159/000358761.

Omalu, B. I., DeKosky, S. T., Minster, R. L., Kamboh, M. I., Hamilton, R. L., & Wecht, C. H. (2005). Chronic traumatic encephalopathy in a National Football League player. *Neurosurgery*, *57*(1), 128–134. discussion 128-134.

O'Meara, E. S., Kukull, W. A., Sheppard, L., Bowen, J. D., McCormick, W. C., Teri, L., & Larson, E. B. (1997). Head injury and risk of Alzheimer's disease by apolipoprotein E genotype. *American Journal of Epidemiology*, *146*(5), 373–384.

Omran, A. R. (2005). The epidemiologic transition: A theory of the epidemiology of population change. *Milbank Quarterly*, *83*(4), 731–757.

Ordonez, L. A. (1979). Biochemical functions of folate in the central nervous system. In M. I. Botez & E. H. Reynolds (Eds.), *Folic acid in neurology, psychiatry, and internal medicine* (pp. 129–145). New York: Raven Press.

Orgogozo, J. M., Dartigues, J. F., Lafont, S., Letenneur, L., Commenges, D., Salamon, R., & Breteler, M. B. (1997). Wine consumption and dementia in the elderly: A prospective community study in the Bordeaux area. *Revue Neurologique*, *153*(3), 185–192.

Osuntokun, B. O., Hendrie, H. C., Ogunniyi, A. O., Hall, K. S., Lekwauwa, U. G., Brittain, H. M., & Rodgers, D. D. (1992). Cross-cultural studies in Alzheimer's disease. *Ethnicity & Disease*, *2*(4), 352–357.

Osuntokun, B. O., Sahota, A., Ogunniyi, A. O., Gureje, O., Baiyewu, O., & Adeyinka, A., et al. (1995). Lack of an association between apolipoprotein E epsilon 4 and Alzheimer's disease in elderly Nigerians. *Annals of Neurology*, *38*(3), 463–465. http://dx.doi.org/10.1002/ana.410380319.

Ott, A., Slooter, A. J., Hofman, A., van Harskamp, F., Witteman, J. C., Van Broeckhoven, C., & Breteler, M. M. (1998). Smoking and risk of dementia and Alzheimer's disease in a population-based cohort study: The Rotterdam Study. *Lancet*, *351*(9119), 1840–1843.

Ott, A., Stolk, R. P., Hofman, A., van Harskamp, F., Grobbee, D. E., & Breteler, M. M. (1996). Association of diabetes mellitus and dementia: The Rotterdam Study. *Diabetologia*, *39*(11), 1392–1397.

Ownby, R. L., Crocco, E., Acevedo, A., John, V., & Loewenstein, D. (2006). Depression and risk for Alzheimer disease: Systematic review, meta-analysis, and metaregression analysis. *Archives of General Psychiatry*, *63*(5), 530–538. http://dx.doi.org/10.1001/archpsyc.63.5.530.

Paganini-Hill, A., & Perez Barreto, M. (2001). Stroke risk in older men and women: Aspirin, estrogen, exercise, vitamins, and other factors. *The Journal of Gender-Specific Medicine: The Official Journal of the Partnership for Women's Health at Columbia*, *4*(2), 18–28.

Pajonk, F. G., Wobrock, T., Gruber, O., Scherk, H., Berner, D., Kaizl, I., & Falkai, P. (2010). Hippocampal plasticity in response to exercise in schizophrenia. *Archives of General Psychiatry*, *67*(2), 133–143. http://dx.doi.org/10.1001/archgenpsychiatry.2009.193.

Palmer, K., Backman, L., Winblad, B., & Fratiglioni, L. (2003). Detection of Alzheimer's disease and dementia in the preclinical phase: Population based cohort study. *BMJ*, *326*(7383), 245.

Palmer, K., Berger, A. K., Monastero, R., Winblad, B., Backman, L., & Fratiglioni, L. (2007). Predictors of progression from mild cognitive impairment to Alzheimer disease. *Neurology*, *68*(19), 1596–1602. http://dx.doi.org/10.1212/01.wnl.0000260968.92345.3f.

Pan, W., Banks, W. A., Fasold, M. B., Bluth, J., & Kastin, A. J. (1998). Transport of brain-derived neurotrophic factor across the blood–brain barrier. *Neuropharmacology*, *37*(12), 1553–1561.

Panay, N., Hamoda, H., Arya, R., Savvas, M., & British Menopause Society & Women's Health Concern, (2013). The 2013 British Menopause Society & Women's Health Concern recommendations on hormone replacement therapy. *Menopause International*, *19*(2), 59–68. http://dx.doi.org/10.1177/1754045313489645.

Paneth, N., & Susser, M. (1995). Early origin of coronary heart disease (the "Barker hypothesis"). *BMJ*, *310*(6977), 411–412.

Pankratz, V. S., Roberts, R. O., Mielke, M. M., Knopman, D. S., Jack, C. R., Jr., Geda, Y. E., & Petersen, R. C. (2015). Predicting the risk of mild cognitive impairment in the Mayo clinic study of aging. *Neurology*, *84*(14), 1433–1442. http://dx.doi.org/10.1212/WNL.0000000000001437.

Papp, K. V., Walsh, S. J., & Snyder, P. J. (2009). Immediate and delayed effects of cognitive interventions in healthy elderly: A review of current literature and future directions. *Alzheimer's & Dementia: The Journal of the Alzheimer's Association*, *5*(1), 50–60. http://dx.doi.org/10.1016/j.jalz.2008.10.008.

Passel, J., Cohn, D. (2008). *U.S. Population Projections 2005–2050. Census Bureau 2011 population estimates*, February.

Patel, A., Rees, S. D., Kelly, M. A., Bain, S. C., Barnett, A. H., & Thalitaya, D., et al. (2011). Association of variants within APOE, SORL1, RUNX1, BACE1 and ALDH18A1 with dementia in Alzheimer's disease in subjects with Down syndrome. *Neuroscience Letters*, *487*(2), 144–148. http://dx.doi.org/10.1016/j.neulet.2010.10.010.

Patel, N. V., Gordon, M. N., Connor, K. E., Good, R. A., Engelman, R. W., Mason, J., & Finch, C. E. (2005). Caloric restriction attenuates Abeta-deposition in Alzheimer transgenic models. *Neurobiology of Aging*, *26*(7), 995–1000. http://dx.doi.org/10.1016/j.neurobiolaging.2004.09.014.

Paternoster, L., Chen, W., & Sudlow, C. L. (2009). Genetic determinants of white matter hyperintensities on brain scans: A systematic assessment of 19 candidate gene polymorphisms in 46 studies in 19,000 subjects. *Stroke*, *40*(6), 2020–2026. http://dx.doi.org/10.1161/STROKEAHA.108.542050.

Pavlik, V. N., Doody, R. S., Massman, P. J., & Chan, W. (2006). Influence of premorbid IQ and education on progression of Alzheimer's disease. *Dementia and Geriatric Cognitive Disorders*, *22*(4), 367–377. http://dx.doi.org/10.1159/000095640.

Payami, H., Montee, K. R., Kaye, J. A., Bird, T. D., Yu, C. E., & Wijsman, E. M., et al. (1994). Alzheimer's disease, apolipoprotein E4, and gender. *JAMA*, *271*(17), 1316–1317.

Paz, I., Seidman, D. S., Danon, Y. L., Laor, A., Stevenson, D. K., & Gale, R. (1993). Are children born small for gestational age at increased risk of short stature? *American Journal of Diseases of Children (1960)*, *147*(3), 337–339.

Peila, R., Rodriguez, B. L., & Launer, L. J. (2002). Type 2 diabetes, APOE gene, and the risk for dementia and related pathologies: The Honolulu-Asia Aging Study. *Diabetes*, *51*(4), 1256–1262.

Pendlebury, S. T., Mariz, J., Bull, L., Mehta, Z., & Rothwell, P. M. (2013). Impact of different operational definitions on mild cognitive impairment rate and MMSE and MoCA performance in transient ischaemic attack and stroke. *Cerebrovascular Diseases (Basel, Switzerland)*, *36*(5–6), 355–362. http://dx.doi.org/10.1159/000355496.

Peres, K., Helmer, C., Amieva, H., Matharan, F., Carcaillon, L., Jacqmin-Gadda, H., & Dartigues, J. F. (2011). Gender differences in the prodromal signs of dementia: Memory complaint and IADL-restriction. A prospective population-based cohort. *Journal of Alzheimer's Disease*, *27*(1), 39–47. http://dx.doi.org/10.3233/JAD-2011-110428.

Perneczky, R., Drzezga, A., Diehl-Schmid, J., Schmid, G., Wohlschlager, A., Kars, S., & Kurz, A. (2006). Schooling mediates brain reserve in Alzheimer's disease: Findings of fluoro-deoxy-glucose-positron emission tomography. *Journal of Neurology, Neurosurgery, and Psychiatry*, *77*(9), 1060–1063. http://dx.doi.org/10.1136/jnnp.2006.094714.

Perneczky, R., Wagenpfeil, S., Lunetta, K. L., Cupples, L. A., Green, R. C., Decarli, C., & Kurz, A. (2010). Head circumference, atrophy, and cognition: Implications for brain reserve in Alzheimer disease. *Neurology*, *75*(2), 137–142. http://dx.doi.org/10.1212/WNL.0b013e3181e7ca97.

Perry, E. K., Perry, R. H., Smith, C. J., Dick, D. J., Candy, J. M., Edwardson, J. A., & Blessed, G. (1987). Nicotinic receptor abnormalities in Alzheimer's and Parkinson's diseases. *Journal of Neurology, Neurosurgery, and Psychiatry*, *50*(6), 806–809.

Perusini, G. (1909). Regarding clinical and peculiar histological psychiatric disorders in very old age. In: F. Nissl & A. Alzheimer (Eds.), *Histologische und Histopathologische Arbeiten* (pp. 297–351). Jena: Verlag G. Fischer.

Peters, R., Beckett, N., Forette, F., Tuomilehto, J., Clarke, R., Ritchie, C., & Bulpitt, C. (2008). Incident dementia and blood pressure lowering in the Hypertension in the Very Elderly Trial cognitive function assessment (HYVET-COG): A double-blind, placebo controlled trial. *Lancet Neurology*, *7*(8), 683–689. http://dx.doi.org/10.1016/S1474-4422(08)70143-1.

Peters, R., Peters, J., Warner, J., Beckett, N., & Bulpitt, C. (2008). Alcohol, dementia and cognitive decline in the elderly: A systematic review. *Age and Ageing*, *37*(5), 505–512. http://dx.doi.org/10.1093/ageing/afn095.

Peters, R., Poulter, R., Warner, J., Beckett, N., Burch, L., & Bulpitt, C. (2008). Smoking, dementia and cognitive decline in the elderly, a systematic review. *BMC Geriatrics*, *8*, 36. http://dx.doi.org/10.1186/1471-2318-8-36.

Petersen, R. B., Nunomura, A., Lee, H. G., Casadesus, G., Perry, G., & Smith, M. A., et al. (2007). Signal transduction cascades associated with oxidative stress in Alzheimer's disease. *Journal of Alzheimer's Disease*, *11*(2), 143–152.

Petersen, R. C. (2004). Mild cognitive impairment as a diagnostic entity. *Journal of Internal Medicine*, *256*(3), 183–194.

Petersen, R. C. (2009). Early diagnosis of Alzheimer's disease: Is MCI too late? *Current Alzheimer Research*, *6*(4), 324–330.

Petersen, R. C. (2010). Does the source of subjects matter?: Absolutely!. *Neurology*, *74*(22), 1754–1755. http://dx.doi.org/10.1212/WNL.0b013e3181e533e7.

Petersen, R. C., Doody, R., Kurz, A., Moh, R. C., Morris, J. C., & Rabins, P. V., et al. (2001). Current concepts in mild cognitive impairment. *Archives of Neurology*, *58*, 1985–1992.

Petersen, R. C., Roberts, R. O., Knopman, D. S., Boeve, B. F., Geda, Y. E., Ivnik, R. J., & Jack, C. R., Jr. (2009). Mild cognitive impairment: Ten years later. *Archives of Neurology*, *66*(12), 1447–1455. http://dx.doi.org/10.1001/archneurol.2009.266.

Petersen, R. C., Smith, G. E., Ivnik, R. J., Tangalos, E. G., Schaid, D. J., Thibodeau, S. N., & Kurland, L. T. (1995). Apolipoprotein E status as a predictor of the development of Alzheimer's disease in memory-impaired individuals. *JAMA*, *273*(16), 1274–1278.

Petersen, R. C., Smith, G. E., Waring, S. C., Ivnik, R. J., Tangalos, E. G., & Kokmen, E. (1999). Mild cognitive impairment: Clinical characterization and outcome. *Archives of Neurology*, *56*, 303–308.

Petersen, R. C., Thomas, R. G., Grundman, M., Bennett, D., Doody, R., Ferris, S., & Thal, L. J. (2005). Vitamin E and donepezil for the treatment of mild cognitive impairment. *The New England Journal of Medicine*, *352*(23), 2379–2388. http://dx.doi.org/10.1056/NEJMoa050151.

Petrovitch, H., White, L. R., Izmirilian, G., Ross, G. W., Havlik, R. J., Markesbery, W., & Launer, L. J. (2000). Midlife blood pressure and neuritic plaques, neurofibrillary tangles, and brain weight at death: The HAAS. Honolulu-Asia aging Study. *Neurobiology of Aging*, *21*(1), 57–62.

Pfeiffer, E. (1975). A short, portable mental status questionnaire for the assessment of organic brain deficit in elderly patients. *Journal of the American Geriatrics Society*, *23*, 433–441.

Pike, C. J., Carroll, J. C., Rosario, E. R., & Barron, A. M. (2009). Protective actions of sex steroid hormones in Alzheimer's disease. *Frontiers in Neuroendocrinology*, *30*(2), 239–258. http://dx.doi.org/10.1016/j.yfrne.2009.04.015.

Pillai, J. A., Hall, C. B., Dickson, D. W., Buschke, H., Lipton, R. B., & Verghese, J. (2011). Association of crossword puzzle participation with memory decline in persons who develop dementia. *Journal of the International Neuropsychological Society*, *17*(6), 1006–1013. http://dx.doi.org/10.1017/S1355617711001111.

Pines, A. (2011). Mid-life smoking and cognition. *Climacteric*, *14*(4), 426–427. http://dx.doi.org/10.3109/13697137.2011.557598.

Plassman, B. L., Havlik, R. J., Steffens, D. C., Helms, M. J., Newman, T. N., Drosdick, D., & Breitner, J. C. (2000). Documented head injury in early adulthood and risk of Alzheimer's disease and other dementias. *Neurology*, *55*(8), 1158–1166.

Plassman, B. L., Langa, K. M., Fisher, G. G., Heeringa, S. G., Weir, D. R., Ofstedal, M. B., & Wallace, R. B. (2007). Prevalence of dementia in the United States: The aging, demographics, and memory study. *Neuroepidemiology*, *29*(1–2), 125–132. http://dx.doi.org/10.1159/000109998.

Podewils, L. J., Guallar, E., Kuller, L. H., Fried, L. P., Lopez, O. L., & Carlson, M., et al. (2005). Physical activity, APOE genotype, and dementia risk: Findings from the Cardiovascular Health Cognition Study. *American Journal of Epidemiology*, *161*(7), 639–651. http://dx.doi.org/10.1093/aje/kwi092.

Polvikoski, T., Sulkava, R., Haltia, M., Kainulainen, K., Vuorio, A., Verkkoniemi, A., & Kontula, K. (1995). Apolipoprotein E, dementia, and cortical deposition of beta-amyloid protein. *The New England Journal of Medicine*, *333*(19), 1242–1247. http://dx.doi.org/10.1056/NEJM199511093331902.

Pomara, N., Willoughby, L. M., Wesnes, K., & Sidtis, J. J. (2004). Increased anticholinergic challenge-induced memory impairment associated with the APOE-epsilon4 allele in the elderly: A controlled pilot study. *Neuropsychopharmacology*, *29*(2), 403–409. http://dx.doi.org/10.1038/sj.npp.1300305.

Population Division Department of Economic and Social Affairs. (2002). *World population ageing: 1950–2050.* <http://www.un.org/esa/population/publications/worldageing19502050/> Accessed 06.11.13.

Posner, H. B., Tang, M. X., Luchsinger, J., Lantigua, R., Stern, Y., & Mayeux, R. (2002). The relationship of hypertension in the elderly to AD, vascular dementia, and cognitive function. *Neurology*, *58*(8), 1175–1181.

Pottala, J. V., Yaffe, K., Robinson, J. G., Espeland, M. A., Wallace, R., & Harris, W. S. (2014). Higher RBC EPA + DHA corresponds with larger total brain and hippocampal volumes: WHIMS-MRI study. *Neurology*, *82*(5), 435–442. http://dx.doi.org/10.1212/WNL.0000000000000080.

Poulton, N. P., & Muir, G. D. (2005). Treadmill training ameliorates dopamine loss but not behavioral deficits in hemi-parkinsonian rats. *Experimental Neurology*, *193*(1), 181–197. http://dx.doi.org/10.1016/j.expneurol.2004.12.006.

Power, M. C., Deal, J., Jack, C. R., Knopman, D. S., Sharrett, A. R., & Mosley, T., et al. (2014). Smoking and white matter hyperintensity grade progression in the Atherosclerosis Risk in Communities (ARIC) Study. *Alzheimer's & Dementia (Abstract)*, *10*(4), 750.

Power, M. C., Weuve, J., Gagne, J. J., McQueen, M. B., Viswanathan, A., & Blacker, D. (2011). The association between blood pressure and incident Alzheimer disease: A systematic review and meta-analysis. *Epidemiology*, *22*(5), 646–659. http://dx.doi.org/10.1097/EDE.0b013e31822708b5.

Prasher, V. P., Farrer, M. J., Kessling, A. M., Fisher, E. M., West, R. J., & Barber, P. C., et al. (1998). Molecular mapping of Alzheimer-type dementia in Down's syndrome. *Annals of Neurology*, *43*(3), 380–383. http://dx.doi.org/10.1002/ana.410430316.

Prentice, R. L., Manson, J. E., Langer, R. D., Anderson, G. L., Pettinger, M., Jackson, R. D., & Rossouw, J. E. (2009). Benefits and risks of postmenopausal hormone therapy when it is initiated soon after menopause. *American Journal of Epidemiology*, *170*(1), 12–23. http://dx.doi.org/10.1093/aje/kwp115.

Prentice, R. L., Sugar, E., Wang, C. Y., Neuhouser, M., & Patterson, R. (2002). Research strategies and the use of nutrient biomarkers in studies of diet and chronic disease. *Public Health Nutrition*, *5*(6A), 977–984. http://dx.doi.org/10.1079/PHN2002382.

Prince, M., Acosta, D., Chiu, H., Scazufca, M., & Varghese, M. (2003). Dementia diagnosis in developing countries: A cross-cultural validation study. *Lancet*, *361*(9361), 909–917. doi:10.1016/S0140-6736(03)12772-9.

Prince, M., Acosta, D., Dangour, A. D., Uauy, R., Guerra, M., Huang, Y., & Rodriguez, G. (2011). Leg length, skull circumference, and the prevalence of dementia in low and middle income countries: A 10/66 population-based cross sectional survey. *International Psychogeriatrics/IPA*, *23*(2), 202–213. http://dx.doi.org/10.1017/S1041610210001274.

Prince, M., Acosta, D., Ferri, C. P., Guerra, M., Huang, Y., Llibre Rodriguez, J. J., & Liu, Z. (2012). Dementia incidence and mortality in middle-income countries, and associations with indicators of cognitive reserve: A 10/66 Dementia Research Group population-based cohort study. *Lancet*, *380*(9836), 50–58. http://dx.doi.org/10.1016/S0140-6736(12)60399-7.

Prince, M., Bryce, R., Albanese, E., Wimo, A., Ribeiro, W., & Ferri, C. P. (2013). The global prevalence of dementia: A systematic review and metaanalysis. *Alzheimer's & Dementia: The Journal of the Alzheimer's Association*, *9*(1), 63–75.e62. http://dx.doi.org/10.1016/j.jalz.2012.11.007.

Prince, M., Prina, M., & Guerchet, M. (2013). *World Alzheimer Report 2013: Journey of caring: An analysis of long-term care for dementia*. London: Alzheimer's Disease International.

Proitsi, P., Lupton, M. K., & Velayudhan, L., et al. (2014). Alleles that increase risk for type 2 diabetes mellitus are not associated with increased risk for Alzheimer's disease. *Neurobiology of Aging*, *35*, 2883.e3–2883.e10.

Qiu, C. (2011). Epidemiological findings of vascular risk factors in Alzheimer's disease: Implications for therapeutic and preventive intervention. *Expert Review of Neurotherapeutics*, *11*(11), 1593–1607. http://dx.doi.org/10.1586/ern.11.146.

Qiu, C., Cotch, M. F., Sigurdsson, S., Jonsson, P. V., Jonsdottir, M. K., Sveinbjrnsdottir, S., & Launer, L. J. (2010). Cerebral microbleeds, retinopathy, and dementia: The AGES-Reykjavik Study. *Neurology*, *75*(24), 2221–2228. http://dx.doi.org/10.1212/WNL.0b013e3182020349.

Qiu, C., Winblad, B., & Fratiglioni, L. (2005). The age-dependent relation of blood pressure to cognitive function and dementia. *Lancet Neurology*, *4*(8), 487–499. http://dx.doi.org/10.1016/S1474-4422(05)70141-1.

Qizilbash, N., Gregson, J., Johnson, M. E., Pearce, N., Douglas, I., Wing, K., & Pocock, S. J. (2015). BMI and risk of dementia in two million people over two decades: A retrospective cohort study. *The Lancet Diabetes & Endocrinology*. http://dx.doi.org/10.1016/S2213-8587(15)00033-9.

Raffaitin, C., Gin, H., Empana, J. P., Helmer, C., Berr, C., Tzourio, C., & Barberger-Gateau, P. (2009). Metabolic syndrome and risk for incident Alzheimer's disease or vascular dementia: The Three-City Study. *Diabetes Care*, *32*(1), 169–174. http://dx.doi.org/10.2337/dc08-0272.

Raiford, K., Anton-Johnson, S., & Haycox, Z., et al. (1994). CERAD part VII: Accuracy of reporting dementia on death certificates of patients with Alzheimer's disease. *Neurology*, *44*, 2208–2209.

Raji, C. A., Erickson, K. I., Lopez, O. L., Kuller, L. H., Gach, H. M., Thompson, P. M., & Becker, J. T. (2014). Regular fish consumption and age-related brain gray matter loss. *American Journal of Preventive Medicine*, *47*(4), 444–451. http://dx.doi.org/10.1016/j.amepre.2014.05.037.

Ramlackhansingh, A. F., Brooks, D. J., Greenwood, R. J., Bose, S. K., Turkheimer, F. E., Kinnunen, K. M., & Sharp, D. J. (2011). Inflammation after trauma: Microglial activation and traumatic brain injury. *Annals of Neurology*, *70*(3), 374–383. http://dx.doi.org/10.1002/ana.22455.

Rapp, S. R., Espeland, M. A., Shumaker, S. A., Henderson, V. W., Brunner, R. L., Manson, J. E., & Investigators, W. (2003). Effect of estrogen plus progestin on global cognitive function in post-menopausal women: The Women's Health Initiative Memory Study: A randomized controlled trial. *JAMA*, *289*(20), 2663–2672. http://dx.doi.org/10.1001/jama.289.20.2663.

Rasmussen, P., Brassard, P., Adser, H., Pedersen, M. V., Leick, L., Hart, E., & Pilegaard, H. (2009). Evidence for a release of brain-derived neurotrophic factor from the brain during exercise. *Experimental Physiology*, *94*(10), 1062–1069. http://dx.doi.org/10.1113/expphysiol.2009.048512.

Ravaglia, G., Forti, P., Lucicesare, A., Pisacane, N., Rietti, E., & Bianchin, M., et al. (2008). Physical activity and dementia risk in the elderly: Findings from a prospective Italian study. *Neurology*, *70*(19 Pt 2), 1786–1794. http://dx.doi.org/10.1212/01.wnl.0000296276.50595.86.

Ravaglia, G., Forti, P., Maioli, F., Martelli, M., Servadei, L., Brunetti, N., & Licastro, F. (2005). Homocysteine and folate as risk factors for dementia and Alzheimer disease. *The American Journal of Clinical Nutrition*, *82*(3), 636–643.

Rebok, G. W., Ball, K., Guey, L. T., Jones, R. N., Kim, H. Y., King, J. W., & ACTIVE Study Group, (2014). Ten-year effects of the advanced cognitive training for independent and vital elderly cognitive training trial on cognition and everyday functioning in older adults. *Journal of the American Geriatrics Society*, *62*(1), 16–24. http://dx.doi.org/10.1111/jgs.12607.

Reed, C. E., & Fenton, S. E. (2013). Exposure to diethylstilbesterol during sensitive life stages: A legacy of heritable health effects. *Birth Defects Research Part C, Embryo Today: Reviews*, *99*(2) http://dx.doi.org/10.1002/bdrc.21035.

Reger, M. A., Watson, G. S., Frey, W. H., II, Baker, L. D., Cholerton, B., Keeling, M. L., & Craft, S. (2006). Effects of intranasal insulin on cognition in memory-impaired older adults: Modulation by APOE genotype. *Neurobiology of Aging*, *27*(3), 451–458. http://dx.doi.org/10.1016/j.neurobiolaging.2005.03.016.

Reijnders, J., van Heugten, C., & van Boxtel, M. (2013). Cognitive interventions in healthy older adults and people with mild cognitive impairment: A systematic review. *Ageing Research Reviews*, *12*(1), 263–275. http://dx.doi.org/10.1016/j.arr.2012.07.003.

Reiman, E. M., Chen, K., Alexander, G. E., Caselli, R. J., Bandy, D., Osborne, D., & Hardy, J. (2004). Functional brain abnormalities in young adults at genetic risk for late-onset alzheimer's dementia. *Proceedings of the National Academy of Sciences of the United States of America*, *101*(1), 284–289. http://dx.doi.org/10.1073/pnas.2635903100.

Reiman, E. M., & Jagust, W. J. (2012). Brain imaging in the study of Alzheimer's disease. *Neuroimage*, *61*(2), 505–516. http://dx.doi.org/10.1016/j.neuroimage.2011.11.075.

Reiman, E. M., Langbaum, J. B., Fleisher, A. S., Caselli, R. J., Chen, K., Ayutyanont, N., & Tariot, P. N. (2011). Alzheimer's prevention initiative: A plan to accelerate the evaluation of presymptomatic treatments. *Journal of Alzheimer's Disease*, *26*(Suppl. 3), 321–329. http://dx.doi.org/10.3233/JAD-2011-0059.

Reiman, E. M., Uecker, A., Caselli, R. J., Lewis, S., Bandy, D., de Leon, M. J., & Thibodeau, S. N. (1998). Hippocampal volumes in cognitively normal persons at genetic risk for Alzheimer's disease. *Annals of Neurology*, *44*(2), 288–291. http://dx.doi.org/10.1002/ana.410440226.

Reisberg, B., Ferris, S. H., de Leon, M. J., & Crook, T. (1982). The Global Deterioration Scale for assessment of primary degenerative dementia. *The American Journal of Psychiatry*, *139*(9), 1136–1139.

Reiss, A. L., Abrams, M. T., Singer, H. S., Ross, J. L., & Denckla, M. B. (1996). Brain development, gender and IQ in children. A volumetric imaging study. *Brain*, *119*(Pt 5), 1763–1774.

Reitz, C., den Heijer, T., van Duijn, C., Hofman, A., & Breteler, M. M. (2007). Relation between smoking and risk of dementia and Alzheimer disease: The Rotterdam Study. *Neurology*, *69*(10), 998–1005. http://dx.doi.org/10.1212/01.wnl.0000271395.29695.9a.

Reitz, C., Jun, G., Naj, A., Rajbhandary, R., Vardarajan, B. N., Wang, L. S., & Mayeux, R. (2013). Variants in the ATP-binding cassette transporter (ABCA7), apolipoprotein E 4,and the risk of late-onset alzheimer disease in African Americans. *JAMA*, *309*(14), 1483–1492. http://dx.doi.org/10.1001/jama.2013.2973.

Reitz, C., Tang, M. X., Schupf, N., Manly, J. J., Mayeux, R., & Luchsinger, J. A. (2010). Association of higher levels of high-density lipoprotein cholesterol in elderly individuals and lower risk of late-onset alzheimer disease. *Archives of Neurology*, *67*(12), 1491–1497. http://dx.doi.org/10.1001/archneurol.2010.297.

Reitz, C., Tang, M. X., Schupf, N., Manly, J. J., Mayeux, R., & Luchsinger, J. A. (2010). A summary risk score for the prediction of Alzheimer disease in elderly persons. *Archives of Neurology*, *67*(7), 835–841. http://dx.doi.org/10.1001/archneurol.2010.136.

Resnick, S. M., Espeland, M. A., Jaramillo, S. A., Hirsch, C., Stefanick, M. L., Murray, A. M., & Davatzikos, C. (2009). Postmenopausal hormone therapy and regional brain volumes: The WHIMS-MRI Study. *Neurology*, *72*(2), 135–142. http://dx.doi.org/10.1212/01.wnl.0000339037.76336.cf.

Resnick, S. M., & Henderson, V. W. (2002). Hormone therapy and risk of Alzheimer disease: A critical time. *JAMA*, *288*(17), 2170–2172.

Reynolds, K., Lewis, B., Nolen, J. D., Kinney, G. L., Sathya, B., & He, J. (2003). Alcohol consumption and risk of stroke: A meta-analysis. *JAMA*, *289*(5), 579–588.

Reynolds, M. D., Johnston, J. M., Dodge, H. H., DeKosky, S. T., & Ganguli, M. (1999). Small head size is related to low Mini-Mental State Examination scores in a community sample of nondemented older adults. *Neurology*, *53*(1), 228–229.

Rice, M.M., Graves A.B., McCurry, S.M., Gibbons, L., Bowen, J., McCormick, W., et al. (October 31–November 3, 1999). Tofu consumption and cognition in older Japanese American men and women. Paper presented at the Third International Symposium on the Role of Soy in Preventing and Treating Chronic Diseases, Washington, DC.

Richard, E., Andrieu, S., Solomon, A., Mangialasche, F., Ahtiluoto, S., Moll van Charante, E. P., & Kivipelto, M. (2012). Methodological challenges in designing dementia prevention trials—The European Dementia Prevention Initiative (EDPI). *Journal of the Neurological Sciences*, *322*(1–2), 64–70. http://dx.doi.org/10.1016/j.jns.2012.06.012.

Richard, E., Van den Heuvel, E., Moll van Charante, E. P., Achthoven, L., Vermeulen, M., & Bindels, P. J., et al. (2009). Prevention of dementia by intensive vascular care (PreDIVA): A cluster-randomized trial in progress. *Alzheimer Disease and Associated Disorders*, *23*(3), 198–204. http://dx.doi.org/10.1097/WAD.0b013e31819783a4.

Richards, M., Hardy, R., Kuh, D., & Wadsworth, M. E. (2001). Birth weight and cognitive function in the British 1946 birth cohort: Longitudinal population based study. *BMJ*, *322*(7280), 199–203.

Richardson, K., Stephan, B. C., Ince, P. G., Brayne, C., Matthews, F. E., & Esiri, M. M. (2012). The neuropathology of vascular disease in the Medical Research Council Cognitive Function and Ageing Study (MRC CFAS). *Current Alzheimer Research*, *9*(6), 687–696.

Rich-Edwards, J. W., & Gillman, M. W. (1997). Commentary: A hypothesis challenged. *BMJ*, *315*(7119), 1348–1349.

Riedel-Heller, S. G., Busse, A., Aurich, C., Matschinger, H., & Angermeyer, M. C. (2001). Incidence of dementia according to DSM-III-R and ICD-10. Results of the Leipzig Longitudinal Study of the Aged (LEILA75+), Part 2. *British Journal of Psychiatry*, *179*, 255–260.

Riggs, J. E. (1992). Cigarette smoking and Parkinson disease: The illusion of a neuroprotective effect. *Clinical Neuropharmacology*, *15*(2), 88–99.

Riley, K. P., Snowdon, D. A., & Markesbery, W. R. (2002). Alzheimer's neurofibrillary pathology and the spectrum of cognitive function: Findings from the Nun Study. *Annals of Neurology*, *51*(5), 567–577. http://dx.doi.org/10.1002/ana.10161.

Rimm, E. B., Stampfer, M. J., Colditz, G. A., Chute, C. G., Litin, L. B., & Willett, W. C. (1990). Validity of self-reported waist and hip circumferences in men and women. *Epidemiology*, *1*(6), 466–473.

Rincon, F., & Wright, C. B. (2013). Vascular cognitive impairment. *Current Opinion in Neurology*, *26*(1), 29–36. http://dx.doi.org/10.1097/WCO.0b013e32835c4f04.

Ritchie, K., Carriere, I., de Mendonca, A., Portet, F., Dartigues, J. F., Rouaud, O., & Ancelin, M. L. (2007). The neuroprotective effects of caffeine: A prospective population study (the Three City Study). *Neurology*, *69*(6), 536–545. http://dx.doi.org/10.1212/01.wnl.0000266670.35219.0c.

Roberts, G. W., Gentleman, S. M., Lynch, A., & Graham, D. I. (1991). Beta A4 amyloid protein deposition in brain after head trauma. *Lancet*, *338*(8780), 1422–1423.

Roberts, G. W., Gentleman, S. M., Lynch, A., Murray, L., Landon, M., & Graham, D. I. (1994). Beta amyloid protein deposition in the brain after severe head injury: Implications for the pathogenesis of Alzheimer's disease. *Journal of Neurology, Neurosurgery, and Psychiatry*, *57*(4), 419–425.

Roberts, J. L., Clare, L., & Woods, R. T. (2009). Subjective memory complaints and awareness of memory functioning in mild cognitive impairment: A systematic review. *Dementia and Geriatric Cognitive Disorders*, *28*(2), 95–109. http://dx.doi.org/10.1159/000234911.

Roberts, J. S., McLaughlin, S. J., & Connell, C. M. (2014). Public beliefs and knowledge about risk and protective factors for Alzheimer's disease. *Alzheimer's & Dementia: The Journal of the Alzheimer's Association*, *10*(5 Suppl.), S381–389. http://dx.doi.org/10.1016/j.jalz.2013.07.001.

Roberts, R. O., Geda, Y. E., Knopman, D. S., Cha, R. H., Pankratz, V. S., & Boeve, B. F., et al. (2008). The Mayo clinic study of aging: Design and sampling, participation, baseline measures and sample characteristics. *Neuroepidemiology*, *30*(1), 58–69.

Roberts, R. O., Knopman, D. S., Mielke, M. M., Cha, R. H., Pankratz, V. S., Christianson, T. J., & Petersen, R. C. (2014). Higher risk of progression to dementia in mild cognitive impairment cases who revert to normal. *Neurology*, *82*(4), 317–325. http://dx.doi.org/10.1212/WNL.0000000000000055.

Rocca, W. A., Cha, R. H., Waring, S. C., & Kokmen, E. (1998). Incidence of dementia and Alzheimer's disease: A reanalysis of data from Rochester, Minnesota, 1975–1984. *American Journal of Epidemiology*, *148*(1), 51–62.

Rocca, W. A., Petersen, R. C., Knopman, D. S., Hebert, L. E., Evans, D. A., Hall, K. S., & White, L. R. (2011). Trends in the incidence and prevalence of Alzheimer's disease, dementia, and cognitive impairment in the United States. *Alzheimer's & Dementia: The Journal of the Alzheimer's Association*, *7*(1), 80–93. http://dx.doi.org/10.1016/j.jalz.2010.11.002.

Rocher, A. B., Chapon, F., Blaizot, X., Baron, J. C., & Chavoix, C. (2003). Resting-state brain glucose utilization as measured by PET is directly related to regional synaptophysin levels: A study in baboons. *Neuroimage*, *20*(3), 1894–1898.

Rogaeva, E., Meng, Y., Lee, J. H., Gu, Y., Kawarai, T., Zou, F., & St George-Hyslop, P. (2007). The neuronal sortilin-related receptor SORL1 is genetically associated with Alzheimer disease. *Nature Genetics*, *39*(2), 168–177. http://dx.doi.org/10.1038/ng1943.

Rogers, J., Kirby, L. C., Hempelman, S. R., Berry, D. L., McGeer, P. L., & Kaszniak, A. W., et al. (1993). Clinical trial of indomethacin in Alzheimer's disease. *Neurology*, *43*(8), 1609–1611.

Roman, G. C., Tatemichi, T. K., Erkinjuntti, T., Cummings, J. L., Masdeu, J. C., & Garcia, J. H., et al. (1993). Vascular dementia: Diagnostic criteria for research studies. Report of the NINDS-AIREN International Workshop. *Neurology*, *43*(2), 250–260.

Romero-Corral, A., Somers, V. K., Sierra-Johnson, J., Thomas, R. J., Collazo-Clavell, M. L., Korinek, J., & Lopez-Jimenez, F. (2008). Accuracy of body mass index in diagnosing obesity in the adult general population. *International Journal of Obesity (2005)*, *32*(6), 959–966. http://dx.doi.org/10.1038/ijo.2008.11.

Ronksley, P. E., Brien, S. E., Turner, B. J., Mukamal, K. J., & Ghali, W. A. (2011). Association of alcohol consumption with selected cardiovascular disease outcomes: A systematic review and meta-analysis. *BMJ*, *342*, d671. http://dx.doi.org/10.1136/bmj.d671.

Roseboom, T., de Rooij, S., & Painter, R. (2006). The Dutch famine and its long-term consequences for adult health. *Early Human Development*, *82*(8), 485–491. http://dx.doi.org/10.1016/j.earlhumdev.2006.07.001.

Rosen, C., Hansson, O., Blennow, K., & Zetterberg, H. (2013). Fluid biomarkers in Alzheimer's disease—current concepts. *Molecular Neurodegeneration*, *8*, 20. http://dx.doi.org/10.1186/1750-1326-8-20.

Roses, A. D., Lutz, M. W., Amrine-Madsen, H., Saunders, A. M., Crenshaw, D. G., Sundseth, S. S., & Reiman, E. M. (2010). A TOMM40 variable-length polymorphism predicts the age of late-onset alzheimer's disease. *The Pharmacogenomics Journal*, *10*(5), 375–384. http://dx.doi.org/10.1038/tpj.2009.69.

Ross, M. G., Desai, M., Khorram, O., McKnight, R. A., Lane, R. H., & Torday, J. (2007). Gestational programming of offspring obesity: A potential contributor to Alzheimer's disease. *Current Alzheimer Research*, *4*(2), 213–217.

Rossouw, J. E., Anderson, G. L., Prentice, R. L., LaCroix, A. Z., Kooperberg, C., Stefanick, M. L., & Writing Group for the Women's Health Initiative Investigators, (2002). Risks and benefits of estrogen plus progestin in healthy postmenopausal women: Principal results from the Women's Health Initiative randomized controlled trial. *JAMA*, *288*(3), 321–333.

Roth, M. (1986). The association of clinical and neurological findings and its bearing on the classification and aetiology of Alzheimer's disease. *British Medical Bulletin*, *42*(1), 42–50.

Rothman, K. J., Greenland, S., & Lash, T. L. (2008). *Modern epidemiology* (3rd ed.). Philadelphia, PA: Wolters Kluwer|Lippincott Williams & Wilkins.

Rovelet-Lecrux, A., Hannequin, D., Raux, G., Le Meur, N., Laquerriere, A., Vital, A., & Campion, D. (2006). APP locus duplication causes autosomal dominant early-onset alzheimer disease with cerebral amyloid angiopathy. *Nature Genetics*, *38*(1), 24–26. http://dx.doi.org/10.1038/ng1718.

Rovio, S., Kareholt, I., Helkala, E. L., Viitanen, M., Winblad, B., Tuomilehto, J., & Kivipelto, M. (2005). Leisure-time physical activity at midlife and the risk of dementia and Alzheimer's disease. *Lancet Neurology*, *4*(11), 705–711. http://dx.doi.org/10.1016/S1474-4422(05)70198-8.

Rubinsztein, D. C., & Easton, D. F. (1999). Apolipoprotein E genetic variation and Alzheimer's disease. A meta-analysis. *Dementia and Geriatric Cognitive Disorders*, *10*(3), 199–209. 17120.

Rudelli, R., Strom, J. O., Welch, P. T., & Ambler, M. W. (1982). Posttraumatic premature Alzheimer's disease. Neuropathologic findings and pathogenetic considerations. *Archives of Neurology*, *39*(9), 570–575.

Ruitenberg, A., Ott, A., van Swieten, J. C., Hofman, A., & Breteler, M. M. (2001). Incidence of dementia: Does gender make a difference? *Neurobiology of Aging*, *22*(4), 575–580.

Ruitenberg, A., van Swieten, J. C., Witteman, J. C. M., Mehta, K. M., van Duijn, C. M., & Hofman, A., et al. (2002). Alcohol consumption and risk of dementia: The Rotterdam Study. *The Lancet*, *359*(9303), 281–286. http://dx.doi.org/10.1016/s0140-6736(02)07493-7.

Rusanen, M., Kivipelto, M., Levalahti, E., Laatikainen, T., Tuomilehto, J., & Soininen, H., et al. (2014). Heart diseases and long-term risk of dementia and Alzheimer's disease: A population-based CAIDE study. *Journal of Alzheimer's Disease*, *42*(1), 183–191. http://dx.doi.org/10.3233/JAD-132363.

Rusanen, M., Kivipelto, M., Quesenberry, C. P., Jr., Zhou, J., & Whitmer, R. A. (2011). Heavy smoking in midlife and long-term risk of Alzheimer disease and vascular dementia. *Archives of Internal Medicine*, *171*(4), 333–339. http://dx.doi.org/10.1001/archinternmed.2010.393.

Rusanen, M., Rovio, S., Ngandu, T., Nissinen, A., Tuomilehto, J., & Soininen, H., et al. (2010). Midlife smoking, apolipoprotein E and risk of dementia and Alzheimer's disease: A population-based cardiovascular risk factors, aging and dementia study. *Dementia and Geriatric Cognitive Disorders*, *30*(3), 277–284. http://dx.doi.org/10.1159/000320484.

Ruscheweyh, R., Willemer, C., Kruger, K., Duning, T., Warnecke, T., Sommer, J., & Floel, A. (2011). Physical activity and memory functions: An interventional study. *Neurobiology of Aging*, *32*(7), 1304–1319. http://dx.doi.org/10.1016/j.neurobiolaging.2009.08.001.

Saczynski, J. S., Beiser, A., Seshadri, S., Auerbach, S., Wolf, P. A., & Au, R. (2010). Depressive symptoms and risk of dementia: The Framingham Heart Study. *Neurology*, *75*(1), 35–41. http://dx.doi.org/10.1212/WNL.0b013e3181e62138.

Saczynski, J. S., Pfeifer, L. A., Masaki, K., Korf, E. S., Laurin, D., & White, L., et al. (2006). The effect of social engagement on incident dementia: The Honolulu-Asia Aging Study. *American Journal of Epidemiology*, *163*(5), 433–440. http://dx.doi.org/10.1093/aje/kwj061.

Sahota, A., Yang, M., Gao, S., Hui, S. L., Baiyewu, O., Gureje, O., & Hendrie, H. C. (1997). Apolipoprotein E-associated risk for Alzheimer's disease in the African-American population is genotype dependent. *Annals of Neurology*, *42*(4), 659–661. http://dx.doi.org/10.1002/ana.410420418.

Salib, E., & Hillier, V. (1997). Head injury and the risk of Alzheimer's disease: A case control study. *International Journal of Geriatric Psychiatry*, *12*(3), 363–368.

Salihu, H. M., Bonnema, S. M., & Alio, A. P. (2009). Obesity: What is an elderly population growing into? *Maturitas*, *63*(1), 7–12. http://dx.doi.org/10.1016/j.maturitas.2009.02.010.

Samieri, C., Okereke, O. I., Devore, E. E., & Grodstein, F. (2013). Long-term adherence to the Mediterranean diet is associated with overall cognitive status, but not cognitive decline, in women. *The Journal of Nutrition*, *143*(4), 493–499. http://dx.doi.org/10.3945/jn.112.169896.

Sano, M., Ernesto, C., Thomas, R. G., Klauber, M. R., Schafer, K., Grundman, M., & Thal, L. J. (1997). A controlled trial of selegiline, alpha-tocopherol, or both as treatment for Alzheimer's disease. The Alzheimer's Disease Cooperative Study. *The New England Journal of Medicine*, *336*(17), 1216–1222. http://dx.doi.org/10.1056/NEJM199704243361704.

Santos, C., Costa, J., Santos, J., Vaz-Carneiro, A., & Lunet, N. (2010). Caffeine intake and dementia: Systematic review and meta-analysis. *Journal of Alzheimer's Disease*, *20*(Suppl. 1), S187–204. http://dx.doi.org/10.3233/JAD-2010-091387.

Santos, C., Lunet, N., Azevedo, A., de Mendonca, A., Ritchie, K., & Barros, H. (2010). Caffeine intake is associated with a lower risk of cognitive decline: A cohort study from Portugal. *Journal of Alzheimer's Disease*, *20*(Suppl 1), S175–185. http://dx.doi.org/10.3233/JAD-2010-091303.

Sapolsky, R. M. (2000). Glucocorticoids and hippocampal atrophy in neuropsychiatric disorders. *Archives of General Psychiatry*, *57*(10), 925–935.

Sato, Y., Nakatsuka, H., Watanabe, T., Hisamichi, S., Shimizu, H., & Fujisaku, S., et al. (1989). Possible contribution of green tea drinking habits to the prevention of stroke. *The Tohoku Journal of Experimental Medicine*, *157*(4), 337–343.

Savva, G. M., Wharton, S. B., Ince, P. G., Forster, G., Matthews, F. E., & Brayne, C. (2009). Age, neuropathology, and dementia. *The New England Journal of Medicine*, *360*(22), 2302–2309. http://dx.doi.org/10.1056/NEJMoa0806142.

Scarmeas, N., Habeck, C. G., Hilton, J., Anderson, K. E., Flynn, J., & Park, A., et al. (2005). APOE related alterations in cerebral activation even at college age. *Journal of Neurology, Neurosurgery, and Psychiatry*, *76*(10), 1440–1444. http://dx.doi.org/10.1136/jnnp.2004.053645.

Scarmeas, N., Levy, G., Tang, M. X., Manly, J., & Stern, Y. (2001). Influence of leisure activity on the incidence of Alzheimer's disease. *Neurology*, *57*(12), 2236–2242.

Scarmeas, N., Luchsinger, J. A., Schupf, N., Brickman, A. M., Cosentino, S., & Tang, M. X., et al. (2009). Physical activity, diet, and risk of Alzheimer disease. *JAMA*, *302*(6), 627–637. http://dx.doi.org/10.1001/jama.2009.1144.

Scarmeas, N., Stern, Y., Mayeux, R., & Luchsinger, J. A. (2006). Mediterranean diet, Alzheimer disease, and vascular mediation. *Archives of Neurology*, *63*(12), 1709–1717. http://dx.doi.org/10.1001/archneur.63.12.noc60109.

Scarmeas, N., Stern, Y., Mayeux, R., Manly, J. J., Schupf, N., & Luchsinger, J. A. (2009). Mediterranean diet and mild cognitive impairment. *Archives of Neurology*, *66*(2), 216–225. http://dx.doi.org/10.1001/archneurol.2008.536.

Scarmeas, N., Stern, Y., Tang, M. X., Mayeux, R., & Luchsinger, J. A. (2006). Mediterranean diet and risk for Alzheimer's disease. *Annals of Neurology*, *59*(6), 912–921. http://dx.doi.org/10.1002/ana.20854.

Schaefer, E. J., Bongard, V., Beiser, A. S., Lamon-Fava, S., Robins, S. J., Au, R., & Wolf, P. A. (2006). Plasma phosphatidylcholine docosahexaenoic acid content and risk of dementia and Alzheimer disease: The Framingham Heart Study. *Archives of Neurology*, *63*(11), 1545–1550. http://dx.doi.org/10.1001/archneur.63.11.1545.

Schierbeck, L. L., Rejnmark, L., Tofteng, C. L., Stilgren, L., Eiken, P., Mosekilde, L., & Jensen, J. E. (2012). Effect of hormone replacement therapy on cardiovascular events in recently postmenopausal women: Randomised trial. *BMJ*, *345*, e6409. http://dx.doi.org/10.1136/bmj.e6409.

Schiffer, T., Schulte, S., Hollmann, W., Bloch, W., & Struder, H. K. (2009). Effects of strength and endurance training on brain-derived neurotrophic factor and insulin-like growth factor 1 in humans. *Hormone and Metabolic Research Hormon- und Stoffwechselforschung Hormones et Metabolisme*, *41*(3), 250–254. http://dx.doi.org/10.1055/s-0028-1093322.

Schmand, B., Eikelenboom, P., & van Gool, W. A. (2011). Value of neuropsychological tests, neuroimaging, and biomarkers for diagnosing Alzheimer's disease in younger and older age cohorts. *Journal of the American Geriatrics Society*, *59*, 1705–1710.

Schmand, B., Smit, J. H., Geerlings, M. I., & Lindeboom, J. (1997). The effects of intelligence and education on the development of dementia. A test of the brain reserve hypothesis. *Psychological Medicine*, *27*(6), 1337–1344.

Schneider, E. B., Sur, S., Raymont, V., Duckworth, J., Kowalski, R. G., Efron, D. T., & Stevens, R. D. (2014). Functional recovery after moderate/severe traumatic brain injury: A role for cognitive reserve? *Neurology*, *82*(18), 1636–1642. http://dx.doi.org/10.1212/WNL.0000000000000379.

Schneider, J. A., Aggarwal, N. T., Barnes, L., Boyle, P., & Bennett, D. A. (2009). The neuropathology of older persons with and without dementia from community versus clinic cohorts. *Journal of Alzheimer's Disease*, *18*(3), 691–701. http://dx.doi.org/10.3233/JAD-2009-1227.

Schneider, J. A., Arvanitakis, Z., Bang, W., & Bennett, D. A. (2007). Mixed brain pathologies account for most dementia cases in community-dwelling older persons. *Neurology*, *69*(24), 2197–2204. http://dx.doi.org/10.1212/01.wnl.0000271090.28148.24.

Schneider, J. A., Arvanitakis, Z., Leurgans, S. E., & Bennett, D. A. (2009). The neuropathology of probable Alzheimer disease and mild cognitive impairment. *Annals of Neurology*, *66*(2), 200–208. http://dx.doi.org/10.1002/ana.21706.

Schneider, J. A., Wilson, R. S., Bienias, J. L., Evans, D. A., & Bennett, D. A. (2004). Cerebral infarctions and the likelihood of dementia from Alzheimer disease pathology. *Neurology*, *62*(7), 1148–1155.

Schneider, L. S., Mangialasche, F., Andreasen, N., Feldman, H., Giacobini, E., Jones, R., & Kivipelto, M. (2014). Clinical trials and late-stage drug development for Alzheimer's disease: An appraisal from 1984 to 2014. *Journal of Internal Medicine*, *275*(3), 251–283. http://dx.doi.org/10.1111/joim.12191.

Schofield, P. W., Jacobs, D., Marder, K., Sano, M., & Stern, Y. (1997). The validity of new memory complaints in the elderly. *Archives of Neurology*, *54*(6), 756–759.

Schofield, P. W., Logroscino, G., Andrews, H. F., Albert, S., & Stern, Y. (1997). An association between head circumference and Alzheimer's disease in a population-based study of aging and dementia. *Neurology*, *49*(1), 30–37.

Schofield, P. W., Marder, K., Dooneief, G., Jacobs, D. M., Sano, M., & Stern, Y. (1997). Association of subjective memory complaints with subsequent cognitive decline in community-dwelling elderly individuals with baseline cognitive impairment. *The American Journal of Psychiatry*, *154*(5), 609–615.

Schofield, P. W., Mosesson, R. E., Stern, Y., & Mayeux, R. (1995). The age at onset of Alzheimer's disease and an intracranial area measurement. A relationship. *Archives of Neurology*, *52*(1), 95–98.

Schofield, P. W., Tang, M., Marder, K., Bell, K., Dooneief, G., Chun, M., & Mayeux, R. (1997). Alzheimer's disease after remote head injury: An incidence study. *Journal of Neurology, Neurosurgery, and Psychiatry*, *62*(2), 119–124.

Schottky, J. (1932). About presenile dementias. *Zeitschrift für die Gesamte Neurologie und Psychiatrie*, *140*, 333–397.

Schrijvers, E. M., Verhaaren, B. F., Koudstaal, P. J., Hofman, A., Ikram, M. A., & Breteler, M. M. (2012). Is dementia incidence declining?: Trends in dementia incidence since 1990 in the Rotterdam Study. *Neurology*, *78*(19), 1456–1463. http://dx.doi.org/10.1212/WNL.0b013e3182553be6.

Schubert, C. R., Carmichael, L. L., Murphy, C., Klein, B. E., Klein, R., & Cruickshanks, K. J. (2008). Olfaction and the 5-year incidence of cognitive impairment in an epidemiological study of older adults. *Journal of the American Geriatrics Society*, *56*(8), 1517–1521. http://dx.doi.org/10.1111/j.1532-5415.2008.01826.x.

Schubert, C. R., Cruickshanks, K. J., Fischer, M. E., Huang, G. H., Klein, B. E., Klein, R., & Nondahl, D. M. (2012). Olfactory impairment in an adult population: The Beaver Dam Offspring Study. *Chemical Senses*, *37*(4), 325–334. http://dx.doi.org/10.1093/chemse/bjr102.

Schubert, C. R., Cruickshanks, K. J., Fischer, M. E., Huang, G. H., Klein, R., Pankratz, N., & Nondahl, D. M. (2013). Odor identification and cognitive function in the Beaver Dam Offspring Study. *Journal of Clinical and Experimental Neuropsychology*, *35*(7), 669–676. http://dx.doi.org/10.1080/13803395.2013.809701.

Schupf, N., Kapell, D., Lee, J. H., Ottman, R., & Mayeux, R. (1994). Increased risk of Alzheimer's disease in mothers of adults with Down's syndrome. *Lancet*, *344*(8919), 353–356.

Schupf, N., & Sergievsky, G. H. (2002). Genetic and host factors for dementia in Down's syndrome. *The British Journal of Psychiatry: The Journal of Mental Science*, *180*, 405–410.

Selhub, J., Jacques, P. F., Bostom, A. G., D'Agostino, R. B., Wilson, P. W., Belanger, A. J., & Rosenberg, I. H. (1995). Association between plasma homocysteine concentrations and extracranial carotid-artery stenosis. *The New England Journal of Medicine*, *332*(5), 286–291. http://dx.doi.org/10.1056/NEJM199502023320502.

Selkoe, D. J. (2013). The therapeutics of Alzheimer's disease: Where we stand and where we are heading. *Annals of Neurology*, *74*(3), 328–336. http://dx.doi.org/10.1002/ana.24001.

Serby, M., Larson, P., & Kalkstein, D. (1991). The nature and course of olfactory deficits in Alzheimer's disease. *The American Journal of Psychiatry*, *148*(3), 357–360.

Serby, M., Mohan, C., Aryan, M., Williams, L., Mohs, R. C., & Davis, K. L. (1996). Olfactory identification deficits in relatives of Alzheimer's disease patients. *Biological Psychiatry*, *39*(5), 375–377. doi:10.1016/0006-3223(95)00472-6.

Seshadri, S., Beiser, A., Au, R., Wolf, P. A., Evans, D. A., Wilson, R. S., & Chui, H. C. (2011). Operationalizing diagnostic criteria for Alzheimer's disease and other age-related cognitive impairment-Part 2. *Alzheimer's & Dementia: The Journal of the Alzheimer's Association*, *7*(1), 35–52. http://dx.doi.org/10.1016/j.jalz.2010.12.002.

Seshadri, S., Beiser, A., Selhub, J., Jacques, P. F., Rosenberg, I. H., D'Agostino, R. B., & Wolf, P. A. (2002). Plasma homocysteine as a risk factor for dementia and Alzheimer's disease. *The New England Journal of Medicine*, *346*(7), 476–483. http://dx.doi.org/10.1056/NEJMoa011613.

Seshadri, S., Wolf, P. A., Beiser, A., Au, R., McNulty, K., & White, R., et al. (1997). Lifetime risk of dementia and Alzheimer's disease. The impact of mortality on risk estimates in the Framingham Study. *Neurology*, *49*(6), 1498–1504.

Seshadri, S., Zornberg, G. L., Derby, L. E., Myers, M. W., Jick, H., & Drachman, D. A. (2001). Postmenopausal estrogen replacement therapy and the risk of Alzheimer disease. *Archives of Neurology*, *58*(3), 435–440.

Shafqat, S. (2008). Alzheimer disease therapeutics: Perspectives from the developing world. *Journal of Alzheimer's Disease*, *15*, 285–287.

Shah, R. S., & Cole, J. W. (2010). Smoking and stroke: The more you smoke the more you stroke. *Expert Review of Cardiovascular Therapy*, *8*(7), 917–932. http://dx.doi.org/10.1586/erc.10.56.

Shalat, S. L., Seltzer, B., Pidcock, C., & Baker, E. L., Jr. (1987). Risk factors for Alzheimer's disease: A case-control study. *Neurology*, *37*(10), 1630–1633.

Shao, H., Breitner, J. C., Whitmer, R. A., Wang, J., Hayden, K., Wengreen, H., & Cache County Investigators, (2012). Hormone therapy and Alzheimer disease dementia: New findings from the Cache County Study. *Neurology*, *79*(18), 1846–1852. http://dx.doi.org/10.1212/WNL.0b013e318271f823.

Sharp, E. S., & Gatz, M. (2011). Relationship between education and dementia: An updated systematic review. *Alzheimer Disease and Associated Disorders*, *25*(4), 289–304. http://dx.doi.org/10.1097/WAD.0b013e318211c83c.

Shaw, P., Lerch, J. P., Pruessner, J. C., Taylor, K. N., Rose, A. B., Greenstein, D., & Giedd, J. N. (2007). Cortical morphology in children and adolescents with different apolipoprotein E gene polymorphisms: An observational study. *Lancet Neurology*, *6*(6), 494–500. http://dx.doi.org/10.1016/S1474-4422(07)70106-0.

Shepardson, N. E., Shankar, G. M., & Selkoe, D. J. (2011). Cholesterol level and statin use in Alzheimer disease: I. Review of epidemiological and preclinical studies. *Archives of Neurology*, *68*(10), 1239–1244. http://dx.doi.org/10.1001/archneurol.2011.203.

Shepardson, N. E., Shankar, G. M., & Selkoe, D. J. (2011). Cholesterol level and statin use in Alzheimer disease: II. Review of human trials and recommendations. *Archives of Neurology*, *68*(11), 1385–1392. http://dx.doi.org/10.1001/archneurol.2011.242.

Sherrington, R., Froelich, S., Sorbi, S., Campion, D., Chi, H., Rogaeva, E. A., & St George-Hyslop, P. H. (1996). Alzheimer's disease associated with mutations in presenilin 2 is rare and variably penetrant. *Human Molecular Genetics*, *5*(7), 985–988.

Sherrington, R., Rogaev, E. I., Liang, Y., Rogaeva, E. A., Levesque, G., Ikeda, M., & St George-Hyslop, P. H. (1995). Cloning of a gene bearing missense mutations in early-onset familial Alzheimer's disease. *Nature*, *375*(6534), 754–760. http://dx.doi.org/10.1038/375754a0.

Shim, Y. S., Yang, D. W., Roe, C. M., Coats, M. A., Benzinger, T. L., Xiong, C., & Morris, J. C. (2015). Pathological correlates of white matter hyperintensities on magnetic resonance imaging. *Dementia and Geriatric Cognitive Disorders*, *39*(1-2), 92–104. http://dx.doi.org/10.1159/000366411.

Shimizu, E., Hashimoto, K., & Iyo, M. (2004). Ethnic difference of the BDNF 196G/A (val66met) polymorphism frequencies: The possibility to explain ethnic mental traits. *American Journal of Medical Genetics Part B, Neuropsychiatric Genetics: The Official Publication of the International Society of Psychiatric Genetics*, *126B*(1), 122–123. http://dx.doi.org/10.1002/ajmg.b.20118.

Shinton, R., & Sagar, G. (1993). Lifelong exercise and stroke. *BMJ*, *307*(6898), 231–234.

Shu, X. O., Yang, G., Jin, F., Liu, D., Kushi, L., Wen, W., & Zheng, W. (2004). Validity and reproducibility of the food frequency questionnaire used in the Shanghai Women's Health Study. *European Journal of Clinical Nutrition*, *58*(1), 17–23. http://dx.doi.org/10.1038/sj.ejcn.1601738.

Shumaker, S. A., Legault, C., Kuller, L., Rapp, S. R., Thal, L., Lane, D. S., & Coker, L. H. (2004). Conjugated equine estrogens and incidence of probable dementia and mild cognitive impairment in postmenopausal women: Women's Health Initiative Memory Study. *JAMA*, *291*(24), 2947–2958. http://dx.doi.org/10.1001/jama.291.24.2947.

Shumaker, S. A., Legault, C., Rapp, S. R., Thal, L., Wallace, R. B., Ockene, J. K., & Wactawski-Wende, J. (2003). Estrogen plus progestin and the incidence of dementia and mild cognitive impairment in postmenopausal women: The Women's Health Initiative Memory Study: A randomized controlled trial. *JAMA*, *289*(20), 2651–2662. http://dx.doi.org/10.1001/jama.289.20.2651.

Signorello, L. B., Munro, H. M., Buchowski, M. S., Schlundt, D. G., Cohen, S. S., & Hargreaves, M. K., et al. (2009). Estimating nutrient intake from a food frequency questionnaire: Incorporating the elements of race and geographic region. *American Journal of Epidemiology*, *170*(1), 104–111. http://dx.doi.org/10.1093/aje/kwp098.

Silva-Gomez, A. B., Rojas, D., Juarez, I., & Flores, G. (2003). Decreased dendritic spine density on prefrontal cortical and hippocampal pyramidal neurons in postweaning social isolation rats. *Brain Research*, *983*(1–2), 128–136.

Singh, B., Parsaik, A. K., Mielke, M. M., Erwin, P. J., Knopman, D. S., & Petersen, R. C., et al. (2014). Association of mediterranean diet with mild cognitive impairment and Alzheimer's disease: A systematic review and meta-analysis. *Journal of Alzheimer's Disease*, *39*(2), 271–282. http://dx.doi.org/10.3233/JAD-130830.

Singh, M., Arseneault, M., Sanderson, T., Murthy, V., & Ramassamy, C. (2008). Challenges for research on polyphenols from foods in Alzheimer's disease: Bioavailability, metabolism, and cellular and molecular mechanisms. *Journal of Agricultural and Food Chemistry*, *56*(13), 4855–4873. http://dx.doi.org/10.1021/jf0735073.

Sjogren, T., Sjogren, H., & Lindgren, A. G. (1952). Morbus Alzheimer and morbus Pick; a genetic, clinical and patho-anatomical study. *Acta Psychiatrica et Neurologica Scandinavica Supplementum*, *82*, 1–152.

Skoog, I., Andreasson, L. A., Landahl, S., & Lernfelt, B. (1998). A population-based study on blood pressure and brain atrophy in 85-year-olds. *Hypertension*, *32*(3), 404–409.

Skoog, I., & Gustafson, D. (2002). Hypertension and related factors in the etiology of Alzheimer's disease. *Annals of the New York Academy of Sciences*, *977*, 29–36.

Skoog, I., Lernfelt, B., Landahl, S., Palmertz, B., Andreasson, L. A., Nilsson, L., & Svanborg, A. (1996). 15-year longitudinal study of blood pressure and dementia. *Lancet*, *347*(9009), 1141–1145.

Slinin, Y., Paudel, M. L., Taylor, B. C., Fink, H. A., Ishani, A., Canales, M. T., & Ensrud, K. E. (2010). 25-Hydroxyvitamin D levels and cognitive performance and decline in elderly men. *Neurology*, *74*(1), 33–41. http://dx.doi.org/10.1212/WNL.0b013e3181c7197b.

Smid, S. D., Maag, J. L., & Musgrave, I. F. (2012). Dietary polyphenol-derived protection against neurotoxic beta-amyloid protein: From molecular to clinical. *Food & Function*, *3*(12), 1242–1250. http://dx.doi.org/10.1039/c2fo30075c.

Smith, A. D., Smith, S. M., de Jager, C. A., Whitbread, P., Johnston, C., Agacinski, G., & Refsum, H. (2010). Homocysteine-lowering by B vitamins slows the rate of accelerated brain atrophy in mild cognitive impairment: A randomized controlled trial. *PLoS One*, *5*(9), e12244. http://dx.doi.org/10.1371/journal.pone.0012244.

Smith, C. (2013). Review: The long-term consequences of microglial activation following acute traumatic brain injury. *Neuropathology and Applied Neurobiology*, *39*(1), 35–44. http://dx.doi.org/10.1111/nan.12006.

Smith, D. (2013). *Stop trying to cure Alzheimer's—And prevent it instead: One of Britain's top dementia experts says we've wasted billions on useless drugs*. Mail Online. <http://www.dailymail.co.uk/health/article-2521024/Stop-trying-cure-Alzheimers-prevent-instead-says-dementia-expert.html> Accessed 19.05.14.

Smith, E. E., Schneider, J. A., Wardlaw, J. M., & Greenberg, S. M. (2012). Cerebral microinfarcts: The invisible lesions. *Lancet Neurology*, *11*(3), 272–282. http://dx.doi.org/10.1016/S1474-4422(11)70307-6.

Smith, G. E., Housen, P., Yaffe, K., Ruff, R., Kennison, R. F., & Mahncke, H. W., et al. (2009). A cognitive training program based on principles of brain plasticity: Results from the Improvement in Memory with Plasticity-based Adaptive Cognitive Training (IMPACT) study. *Journal of the American Geriatrics Society*, *57*(4), 594–603. http://dx.doi.org/10.1111/j.1532-5415.2008.02167.x.

Smith, P. J., Blumenthal, J. A., Hoffman, B. M., Cooper, H., Strauman, T. A., Welsh-Bohmer, K., & Sherwood, A. (2010). Aerobic exercise and neurocognitive performance: A meta-analytic review of randomized controlled trials. *Psychosomatic Medicine*, *72*(3), 239–252. http://dx.doi.org/10.1097/PSY.0b013e3181d14633.

Smyth, K. A., Fritsch, T., Cook, T. B., McClendon, M. J., Santillan, C. E., & Friedland, R. P. (2004). Worker functions and traits associated with occupations and the development of AD. *Neurology*, *63*(3), 498–503.

Snowdon, D. A. (2001). *Aging with grace*. New York: Bantum Books.

Snowdon, D. A., Greiner, L. H., & Markesbery, W. R. (2000). Linguistic ability in early life and the neuropathology of Alzheimer's disease and cerebrovascular disease. Findings from the Nun Study. *Annals of the New York Academy of Sciences*, *903*, 34–38.

Snowdon, D. A., Greiner, L. H., Mortimer, J. A., Riley, K. P., Greiner, P. A., & Markesbery, W. R. (1997). Brain infarction and the clinical expression of Alzheimer disease. The Nun Study. *JAMA*, *277*(10), 813–817.

Snowdon, D. A., Kemper, S. J., Mortimer, J. A., Greiner, L. H., Wekstein, D. R., & Markesbery, W. R. (1996). Linguistic ability in early life and cognitive function and Alzheimer's disease in late life. Findings from the Nun Study. *JAMA*, *275*(7), 528–532.

Snowdon, D. A., Tully, C. L., Smith, C. D., Riley, K. P., & Markesbery, W. R. (2000). Serum folate and the severity of atrophy of the neocortex in Alzheimer disease: Findings from the Nun study. *The American Journal of Clinical Nutrition*, *71*(4), 993–998.

Sofi, F., Macchi, C., Abbate, R., Gensini, G. F., & Casini, A. (2010). Effectiveness of the Mediterranean diet: Can it help delay or prevent Alzheimer's disease? *Journal of Alzheimer's Disease*, *20*(3), 795–801. http://dx.doi.org/10.3233/JAD-2010-1418.

Sohrabji, F., & Lewis, D. K. (2006). Estrogen-BDNF interactions: Implications for neurodegenerative diseases. *Frontiers in Neuroendocrinology*, *27*(4), 404–414. http://dx.doi.org/10.1016/j.yfrne.2006.09.003.

Sole-Padulles, C., Bartres-Faz, D., Junque, C., Vendrell, P., Rami, L., Clemente, I. C., & Molinuevo, J. L. (2009). Brain structure and function related to cognitive reserve variables in normal aging, mild cognitive impairment and Alzheimer's disease. *Neurobiology of Aging*, *30*(7), 1114–1124. http://dx.doi.org/10.1016/j.neurobiolaging.2007.10.008.

Solfrizzi, V., D'Introno, A., Colacicco, A. M., Capurso, C., Del Parigi, A., Baldassarre, G., & Panza, F. (2007). Alcohol consumption, mild cognitive impairment, and progression to dementia. *Neurology*, *68*(21), 1790–1799. http://dx.doi.org/10.1212/01.wnl.0000262035.87304.89.

Solomon, A., Kivipelto, M., Wolozin, B., Zhou, J., & Whitmer, R. A. (2009). Midlife serum cholesterol and increased risk of Alzheimer's and vascular dementia three decades later. *Dementia and Geriatric Cognitive Disorders*, *28*(1), 75–80. http://dx.doi.org/10.1159/000231980.

Solomon, A., & Soininen, H. (2015). Dementia: Risk prediction models in dementia prevention. *Nature Reviews Neurology*. http://dx.doi.org/10.1038/nrneurol.2015.81.

Solomon, C. G., & Manson, J. E. (1997). Obesity and mortality: A review of the epidemiologic data. *The American Journal of Clinical Nutrition*, *66*(4 Suppl.), 1044S–1050S.

Soni, M., Rahardjo, T. B., Soekardi, R., Sulistyowati, Y., Lestariningsih, Yesufu-Udechuku, A., & Hogervorst, E. (2014). Phytoestrogens and cognitive function: A review. *Maturitas*, *77*(3), 209–220. http://dx.doi.org/10.1016/j.maturitas.2013.12.010.

Sonnen, J. A., Larson, E. B., Brickell, K., Crane, P. K., Woltjer, R., & Montine, T. J., et al. (2009). Different patterns of cerebral injury in dementia with or without diabetes. *Archives of Neurology*, *66*(3), 315–322. http://dx.doi.org/10.1001/archneurol.2008.579.

Sonnen, J. A., Larson, E. B., Crane, P. K., Haneuse, S., Li, G., Schellenberg, G. D., & Montine, T. J. (2007). Pathological correlates of dementia in a longitudinal, population-based sample of aging. *Annals of Neurology*, *62*(4), 406–413. http://dx.doi.org/10.1002/ana.21208.

Sonnen, J. A., Larson, E. B., Haneuse, S., Woltjer, R., Li, G., Crane, P. K., & Montine, T. J. (2009). Neuropathology in the adult changes in thought study: A review. *Journal of Alzheimer's Disease*, *18*(3), 703–711. http://dx.doi.org/10.3233/JAD-2009-1180.

Sorensen, H. T., Sabroe, S., Rothman, K. J., Gillman, M., Steffensen, F. H., & Fischer, P., et al. (1999). Birth weight and length as predictors for adult height. *American Journal of Epidemiology*, *149*(8), 726–729.

Soya, H., Nakamura, T., Deocaris, C. C., Kimpara, A., Iimura, M., Fujikawa, T., & Nishijima, T. (2007). BDNF induction with mild exercise in the rat hippocampus. *Biochemical and Biophysical Research Communications*, *358*(4), 961–967. http://dx.doi.org/10.1016/j.bbrc.2007.04.173.

Sparks, D. L., Scheff, S. W., Hunsaker, J. C., III, Liu, H., Landers, T., & Gross, D. R. (1994). Induction of Alzheimer-like beta-amyloid immunoreactivity in the brains of rabbits with dietary cholesterol. *Experimental Neurology*, *126*(1), 88–94. http://dx.doi.org/10.1006/exnr.1994.1044.

Sparks, D. L., Scheff, S. W., Liu, H., Landers, T. M., Coyne, C. M., & Hunsaker, J. C., III (1995). Increased incidence of neurofibrillary tangles (NFT) in non-demented individuals with hypertension. *Journal of the Neurological Sciences*, *131*(2), 162–169.

Sperling, R. A., Rentz, D. M., Johnson, K. A., Karlawish, J., Donohue, M., & Salmon, D. P., et al. (2014). The A4 study: Stopping AD before symptoms begin? *Science Translational Medicine*, *6*(228), 228fs213. http://dx.doi.org/10.1126/scitranslmed.3007941.

Spitzer, R. L., Williams, J. B., & Skodol, A. E. (1980). DSM-III: The major achievements and an overview. *The American Journal of Psychiatry*, *137*(2), 151–164.

Sprague, B. L., Trentham-Dietz, A., & Cronin, K. A. (2012). A sustained decline in postmenopausal hormone use: Results from the National Health and Nutrition Examination Survey, 1999–2010. *Obstetrics and Gynecology*, *120*(3), 595–603. http://dx.doi.org/10.1097/AOG.0b013e318265df42.

Staff, R. T., Murray, A. D., Ahearn, T. S., Mustafa, N., Fox, H. C., & Whalley, L. J. (2012). Childhood socioeconomic status and adult brain size: Childhood socioeconomic status influences adult hippocampal size. *Annals of Neurology*, *71*(5), 653–660. http://dx.doi.org/10.1002/ana.22631.

Staff, R. T., Murray, A. D., Deary, I. J., & Whalley, L. J. (2004). What provides cerebral reserve? *Brain*, *127*(Pt 5), 1191–1199. http://dx.doi.org/10.1093/brain/awh144.

Stamm, J. M., Bourlas, A. P., Baugh, C. M., Fritts, N. G., Daneshvar, D. H., Martin, B. M., & Stern, R. A. (2015). Age of first exposure to football and later-life cognitive impairment in former NFL players. *Neurology*. http://dx.doi.org/10.1212/WNL.0000000000001358.

Steffens, D. C., Plassman, B. L., Helms, M. J., Welsh-Bohmer, K. A., Saunders, A. M., & Breitner, J. C. (1997). A twin study of late-onset depression and apolipoprotein E epsilon 4 as risk factors for Alzheimer's disease. *Biological Psychiatry*, *41*(8), 851–856. http://dx.doi.org/10.1016/S0006-3223(96)00247-8.

Stein, T. D., Alvarez, V. E., & McKee, A. C. (2014). Chronic traumatic encephalopathy: A spectrum of neuropathological changes following repetitive brain trauma in athletes and military personnel. *Alzheimers Research & Therapy*, *6*(1), 4. http://dx.doi.org/10.1186/alzrt234.

Stelzmann, R. A., Schnitzlein, H. N., & Murtagh, F. R. (1995). An English translation of Alzheimer's 1907 Paper, "Uber eine eigenartige Erkankung der Hirnrinde". *Clinical Anatomy*, *8*, 429–431.

Stern, Y. (2002). What is cognitive reserve? Theory and research application of the reserve concept. *Journal of the International Neuropsychological Society*, *8*(3), 448–460.

Stern, Y. (2012). Cognitive reserve in ageing and Alzheimer's disease. *Lancet Neurology*, *11*(11), 1006–1012. http://dx.doi.org/10.1016/S1474-4422(12)70191-6.

Stern, Y., Alexander, G. E., Prohovnik, I., & Mayeux, R. (1992). Inverse relationship between education and parietotemporal perfusion deficit in Alzheimer's disease. *Annals of Neurology*, *32*(3), 371–375. http://dx.doi.org/10.1002/ana.410320311.

Stern, Y., Alexander, G. E., Prohovnik, I., Stricks, L., Link, B., & Lennon, M. C., et al. (1995). Relationship between lifetime occupation and parietal flow: Implications for a reserve against Alzheimer's disease pathology. *Neurology*, *45*(1), 55–60.

Stern, Y., Gurland, B., Tatemichi, T. K., Tang, M. X., Wilder, D., & Mayeux, R. (1994). Influence of education and occupation on the incidence of Alzheimer's disease. *JAMA*, *271*(13), 1004–1010.

Stern, Y., Tang, M. X., Denaro, J., & Mayeux, R. (1995). Increased risk of mortality in Alzheimer's disease patients with more advanced educational and occupational attainment. *Annals of Neurology*, *37*(5), 590–595. http://dx.doi.org/10.1002/ana.410370508.

Stevens, J., Cai, J., Pamuk, E. R., Williamson, D. F., Thun, M. J., & Wood, J. L. (1998). The effect of age on the association between body-mass index and mortality. *The New England Journal of Medicine*, *338*(1), 1–7. http://dx.doi.org/10.1056/NEJM199801013380101.

Stevenson, J. C., & Whitehead, M. I. (2002). Hormone replacement therapy. *BMJ*, *325*(7356), 113–114.

Stewart, R., Masaki, K., Xue, Q. L., Peila, R., Petrovitch, H., & White, L. R., et al. (2005). A 32-year prospective study of change in body weight and incident dementia: The Honolulu-Asia Aging Study. *Archives of Neurology*, *62*(1), 55–60. http://dx.doi.org/10.1001/archneur.62.1.55.

Stewart, W. F., Kawas, C., Corrada, M., & Metter, E. J. (1997). Risk of Alzheimer's disease and duration of NSAID use. *Neurology*, *48*(3), 626–632.

Straub, R. H. (2007). The complex role of estrogens in inflammation. *Endocrine Reviews*, *28*(5), 521–574. http://dx.doi.org/10.1210/er.2007-0001.

Strittmatter, W. J., Saunders, A. M., Schmechel, D., Pericak-Vance, M., Enghild, J., & Salvesen, G. S., et al. (1993). Apolipoprotein E: High-avidity binding to beta-amyloid and increased frequency of type 4 allele in late-onset familial Alzheimer disease. *Proceedings of the National Academy of Sciences of the United States of America*, *90*(5), 1977–1981.

Strozyk, D., Blennow, K., White, L. R., & Launer, L. J. (2003). CSF Abeta 42 levels correlate with amyloid-neuropathology in a population-based autopsy study. *Neurology*, *60*(4), 652–656.

Sumowski, J. F., Chiaravalloti, N., Krch, D., Paxton, J., & Deluca, J. (2013). Education attenuates the negative impact of traumatic brain injury on cognitive status. *Archives of Physical Medicine and Rehabilitation*, *94*(12), 2562–2564. http://dx.doi.org/10.1016/j.apmr.2013.07.023.

Sun, A. Y., Wang, Q., Simonyi, A., & Sun, G. Y. (2008). Botanical phenolics and brain health. *Neuromolecular Medicine*, *10*(4), 259–274. http://dx.doi.org/10.1007/s12017-008-8052-z.

Sundman, M. H., Hall, E. E., & Chen, N. K. (2014). Examining the relationship between head trauma and neurodegenerative disease: A review of epidemiology, pathology and neuroimaging techniques. *Journal of Alzheimers Disease & Parkinsonism*, *4*. http://dx.doi.org/10.4172/2161-0460.1000137.

Sundstrom, A., Nilsson, L. G., Cruts, M., Adolfsson, R., Van Broeckhoven, C., & Nyberg, L. (2007). Increased risk of dementia following mild head injury for carriers but not for non-carriers of the APOE epsilon4 allele. *International Psychogeriatrics/IPA*, *19*(1), 159–165. http://dx.doi.org/10.1017/S1041610206003498.

Swardfager, W., Lanctot, K., Rothenburg, L., Wong, A., Cappell, J., & Herrmann, N. (2010). A meta-analysis of cytokines in Alzheimer's disease. *Biological Psychiatry*, *68*(10), 930–941. http://dx.doi.org/10.1016/j.biopsych.2010.06.012.

Szekely, C. A., Breitner, J. C., Fitzpatrick, A. L., Rea, T. D., Psaty, B. M., & Kuller, L. H., et al. (2008). NSAID use and dementia risk in the Cardiovascular Health Study: Role of APOE and NSAID type. *Neurology*, *70*(1), 17–24. http://dx.doi.org/10.1212/01.wnl.0000284596.95156.48.

Szekely, C. A., Green, R. C., Breitner, J. C., Ostbye, T., Beiser, A. S., Corrada, M. M., & Zandi, P. P. (2008). No advantage of A beta 42-lowering NSAIDs for prevention of Alzheimer dementia in six pooled cohort studies. *Neurology*, *70*(24), 2291–2298. http://dx.doi.org/10.1212/01.wnl.0000313933.17796.f6.

Szekely, C. A., Thorne, J. E., Zandi, P. P., Ek, M., Messias, E., & Breitner, J. C., et al. (2004). Nonsteroidal anti-inflammatory drugs for the prevention of Alzheimer's disease: A systematic review. *Neuroepidemiology*, *23*(4), 159–169. http://dx.doi.org/10.1159/000078501.

Szekely, C. A., & Zandi, P. P. (2010). Non-steroidal anti-inflammatory drugs and Alzheimer's disease: The epidemiological evidence. *CNS & Neurological Disorders Drug Targets*, *9*(2), 132–139.

Taaffe, D. R., Irie, F., Masaki, K. H., Abbott, R. D., Petrovitch, H., & Ross, G. W., et al. (2008). Physical activity, physical function, and incident dementia in elderly men: The Honolulu-Asia

Aging Study. *The Journals of Gerontology Series A, Biological Sciences and Medical Sciences, 63*(5), 529–535.

Tan, Z. S., Harris, W. S., Beiser, A. S., Au, R., Himali, J. J., Debette, S., & Seshadri, S. (2012). Red blood cell omega-3 fatty acid levels and markers of accelerated brain aging. *Neurology, 78*(9), 658–664. http://dx.doi.org/10.1212/WNL.0b013e318249f6a9.

Tan, Z. S., Seshadri, S., Beiser, A., Wilson, P. W., Kiel, D. P., Tocco, M., & Wolf, P. A. (2003). Plasma total cholesterol level as a risk factor for Alzheimer disease: The Framingham Study. *Archives of Internal Medicine, 163*(9), 1053–1057. http://dx.doi.org/10.1001/archinte.163.9.1053.

Tang, M. X., Cross, P., Andrews, H., Jacobs, D. M., Small, S., Bell, K., & Mayeux, R. (2001). Incidence of AD in African-Americans, Caribbean Hispanics, and Caucasians in northern Manhattan. *Neurology, 56*(1), 49–56.

Tang, M. X., Maestre, G., Tsai, W. Y., Liu, X. H., Feng, L., Chung, W. Y., & Mayeux, R. (1996). Effect of age, ethnicity, and head injury on the association between APOE genotypes and Alzheimer's disease. *Annals of the New York Academy of Sciences, 802*, 6–15.

Tang, M. X., Maestre, G., Tsai, W. Y., Liu, X. H., Feng, L., Chung, W. Y., & Mayeux, R. (1996). Relative risk of Alzheimer disease and age-at-onset distributions, based on APOE genotypes among elderly African Americans, Caucasians, and Hispanics in New York City. *American Journal of Human Genetics, 58*(3), 574–584.

Tangney, C. C., Aggarwal, N. T., Li, H., Wilson, R. S., Decarli, C., & Evans, D. A., et al. (2011). Vitamin B12, cognition, and brain MRI measures: A cross-sectional examination. *Neurology, 77*(13), 1276–1282. http://dx.doi.org/10.1212/WNL.0b013e3182315a33.

Tangney, C. C., Kwasny, M. J., Li, H., Wilson, R. S., Evans, D. A., & Morris, M. C. (2011). Adherence to a Mediterranean-type dietary pattern and cognitive decline in a community population. *The American Journal of Clinical Nutrition, 93*(3), 601–607. http://dx.doi.org/10.3945/ajcn.110.007369.

Tardif, S., & Simard, M. (2011). Cognitive stimulation programs in healthy elderly: A review. *International Journal of Alzheimer's Disease, 2011*, 378934. http://dx.doi.org/10.4061/2011/378934.

The 3C Study Group (2003). Vascular factors and risk of dementia: Design of the Three-City Study and baseline characteristics of the study population. *Neuroepidemiology, 22*(6), 316–325.

Thies, W., & Bleiler, L. (2011). 2011 Alzheimer's disease facts and figures. *Alzheimer's & Dementia: The Journal of the Alzheimer's Association, 7*(2), 208–244. http://dx.doi.org/10.1016/j.jalz.2011.02.004.

Thorndike, E. L. (1921). *The teacher's word book.* New York: Columbia University.

Tjonneland, A., Gronbaek, M., Stripp, C., & Overvad, K. (1998). Wine intake and diet in a random sample of 48,763 Danish men and women. *The American Journal of Clinical Nutrition, 69*, 46–54.

Toledo, J. B., Shaw, L. M., & Trojanowski, J. Q. (2013). Plasma amyloid beta measurements—A desired but elusive Alzheimer's disease biomarker. *Alzheimers Research & Therapy, 5*(2), 8. http://dx.doi.org/10.1186/alzrt162.

Tombaugh, T. N., & McIntyre, N. J. (1992). The mini-mental state examination: A comprehensive review. *Journal of the American Geriatrics Society, 40*(9), 922–935.

Tomlinson, B. E., Blessed, G., & Roth, M. (1968). Observations on the brains of non-demented old people. *Journal of the Neurological Sciences, 7*(2), 331–356.

Tomlinson, B. E., Blessed, G., & Roth, M. (1970). Observations on the brains of demented old people. *Journal of the Neurological Sciences, 11*(3), 205–242.

Tramo, M. J., Loftus, W. C., Stukel, T. A., Green, R. L., Weaver, J. B., & Gazzaniga, M. S. (1998). Brain size, head size, and intelligence quotient in monozygotic twins. *Neurology, 50*(5), 1246–1252.

Trejo, J. L., Carro, E., & Torres-Aleman, I. (2001). Circulating insulin-like growth factor I mediates exercise-induced increases in the number of new neurons in the adult hippocampus. *The Journal of Neuroscience*, *21*(5), 1628–1634.

Trichopoulou, A., Costacou, T., Bamia, C., & Trichopoulos, D. (2003). Adherence to a Mediterranean diet and survival in a Greek population. *The New England Journal of Medicine*, *348*(26), 2599–2608. http://dx.doi.org/10.1056/NEJMoa025039.

Truelsen, T., Thudium, D., & Gronbaek, M. (2002). Amount and type of alcohol and risk of dementia: The Copenhagen City Heart Study. *Neurology*, *59*(9), 1313–1319.

Tschanz, J. T., Treiber, K., Norton, M. C., Welsh-Bohmer, K. A., Toone, L., Zandi, P. P., & Cache County Study Group, (2005). A population study of Alzheimer's disease: Findings from the Cache County Study on memory, health, and aging. *Care Management Journals: Journal of Case Management; The Journal of Long Term Home Health Care*, *6*(2), 107–114.

Uauy, R., & Dangour, A. D. (2006). Nutrition in brain development and aging: Role of essential fatty acids. *Nutrition Reviews*, *64*(5 Pt 2), S24–33. discussion S72-91.

Ueland, P. M., & Refsum, H. (1989). Plasma homocysteine, a risk factor for vascular disease: Plasma levels in health, disease, and drug therapy. *The Journal of Laboratory and Clinical Medicine*, *114*(5), 473–501.

United States General Accounting Office. (1998). *Alzheimer's disease: Estimates of prevalence in the United States*. Washington, DC: United States General Accounting Office.

US Department of Health Education and Welfare, National Center for Health Statistics (1967). *Eighth revision international classification of diseases adapted for use in the United States*. Public Health Service Publication No. 1693. Washington, DC: U.S. Government Printing Office.

Vagelatos, N. T., & Eslick, G. D. (2013). Type 2 diabetes as a risk factor for Alzheimer's disease: The confounders, interactions, and neuropathology associated with this relationship. *Epidemiologic Reviews*. http://dx.doi.org/10.1093/epirev/mxs012.

Valenzuela, M. J., & Sachdev, P. (2006). Brain reserve and dementia: A systematic review. *Psychological Medicine*, *36*(4), 441–454. http://dx.doi.org/10.1017/S0033291705006264.

Valkanova, V., Eguia Rodriguez, R., & Ebmeier, K. P. (2014). Mind over matter—What do we know about neuroplasticity in adults? *International Psychogeriatrics/IPA*, *26*(6), 891–909. http://dx.doi.org/10.1017/S1041610213002482.

van der Flier, W. M., van Buchem, M. A., Weverling-Rijnsburger, A. W. E., Mutsaers, E. R., Bollen, E. L. E. M., & Admiraal-Behloul, F., et al. (2004). Memory complaints in patients with normal cognition are associated with smaller hippocampal volumes. *Journal of Neurology*, *251*, 671–675.

van der Zwaluw, N. L., Dhonukshe-Rutten, R. A., van Wijngaarden, J. P., Brouwer-Brolsma, E. M., van de Rest, O., In 't Veld, P. H., & de Groot, L. C. (2014). Results of 2-year vitamin B treatment on cognitive performance: Secondary data from an RCT. *Neurology*. http://dx.doi.org/10.1212/WNL.0000000000001050.

van Duijn, C., Stijnen, T., & Hofman, A. (1991). Risk Factors for Alzheimer's disease: Overview of the EURODEM Collaborative Re-Analysis of Case-Control studies. *International Journal of Epidemiology*, *20*(2 (Suppl. 2)), S4–S11.

van Duijn, C. M., Clayton, D., Chandra, V., Fratiglioni, L., Graves, A. B., & Heyman, A., et al. (1991). Familial aggregation of Alzheimer's disease and related disorders: A collaborative Re-Analayis of Case-Control studies. *International Journal of Epidemiology*, *20*(Suppl. 2), S13–20.

van Duijn, C. M., Tanja, T. A., Haaxma, R., Schulte, W., Saan, R. J., Lameris, A. J., & Hofman, A. (1992). Head trauma and the risk of Alzheimer's disease. *American Journal of Epidemiology*, *135*(7), 775–782.

van Gelder, B. M., Buijsse, B., Tijhuis, M., Kalmijn, S., Giampaoli, S., & Nissinen, A., et al. (2007). Coffee consumption is inversely associated with cognitive decline in elderly European men: The FINE study. *European Journal of Clinical Nutrition*, *61*(2), 226–232. http://dx.doi.org/10.1038/sj.ejcn.1602495.

van Gelder, B. M., Tijhuis, M., Kalmijn, S., Giampaoli, S., Nissinen, A., & Kromhout, D. (2006). Marital status and living situation during a 5-year period are associated with a subsequent 10-year cognitive decline in older men: The FINE study. *The Journals of Gerontology Series B, Psychological Sciences and Social Sciences*, *61*(4), P213–219.

Vanhanen, M., Koivisto, K., Moilanen, L., Helkala, E. L., Hanninen, T., Soininen, H., & Kuusisto, J. (2006). Association of metabolic syndrome with Alzheimer disease: A population-based study. *Neurology*, *67*(5), 843–847. http://dx.doi.org/10.1212/01.wnl.0000234037.91185.99.

van Oijen, M., de Jong, F. J., Hofman, A., Koudstaal, P. J., & Breteler, M. M. (2007). Subjective memory complaints, education, and risk of Alzheimer's disease. *Alzheimer's & Dementia: The Journal of the Alzheimer's Association*, *3*(2), 92–97. http://dx.doi.org/10.1016/j.jalz.2007.01.011.

van Praag, H., Christie, B. R., Sejnowski, T. J., & Gage, F. H. (1999). Running enhances neurogenesis, learning, and long-term potentiation in mice. *Proceedings of the National Academy of Sciences of the United States of America*, *96*(23), 13427–13431.

van Praag, H., Shubert, T., Zhao, C., & Gage, F. H. (2005). Exercise enhances learning and hippocampal neurogenesis in aged mice. *The Journal of Neuroscience*, *25*(38), 8680–8685. http://dx.doi.org/10.1523/JNEUROSCI.1731-05.2005.

Veeraswamy, S., Vijayam, B., Gupta, V. K., & Kapur, A. (2012). Gestational diabetes: The public health relevance and approach. *Diabetes Research and Clinical Practice*, *97*(3), 350–358. http://dx.doi.org/10.1016/j.diabres.2012.04.024.

Vega, J. N., & Newhouse, P. A. (2014). Mild cognitive impairment: Diagnosis, longitudinal course, and emerging treatments. *Current Psychiatry Reports*, *16*(10), 490. http://dx.doi.org/10.1007/s11920-014-0490-8.

Vellas, B., Carrie, I., Gillette-Guyonnet, S., Touchon, J., Dantoine, T., & Dartigues, J. F., et al. (2014). MAPT study: A multidomain approach for preventing Alzheimer's disease: Design and baseline data. *Journal of Prevention of Alzheimer's Disease*, *1*(1), 13–22.

Vemuri, P., Wiste, H. J., Weigand, S. D., Shaw, L. M., Trojanowski, J. Q., Weiner, M. W., & Alzheimer's Disease Neuroimaging Initiative, (2009). MRI and CSF biomarkers in normal, MCI, and AD subjects: predicting future clinical change. *Neurology*, *73*(4), 294–301. http://dx.doi.org/10.1212/WNL.0b013e3181af79fb.

Verghese, J., Lipton, R. B., Katz, M. J., Hall, C. B., Derby, C. A., Kuslansky, G., & Buschke, H. (2003). Leisure activities and the risk of dementia in the elderly. *The New England Journal of Medicine*, *348*(25), 2508–2516. http://dx.doi.org/10.1056/NEJMoa022252.

Vidarsdottir, H., Fang, F., Chang, M., Aspelund, T., Fall, K., Jonsdottir, M. K., & Valdimarsdottiru, U. (2014). Spousal loss and cognitive function in later life: A 25-year follow-up in the AGES-Reykjavik study. *American Journal of Epidemiology*, *179*(6), 674–683. http://dx.doi.org/10.1093/aje/kwt321.

Viola, K. L., Sbarboro, J., Sureka, R., De, M., Bicca, M. A., Wang, J., & Klein, W. L. (2015). Towards non-invasive diagnostic imaging of early-stage Alzheimer's disease. *Nature Nanotechnology*, *10*(1), 91–98. http://dx.doi.org/10.1038/nnano.2014.254.

Viswanathan, A., Rocca, W. A., & Tzourio, C. (2009). Vascular risk factors and dementia: How to move forward? *Neurology*, *72*(4), 368–374. http://dx.doi.org/10.1212/01.wnl.0000341271.90478.8e.

Vital, T. M., Stein, A. M., de Melo Coelho, F. G., Arantes, F. J., Teodorov, E., & Santos-Galduroz, R. F. (2014). Physical exercise and vascular endothelial growth factor (VEGF) in elderly: A systematic review. *Archives of Gerontology and Geriatrics*, *59*(2), 234–239. http://dx.doi.org/10.1016/j.archger.2014.04.011.

von Schacky, C. (2014). Omega-3 index and cardiovascular health. *Nutrients*, *6*(2), 799–814. http://dx.doi.org/10.3390/nu6020799.

Vythilingam, M., Heim, C., Newport, J., Miller, A. H., Anderson, E., Bronen, R., & Bremner, J. D. (2002). Childhood trauma associated with smaller hippocampal volume in women with major depression. *The American Journal of Psychiatry*, *159*(12), 2072–2080.

Wacholder, S., McLaughlin, J. K., Silverman, D. T., & Mandel, J. S. (1992). Selection of controls in case-control studies. I. Principles. *American Journal of Epidemiology*, *135*(9), 1019–1028.

Walsh, D. M., & Selkoe, D. J. (2007). A beta oligomers—A decade of discovery. *Journal of Neurochemistry*, *101*(5), 1172–1184. http://dx.doi.org/10.1111/j.1471-4159.2006.04426.x.

Wang, H. X., Fratiglioni, L., Frisoni, G. B., Viitanen, M., & Winblad, B. (1999). Smoking and the occurrence of Alzheimer's disease: Cross-sectional and longitudinal data in a population-based study. *American Journal of Epidemiology*, *149*(7), 640–644.

Wang, H. X., Wahlin, A., Basun, M. D., Fastbom, J., Winblad, B., & Fratiglioni, L. (2001). Vitamin B12 and folate in relation to the development of Alzheimer's disease. *Neurology*, *56*, 1188–1194.

Wang, J., Ho, L., Qin, W., Rocher, A. B., Seror, I., Humala, N., & Pasinetti, G. M. (2005). Caloric restriction attenuates beta-amyloid neuropathology in a mouse model of Alzheimer's disease. *The FASEB Journal: Official Publication of the Federation of American Societies for Experimental Biology*, *19*(6), 659–661. http://dx.doi.org/10.1096/fj.04-3182fje.

Wang, J., Ho, L., Zhao, Z., Seror, I., Humala, N., Dickstein, D. L., & Pasinetti, G. M. (2006). Moderate consumption of Cabernet Sauvignon attenuates Abeta neuropathology in a mouse model of Alzheimer's disease. *The FASEB Journal: Official Publication of the Federation of American Societies for Experimental Biology*, *20*(13), 2313–2320. http://dx.doi.org/10.1096/fj.06-6281com.

Wang, J., Tan, L., Wang, H. F., Tan, C. C., Meng, X. F., Wang, C., & Yu, J. T. (2014). Anti-inflammatory drugs and risk of Alzheimer's disease: An updated systematic review and meta-analysis. *Journal of Alzheimer's Disease*. http://dx.doi.org/10.3233/JAD-141506.

Wang, J., Varghese, M., Ono, K., Yamada, M., Levine, S., Tzavaras, N., & Pasinetti, G. M. (2014). Cocoa extracts reduce oligomerization of amyloid-beta: Implications for cognitive improvement in Alzheimer's disease. *Journal of Alzheimer's Disease*, *41*(2), 643–650. http://dx.doi.org/10.3233/JAD-132231.

Wang, L., van Belle, G., Crane, P. K., Kukull, W. A., Bowen, J. D., & McCormick, W. C., et al. (2004). Subjective memory deterioration and future dementia in people aged 65 and older. *Journal of the American Geriatrics Society*, *52*(12), 2045–2051. http://dx.doi.org/10.1111/j.1532-5415.2004.52568.x.

Ward, D. D., Summers, M. J., Saunders, N. L., Janssen, P., Stuart, K. E., & Vickers, J. C. (2014). APOE and BDNF Val66Met polymorphisms combine to influence episodic memory function in older adults. *Behavioural Brain Research*, *271*, 309–315. http://dx.doi.org/10.1016/j.bbr.2014.06.022.

Warner, M. D., Peabody, C. A., Flattery, J. J., & Tinklenberg, J. R. (1986). Olfactory deficits and Alzheimer's disease. *Biological Psychiatry*, *21*(1), 116–118.

Weiner, H. L., & Selkoe, D. J. (2002). Inflammation and therapeutic vaccination in CNS diseases. *Nature*, *420*(6917), 879–884. http://dx.doi.org/10.1038/nature01325.

Weiner, M. W., Veitch, D. P., Aisen, P. S., Beckett, L. A., Cairns, N. J., Green, R. C., & Trojanowski, J. Q. (2013). The Alzheimer's disease neuroimaging initiative: A review of papers published since its inception. *Alzheimer's & Dementia: The Journal of the Alzheimer's Association*, *9*(5), e111–194. http://dx.doi.org/10.1016/j.jalz.2013.05.1769.

Weintraub, S., Wicklund, A. H., & Salmon, D. P. (2012). The neuropsychological profile of Alzheimer disease. *Cold Spring Harbor Perspectives Medicine*, *2*(4), a006171. http://dx.doi.org/10.1101/cshperspect.a006171.

Weisman, D., Cho, M., Taylor, C., Adame, A., Thal, L. J., & Hansen, L. A. (2007). In dementia with Lewy bodies, Braak stage determines phenotype, not Lewy body distribution. *Neurology*, *69*(4), 356–359. http://dx.doi.org/10.1212/01.wnl.0000266626.64913.0f.

Weissman, M. M., Myers, J. K., Tischler, G. L., Holzer, C. E., III, et al., Leaf, P. J., & Orvaschel, H., et al. (1985). Psychiatric disorders (DSM-III) and cognitive impairment among the elderly in a U.S. urban community. *Acta psychiatrica Scandinavica*, *71*(4), 366–379.

Wengreen, H., Munger, R. G., Cutler, A., Quach, A., Bowles, A., Corcoran, C., & Welsh-Bohmer, K. A. (2013). Prospective study of Dietary Approaches to Stop Hypertension- and Mediterranean-style dietary patterns and age-related cognitive change: The Cache County Study on Memory, Health and Aging. *The American Journal of Clinical Nutrition*, *98*(5), 1263–1271. http://dx.doi.org/10.3945/ajcn.112.051276.

Weuve, J., Hebert, L. E., Scherr, P. A., & Evans, D. A. (2014). Deaths in the United States among persons with Alzheimer's disease (2010–2050). *Alzheimer's & Dementia: The Journal of the Alzheimer's Association*, *10*(2), e40–46. http://dx.doi.org/10.1016/j.jalz.2014.01.004.

Whalley, L. J., Dick, F. D., & McNeill, G. (2006). A life-course approach to the aetiology of late-onset dementias. *Lancet neurology*, *5*(1), 87–96. http://dx.doi.org/10.1016/S1474-4422(05)70286-6.

White, L. (1997). Alzheimer's disease: The evolution of a diagnosis. *Public Health Reports*, *112*(6), 495–496.

White, L. (2009). Brain lesions at autopsy in older Japanese-American men as related to cognitive impairment and dementia in the final years of life: A summary report from the Honolulu-Asia aging study. *Journal of Alzheimer's Disease*, *18*(3), 713–725. http://dx.doi.org/10.3233/JAD-2009-1178.

White, L., Petrovitch, H., Ross, G. W., Masaki, K. H., Abbott, R. D., Teng, E. L., & Curb, J. D. (1996). Prevalence of dementia in older Japanese-American men in Hawaii: The Honolulu-Asia Aging Study. *JAMA*, *276*(12), 955–960.

White, L., Small, B. J., Petrovitch, H., Ross, G. W., Masaki, K., Abbott, R. D., & Markesbery, W. (2005). Recent clinical-pathologic research on the causes of dementia in late life: update from the Honolulu-Asia Aging Study. *Journal of Geriatric Psychiatry and Neurology*, *18*(4), 224–227. http://dx.doi.org/10.1177/0891988705281872.

White, L. R., Petrovitch, H., Ross, G. W., Masaki, K., Hardman, J., Nelson, J., & Markesbery, W. (2000). Brain aging and midlife tofu consumption. *Journal of the American College of Nutrition*, *19*(2), 242–255.

Whitmer, R. A., Gunderson, E. P., Barrett-Connor, E., Quesenberry, C. P., Jr., & Yaffe, K. (2005). Obesity in middle age and future risk of dementia: A 27 year longitudinal population based study. *BMJ*, *330*(7504), 1360. http://dx.doi.org/10.1136/bmj.38446.466238.E0.

Whitmer, R. A., Gustafson, D. R., Barrett-Connor, E., Haan, M. N., Gunderson, E. P., & Yaffe, K. (2008). Central obesity and increased risk of dementia more than three decades later. *Neurology*, *71*(14), 1057–1064. http://dx.doi.org/10.1212/01.wnl.0000306313.89165.ef.

Whitmer, R. A., Quesenberry, C. P., Zhou, J., & Yaffe, K. (2011). Timing of hormone therapy and dementia: The critical window theory revisited. *Annals of neurology*, *69*(1), 163–169. http://dx.doi.org/10.1002/ana.22239.

Whitmer, R. A., Sidney, S., Selby, J., Johnston, S. C., & Yaffe, K. (2005). Midlife cardiovascular risk factors and risk of dementia in late life. *Neurology*, *64*(2), 277–281. http://dx.doi.org/10.1212/01.WNL.0000149519.47454.F2.

Whitwell, J. L., Josephs, K. A., Murray, M. E., Kantarci, K., Przybelski, S. A., Weigand, S. D., & Jack, C. R., Jr. (2008). MRI correlates of neurofibrillary tangle pathology at autopsy: A voxel-based morphometry study. *Neurology*, *71*(10), 743–749. http://dx.doi.org/10.1212/01.wnl.0000324924.91351.7d.

Wikipedia The Free Encyclopedia. Jeanne Calment. Retrieved 4 April, 2014.

Willett, W. C. (2013). *Nutritional epidemiology*. New York: Oxford University Press.

Willette, A. A., Xu, G., Johnson, S. C., Birdsill, A. C., Jonaitis, E. M., Sager, M. A., & Bendlin, B. B. (2013). Insulin resistance, brain atrophy, and cognitive performance in late middle-aged adults. *Diabetes Care*, *36*(2), 443–449. http://dx.doi.org/10.2337/dc12-0922.

Willey, J., Khan, E., Cespedes, S., Moon, Y. P., Rundek, T., & Cheung, K., et al. (2014). Attributable risks of hypertension and diabetes for stroke, myocardial infarction and vascular death in the Northern Manhattan Study. *Circulation*, *129*, AP172.

Williams, D. B., Annegers, J. F., Kokmen, E., O'Brien, P. C., & Kurland, L. T. (1991). Brain injury and neurologic sequelae: a cohort study of dementia, parkinsonism and amyotrophic lateral sclerosis. *Neurology*, *41*(10), 1554–1557.

Williams, J. W., Plassman, B. L., Burke, J., Holsinger, T., & Benjamin, S. (2010). Preventing Alzheimer's disease and cognitive decline. In *Evidence report/technology assessment, No. 93*. Rockville, MD: Agency for Healthcare Research and Quality.

Williams, R. J., & Spencer, J. P. (2012). Flavonoids, cognition, and dementia: Actions, mechanisms, and potential therapeutic utility for Alzheimer disease. *Free Radical Biology & Medicine*, *52*(1), 35–45. http://dx.doi.org/10.1016/j.freeradbiomed.2011.09.010.

Williamson, J. D., Launer, L. J., Bryan, R. N., Coker, L. H., Lazar, R. M., Gerstein, H. C., & Action to Control Cardiovascular Risk in Diabetes Memory in Diabetes Investigators, (2014). Cognitive function and brain structure in persons with type 2 diabetes mellitus after intensive lowering of blood pressure and lipid levels: A randomized clinical trial. *JAMA Internal Medicine*, *174*(3), 324–333. http://dx.doi.org/10.1001/jamainternmed.2013.13656.

Willis, S. L., Tennstedt, S. L., Marsiske, M., Ball, K., Elias, J., Koepke, K. M., & ACTIVE Study Group (2006). Long-term effects of cognitive training on everyday functional outcomes in older adults. *JAMA*, *296*(23), 2805–2814. http://dx.doi.org/10.1001/jama.296.23.2805.

Wilson, R. S., Arnold, S. E., Schneider, J. A., Boyle, P. A., Buchman, A. S., & Bennett, D. A. (2009). Olfactory impairment in presymptomatic Alzheimer's disease. *Annals of the New York Academy of Sciences*, *1170*, 730–735. http://dx.doi.org/10.1111/j.1749-6632.2009.04013.x.

Wilson, R. S., Arnold, S. E., Schneider, J. A., Tang, Y., & Bennett, D. A. (2007). The relationship between cerebral Alzheimer's disease pathology and odour identification in old age. *Journal of Neurology, Neurosurgery, and Psychiatry*, *78*(1), 30–35. http://dx.doi.org/10.1136/jnnp.2006.099721.

Wilson, R. S., Bennett, D. A., Bienias, J. L., Aggarwal, N. T., Mendes De Leon, C. F., Morris, M. C., & Evans, D. A. (2002). Cognitive activity and incident AD in a population-based sample of older persons. *Neurology*, *59*(12), 1910–1914.

Wilson, R. S., Capuano, A. W., Boyle, P. A., Hoganson, G. M., Hizel, L. P., Shah, R. C., & Bennett, D. A. (2014). Clinical-pathologic study of depressive symptoms and cognitive decline in old age. *Neurology*, *83*(8), 702–709. http://dx.doi.org/10.1212/WNL.0000000000000715.

Wilson, R. S., Hoganson, G. M., Rajan, K. B., Barnes, L. L., Mendes de Leon, C. F., & Evans, D. A. (2010). Temporal course of depressive symptoms during the development of Alzheimer disease. *Neurology*, *75*(1), 21–26. http://dx.doi.org/10.1212/WNL.0b013e3181e620c5.

Wilson, R. S., Krueger, K. R., Arnold, S. E., Schneider, J. A., Kelly, J. F., Barnes, L. L., & Bennett, D. A. (2007). Loneliness and risk of Alzheimer disease. *Archives of General Psychiatry*, *64*(2), 234–240. http://dx.doi.org/10.1001/archpsyc.64.2.234.

Wilson, R. S., Mendes De Leon, C. F., Barnes, L. L., Schneider, J. A., Bienias, J. L., & Evans, D. A., et al. (2002). Participation in cognitively stimulating activities and risk of incident Alzheimer disease. *JAMA*, *287*(6), 742–748.

Wilson, R. S., Scherr, P. A., Bienias, J. L., Mendes de Leon, C. F., Everson-Rose, S. A., & Bennett, D. A., et al. (2005). Socioeconomic characteristics of the community in childhood and cognition in old age. *Experimental Aging Research*, *31*(4), 393–407. http://dx.doi.org/10.1080/03610730500206683.

Wilson, R. S., Scherr, P. A., Schneider, J. A., Tang, Y., & Bennett, D. A. (2007). Relation of cognitive activity to risk of developing Alzheimer disease. *Neurology*, *69*(20), 1911–1920. http://dx.doi.org/10.1212/01.wnl.0000271087.67782.cb.

Wilson, R. S., Yu, L., Trojanowski, J. Q., Chen, E. Y., Boyle, P. A., & Bennett, D. A., et al. (2013). TDP-43 pathology, cognitive decline, and dementia in old age. *JAMA Neurology*, *70*(11), 1418–1424. http://dx.doi.org/10.1001/jamaneurol.2013.3961.

Wimo, A., & Prince, M. (2010). The global economic impact of dementia. In *World Alzheimer report 2010*. London: Alzheimer's Disease International.

Winnock, M., Letenneur, L., Jacqmin-Gadda, H., Dallongeville, J., Amouyel, P., & Dartigues, J. F. (2002). Longitudinal analysis of the effect of apolipoprotein E epsilon4 and education on cognitive performance in elderly subjects: The PAQUID study. *Journal of Neurology, Neurosurgery, and Psychiatry*, *72*(6), 794–797.

Wirdefeldt, K., Adami, H. O., Cole, P., Trichopoulos, D., & Mandel, J. (2011). Epidemiology and etiology of Parkinson's disease: A review of the evidence. *European Journal of Epidemiology*, *26*(Suppl. 1), S1–58. http://dx.doi.org/10.1007/s10654-011-9581-6.

Wirth, M., Villeneuve, S., La Joie, R., Marks, S. M., & Jagust, W. J. (2014). Gene-environment interactions: Lifetime cognitive activity, APOE genotype, and beta-amyloid burden. *The Journal of Neuroscience*, *34*(25), 8612–8617. http://dx.doi.org/10.1523/JNEUROSCI.4612-13.2014.

Wisniewski, T., Dowiat, W. K., Buxbaum, J. D., Khorkova, O., Efthimiopoulos, S., & Kulcyzcki, J., et al. (1998). A novel Polish presenilin-1 mutation (P117L) is associated with familial Alzheimer's disease and leads to death as early as the age of 28 years. *Neuroreport*, *9*(2), 217–221.

Witte, A. V., Fobker, M., Gellner, R., Knecht, S., & Floel, A. (2009). Caloric restriction improves memory in elderly humans. *Proceedings of the National Academy of Sciences of the United States of America*, *106*(4), 1255–1260. http://dx.doi.org/10.1073/pnas.0808587106.

Wolf, H., Julin, P., Gertz, H. J., Winblad, B., & Wahlund, L. O. (2004). Intracranial volume in mild cognitive impairment, Alzheimer's disease and vascular dementia: Evidence for brain reserve? *International Journal of Geriatric Psychiatry*, *19*(10), 995–1007. http://dx.doi.org/10.1002/gps.1205.

Wolf, H., Kruggel, F., Hensel, A., Wahlund, L. O., Arendt, T., & Gertz, H. J. (2003). The relationship between head size and intracranial volume in elderly subjects. *Brain Research*, *973*(1), 74–80.

Wolf, P. A., Beiser, A., Elias, M. F., Au, R., Vasan, R. S., & Seshadri, S. (2007). Relation of obesity to cognitive function: Importance of central obesity and synergistic influence of concomitant hypertension. The Framingham Heart Study. *Current Alzheimer Research*, *4*(2), 111–116.

Wolf, P. A., D'Agostino, R. B., Kannel, W. B., Bonita, R., & Belanger, A. J. (1988). Cigarette smoking as a risk factor for stroke. The Framingham Study. *JAMA*, *259*(7), 1025–1029.

Women's Health Initiative Study Group (1998). Design of the Women's Health Initiative clinical trial and observational study. *Controlled Clinical Trials*, *19*(1), 61–109.

Woollett, K., & Maguire, E. A. (2011). Acquiring "the Knowledge" of London's layout drives structural brain changes. *Current Biology*, *21*(24), 2109–2114. http://dx.doi.org/10.1016/j.cub.2011.11.018.

Wrann, C. D., White, J. P., Salogiannnis, J., Laznik-Bogoslavski, D., Wu, J., Ma, D., & Spiegelman, B. M. (2013). Exercise induces hippocampal BDNF through a PGC-1alpha/FNDC5 pathway. *Cell Metabolism*, *18*(5), 649–659. http://dx.doi.org/10.1016/j.cmet.2013.09.008.

Wyss-Coray, T., & Rogers, J. (2012). Inflammation in Alzheimer disease-a brief review of the basic science and clinical literature. *Cold Spring Harbor Perspectives Medicine*, *2*(1), a006346. http://dx.doi.org/10.1101/cshperspect.a006346.

Xu, Z. Q., Zhang, L. Q., Wang, Q., Marshall, C., Xiao, N., Gao, J. Y., & Xiao, M. (2013). Aerobic exercise combined with antioxidative treatment does not counteract moderate- or mid-stage Alzheimer-like pathophysiology of APP/PS1 mice. *CNS Neuroscience & Therapeutics*, *19*(10), 795–803. http://dx.doi.org/10.1111/cns.12139.

Yaffe, K., Ackerson, L., Kurella Tamura, M., Le Blanc, P., Kusek, J. W., Sehgal, A. R., & Go, A. S. (2010). Chronic kidney disease and cognitive function in older adults: findings from the chronic renal insufficiency cohort cognitive study. *Journal of the American Geriatrics Society*, *58*(2), 338–345. http://dx.doi.org/10.1111/j.1532-5415.2009.02670.x.

Yaffe, K., Barnes, D., Nevitt, M., Lui, L. Y., & Covinsky, K. (2001). A prospective study of physical activity and cognitive decline in elderly women: Women who walk. *Archives of Internal Medicine*, *161*(14), 1703–1708.

Yaffe, K., Barrett-Connor, E., Lin, F., & Grady, D. (2002). Serum lipoprotein levels, statin use, and cognitive function in older women. *Archives of Neurology*, *59*(3), 378–384.

Yaffe, K., Laffan, A. M., Harrison, S. L., Redline, S., Spira, A. P., Ensrud, K. E., & Stoneu, K. L. (2011). Sleep-disordered breathing, hypoxia, and risk of mild cognitive impairment and dementia in older women. *JAMA*, *306*(6), 613–619. http://dx.doi.org/10.1001/jama.2011.1115.

Yaffe, K., Sawaya, G., Lieberburg, I., & Grady, D. (1998). Estrogen therapy in postmenopausal women: Effects on cognitive function and dementia. *JAMA*, *279*(9), 688–695.

Yamada, M., Kasagi, F., Mimori, Y., Miyachi, T., Ohshita, T., & Sasaki, H. (2009). Incidence of dementia among atomic-bomb survivors—Radiation Effects Research Foundation Adult Health Study. *Journal of the Neurological Sciences*, *281*(1–2), 11–14. http://dx.doi.org/10.1016/j.jns.2009.03.003.

Yamada, M., Sasaki, H., Mimori, Y., Kasagi, F., Sudoh, S., Ikeda, J., & Kodama, K. (1999). Prevalence and risks of dementia in the Japanese population: RERF's adult health study Hiroshima subjects. Radiation Effects Research Foundation. *Journal of the American Geriatrics Society*, *47*(2), 189–195.

Yates, P. A., Desmond, P. M., Phal, P. M., Steward, C., Szoeke, C., Salvado, O., & Rowe, C. C. (2014). Incidence of cerebral microbleeds in preclinical Alzheimer disease. *Neurology*, *82*(14), 1266–1273. http://dx.doi.org/10.1212/WNL.0000000000000285.

Yoshitake, T., Kiyohara, Y., Kato, I., Ohmura, T., Iwamoto, H., & Nakayama, K., et al. (1995). Incidence and risk factors of vascular dementia and Alzheimer's disease in a defined elderly Japanese population: The Hisayama Study. *Neurology*, *45*(6), 1161–1168.

Young, L. R., & Nestle, M. (2002). The contribution of expanding portion sizes to the US obesity epidemic. *American Journal of Public Health*, *92*(2), 246–249.

Yu, F., Xu, B., Song, C., Ji, L., & Zhang, X. (2013). Treadmill exercise slows cognitive deficits in aging rats by antioxidation and inhibition of amyloid production. *Neuroreport*, *24*(6), 342–347. http://dx.doi.org/10.1097/WNR.0b013e3283606c5e.

Zandi, P. P., Anthony, J. C., Hayden, K. M., Mehta, K., Mayer, L., & Breitner, J. C., et al. (2002). Reduced incidence of AD with NSAID but not H2 receptor antagonists: The Cache County Study. *Neurology*, *59*(6), 880–886.

Zandi, P. P., Anthony, J. C., Khachaturian, A. S., Stone, S. V., Gustafson, D., Tschanz, J. T., & Breitner, J. C. (2004). Reduced risk of Alzheimer disease in users of antioxidant vitamin supplements: The Cache County Study. *Archives of Neurology*, *61*(1), 82–88. http://dx.doi.org/10.1001/archneur.61.1.82.

Zandi, P. P., Sparks, D. L., Khachaturian, A. S., Tschanz, J., Norton, M., Steinberg, M., & Breitner, J. C. (2005). Do statins reduce risk of incident dementia and Alzheimer disease? The Cache County Study. *Archives of General Psychiatry*, *62*(2), 217–224. http://dx.doi.org/10.1001/archpsyc.62.2.217.

Zhang, M., Katzman, R., & Salmon, D., et al. (1990). The prevalence of dementia and Alzheimer's disease in Shanghai, China: Impact of age, gender and education. *Annals of Neurology*, *27*, 428–437.

Zhang, Y., Schuff, N., Jahng, G. H., Bayne, W., Mori, S., Schad, L., & Weiner, M. W. (2007). Diffusion tensor imaging of cingulum fibers in mild cognitive impairment and Alzheimer disease. *Neurology*, *68*(1), 13–19. http://dx.doi.org/10.1212/01.wnl.0000250326.77323.01.

Zhang, Z., Gu, D., & Hayward, M. D. (2008). Early life influences on cognitive impairment among oldest old Chinese. *The Journals of Gerontology Series B, Psychological Sciences and Social Sciences*, *63*(1), S25–33.

Zhao, C., Teng, E. M., Summers, R. G., Jr., Ming, G. L., & Gage, F. H. (2006). Distinct morphological stages of dentate granule neuron maturation in the adult mouse hippocampus. *The Journal of Neuroscience*, *26*(1), 3–11. http://dx.doi.org/10.1523/JNEUROSCI.3648-05.2006.

Zhou, W., Xu, D., Peng, X., Zhang, Q., Jia, J., & Crutcher, K. A. (2008). Meta-analysis of APOE4 allele and outcome after traumatic brain injury. *Journal of Neurotrauma*, *25*(4), 279–290. http://dx.doi.org/10.1089/neu.2007.0489

Index

Note: Page numbers followed by "*f*" and "*t*" refer to figures and tables, respectively.